Edited by
Christoph Sotriffer

Virtual Screening

Methods and Principles in Medicinal Chemistry

Previous Volumes of this Series:

Rautio, Jarkko (Ed.)

Prodrugs and Targeted Delivery

Towards Better ADME Properties

2011

ISBN: 978-3-527-32603-7

Vol. 47

Smit, Martine J. / Lira, Sergio A. / Leurs, Rob (Eds.)

Chemokine Receptors as Drug Targets

2011

ISBN: 978-3-527-32118-6

Vol. 46

Ghosh, Arun K. (Ed.)

Aspartic Acid Proteases as Therapeutic Targets

2010

ISBN: 978-3-527-31811-7

Vol. 45

Ecker, Gerhard F. / Chiba, Peter (Eds.)

Transporters as Drug Carriers

Structure, Function, Substrates

2009

ISBN: 978-3-527-31661-8

Vol. 44

Faller, Bernhard / Urban, Laszlo (Eds.)

Hit and Lead Profiling

Identification and Optimization of Drug-like Molecules

2009

ISBN: 978-3-527-32331-9

Vol. 43

Sippl, Wolfgang / Jung, Manfred (Eds.)

Epigenetic Targets in Drug Discovery

2009

ISBN: 978-3-527-32355-5

Vol. 42

Todeschini, Roberto / Consonni, Viviana

Molecular Descriptors for Chemoinformatics

Volume I: Alphabetical Listing / Volume II: Appendices, References

2009

ISBN: 978-3-527-31852-0

Vol. 41

van de Waterbeemd, Han / Testa, Bernard (Eds.)

Drug Bioavailability

Estimation of Solubility, Permeability, Absorption and Bioavailability

Second, Completely Revised Edition

2008

ISBN: 978-3-527-32051-6

Vol. 40

Ottow, Eckhard / Weinmann, Hilmar (Eds.)

Nuclear Receptors as Drug Targets

2008

ISBN: 978-3-527-31872-8

Vol. 39

Vaz, Roy J. / Klabunde, Thomas (Eds.)

Antitargets

Prediction and Prevention of Drug Side Effects

2008

ISBN: 978-3-527-31821-6

Vol. 38

Edited by
Christoph Sotriffer

Virtual Screening

Principles, Challenges, and Practical Guidelines

WILEY-VCH

WILEY-VCH Verlag GmbH & Co. KGaA

Series Editors

Prof. Dr. Raimund Mannhold
Molecular Drug Research Group
Heinrich-Heine-Universität
Universitätsstrasse 1
40225 Düsseldorf
Germany
mannhold@uni-duesseldorf.de

Prof. Dr. Hugo Kubinyi
Donnersbergstrasse 9
67256 Weisenheim am Sand
Germany
kubinyi@t-online.de

Prof. Dr. Gerd Folkers
Collegium Helveticum
STW/ETH Zurich
8092 Zurich
Switzerland
folkers@collegium.ethz.ch

Volume Editor

Prof. Dr. Christoph Sotriffer
University of Würzburg
Institute of Pharmacy and Food Chemistry
Am Hubland
97074 Würzburg
Germany

Cover Description
Virtual screening is a process of hierarchical filtering, searching compounds from chemical space that are suitable for interaction with targets from biological space. – The illustrated hit stems from a virtual screening study conducted by Brenk et al. (2003), which is discussed in chapters 10 and 12 of this book. (Support by Dr. Matthias Zentgraf in preparation of this graph is gratefully acknowledged.)

Library of Congress Card No.: applied for

British Library Cataloguing-in-Publication Data
A catalogue record for this book is available from the British Library.

Bibliographic information published by the Deutsche Nationalbibliothek
The Deutsche Nationalbibliothek lists this publication in the Deutsche Nationalbibliografie; detailed bibliographic data are available on the Internet at http://dnb.d-nb.de.

Typesetting Thomson Digital, Noida, India
Printing and Binding Strauss GmbH, Mörlenbach
Cover Design Schulz Grafik-Design, Fußgönheim

Printed in the Federal Republic of Germany
Printed on acid-free paper

ISBN: 978-3-527-32636-5

Dedicated with love

to Edith, Mathilde, Jonathan, and Therese

Contents

Virtual Screening. Edited by C. Sotriffer

ISBN: 978-3-527-32636-5

List of Contributors

Éric Arnoult
Janssen-Cilag S.A.
Campus de Maigremont
BP 615
27106 Val de Reuil Cedex
France

Jürgen Bajorath
Rheinische Friedrich-Wilhelms-Universität
Department of Life Science Informatics
B-IT, LIMES Program Unit Chemical Biology and Medicinal Chemistry
Dahlmannstr. 2
53113 Bonn
Germany

Daniele Bemporad
Janssen Pharmaceutical N.V.
Johnson & Johnson Pharmaceutical Research and Development
Turnhoutseweg 30
2340 Beerse
Belgium

Markus Boehm
Pfizer Pharma Therapeutics R & D
Worldwide Medicinal Chemistry
Eastern Point Rd
Groton, CT 06340
USA

Christophe Buyck
Tibotec BVBA
Turnhoutseweg 30
2340 Beerse
Belgium

Amedeo Caflisch
University of Zurich
Department of Biochemistry
Winterthurerstrasse 190
8057 Zurich
Switzerland

Claudio N. Cavasotto
University of Texas at Houston
School of Biomedical Informatics
7000 Fannin, Ste. 600
Houston, TX 77030
USA

Jason C. Cole
University of Cambridge
Crystallographic Data Centre
12 Union Road
Cambridge CB2 1EZ
UK

Maxwell D. Cummings
Tibotec BVBA
Turnhoutseweg 30
2340 Beerse
Belgium

Virtual Screening. Edited by C. Sotriffer

ISBN: 978-3-527-32636-5

Ralf Heinke
Martin-Luther University of Halle-Wittenberg
Department of Pharmaceutical Chemistry
Wolfgang-Langenbeck-Str. 4
06120 Halle
Germany

Angela M. Henzler
Universität Hamburg
Zentrum für Bioinformatik
Bundesstraße 43
20146 Hamburg
Germany

Trevor Howe
Janssen Pharmaceutical N.V.
Johnson & Johnson Pharmaceutical Research and Development
Turnhoutseweg 30
2340 Beerse
Belgium

Danzhi Huang
University of Zurich
Department of Biochemistry
Winterthurerstrasse 190
8057 Zurich
Switzerland

Manfred Jung
Albert-Ludwigs-University of Freiburg
Institute of Pharmaceutical Sciences
Stefan-Meier-Str. 31
79104 Freiburg
Germany

György M. Keserű
Gedeon Richter plc.
P.O.B. 27
1475 Budapest
Hungary

Johannes Kirchmair
University of Innsbruck
Faculty of Chemistry and Pharmacy and Center for Molecular Biosciences (CMBI)
Departments of Theoretical Chemistry and Pharmaceutical Chemistry
Innrain 52
6020 Innsbruck
Austria

Róbert Kiss
Heriot-Watt University
Edinburgh Campus
Edinburgh EH14 4AS
UK

and

Gedeon Richter plc.
P.O.B. 27
1475 Budapest
Hungary

Herbert Koeppen
Boehringer Ingelheim Pharma GmbH & Co. KG
Department of Lead Discovery
Birkendorfer Str. 65
88397 Biberach an der Riss
Germany

Oliver Korb
University of Cambridge
Crystallographic Data Centre
12 Union Road
Cambridge CB2 1EZ
UK

Jan Kriegl
Boehringer Ingelheim Pharma GmbH & Co. KG
Department of Lead Discovery
Birkendorfer Str. 65
88397 Biberach an der Riss
Germany

Thierry Langer
Prestwick Chemical Inc.
Blvd Gonthier d'Andernach,
67 400 Illkirch
France

Uta Lessel
Boehringer Ingelheim Pharma GmbH & Co. KG
Department of Lead Discovery
Birkendorfer Str. 65
88397 Biberach an der Riss
Germany

John Liebeschuetz
University of Cambridge
Crystallographic Data Centre
12 Union Road
Cambridge CB2 1EZ
UK

Klaus R. Liedl
University of Innsbruck
Faculty of Chemistry and Pharmacy and Center for Molecular Biosciences (CMBI)
Department of Theoretical Chemistry
Innrain 52
6020 Innsbruck
Austria

Patrick Markt
University of Innsbruck
Institute of Pharmacy
Innrain 52
6020 Innsbruck
Austria

Hans Matter
Sanofi-Aventis Deutschland GmbH
Structure, Design & Informatics
LG-CR, Building G 878
65926 Frankfurt at Main
Germany

Maria A. Miteva
University Paris Diderot
Inserm UMR-S 973, MTi
CDithem Platform
35 Rue Hélène Brion
75013 Paris
France

Tjelvar S.G. Olsson
University of Cambridge
Crystallographic Data Centre
12 Union Road
Cambridge CB2 1EZ
UK

Matthias Rarey
Universität Hamburg
Zentrum für Bioinformatik
Bundesstraße 43
20146 Hamburg
Germany

Didier Rognan
Structural Chemogenomics Group
Laboratory of Therapeutic Innovation
UMR 7200 CNRS-UdS
74 route du Rhin
67400 Illkirch
France

Daniela Schuster
University of Innsbruck
Institute of Pharmacy
Innrain 52
6020 Innsbruck
Austria

Wolfgang Sippl
Martin-Luther University of Halle-Wittenberg
Department of Pharmaceutical Chemistry
Wolfgang-Langenbeck-Str. 4
06120 Halle
Germany

Christoph Sotriffer
University of Würzburg
Institute of Pharmacy and Food Chemistry
Am Hubland
97074 Würzburg
Germany

Olivier Sperandio
University Paris Diderot
Inserm UMR-S 973, MTi
CDithem Platform
35 Rue Hélène Brion
75013 Paris
France

Gudrun M. Spitzer
University of Innsbruck
Faculty of Chemistry and Pharmacy and Center for Molecular Biosciences (CMBI)
Department of Theoretical Chemistry
Innrain 52
6020 Innsbruck
Austria

Dagmar Stumpfe
Rheinische Friedrich-Wilhelms-Universität
Department of Life Science Informatics
B-IT, LIMES Program Unit Chemical Biology and Medicinal Chemistry
Dahlmannstr. 2
53113 Bonn
Germany

Christofer S. Tautermann
Boehringer Ingelheim Pharma GmbH & Co. KG
Department of Lead Discovery
Birkendorfer Str. 65
88397 Biberach an der Riss
Germany

Gary Tresadern
Janssen-Cilag S.A.
Johnson & Johnson Pharmaceutical Research & Development
Calle Jarama 75
Poligono Industrial
45007 Toledo
Spain

Urszula Uciechowska
Martin-Luther University of Halle-Wittenberg
Department of Pharmaceutical Chemistry
Wolfgang-Langenbeck-Str. 4
06120 Halle
Germany

Bruno O. Villoutreix
University Paris Diderot
Inserm UMR-S 973, MTi
CDithem Platform
35 Rue Hélène Brion
75013 Paris
France

Ann M. Vos
Tibotec BVBA
Turnhoutseweg 30
2340 Beerse
Belgium

Jörg K. Wegner
Tibotec BVBA
Turnhoutseweg 30
2340 Beerse
Belgium

Bernd Wellenzohn
Boehringer Ingelheim Pharma GmbH
& Co. KG
Department of Lead Discovery
Birkendorfer Str. 65
88397 Biberach an der Riss
Germany

Preface

In an early definition by Walters, Stahl, and Murcko [1], virtual screening (VS) is described as the "Use of high-performance computing to analyze large databases of chemical compounds in order to identify possible drug candidates."

Virtual screening has become an integral part of the drug discovery process. It has largely been a numbers game focusing on questions like how can we filter down the enormous chemical space of over 10^{60} conceivable compounds to a manageable number that can be synthesized or purchased and tested. Although filtering the entire chemical universe might be a fascinating question, more practical VS scenarios focus on designing and optimizing targeted combinatorial libraries and enriching libraries of available compounds from in-house compound repositories or vendor offerings.

The purpose of virtual screening is to come up with hits of novel chemical structure that bind to the macromolecular target of interest. Thus, success of a virtual screen is defined in terms of finding interesting new scaffolds rather than many hits. Interpretations of VS accuracy should therefore be considered with caution. Low hit rates of interesting scaffolds are clearly preferable over high hit rates of already known scaffolds.

In a logical and didactic way, this volume is organized in four parts covering principles, challenges, practical guidelines, and case studies under different scenarios. Chapters of Part One are dedicated to virtual screening of chemical space, processing of small molecule databases for virtual screening, ligand-based and target-based virtual screening, virtual screening with 3D pharmacophore models, and docking methods. Challenges discussed in Part Two comprise affinity prediction, fragment-based approaches, handling of protein flexibility, as well as consideration of water and solvation effects, as well as parallel virtual screening for compound profiling and prediction of off-target effects. Finally, strategies, recommendations, and caveats for applying virtual screening methodology are given and many success stories are described.

As an add-on value, this volume contains two appendices. A brief tabular compilation, including classification, short description, references, and links, gives a very informative software overview. Beyond it, successful virtual screening application studies for pharmacological targets are tabulated.

Virtual Screening. Edited by C. Sotriffer

ISBN: 978-3-527-32636-5

We are very grateful to Christoph Sotriffer who assembled a team of leading experts to discuss all above-mentioned aspects. This book is well suited both for all practitioners in medicinal chemistry and for graduate students who want to learn how to apply virtual screening methodology. We are also grateful to Frank Weinreich and Nicola Oberbeckmann-Winter for their ongoing support and enthusiasm for our series "Methods and Principles in Medicinal Chemistry."

October 2010

Raimund Mannhold, Düsseldorf
Hugo Kubinyi, Weisenheim am Sand
Gerd Folkers, Zürich

Reference

1 Walters, W.P., Stahl, M.T., and Murcko, M.A. (1998) Virtual screening: an overview. *Drug Discovery Today*, **3**, 160–178.

A Personal Foreword

Seek, and you will find.

Drug discovery in general and virtual screening in particular is a matter of searching. Often compared with looking for the needle in the haystack, virtual screening is an attempt to identify molecules with very particular properties by scanning through large pools of chemical compounds. As with any search, it makes sense to clarify a few questions before starting: *What* do I actually look for? *Where* should I search? *How* should the search be carried out? None of these questions is as trivial as it initially sounds – that is why an entire book can be dedicated to virtual screening.

Indeed, while the general concept is very simple, turning virtual screening into a practically useful method is much more complex. First of all, the object of the search, the intended goal must be defined. Obviously, in the context of drug discovery it is always a bioactive molecule, be it an enzyme inhibitor, a receptor agonist or an antagonist, or a disruptor of macromolecular complexes. The essential question, however, is which molecular property determines the bioactivity and provides a suitable discrimination between objects showing this activity and those that do not. The entire search makes sense only if such relevant and discriminating properties can be defined. Concepts of molecular similarity and models of molecular recognition are required in this context. In practice, the issue is further complicated by the fact that bioactivity alone is not sufficient for a virtual screening hit to be of value in drug discovery projects. Many additional criteria, such as synthetic accessibility and a suitable pharmacokinetic profile, must be met. Virtual screening must also take such boundary conditions into account.

This leads to the second issue: the area in which the search should be carried out. Simply going through the entire collection of all hitherto synthesized or isolated chemical compounds is certainly not the best idea. Again, criteria must be defined to set reasonable boundaries to the search. On the other hand, the big advantage of *virtual* over experimental screening is the possibility to extend the search to new areas of chemical space, as characterized, for example, by virtual combinatorial libraries. There are many good reasons for following such a route, but the danger of inadvertently just increasing the haystack (without many more needles in it) should not be overlooked.

Virtual Screening. Edited by C. Sotriffer

ISBN: 978-3-527-32636-5

The third issue deals with the technology itself. Which strategies and which tools are available for carrying out efficient searches? Due to the multifaceted nature of virtual screening, this touches many fields of the computational disciplines involved, from chemo- and bioinformatics to molecular modeling and computational chemistry. In fact, virtual screening is not a single method, but rather a process or workflow, a combination of multiple approaches. Thinking of virtual screening as a hierarchical filtering procedure is probably the most common view, as appreciated by the illustration chosen for the cover of this book. This view of hierarchical filtering has been propagated in particular by Gerhard Klebe, one of the pioneers of structure-based virtual screening, whose lab I had the pleasure to join back in the year 2000. It was also there that I personally came in touch with virtual screening. By then it was still a nascent technique, with just a few dozen publications available. But the impressive results that appeared in the literature have paved the way for fast dissemination of the technology, with hundreds of applications and a wealth of methodological developments in the past 10 years. In this sense, virtual screening has matured to a standard technique of early drug discovery, widely applied in industry and academia, and there is certainly no doubt today that this technique works and that it delivers practically useful results.

Nevertheless, success is not guaranteed, and many limitations exist that certainly preclude a simple "black-box-like" application. Using virtual screening is easy nowadays, with many dedicated software tools and databases freely available to anyone. Applying it correctly, however, is not as straightforward, and even published studies sometimes raise doubts whether the chosen settings and procedures can really be expected to deliver meaningful results. Besides internal method validation, experimental confirmation would be mandatory, but this is not always readily accessible and sometimes not carried out with sufficient detail and care. On the other hand, even very cautious application of the best possible techniques can lead to results that upon experimental validation disprove the original design hypothesis, for example, with respect to a certain requested interaction or binding mode. There is, in fact, a gray area in virtual screening where good results and valuable hits are obtained, but not for the right (or expected) reasons. One may attribute this to the fact that the filtering steps simply serve to eliminate all compounds with completely unsuitable properties. This increases the hit rate in the set of molecules that passed the filters and may lead to the discovery of actives even though the details of their interaction and their score are not correctly estimated. For many practical purposes, this may even be acceptable, but the scientific claim of the method certainly is to reliably predict active compounds on a rational basis of molecular similarity and correct assumptions about the underlying protein–ligand interactions.

These considerations bring me to my motivation for compiling this book: instead of focusing purely on the identification of active compounds, it is the question which underlying models, concepts, and procedures enable us to succeed in this endeavor. My feeling was that this should be of interest for the user and the developer alike. Accordingly, the goal was to arrange a book that on the one hand outlines the essential features for a successful practical application of virtual screening and on the other hand discusses the underlying hypotheses and limitations that are essential for a more complete understanding and also takes a step toward refined methods and an improved virtual screening technology.

With this intention in mind, I chose to outline the book in four major parts: principles, challenges, practical guidelines, and case studies under different scenarios. The Part One, "Principles," illustrates the main concepts of virtual screening and its fundamental techniques and discusses the essential aspects of their successful application. As virtual screening requires a collection of compounds that bears the reasonable chance to contain molecules with the requested properties, attention is first paid to the underlying data. Simply screening the available corporate compound database is certainly the most straightforward approach, but success is by no means guaranteed since the collection may be heavily biased toward certain chemotypes with relatively limited diversity. To proceed more systematically, it makes sense to think about compound databases in terms of chemical space, that is, the entire collection of all possible molecules. Which regions are of relevance for drug discovery in general and for my specific target in particular? How well are these regions covered by real, already existing compounds? And how could the search be expanded into unexplored areas by means of virtual compound libraries? The first chapter is dedicated to these more fundamental issues of search spaces, whereas the second chapter focuses on the more practical aspects related to compound databases. Chemical structures must be represented in a format that conveys all required information in an unambiguous way and is amenable to rapid processing by many different software tools. On the other hand, the stereochemistry, tautomers, and different protonation states need to be considered. Furthermore, it may be advantageous to generate multiple conformers of each molecule. Once it is clear *how* structures should be represented and stored, the question arises *which* structures actually need to be processed. As illustrated in detail in this chapter, a raw database should normally be prefiltered to eliminate all compounds that are highly unlikely to be of practical use in a drug discovery project.

Once the search databases are set up, screening can start even in the absence of a 3D target structure, provided that at least one active ligand is known. Accordingly, in Chapter 3, ligand-based virtual screening is introduced. This class of methods is based on molecular similarity, which is the general assumption that similar molecules exhibit similar binding properties for a given target. As simple as this sounds, it is unfortunately not clear in which terms this similarity should be measured and which molecular properties are the best predictors of similarity in terms of binding affinity. Therefore, a discussion of descriptors and similarity measures lies at the heart of this chapter, before the screening based on such similarity measures is described. In this context, attention is also paid both to the selection of the reference ligand for the search and to the machine-learning approaches that can be applied if multiple active and inactive ligands are available.

If structural information about the target is available, structure-based (i.e., target-based) virtual screening can be applied. It is the second large class of approaches, either used as an alternative to ligand-based screening or in combination with it. Before describing in later chapters the techniques that use protein structure information, Chapter 4 analyzes the quality of the underlying experimental data and shows how such data must be handled in order to avoid potential pitfalls. The focus here is on protein crystal structures and the possible errors and limitations of the corresponding structural data. This is coupled with a detailed discussion how an appropriate protein structure can be selected and how it should be set up for virtual screening.

Chapter 5 is naturally suited to make the transition from ligand-based to target-based virtual screening, as it deals with 3D pharmacophore models. Such models can be generated either from a set of active ligands or from the structure of a binding site (ideally complexed with a ligand) or from the combination of both. Particular attention should be paid to model validation, as discussed in detail in this chapter. Enrichment assessments and enrichment metrics are illustrated, and these aspects are relevant not only for pharmacophore-based techniques but also for virtual screening in general. Since no chapter is dedicated exclusively to validation aspects, this section is a "must read" for anyone not yet familiar with validation of virtual screening procedures. The second half of Chapter 5 is dedicated to the screening techniques based on pharmacophore models and to the postprocessing of screening hits. A broad range of application examples concludes this chapter.

Moving on to the core technique of target-based virtual screening, Chapter 6 of Part One is dedicated to docking methods. The fundamentals of molecular docking as a process of sampling and scoring are introduced, before going through the docking-based virtual screening workflow, with ligand and protein setup, choice of the docking program and its application, and postprocessing of the docking results. Finally, recent advances of the docking field are summarized, including those related to the enduring issue of protein flexibility and the role of water, two topics that already point to the next part of the book.

In Part Two, three of the most frequently encountered challenges in structure-based virtual screening are analyzed in detail: the first about scoring (Chapter 7), the second about protein flexibility (Chapters 8 and 9), and the third about the consideration of water and solvation effects (Chapter 10). All three issues are closely related to each other since protein flexibility and water molecules directly affect the scoring of protein–ligand complexes. With an ideal scoring method at hand, docking and structure-based virtual screening would reduce to a pure search problem. Nonbinders could be clearly distinguished from binders, the binders could be correctly ranked by affinity, and this ranking would be based on the correct docking pose. Unfortunately, none of these ultimate goals has been reached so far. In particular, the discrimination of nonbinders and the ranking of binders are still not possible with sufficient reliability. The chapter on scoring functions describes available approaches, their limitations, recent developments, and the general strategies and recommendations for their application in virtual screening.

Protein flexibility as the second major challenge is discussed in two separate chapters. The first is dedicated primarily to the algorithmic description of the methods available for handling protein flexibility, based on a new classification of the different approaches. The second chapter focuses on their application in high-throughput docking and virtual screening. As these chapters illustrate, a multitude of different approaches are already available for at least partial consideration of protein flexibility, but taking full account of all ligand and protein degrees of freedom and of the mutual adaptation between the binding partners is still out of reach for practical application in virtual screening. Accordingly, one should carefully select the most appropriate approach, depending on the known properties and the available data of the target system, and one should be aware that "surprises" may occur as long as flexible systems are not treated fully flexibly.

Similar considerations apply to water molecules, given that the accurate prediction of water-mediated effects is still not possible. Again, the main problems are scoring and the dynamic nature of water interactions. Nevertheless, as illustrated in Chapter 10, many methods for analyzing water molecules in protein binding sites are available and water-sensitive virtual screening can be carried out. Even though perfect predictions are out of reach, careful consideration of the current knowledge about water molecules can certainly improve the outcome of virtual screening studies.

Despite all the challenges and limitations, impressive results can be obtained with virtual screening, as illustrated in Part Three, dedicated to "Applications and Practical Guidelines." Strategies, recommendations, and caveats for applied virtual screening are summarized in Chapter 11. Focusing on ligand-based approaches, this chapter discusses the main aspects affecting the outcome of ligand-based virtual screening, outlines the applicability domain, and comments on opportunities and intrinsic limitations. This is followed in Chapter 12 by a summary of selected applications and success stories of prospective virtual screening. Here, particular emphasis is placed on workflow comparison. Both ligand-based and structure-based studies are presented, and illustrations are given for the fact that these two branches of virtual screening should not be seen as competing: it is rather their combination that may enhance hit rates. Further application examples and a more detailed discussion of particular case studies and practical aspects are provided in the next five chapters of Part Four, dedicated to virtual screening under different scenarios. As the first scenario, ligand-based application studies are presented and discussed (Chapter 13). In the absence of a target structure, an alternative scenario consists of homology modeling and the use of the resulting models for structure-based virtual screening; this is discussed in depth in Chapters 14 and 15. Similar to structure-based virtual screening using experimentally determined structures, the studies discussed primarily focus on small-molecule binding sites. In contrast, Chapter 16 is dedicated to the emerging field of protein–protein interactions and how target-based virtual screening can be used to identify modulators of such interactions. Finally, Chapter 17 describes how fragment-based approaches may be used in virtual screening and illustrates how these techniques can lead to the detection of small bioactive compounds.

All application studies mentioned throughout the book are summarized in a tabular compilation in the Appendix. The same is true for all cited programs, tools, and databases for virtual screening. Each entry in the tables contains a reference to the literature or a web site address. In fact, the tables were compiled with the explicit hope that the reader and the user may find them helpful for rapidly retrieving further information.

Editing this book was a valuable experience for me. It was a real pleasure to get in touch with all the scientists from industry and academia who contributed to this volume. Their willingness to share their knowledge and experience in virtual screening in the form of this book was essential for making this project come true. I am, therefore, deeply indebted to all authors for their contributions and their cooperation. I also thank the members of my group at the University of Würzburg for their help, in particular with respect to the preparation of the Appendix.

The book would not have been realized in this form without the kind invitation, the encouragement, and the valuable suggestions of the series editors. Their support is gratefully acknowledged. Finally, I also want to thank Dr. Frank Weinreich and Dr. Nicola Oberbeckmann-Winter from Wiley-VCH in Weinheim for their very pleasant collaboration and support during all steps of editing this volume.

May all readers find what they search – in virtual screening and in this book!

October 2010 *Christoph Sotriffer*, Würzburg

Part One
Principles

Virtual Screening. Edited by C. Sotriffer

ISBN: 978-3-527-32636-5

1
Virtual Screening of Chemical Space: From Generic Compound Collections to Tailored Screening Libraries

Markus Boehm

1.1
Introduction

Today's challenge of making the drug discovery process more efficient remains unchanged. The need for developing safe and innovative drugs, under the increasing pressure of speed and cost reduction, has shifted the focus toward improving the early discovery phase of lead identification and optimization. "Fail early, fail fast, and fail cheap" has often been quoted as the key principle contributing to the overall efficiency gain in drug discovery. While high-throughput screening (HTS) of large compound libraries is still the major source for discovering novel hits in the pharmaceutical industry, virtual screening has made an increasing impact in many areas of the lead identification process and has evolved into an established computational technology in modern drug discovery over the past 10 years.

Traditionally, virtual screening is conducted simply by searching the company proprietary database of its compound collections, and this approach continues to be a mainstream application. However, the continuous development of novel and more sophisticated virtual screening methods has opened up the possibility to search also for compounds that do not necessarily exist in physical form in a screening collection. Such compounds can be obtained either from a multitude of external sources, such as compound libraries from commercial vendors, or from public or commercial databases. Even more, virtual screening can deal with molecules that purely exist as virtual entities derived from *de novo* design ideas or enumeration of combinatorial libraries. Taken to its extreme, any molecule conceivable by the human mind can in theory be evaluated by virtual screening. This has led to the concept of chemical space comprising the entire collection of all possible molecules – real and imaginary – that could be created. Since such a chemical space is huge, it is crucial for the success of drug discovery to identify those regions in chemical space that contain molecules of oral druglike quality that are likely to be biologically active. Virtual screening has the unique capability of not only searching the small fraction of chemical space occupied by compounds in existing screening collections but also exploring new and so far

Virtual Screening. Edited by C. Sotriffer

ISBN: 978-3-527-32636-5

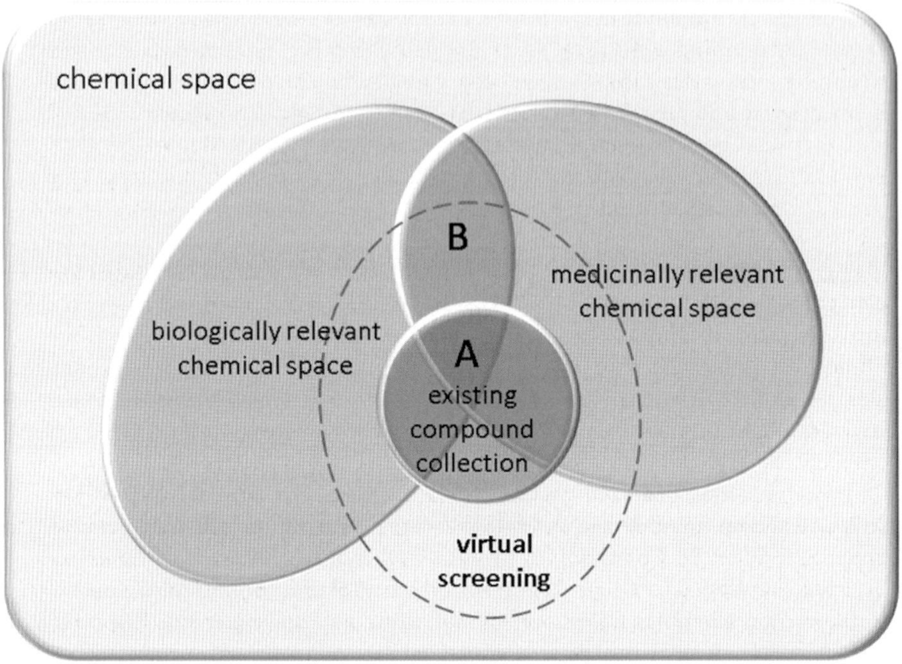

Figure 1.1 Regions of biologically and medicinally relevant chemical space within the continuum of chemical space. Only a small portion of chemical space has been sampled by existing compound collections, which led to the discovery of drugs (A). Virtual screening has the unique opportunity to expand into unexplored chemical space to find new pockets of space where drugs are likely to be discovered (B).

undiscovered regions (Figure 1.1). The challenge for the future is to better define and systematically explore those promising areas in chemical space.

1.2 Concepts of Chemical Space

Despite the fact that the term *chemical space* has received widespread attention in drug discovery, only few concrete definitions have been proposed. Lipinski suggested that chemical space "can be viewed as being analogous to the cosmological universe in its vastness, with chemical compounds populating space instead of stars" [1]. More concrete, chemical space can be defined as the entire collection of all meaningful chemical compounds, typically restricted to small organic molecules [2]. To navigate through the vastness of chemical space, compounds can be mapped onto the coordinates of a multidimensional descriptor space. Each dimension represents various properties describing the molecules, such as physicochemical or topological properties, molecular fingerprints, or similarity to a given reference compound [3]. Depending on the particular descriptor and property set used for defining a chemical space, the representation of compounds in this chemical space varies. Thus, the relative distribution of molecules within the chemical space and the relationship between them strongly depend on the chosen descriptor set. The consequence of this is that changes in chemical representation of molecules are likely to result in changes in their neighborhood relationship. This aspect is important to keep in mind when it comes to measuring diversity or similarity within a set of molecules.

How vast is chemical space? Various estimates of the size of chemical space have been proposed. The number of all possible, small organic compounds ranges anywhere from 10^{18} to 10^{180} molecules [4]. The first attempt to systematically enumerate all molecules of up to 13 heavy atoms applying basic chemical feasibility rules resulted in less than 10^{9} structures [5]. However, with every additional heavy atom the number of possible structures grows exponentially due to the combinatorial explosion of enumeration. Thus, it is estimated that with less than 30 heavy atoms more than 10^{63} molecules with a molecular weight of less than 500 can be generated, predicted to be stable at room temperature and stable toward oxygen and water [6]. Compared to the estimated number of atoms in the entire observable universe (10^{80}), it seems that for all practical purposes chemical space is infinite and any attempt to fully capture it even with computational methods appears to be futile. Even more, in contrast to the number of compounds in a typical screening collection of large pharmaceutical companies (10^{6}) it becomes clearly obvious that only a tiny fraction of chemical space is examined.

One might ask why hit identification in drug discovery is successful, despite the fact that only a very limited set of compounds within the entire chemical space is being probed. It has been hypothesized that existing screening collections are not just randomly selected from chemical space, but are already enriched with molecules that are likely to be recognized by biological targets [7]. Many synthesized compounds have been derived from natural products, metabolites, protein substrates, natural ligands, and other biogenic molecules. Hence, a certain "biogenic bias" is inherently built into existing screening libraries resulting in an increased chance of finding active hits. This observation indicates that, given the vast and infinite size of chemical space, the goal should not be to exhaustively sample the entire space but to identify those regions that contain compounds likely to be active against biological targets (biologically relevant chemical space).

Another limiting factor is that not all biologically active molecules have the desired physicochemical properties required for oral drugs. There are many aspects important for a biologically active compound to become a safe and orally administered drug, such as absorption, permeability, metabolic stability, or toxicity. The concept of *druglikeness* has been introduced to determine the characteristics necessary for a drug likely to be successful. Over time, this has been further extended toward leadlike criteria with more stringent rules and guidelines recommended for compounds in a screening collection (Section 1.3). It is generally assumed that molecules have an increased chance to be successfully developed into a medicine when they satisfy lead- and druglike criteria (medicinally relevant chemical space).

Unfortunately, not much is known about the size and regions of biologically and medicinally relevant chemical space. Current definitions of such relevant spaces often rely on the knowledge of existing, mostly orally administered drugs, and are limited by the chemical diversity of historical screening collections and by the biological diversity of known druggable targets. On one side, the data accumulated so far suggest that compounds active against certain target families (e.g., GPCRs, kinases, etc.) tend to cluster together in specific regions of chemical space [8]. For individual targets from those families, the relevant chemical space seems to be well defined, and the likelihood of finding drugs in these defined regions is high (Section 1.5). On the other side, there are many target classes that have been deemed as difficult or undruggable, such as certain proteases or phosphatases. Also, a fairly unresolved area in drug discovery is the identification of small molecule modulators of protein–protein interactions in biological signaling cascades [9]. It is assumed that the chemical space represented by traditional screening collections is inadequate to successfully tackle these "tough targets," and new regions of chemical space need to be explored. Possible sources of chemical matter potentially occupying such unexplored regions of space can be derived from natural products or through emerging technologies such as diversity-oriented synthesis for generating natural product-like combinatorial libraries (Section 1.4).

1.3
Concepts of Druglikeness and Leadlikeness

It has been demonstrated that the lead development stage contributes 40% to the overall attrition rate throughout the whole drug development process, beginning from the first assay development to final registration [10]. Therefore, it is assumed that significant improvements can be realized in the early phase of lead identification and development. In-depth analysis of marketed oral drugs led to the introduction of druglikeness that defines the physicochemical properties that determine key issues of drug development, such as absorption and permeability. Lipinski's influential analysis of compounds failing to become orally administered drugs resulted in the well-known "rule of five" [11]. In short, the rule predicts that poor absorption or permeation of a drug is more likely to occur when there are more than 5 H-bond donors, 10 H-bond acceptors, the molecular weight is greater than 500, and the calculated log P is greater than 5 (Table 1.1). The concept of *druglikeness* has been widely accepted and embraced by scientists in drug discovery nowadays, with many variations and extensions of the original rules, and it has served its purpose well to help optimize pharmacokinetic properties of drug candidate molecules [12, 13].

The rules defining druglikeness, however, should not necessarily be applied to lead molecules. One of the reasons is the observation that, on average, compounds in comparison to their initial leads become larger and more complex during the lead optimization phase, and the associated physicochemical properties (e.g., molecular weight, calculated log P, etc.) increase accordingly [14, 15]. To ensure

Table 1.1 Comparison of properties typically used for leadlikeness and druglikeness criteria.

Properties	Leadlikeness	Druglikeness
Molecular weight (MW)	≤350	≤500
Lipophilicity (clog *P*)	≤3.0	≤5.0
H-bond donor (sum of NH and OH)	≤3	≤5
H-bond acceptor (sum of N and O)	≤8	≤10
Polar surface area (PSA)	≤120 Å^2	≤150 Å^2
Number of rotatable bonds	≤8	≤10
Structural filters	Reactive groups Warhead-containing agents Frequent hitters Promiscuous inhibitors	

that the properties of an optimized compound remain within druglike space, the criteria for *leadlikeness* have been more narrowly defined to accommodate the expected growth during drug optimization (Table 1.1). Complementary to the comparison of drug and lead pairs from historical data, Hann *et al.* analyzed in a more theoretical approach, using a simplified ligand–receptor interaction model, how the probability of finding a hit varies with the complexity of a molecule [16]. The model shows that the probability of observing a "useful interaction event" decreases when molecules become increasingly complex. This suggests that less complex molecules, in accordance with leadlike criteria, are more likely to turn into hits (albeit weaker) serving as common starting points for the successful discovery of drugs.

Another aspect underlining the importance of leadlike properties is associated with the fundamental shift in the screening paradigm in drug discovery from functional biological assays to biochemical assays. While biological assays measure a true biological activity, biochemical assays are designed to measure specific molecular interactions between a compound and its target. Biochemical assays are highly sensitive assays, well suited for screening compounds in a high-throughput fashion, but due to their artificial nature they are also susceptible to compound interference resulting in false positive hits. It has been suggested that compounds with leadlike properties also interact with their targets in a leadlike manner, that is, by noncovalent binding through hydrogen bonds, hydrophobic interactions, and monoionic bonding [17]. In general, such desirable interaction types result in reversible, time-independent, and competitive binding characteristics allowing the generation of meaningful structure–activity data. In contrast, nonleadlike compounds tend to bind to their target in nonleadlike ways, such as forming covalent, chelate, or polyionic bonds. Thus, nonleadlike compounds are more prone to generating artifact data in biochemical assays.

Among the well-known offenders with nonleadlike properties are protein-reactive compounds, warhead-containing agents, frequent hitters, and aggregator compounds (Table 1.1) [18]. Computationally, the elimination of reactive and warhead-containing compounds can be accomplished by applying various sets of substructure filters [17, 19]. Frequent hitters can be identified by statistical models or other virtual screening methods [20]. Aggregator compounds have been described as being promiscuous inhibitors by forming aggregates in solution, resulting in nonspecific binding and interference with the biochemical assay [21]. However, they are difficult to predict computationally and require additional biophysical methods (e.g., light scattering experiments) or modifications of the biochemical assay (e.g., addition of detergent or protein serum) to support their detection experimentally [22]. Exacerbating the problem, the interference of compounds in biochemical screens resulting in artifact data mostly depends on the individual assay conditions, which makes it difficult to develop generally applicable rules for detecting potential false positives across different assays.

The ultimate goal of identifying compounds with leadlike properties is to design high-quality screening libraries, whether it is for experimental or virtual screening purposes [23]. From a practical standpoint, it appears that leadlike criteria are more straightforward to implement by applying rules to filter out nonleadlike compounds, with the aim of enriching the compound collection with leadlike matter. In other words, one can agree on which compounds not to screen, but the question which compounds to screen often leads to lengthy debates among experienced medicinal chemists.

1.4 Diversity-Based Libraries

Since the advent of large-scale combinatorial chemistry in drug discovery coupled with high-speed parallel synthesis of thousands of compounds, the concept of *molecular diversity* has increasingly gained importance. When little or nothing is known about the biological target, it is often assumed that screening a compound library as diverse as possible maximizes the chance of finding active hits. Moreover, the continuous addition of compounds to the screening file, either from internal combinatorial library efforts or through purchase of external compound collections, is most valuable when the underlying overall diversity can be expanded. At the same time, there is an ever-growing pressure to reduce costs by decreasing the number of compounds that need to be screened while simultaneously maintaining diversity. Hence, well-defined strategies for the optimal design of *diversity-based libraries* are necessary.

1.4.1 Concepts of Molecular Diversity

The generally accepted understanding of molecular diversity is a quantitative description of dissimilarity between molecules in a given set of compounds. The exact interpretation of this concept, however, has created quite a heated debate in the scientific literature [24]. For example, Roth fervently advocated that *per se* "there is no such thing as diversity" [25]. Diversity of chemical structure does not necessarily imply diversity of biological activity. In order to be meaningful, diversity can only be applied within a frame of reference, that is, the biological assay. Hence, structural diversity of compounds should be interpreted only with respect to their relative effect in biological screens. Finding descriptors for biological activity is necessary to describe the diversity of biological activities for compounds present in a library. Unfortunately, it is often difficult or impossible to predict in advance which descriptors are most effective in a given situation. While it remains to be a matter of subjectivity what makes a compound set diverse and how to quantify diversity, or if one compound set is more diverse than another, the minimum value gained by a diversity application is the elimination of redundancy within a screening set. A diverse set of compounds should contain only nonredundant molecules that simultaneously span a wide range of properties covering the chemical space.

The basis of removing redundancy from a compound set is formed by the general belief that similar molecules typically exhibit similar biological activities. This concept has been defined as the *similarity property principle* or neighborhood behavior, and is the fundamental assumption behind all similarity and diversity applications [26]. Although generally accepted, one can quickly find arguments against this principle, as there are many examples described where subtle modifications of a compound can lead to dramatic changes in activity (activity cliffs, "magic methyl," etc.) or major changes in the molecular structure not resulting in significant activity differences (flat SAR). From a statistical point of view, however, it has been demonstrated that a set of compounds similar to an active hit contains a higher number of actives compared to a random set, thus increasing the probability of finding actives [27]. Various groups have analyzed large activity data sets and came to the conclusion that on average there is a 30% chance that a compound within a certain similarity cutoff (Tanimoto coefficient $\geq$0.85 using Daylight fingerprints) to an active hit is itself active [28, 29]. The backside of this finding is that diversity methods selecting a representative compound within a subset of similar compounds incur a 70% chance of picking an inactive compound and excluding compounds that might have had activity. Exacerbating the effect, diversity selections often tend to more aggressively reduce the size of screening sets by loosening similarity criteria beyond the range where the similarity property principle is applicable. This might lead to a decreased coverage of biological space, limiting the chance of finding actives within the chosen subset.

1.4.2 Descriptor-Based Diversity Selection

Various strategies for the design of diversity-based screening collections have been proposed. Before initiating the selection process, some more fundamental questions should be addressed. For instance, it is often unclear how large a screening library should be and how many cluster representatives need to be selected. Using fingerprints and default similarity cutoffs for clustering (see above) and assuming the presence of actives in a cluster, there is only a 30% probability of identifying an active hit when a single representative per cluster is chosen. The selection of five compounds per cluster increases the chance of finding actives to 80% [28]. This finding suggests the selection of multiple representatives per cluster to increase the likelihood of uncovering actives. However, this comes at the expense of including fewer clusters during the selection process.

A mathematical model was developed by Harper *et al.* to provide a more quantitative framework for assessing the optimal parameters of a screening collection and their effect on the probability of producing lead series in a given biological assay [30]. For each cluster in a screening collection, the percentage of compounds expected to hit the biological target, as well as the probability of an existing lead molecule in the cluster, is empirically estimated. According to the model, the expected number of lead series per screen ("lead discovery rate") increases linearly with the number of compounds in a screening library. However, the probability of finding one or more lead series in a given screen does not grow proportionally with the size of the library. For instance, it was estimated that an average hit rate of 1.2 leads per screen is required to find at least one lead on 70% of screens. To increase the proportion of screens identifying leads to 80% and beyond requires a sharp increase in the number of compounds to be screened. This result of diminishing returns has been experienced by many companies when their screening collections have dramatically increased in size, but it has not translated into a proportional increase in successful screening campaigns. One of the main conclusions from the analysis is that, in order to increase the chance of finding lead series, a screening library of a given size should contain as many diverse clusters as possible, ideally with only one or few representatives per cluster. Increasing the number of compounds per cluster at the cost of decreasing the number of clusters ultimately lowers the likelihood of finding leads.

In principle, there are three main steps required to carry out diversity-based subset selections: (1) the calculation of descriptors representing the compound structures, (2) a quantitative method to describe the similarity or dissimilarity of molecules in relationship to each other, and (3) selection methods to identify compounds based on their similarity or dissimilarity values that best represent the entire compound set. In the following, the three steps are described in more detail.

Numerous descriptors encoding molecular properties with varying degrees of information content and complexity have been developed [31]. The current version of the Dragon software alone calculates over 3200 molecular descriptors [32]. The many different representations can be classified according to the type of information they encode [4, 33]. Whole-molecule descriptors represent different properties of a molecule in a single number, such as molecular weight or calculated log P. Descriptors derived from 2D representations of molecules include topological indices, which describe a structure according to its size and shape by a single number, and fingerprint-based descriptors, characterizing molecules by their substructural features. Graph-based molecular descriptors attempt to reduce the molecular complexity while capturing the overall information content of the molecular topology and properties. Descriptors derived from the 3D structure of molecules consist of fingerprint-based descriptors and other more complex representations, encoding properties such as shape or pharmacophore information of a molecule.

In order to quantify the degree of similarity or dissimilarity between two compounds, various similarity coefficients have been developed for different applications, many of them widely used for chemical similarity searching [34]. Several groups compared the performance of different similarity coefficients in combination with various fingerprint types, and it was often found that the Tanimoto coefficient markedly outperformed other similarity measures, making it the similarity coefficient of choice for fingerprint-based similarity searching [35].

Methods for selecting diverse subsets from a compound collection include (1) dissimilarity-based compound selection, (2) clustering, (3) partitioning, and (4) the use of optimization approaches, and are discussed in the following. Dissimilarity-based methods involve the selection of compound sets that maximize the dissimilarity between pairs of molecules [36]. In an iterative fashion, those molecules from a compound collection that are mostly dissimilar to the already selected compounds from the subset are added to the subset. The MaxMin selection technique and the sphere exclusion algorithm are the preferred methods of choice among dissimilarity-based methods [37, 38]. Clustering methods involve the identification of groups of compounds such that compounds within a cluster are highly similar whereas compounds from different clusters are dissimilar. Choosing one or only few representatives per cluster, usually the cluster centroids, has been demonstrated to be the best strategy for designing a highly diverse subset to maximize the chances of hit identification. Many different clustering algorithms have been developed, and they can be divided into hierarchical and nonhierarchical methods [39]. Since clustering is based on relative similarities of molecules to each other and not on an absolute scale in chemical space, it is often difficult to compare two different data sets, which is required, for instance, when purchasing new compound collections. In contrast, partitioning or cell-based methods provide an absolute measure of compounds in terms of their location in chemical space, spanned by a predefined descriptor set [40]. A low-dimensional descriptor space is required, where descriptors are mapped onto each axis of the chemical space by binning (partitioning) the range of their values into a set of cells. Molecules that fall into the same cells can be considered similar, and a diverse subset of compounds is selected by taking one or a few representatives from each cell. Pearlman's well-known BCUT descriptors, typically mapped into a six-dimensional space, were developed for the use in partitioning-based approaches [41]. A chemical global positioning system, ChemGPS, was introduced to provide a low-dimensional chemical space as a frame of reference suitable for diversity analysis [42]. A set of 72 descriptors was condensed into a nine-dimensional space by means of principal component analysis. Finally, optimization-based approaches use genetic algorithms or simulated annealing to efficiently sample large chemical spaces [43, 44].

1.4.3 Scaffold-Based Diversity Selection

An alternative approach to describe the diversity of a compound collection has been realized by the classification of molecules according to their underlying scaffolds. Compared to methods using traditional descriptors such as fingerprints, scaffold classification methods provide a different view of comparing databases of compounds. Scaffold diversity and coverage, as well as over- or underrepresented regions of scaffold space, can be easily assessed across different data sets, such as publicly or commercially available screening collections [45]. Scaffold analysis is also applied to HTS data to retrieve more chemically intuitive clustering results [46]. Finally, classification of compounds according to their scaffolds can help identify privileged structures and serve as a starting point for designing scaffold-focused libraries (Section 1.5) [47, 48].

Although there is no exact definition for a molecular scaffold, it generally refers to a common structural core motif. Scaffolds often resemble the chemotypes of molecules, which medicinal chemists use to categorize compounds into chemical series. Bemis and Murcko have introduced the widely used classification of compounds according to their molecular framework [49]. The molecular framework of a compound, also referred to as "Murcko scaffold," is formed by deleting all terminal acyclic side-chain atoms from the original molecule. In addition, all atom and bond types can be removed to arrive at the graph framework of the molecule. The removal of linker length and ring size information results in the reduced graph representation of the molecule. The feature tree descriptor used in FTrees is a popular example where compounds are described by a graph (tree) that represents each molecular fragment and functional group (feature) as a node and their connectivity as edges [50]. This reduces the molecular descriptor complexity while still maintaining the overall topology and property information, making this descriptor ideal for scaffold hopping searches [51]. In a related approach, "molecular equivalence indices" (MEQI) classify molecules with respect to a variety of structural features and topological shapes, which can be used to hierarchically classify compound sets into classes of chemotypes [52]. Recently, a hierarchical classification system, Scaffold Tree, has been described [53]. Each level of the hierarchy consists of well-defined chemical substructures by iteratively removing rings from the molecular framework. Prioritization rules ensure that peripheral rings are removed first to achieve unique classification trees. Besides the benefit of its visually intuitive presentation of the scaffold tree, potential applications of this method are the detection of potential chemical series from screening hits on the basis of their hierarchical classification and the retrosynthetic combinatorial analysis of library compounds to identify the scaffolds that have been most likely used. The idea of a hierarchical classification of scaffolds has been expanded to incorporate the biological space associated with the compounds. The program Scaffold Hunter has been developed both to analyze the complex relationship of structure and activity data and to identify scaffolds of compounds likely to contain the desired biological activity [54, 55]. Analogous to the Scaffold Tree approach, scaffolds are hierarchically organized, however, using activity data as the key selection criterion during the structural deconstruction and tree building process. Scaffolds that share activity with their neighboring scaffolds in the hierarchical tree but are not represented by compounds in the data set are identified. Such virtual scaffolds can serve as starting points for the discovery of new biologically relevant scaffolds.

1.4.4 Sources of Diversity

Besides the established sources of obtaining diversity, mainly from historic compound collections, publicly or commercially available compound libraries, and natural products, novel approaches toward expanding diversity have been described in the recent literature.

The systematic enumeration of all possible organic molecules of up to 11 atoms of C, N, O, and F, applying simple valence, chemical stability, and synthetic feasibility rules, has been reported [56]. A total of 26.4 million compounds were generated and collected in a chemical universe database (GDB-11). An extended version (GDB-13) has been published that contains 970 million molecules of up to 13 atoms of C, N, O, S, and Cl enumerated in a similar manner, making it the largest database of publicly available virtual molecules [5]. It contains a vast number of unexplored structures and provides a new source for design ideas to identify bioactive small molecules and scaffolds. The first successful application of the GDB discovering a novel class of NMDA glycine site inhibitors has been recently reported [57].

Bioactive molecules have been shown to contain only a limited number of unique ring systems. For that reason, in analogy to the chemical universe of the GDB, several groups have explored the ring universe to identify novel ring systems and heteroaromatic scaffolds. A comprehensive collection of more than 40 000 different rings extracted from the CAS registry has been classified into ring systems on the basis of their topology, and it was shown that the distribution of rings is not continuous but contains many significant voids [58]. A drug ring database containing ring systems from proprietary and commercial compound collections has been developed as a source for scaffold replacement design [59]. Generating a database of over 600 000 heteroaromatic ring scaffolds, the comparison to scaffolds associated with biological activity revealed that bioactive scaffolds are very sparsely distributed, forming well-defined "bioactivity islands" in virtual scaffold space [60]. It is, however, unclear if biological activity is truly limited to only such small region of ring space, or if most ring systems are simply not synthetically accessible and thus have never been prepared. To overcome this limitation, the future challenge is to actively develop novel synthetic routes to prepare molecules with so far unexplored ring systems. A "virtual exploratory heterocyclic library" (VEHICLe) of almost 25 000 ring systems was created, containing a complete enumerated set of heteroaromatic rings, with rings being removed that are likely to be synthetically unfeasible according to a set of empirical rules [61]. Interestingly, the authors find that only 1700 of them (7%) have been published, and of these only a small percentage is routinely used in the synthesis of druglike molecules. They highlight many simple and apparently tractable heterocycles that have not been described in the literature so far and put out a "challenge to creative organic chemists to either make them or explain why they cannot be made."

It has been argued that the trend in drug discovery over the past decade toward achiral, aromatic compounds, presumably due to their amenability to high-throughput synthetic approaches, may have contributed to a higher failure rate of drug development candidates [62]. Concurrently, it has been reported that the complexity of a molecule is a key criterion determining the success of the drug candidate [63]. The increase in molecular complexity, measured as the extent of bond saturation and the number of chiral centers, has been demonstrated to correlate with an overall improved compound developability. Changes in molecular complexity affect the three-dimensional shape of a compound, which might lead to improved interactions with the target receptor. The resulting improved potency and selectivity profile ultimately increases the chance of a successful drug candidate. Although aromatic rings and achiral centers still dominantly define classical drug structures, this might suggest a trend away from flat aromatic structures toward more complex molecules.

In the recent past, natural products and natural product-like molecules that lie outside the range of traditional "rule of five" druglike space have gained renewed interest in drug discovery [64, 65]. Technological advances have enabled the combination of approaches that leverage the unique diversity of building blocks from natural product sources with the strength of combinatorial library design. The diversity-oriented synthesis (DOS) approach allows the rapid synthesis of chemical libraries containing structurally complex molecules with a range of scaffold variations and chiral centers, creating a broad distribution of diverse compounds capable of binding a range of biological targets [66]. The main emphasis of natural product-like drug discovery so far, however, is on the identification of novel tool compounds to probe the target of interest and support further pharmacological *in vitro* studies, not on the development of oral drugs [67, 68]. Finally, macrocyclic molecules (containing a ring of seven or more atoms) represent another emerging structural class outside of classical oral druglike space, with a strong potential for historically difficult targets such as protein–protein interactions [69]. Macrocycles are capable of forming high-affinity interactions with the shallow contact surfaces that are typical for interfaces involved in protein–protein interactions. Due to their intrinsic conformational constraint, they can position arrays of functional groups across a wide interaction area, without the penalty of introducing multiple rotatable bonds.

Virtual screening provides an excellent opportunity to explore large databases of virtual small molecules and ring systems as highlighted above, supporting the design of combinatorial libraries with novel scaffolds or ring systems, or can be employed for tasks such as bioisosteric replacement design and scaffold hopping. However, in order to increase the chance of successfully synthesizing molecules proposed by virtual screening methods, more effort has to be put into the development of predictive methods to account for chemical feasibility. Not only should it include if a particular compound can be synthesized but it should also include if it can be rapidly followed up (i.e., chemically enabled) with analogues during lead optimization in a medicinal chemistry campaign. Computational approaches to assess synthetic accessibility have been described in the literature, mainly based on retrosynthetic or complexity-based analysis of molecules [70, 71].

1.5 Focused Libraries

Random screening of compound libraries in a high-throughput fashion is the major source of finding new leads in drug discovery when little or nothing is known about a target. Modern HTS technologies can routinely screen millions of compounds in a few weeks. However, in certain screening paradigms this approach may not always be feasible. For instance, the assay format cannot be scaled up to HTS format or only a low-throughput cell-based assay is available. In this situation, it is necessary to reduce the number of compounds to be screened, and the selection of diversity-based compound subsets is a viable option (Section 1.4). At the beginning of a new drug discovery project, it is often likely that information already exists to jump-start the program. When sufficient knowledge about a drug target is available, the design of targeted or *focused libraries* is possible. Various computational methods can "focus" the selection of compounds toward individual targets or entire target classes. The growing amount of knowledge for many drug targets and known drugs has resulted in an increased number of publications that describe new methods for the design of target and target family-focused libraries. Consequently, the screening of moderately sized (10^4–10^5) focused libraries has emerged as a promising alternative and efficient approach for lead identification.

1.5.1 Concepts of Focused Design

In their seminal work, Hopkins and coworkers mapped the entire known pharmacological space (biologically relevant chemical space) on the basis of a comprehensive collection of literature data [8]. This compound-centric view allowed them to identify targets for which drugs and chemical tools have been discovered, and how they are related to each other. Not surprisingly, the most densely populated target families represent attractive gene families that are actively pursued in drug discovery, notably kinases, GPCRs, ion channels, proteases, phosphatases, and nuclear hormone receptors. These multimember gene families, which account for more than 50% of the known human druggable genome, are also the prime candidates for targeted library design efforts due to their family-wide similarities in molecular recognition or enzymatic mechanisms.

A certain amount of prior knowledge about members of the target families is required for the successful design of focused libraries. Increased efforts in collecting and annotating pharmacological data of molecules are undertaken (Section 1.7). The availability of an ever-growing number of protein structures in the Protein Data Bank (PDB) facilitates the generation of structure-based knowledge of target classes.

Depending on the type and amount of information available for a target family, one can apply ligand-based, structure-based, or chemogenomics approaches for the design of focused libraries, or ideally all methods can be combined in a complementary fashion [72]. Interestingly, while GPCRs represent the second largest gene family (after kinases), they almost completely lack any structural information due to their membrane-bound nature. Only recently, the first crystal structures of human GPCR targets (β_2 adrenergic, A_{2a} adenosine receptors) have been solved. Hence, the design of GPCR focused libraries in the past was often limited to ligand-based methods. The development of refined homology models and prediction of ligand binding modes start to compensate for the lack of GPCR structures, making structure-based methods more amenable to focused library design [73].

1.5.2
Ligand-Based Focused Design

The use of simple molecular properties has been demonstrated to construct models that discriminate compounds belonging to different target families. Depending on their target family, bioactive molecules show differences in their physicochemical properties [74, 75]. These variations can be used either as simple descriptor-based guidelines or to develop predictive models that focus the composition of chemical libraries toward a particular target family. For example, a neural network model was constructed on the basis of a small set of physicochemical properties to categorize compounds as GPCR-like or non-GPCR-like [76]. According to the model, GPCR-like compounds tend to be less flexible, less polar, and more hydrophobic compared to non-GPCR-like molecules. Other classification methods have been applied as well, such as Bayesian models, recursive partitioning, self-organizing maps (SOM), and other machine learning systems, in combination with various 2D or 3D descriptors [77, 78]. BCUT descriptors not only are being used for diversity-based subset selections (Section 1.4) but have also been employed to design focused libraries [79]. Instead of selecting diverse representatives from each cell in the low-dimensional descriptor space, compounds from "promising cells" are chosen that contain known active ligands.

Following a pharmacophore approach, a consensus 3D pharmacophore fingerprint based on a set of known GPCR ligands was created, which was subsequently used for building GPCR focused libraries [80]. Using a four-point pharmacophore fingerprint as a measure for similarity, GPCR-specific pharmacophores were identified and applied toward the design of focused libraries [81]. Particularly for large target families where a wealth of data exists, such as kinases and GPCRs, known ligands can be used to define queries to search against compound collections using substructure and similarity searches, and identified molecules can be compiled into focused screening collections [82, 83].

The notion that compounds with a benzodiazepine core were active as ligands against a variety of GPCRs, such as central and peripheral benzodiazepine, kappa opioid, and CCK receptors, has led to the *privileged structure* concept [84]. The observed activity crossover of a single compound to multiple targets of the same gene family implies that an underlying molecular scaffold is "privileged" to lend its activity to more than one receptor. The privileged structure concept has appeared more frequently in the recent literature and is interpreted in two different flavors [48]. In a strict sense, privileged structures should be defined as substructures with a proven correlation to a particular target family, based on specifically defined key structural elements that account for a commonality in molecular recognition across the target family members. In a broader context, privileged structures are interpreted as substructures emerging in compounds that showed effects on multiple target proteins, irrespective of their underlying target families. It is unknown why these fragments bind with higher than average frequency to multiple targets, and often there is no clear dividing line between privileged structures and promiscuous binders. Nevertheless, an increasing number of scaffolds have been described as privileged structures, mainly for GPCR and kinase targets, including indoles, biphenyls, benzopyranes, aryl piperazines, or aminopyrimidines [85].

Several groups have carried out fragmentation analyses of compounds active against target families, and the observed frequently recurring fragments were used as input for the design of focused libraries. In one of the first studies, a "retrosynthetic combinatorial analysis procedure" (RECAP) was developed using a limited set of defined fragmentation rules to identify privileged substructural elements [86]. Novel kinase inhibitors were designed in a reconstructive approach by fragmentation of known inhibitors and *de novo* assembly of fragments based on predictive models. The authors noted that while this approach worked well in designing active molecules, it remains to be challenging to also find selective kinase inhibitors [87]. A similar "virtual fragment linking" approach validated across a variety of different target classes has also been reported [88]. A combination of virtual and experimental (NMR, biochemical) screening methods was employed to identify novel scaffolds for the design of kinase-targeted libraries [89].

These and other reports give evidence of frequently occurring substructural elements connected to activity across a diverse panel of proteins. However, it is still debatable if such privileged structures are truly privileged in a selective manner against specific target families [90]. For instance, it is possible that fragments occurring with high frequency are simply elements of druglike, easy to synthesize, and therefore overrepresented molecules in compound collections. More thorough analyses are required that study the selectivity of privileged structures against target families and consider only statistically significant fragments by normalizing their occurrences in active compounds versus mere incidence in the screening libraries.

1.5.3
Structure-Based Focused Design

Compared to ligand-based approaches, the use of structure-based methods has received less attention in the past, mainly due to their limited applicability to target classes with available protein structures and also because some of the methods such as docking still involve computationally intensive processes. Nevertheless, for certain target classes, particularly for kinases, significant amount of structural information is available, making structure-based approaches a viable option for compound selection and focused library design. The publication of the first human GPCR crystal structures, as well as the development of more refined homology models in combination with site-directed mutagenesis data and ligand structure–activity relationships (SAR), has also advanced the design of structure-based focused libraries for GPCR targets.

Protein–ligand docking and pharmacophore searching are the two main structure-based techniques for searching a large number of compounds to design focused libraries. Fast high-throughput docking methods allow the evaluation of large virtual libraries in a protein binding pocket, followed by the selection of compounds according to their docking scores. Due to the limited accuracy of scoring functions in general, it is advisable to also maintain a certain amount of diversity within the selected subset to facilitate the detection of potential new binding modes not predicted by docking [91]. The docking of combinatorial libraries based on a selected number of scaffolds, linkers, and functional groups allowed the design and synthesis of a target-focused virtual library while optimizing size versus diversity [47]. For designing a kinase-focused library, various scaffolds were prioritized by docking small virtual libraries generated around each core. Scaffolds that led to consistently docked structures according to cluster analysis were selected [92]. By docking privileged fragments derived from fragmentation of known kinase inhibitors into their respective protein binding pockets, both ligand-based and structural information was combined to assemble novel scaffold libraries for a kinase-focused library [93].

1.5.4
Chemogenomics Approaches

A new strategy in drug discovery termed *chemogenomics* has been defined as the investigation of classes of compounds against families of functionally related proteins [94]. It provides a unique approach to organize targets according to their gene families and discover ligands for related targets in a systematic manner, thus enhancing the efficiency of the drug discovery process [95]. Analogous to the similarity property principle (i.e., similar chemical structures share similar biological activities), the underlying assumption of chemogenomics is that similar biological structures share similar ligands. Indeed, it has often been observed that compounds active against one protein also show activity against other members of the same gene family. Chemogenomics attempts to link chemical structures of bioactive molecules and their effect on entire targets classes. Ultimately, insights into this relationship enable the rational design of focused libraries against one or multiple gene family members. Since the success of identifying and exploiting these links depends on the availability of structural and biological data for a larger number of targets, chemogenomics methods have been applied largely to not only major gene families, GPCRs and kinases mainly, but also proteases, nuclear hormone receptors, and ion channels.

Due to the lack of protein structures, similarities among GPCR targets have been mainly explored by sequence-based methods. The conventional approach of mapping the homology between GPCRs in a phylogenetic tree analysis employs full protein sequences. More relevant from a drug design perspective, however, is the comparison of targets based on their ligand recognition. Several groups have identified putative ligand binding sites within the transmembrane region of GPCRs [96, 97]. The relevant amino acids defining the pockets (20–50 residues) can be represented by their physicochemical properties (charged, polar, hydrophobic, aromatic, etc.) and are converted into bit strings unique for each receptor. This enables a straightforward comparison of ligand binding sites of targets across the entire gene family. Similarly, "structural interaction fingerprints" (SIFt) were developed for kinase binding sites, based on fingerprints derived from physicochemical properties of selected binding site residues [98].

This approach can be applied to find novel sources of ligands for GPCRs without existing leads by first evaluating similar GPCRs for which ligands are known. For example, active compounds for the CRTH2 receptor were identified by screening ligands from the structurally related AT1 and AT2 receptors [99]. Notably, the close relationship between the CRTH2 and AT1/AT2 receptors was not revealed by their full-length sequence homology. Small molecule antagonists for SSTR5 were identified by starting with a known histamine H1 antagonist, after a chemogenomics analysis had shown a close similarity between SSTR5 and opioid, histamine, dopamine, and serotonin receptors [100]. The same strategy has also been proposed to identify ligands for several orphan GPCRs [97].

A more elaborate chemogenomics approach, "thematic analysis," has been developed by Biofocus to better characterize the binding regions across a range of different GPCRs [101]. The putative ligand interaction site is divided into separate microenvironments with well-defined properties for each subsite (themes) and paired with matching fragments (motifs) based on known ligand structures. Combined, these thematic fingerprints can be used to classify new GPCRs and to design libraries focused on particular GPCR subclasses. A similar concept termed "chemoprint" has been applied to GPCRs by systematically annotating key interaction pairs of ligand fragments and their putative protein binding residues [102]. It is worth noting that in combination with homology modeling, the authors have established a method for deriving sequence-based 3D pharmacophore models for a wide range of GPCR targets, useful for virtual screening and focused library design.

A ligand-centric view of chemogenomics is the classification of biological targets based on activity profiles of diverse ligands [103]. These affinity fingerprints can then serve as a measure of protein similarity. It has been demonstrated that clustering of kinases based on their ligand SAR is different from the sequence-based clustering [104]. Both ligand- and structure-based classifications are often complementary and provide alternative views of the same protein family. The BioPrint database from Cerep comprises activity profiles of chemical structures experimentally measured across a large number of targets. Using experimental binding data generated from 2000 druglike compounds on 40 GPCR targets, a global QSAR model employing pharmacophore features relevant to GPCR binding characteristics has been developed and applied to design GPCR focused libraries [105].

1.6 Virtual Combinatorial Libraries and Fragment Spaces

With today's computational resources it is usually not a problem to exhaustively search compounds from corporate collections, vendor libraries, or small combinatorial libraries, which typically range in the order of 10^5–10^7 molecules. However, for large virtual combinatorial libraries and collections thereof, it becomes quickly unfeasible to enumerate all possible virtual molecules in advance due to combinatorial explosion. Consequently, there has been an increasing interest in computational methods to find alternative ways to systematically search large virtual combinatorial libraries, allowing a dramatic expansion of unexplored chemical space.

A solution to the problem is to encode molecules of virtual combinatorial libraries not as enumerated products, but rather to keep them in their unenumerated form as building blocks (fragments), together with linkage rules for how to combine them. The efficiency of searching virtual combinatorial libraries in their *fragment space* representation compared to their enumerated products is easily explained by the different numbers of molecules that have to be processed during a similarity search. For instance, if a two-component combinatorial library with 1000 building blocks each is searched in its enumerated form, one million product structures have to be compared to a given query. In contrast, only 2000 monomers have to be evaluated in their corresponding fragment space. Extending this comparison to large sets of combinatorial libraries, the number of products can by far exceed 10^{12} possible virtual products, making a systematic enumeration unfeasible, whereas searching in the equivalent fragment space keeps the number still at a manageable size.

A large fragment space encoding over 10^{13} possible product structures has been created at Pfizer by taking a collection of 358 combinatorial libraries based on proprietary validated reaction protocols [106]. This fragment space can be systematically explored with the similarity search program FTrees-FS (extension of FTrees) that does not require the upfront enumeration of product structures [50, 107]. The result is a list of virtual products similar to the search query, synthetically accessible by one or more of the reaction protocols stored in the fragment space. Grouping the virtual hits by their synthetic protocols allows a fast follow-up design of focused libraries. A similar fragment space based on feature tree descriptors spanning 10^{11} potential products was generated using proprietary reaction protocols [108]. The selection of diverse sets of input reagents enabled both diverse and focused decorations of the central scaffolds identified by the search. In a related approach, a "monomer-based similarity searching" (MoBSS) method has been developed using atom pair descriptors [109]. To avoid time-consuming product enumeration, the descriptors are generated from the monomers of virtual combinatorial libraries collected in a fragment space. Since atom pair descriptors computed from interatomic distances lend themselves to pairwise additivity, product atom pairs can be rapidly computed from those of the constituent monomers through an arithmetic manipulation.

Fragment spaces have also been assembled by rule-based fragmentation of drug molecules. To build such a space, the RECAP program has been applied to drugs from the World Drug Index (WDI) and other druglike molecule collections [86, 110]. Applying a set of retrosynthetic rules, the drug molecules are disconnected into their individual fragments, and together with their associated link types they are incorporated into the fragment space. The large variety of generated fragments combined with a countless number of possible recombinations based on a limited set of connection rules permits a high degree of diversity of virtual products. However, this comes at the expense of their synthetic feasibility, which in contrast to hits from combinatorial fragment spaces is often unknown [111]. Predictive methods to assess synthetic feasibility of virtual *de novo* molecules have been proposed [112].

The calculation of "basis products" is an efficient way of representing large combinatorial libraries by strategically selecting subsets of compounds without complete enumeration. They are derived by enumerating one building block at a time while holding all other reaction components fixed, and this is consecutively repeated for all other building blocks. In the case of a two-component reaction with 1000 monomers each, only 1999 basis products have to be enumerated (A_1B_1, A_2B_1, A_3B_1, ..., $A_{1000}B_1$, A_1B_2, A_1B_3, ..., A_1B_{1000}). This way, any virtual product in the combinatorial library is represented by a set of basis products (e.g., A_3B_7 represented by A_3B_1 and A_1B_7). Basis products can be used in the same way as enumerated combinatorial library products, such as property filtering or docking [113]. However, the underlying assumption and limitation of this approach is that properties or docking scores from the various building blocks behave in an additive manner. A large number of virtual combinatorial libraries were also efficiently encoded by Bayesian modeling [114]. Representative members from a large number of combinatorial libraries are used to derive a multicategory Bayesian model. The resulting "Bayesian idea generator" (BIG) allows to predict the likelihood of a given compound belonging to a certain combinatorial library. Several top-ranking libraries are suggested and prioritized according to their Bayesian score.

Virtual combinatorial libraries can also be explored by structure-based virtual screening methods without prior enumeration. Docking of large virtual combinatorial libraries is offered by many docking programs, such as DREAM++, FlexX^c, CombiDOCK, and CombiGlide, among others [115]. Typically, the library templates are placed in the binding pocket, and each subsite is individually probed by docking the various R-groups of the library. Compounds with the highest scoring R-group combinations are selected and synthesized as part of the focused library. Notably, the FlexNovo software is capable of directly accessing fragment spaces generated as described above [116].

1.7
Databases of Chemical and Biological Information

Numerous databases of chemical structures, biological targets, and bioactivity data relevant for drug discovery have emerged in recent years. They are a unique source both for generating new ideas to identify chemical matter and for providing information-rich content for chemical and biological targets. Besides traditional compound databases with a large number of diverse chemical structures, there is an increased interest in annotated compound libraries aiming at capturing information to establish relationships between chemical matter and their biological function [117]. All relevant databases have been extensively reviewed in the literature. In the following, representative public and commercial databases relevant for drug discovery are highlighted (Table 1.2).

ZINC is a free database of commercially available compounds that in its current version contains over 13 million purchasable compounds from vendor catalogs [118]. Multiple formats are provided to fit the needs for various virtual screening applications such as substructure and similarity searches, property filtering, and docking. Subsets of druglike, leadlike, and fragment compounds have been generated and can be accessed separately. Similarly, ChemDB is a chemical database of over 5 million small molecules collected from electronic catalogs of commercial vendors. In addition, computational reaction models enable searches through virtual chemical space by predicting hypothetical products synthetically accessible from building blocks contained in the database [119]. Web-based chemistry search engines are capable of mining a large number of molecules from various public data repositories, such as ChemSpider (20 million) and eMolecules (7 million), the latter also offering databases for download to be used for virtual screening.

PubChem is a component of the NIH Molecular Libraries Roadmap Initiative providing information on biological activities of small molecules. It is organized as three interconnected databases, containing chemical samples from a variety of sources (PubChem Substance), compound information related to substances such as physicochemical properties and descriptors for similarity searching (PubChem Compound), and bioactivity data of chemical substances (PubChem BioAssay). The dynamically growing primary databases contain over 61 million records of chemical substances, 25 million unique compound structures, and bioactivity data from more than 1600 assays. Data mining approaches to create representative subsets for virtual screening purposes [120] and cross-assay analyses of bioactivity data to study polypharmacology behavior in the PubChem collection [121] have been described. Other publicly available compound databases annotated with biological data are ChemBank with over 1.2 million chemicals [122] and DrugBank covering almost 4800 drugs [123].

Several commercial databases of annotated compound libraries exist, mostly compiled from literature and patent sources. The StARLITe database (now ChEMBL) is a large collection of chemicals mined from literature, including target and bioactivity information for 500 000 compounds. The WOMBAT (World of Molecular Bioactivity) database from Sunset Molecular contains 300 000 molecular entries associated with biological activities and target information [124]. Jubilant BioSys, GVK Bio, and Aureus Pharma are commercial providers of large target-centric compound databases, focusing mostly on large target classes such as kinases, GPCRs, nuclear hormone receptors, or ion channels. The databases integrate chemical structures with activity data and target information collected from literature and published patents.

Nowadays, more than 60% of new chemical substances entering the Chemical Abstract Service (CAS) registry are sourced from patents. Thus, in addition to

Table 1.2 Representative databases of chemical and biological information relevant for drug discovery.

Database	Provider	Coverage	Website
ChemSpider	RSC	20 million chemicals	http://www.chemspider.com
eMolecules	eMolecules Inc.	7 million chemicals	http://www.emolecules.com
ZINC 8	UCSF	13 million chemicals	http://zinc.docking.org
ChemDB	UC Irvine	5 million chemicals	http://cdb.ics.uci.edu
ChemBank	Broad Institute	1.2 million chemicals	http://chembank.broadinstitute.org
DrugBank	University Alberta	4800 drugs; 2500 targets	http://www.drugbank.ca
PubChem	NIH Molecular Libraries Roadmap Initiative	61 million substances; 25 million chemicals; 1600 bioassays	http://pubchem.ncbi.nlm.nih.gov
ChEMBL (StARLITe)	EMBL-EBI (Inpharmatica)	500 000 chemicals; 5000 targets	http://www.ebi.ac.uk/chembldb
WOMBAT 2009.1	Sunset Molecular	300 000 chemicals; 2000 targets	http://www.sunsetmolecular.com
BioPrint	Cerep	2500 drugs; 159 bioassays	http://www.cerep.fr
ChemBioBase	Jubilant Biosys	2 million chemicals; 1500 targets	http://www.jubilantbiosys.com
MedChem	GVK Bio	1 million chemicals; 5600 targets	http://www.gvkbio.com
Target inhibitor	GVK Bio	3.5 million chemicals (patent and literature)	http://www.gvkbio.com
AurSCOPE	Aureus Pharma	500 000 chemicals; 1.7 million activities	http://www.aureus-pharma.com

capturing information from literature and available compound databases, the mining of chemical and biological data from the patent literature is attracting considerable attention. Not only does it provide a mostly untapped source of ideas for new lead generation but it also allows to identify regions in chemical space already investigated. The use of text analytics tools is an efficient way to mine the drug and patent literature [125]. Researchers at IBM have developed a system that enables the user to mine patents from the US Patent corpus [126]. A chemical annotator recognizes and extracts chemical entities in patent documents, and a name-to-structure converter generates molecular structures that are stored in a database for similarity searching. The authors were able to index 3.6 million unique chemical structures from 4.4 million patents. A similar patent database, SureChem from Reel Two, was created by extracting all chemical names from the full text of US, EPO, JP, and WO patents and contains 11 million unique chemical structures covering 18 million patents.

A limiting factor is that text analytics methods are largely confined to specific compounds exemplified in the patents, which are only a small portion of the theoretically possible chemical structures represented in the Markush claim. The improved access to searchable databases of Markush structures and the development of sophisticated chemoinformatics tools to efficiently mine and enumerate the potentially billions of claimed chemical structures are the next logical steps toward capturing the vast chemical space contained in the patent corpus [127, 128].

1.8
Conclusions and Outlook

Virtual screening increasingly impacts the hit finding process in drug discovery by preselecting compounds for biological evaluation. Due to a high false positive rate associated with most virtual screening methods, the selection of only few cherry-picked compounds to identify active molecules ("needle in the haystack") is often less likely to be successful. It rather plays to its strength when virtual screening is applied in the context of narrowing down the number of compounds to be tested by enriching screening sets with drug- and leadlike compounds likely to be active, that is, molecules in biologically and medicinally relevant chemical space. Eliminating compounds with nondruglike and nonleadlike properties from a screening collection is often not considered as virtual screening, but it is a crucial factor contributing to the overall success of high-quality lead identification. Reducing the number of compounds for efficient biological testing can be accomplished by carefully applying diversity-based selection criteria. The design of focused libraries targeting a specific protein or protein family is a proven method of choice to increase the chances of finding active leads. The unique capability of virtual screening to search compounds in their virtual form not only allows access to the small fraction of chemical space represented by existing screening libraries but also allows to expand into other regions of chemical space (Figure 1.2). Virtual screening of compound collections from external sources (vendors, patents, and literature), the design of large virtual combinatorial libraries and their efficient representation as frag-

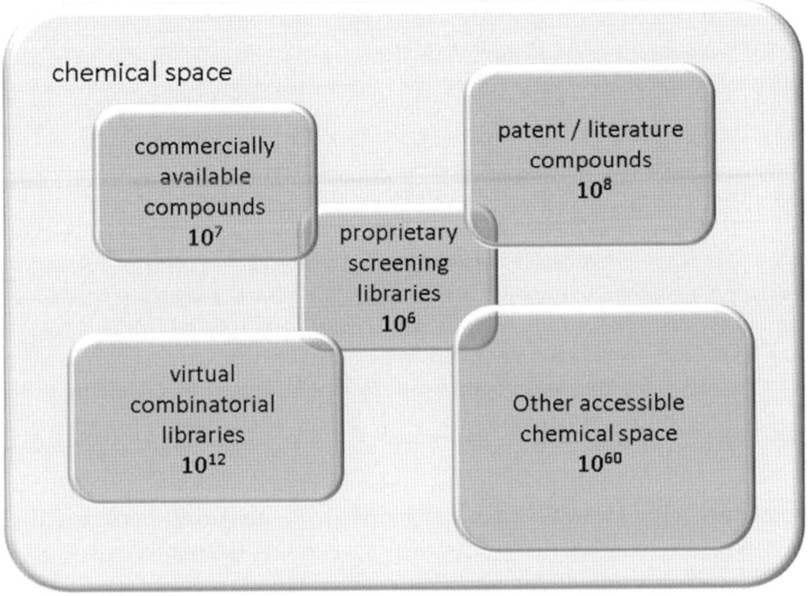

Figure 1.2 Virtual screening has the capability to expand searches outside of typical screening libraries (amenable to HTS) into new dimensions of chemical space. The various sources of accessible chemical spaces are described throughout the text. Typical or estimated numbers of compounds are highlighted in bold.

ment spaces, or recently emerging alternative sources of diverse chemical matter (*de novo* enumerated small molecules or ring scaffolds) offer plenty of opportunities. However, the future challenge remains to more reliably predict biological activity and chemical feasibility of compounds being proposed for synthesis. Ultimately, the goal of next-generation virtual screening methods is the identification and systematic exploration of truly synthetically accessible and biologically and medicinally relevant chemical space.

1.9 Glossary

Chemical library	Collection of chemical compounds.
Chemical space	Collection of all possible meaningful compounds, typically restricted to small organic molecules.
Chemogenomics	Discovery and description of classes of compounds against families of functionally related proteins.
Combinatorial chemistry	Generation of large collections of compound libraries by systematic combination of smaller building blocks. Large virtual combinatorial libraries are often created in the form of fragment spaces.

Diversity-based library	Compound library designed to create a maximally diverse collection of compounds to cover a broad range of protein classes, especially when they are unknown or difficult to target.
Druglikeness	Physicochemical properties to improve the likelihood of success in drug development.
Focused library	Compound library designed around selected, often privileged scaffolds tailored toward targeting specific protein families (GPCRs, kinases, etc.).
Fragment space	Chemical space representation where molecules are encoded as building blocks (fragments) and linkage rules.
Leadlikeness	Criteria for ideal lead molecules that serve as a basis for further chemical optimization in a medicinal chemistry campaign.
Molecular diversity	Quantitative description how different molecules are from each other in a compound collection.
Privileged structure	A single molecular framework or frequently occurring fragment able to provide ligands for multiple receptors, often within a protein family.
Similarity property principle	Fundamental assumption that similar compounds typically exhibit similar biological activity; also referred to as neighborhood behavior.

Acknowledgment

The author would like to thank David Hepworth for fruitful discussions and critical reading of the manuscript.

References

1 Lipinski, C. and Hopkins, A. (2004) Navigating chemical space for biology and medicine. *Nature*, **432**, 855–861.
2 Dobson, C.M. (2004) Chemical space and biology. *Nature*, **432**, 824–828.
3 Medina-Franco, J.L., Martinez-Mayorga, K., Giulianotti, M.A., Houghten, R.A., and Pinilla, C. (2008) Visualization of the chemical space in drug discovery. *Current Computer-Aided Drug Design*, **4**, 322–333.
4 Gorse, A.D. (2006) Diversity in medicinal chemistry space. *Current Topics in Medicinal Chemistry*, **6**, 3–18.
5 Blum, L.C. and Reymond, J.L. (2009) 970 million druglike small molecules for virtual screening in the chemical universe database GDB-13. *Journal of the American Chemical Society*, **131**, 8732–8733.
6 Bohacek, R.S., McMartin, C., and Guida, W.C. (1996) The art and practice of structure-based drug design: a molecular modeling perspective. *Medicinal Research Reviews*, **16**, 3–50.
7 Hert, J., Irwin, J.J., Laggner, C., Keiser, M.J., and Shoichet, B.K. (2009) Quantifying biogenic bias in screening libraries. *Nature Chemical Biology*, **5**, 479–483.
8 Paolini, G.V., Shapland, R.H., van Hoorn, W.P., Mason, J.S., and Hopkins, A.L. (2006) Global mapping of pharmacological space. *Nature Biotechnology*, **24**, 805–815.

9 Arkin, M.R. and Wells, J.A. (2004) Small-molecule inhibitors of protein–protein interactions: progressing towards the dream. *Nature Reviews. Drug Discovery*, **3**, 301–317.

10 Milne, G.M. (2003) Pharmaceutical productivity: the imperative for new paradigms. *Annual Reports in Medicinal Chemistry*, **38**, 383–396.

11 Lipinski, C.A., Lombardo, F., Dominy, B.W., and Feeney, P.J. (1997) Experimental and computational approaches to estimate solubility and permeability in drug discovery and development settings. *Advanced Drug Delivery Reviews*, **23**, 3–25.

12 Leeson, P.D. and Springthorpe, B. (2007) The influence of drug-like concepts on decision-making in medicinal chemistry. *Nature Reviews. Drug Discovery*, **6**, 881–890.

13 Vistoli, G., Pedretti, A., and Testa, B. (2008) Assessing drug-likeness: what are we missing? *Drug Discovery Today*, **13**, 285–294.

14 Teague, S.J., Davis, A.M., Leeson, P.D., and Oprea, T. (1999) The design of leadlike combinatorial libraries. *Angewandte Chemie. International Edition in English*, **38**, 3743–3748.

15 Keserü, G.M. and Makara, G.M. (2009) The influence of lead discovery strategies on the properties of drug candidates. *Nature Reviews. Drug Discovery*, **8**, 203–212.

16 Hann, M.M., Leach, A.R., and Harper, G. (2001) Molecular complexity and its impact on the probability of finding leads for drug discovery. *Journal of Chemical Information and Computer Sciences*, **41**, 856–864.

17 Rishton, G.M. (2003) Nonleadlikeness and leadlikeness in biochemical screening. *Drug Discovery Today*, **8**, 86–96.

18 Rishton, G.M. (2008) Molecular diversity in the context of leadlikeness: compound properties that enable effective biochemical screening. *Current Opinion in Chemical Biology*, **12**, 340–351.

19 Rishton, G.M. (1997) Reactive compounds and *in vitro* false positives in HTS. *Drug Discovery Today*, **2**, 382–384.

20 Roche, O., Schneider, P., Zuegge, J., Guba, W., Kansy, M., Alanine, A., Bleicher, K., Danel, F., Gutknecht, E.M., Rogers-Evans, M., Neidhart, W., Stalder, H., Dillon, M., Sjogren, E., Fotouhi, N., Gillespie, P., Goodnow, R., Harris, W., Jones, P., Taniguchi, M., Tsujii, S., von der Saal, W., Zimmermann, G., and Schneider, G. (2002) Development of a virtual screening method for identification of "frequent hitters" in compound libraries. *Journal of Medicinal Chemistry*, **45**, 137–142.

21 McGovern, S.L., Helfand, B.T., Feng, B., and Shoichet, B.K. (2003) A specific mechanism of nonspecific inhibition. *Journal of Medicinal Chemistry*, **46**, 4265–4272.

22 Feng, B.Y., Simeonov, A., Jadhav, A., Babaoglu, K., Inglese, J., Shoichet, B.K., and Austin, C.P. (2007) A high-throughput screen for aggregation-based inhibition in a large compound library. *Journal of Medicinal Chemistry*, **50**, 2385–2390.

23 Hann, M.M. and Oprea, T.I. (2004) Pursuing the leadlikeness concept in pharmaceutical research. *Current Opinion in Chemical Biology*, **8**, 255–263.

24 Martin, Y.C. (2001) Diverse viewpoints on computational aspects of molecular diversity. *Journal of Combinatorial Chemistry*, **3**, 231–250.

25 Roth, H.J. (2005) There is no such thing as 'diversity'! *Current Opinion in Chemical Biology*, **9**, 293–295.

26 Johnson, M.A. and Maggiora, G.M. (1990) *Concepts and Applications of Molecular Similarity*, John Wiley & Sons, Inc., New York.

27 Patterson, D.E., Cramer, R.D., Ferguson, A.M., Clark, R.D., and Weinberger, L.E. (1996) Neighborhood behavior: a useful concept for validation of "molecular diversity" descriptors. *Journal of Medicinal Chemistry*, **39**, 3049–3059.

28 Martin, Y.C., Kofron, J.L., and Traphagen, L.M. (2002) Do structurally similar molecules have similar biological activity? *Journal of Medicinal Chemistry*, **45**, 4350–4358.

29 Muchmore, S.W., Debe, D.A., Metz, J.T., Brown, S.P., Martin, Y.C., and Hajduk,

P.J. (2008) Application of belief theory to similarity data fusion for use in analog searching and lead hopping. *Journal of Chemical Information and Modeling*, **48**, 941–948.

30 Harper, G., Pickett, S.D., and Green, D.V. (2004) Design of a compound screening collection for use in high throughput screening. *Combinatorial Chemistry and High Throughput Screening*, **7**, 63–70.

31 Todeschini, R. (2009) *Molecular Descriptors for Cheminformatics*, Wiley-VCH Verlag GmbH, Weinheim.

32 Todeschini, R. (2009) Dragon descriptors. Talete srl, Milan, Italy.

33 Gillet, V.J., Willett, P., John, B.T., and David, J.T. (2007) Compound selection using measures of similarity and dissimilarity, in *Comprehensive Medicinal Chemistry II*, Elsevier, Oxford, pp. 167–192.

34 Holliday, J.D., Hu, C.Y., and Willett, P. (2002) Grouping of coefficients for the calculation of inter-molecular similarity and dissimilarity using 2D fragment bit-strings. *Combinatorial Chemistry and High Throughput Screening*, **5**, 155–166.

35 Chen, X. and Reynolds, C.H. (2002) Performance of similarity measures in 2D fragment-based similarity searching: comparison of structural descriptors and similarity coefficients. *Journal of Chemical Information and Computer Sciences*, **42**, 1407–1414.

36 Willett, P. (1999) Dissimilarity-based algorithms for selecting structurally diverse sets of compounds. *Journal of Computational Biology*, **6**, 447–457.

37 Ashton, M., Barnard, J., Casset, F., Charlton, M., Downs, G., Gorse, D., Holliday, J., Lahana, R., and Willett, P. (2002) Identification of diverse database subsets using property-based and fragment-based molecular descriptions. *Quantitative Structure–Activity Relationship*, **21**, 598–604.

38 Gobbi, A. and Lee, M.L. (2003) DISE: directed sphere exclusion. *Journal of Chemical Information and Computer Sciences*, **43**, 317–323.

39 Downs, G.M. and Barnard, J.M. (2003) Clustering methods and their uses in computational chemistry, in *Reviews in Computational Chemistry*, vol. **18** (eds B. Kenny and D.B.B. Lipkowitz), John Wiley & Sons, Inc., New York, pp. 1–40.

40 Lewis, R.A., Mason, J.S., and McLay, I.M. (1997) Similarity measures for rational set selection and analysis of combinatorial libraries: the diverse property-derived (DPD) approach. *Journal of Chemical Information and Computer Sciences*, **37**, 599–614.

41 Pearlman, R.S. and Smith, K.M. (1999) Metric validation and the receptor-relevant subspace concept. *Journal of Chemical Information and Computer Sciences*, **39**, 28–35.

42 Oprea, T.I. and Gottfries, J. (2001) Chemography: the art of navigating in chemical space. *Journal of Combinatorial Chemistry*, **3**, 157–166.

43 Gillet, V.J., Willett, P., Bradshaw, J., and Green, D.V.S. (1998) Selecting combinatorial libraries to optimize diversity and physical properties. *Journal of Chemical Information and Computer Sciences*, **39**, 169–177.

44 Agrafiotis, D.K. (2002) Multiobjective optimization of combinatorial libraries. *Journal of Computer-Aided Molecular Design*, **16**, 335–356.

45 Krier, M., Bret, G., and Rognan, D. (2006) Assessing the scaffold diversity of screening libraries. *Journal of Chemical Information and Modeling*, **46**, 512–524.

46 Harper, G. and Pickett, S.D. (2006) Methods for mining HTS data. *Drug Discovery Today*, **11**, 694–699.

47 Krier, M., Araujo-Junior, J.X., Schmitt, M., Duranton, J., Justiano-Basaran, H., Lugnier, C., Bourguignon, J.J., and Rognan, D. (2005) Design of small-sized libraries by combinatorial assembly of linkers and functional groups to a given scaffold: application to the structure-based optimization of a phosphodiesterase 4 inhibitor. *Journal of Medicinal Chemistry*, **48**, 3816–3822.

48 Muller, G. (2003) Medicinal chemistry of target family-directed masterkeys. *Drug Discovery Today*, **8**, 681–691.

49 Bemis, G.W. and Murcko, M.A. (1996) The properties of known drugs. 1. Molecular frameworks. *Journal of Medicinal Chemistry*, **39**, 2887–2893.

50 Rarey, M. and Dixon, J.S. (1998) Feature trees: a new molecular similarity measure based on tree matching. *Journal of Computer-Aided Molecular Design*, **12**, 471–490.

51 Martin, Y.C. and Muchmore, S. (2009) Beyond QSAR: lead hopping to different structures. *QSAR & Combinatorial Science*, **28**, 797–801.

52 Xu, Y.J. and Johnson, M. (2002) Using molecular equivalence numbers to visually explore structural features that distinguish chemical libraries. *Journal of Chemical Information and Computer Sciences*, **42**, 912–926.

53 Schuffenhauer, A., Ertl, P., Roggo, S., Wetzel, S., Koch, M.A., and Waldmann, H. (2007) The scaffold tree: visualization of the scaffold universe by hierarchical scaffold classification. *Journal of Chemical Information and Modeling*, **47**, 47–58.

54 Wetzel, S., Klein, K., Renner, S., Rauh, D., Oprea, T.I., Mutzel, P., and Waldmann, H. (2009) Interactive exploration of chemical space with Scaffold Hunter. *Nature Chemical Biology*, **5**, 581–583.

55 Renner, S., van Otterlo, W.A., Dominguez Seoane, M., Mocklinghoff, S., Hofmann, B., Wetzel, S., Schuffenhauer, A., Ertl, P., Oprea, T.I., Steinhilber, D., Brunsveld, L., Rauh, D., and Waldmann, H. (2009) Bioactivity-guided mapping and navigation of chemical space. *Nature Chemical Biology*, **5**, 585–592.

56 Fink, T. and Reymond, J.L. (2007) Virtual exploration of the chemical universe up to 11 atoms of C, N, O, F: assembly of 26.4 million structures (110.9 million stereoisomers) and analysis for new ring systems, stereochemistry, physicochemical properties, compound classes, and drug discovery. *Journal of Chemical Information and Modeling*, **47**, 342–353.

57 Nguyen, K.T., Syed, S., Urwyler, S., Bertrand, S., Bertrand, D., and Reymond, J.L. (2008) Discovery of NMDA glycine site inhibitors from the chemical universe database GDB. *ChemMedChem*, **3**, 1520–1524.

58 Lipkus, A.H. (2001) Exploring chemical rings in a simple topological-descriptor space. *Journal of Chemical Information and Computer Sciences*, **41**, 430–438.

59 Lewell, X.Q., Jones, A.C., Bruce, C.L., Harper, G., Jones, M.M., McLay, I.M., and Bradshaw, J. (2003) Drug rings database with web interface. A tool for identifying alternative chemical rings in lead discovery programs. *Journal of Medicinal Chemistry*, **46**, 3257–3274.

60 Ertl, P., Jelfs, S., Muhlbacher, J., Schuffenhauer, A., and Selzer, P. (2006) Quest for the rings. *In silico* exploration of ring universe to identify novel bioactive heteroaromatic scaffolds. *Journal of Medicinal Chemistry*, **49**, 4568–4573.

61 Pitt, W.R., Parry, D.M., Perry, B.G., and Groom, C.R. (2009) Heteroaromatic rings of the future. *Journal of Medicinal Chemistry*, **52**, 2952–2963.

62 Ritchie, T.J. and Macdonald, S.J.F. (2009) The impact of aromatic ring count on compound developability: are too many aromatic rings a liability in drug design? *Drug Discovery Today*, **14**, 1011–1020.

63 Lovering, F., Bikker, J., and Humblet, C. (2009) Escape from flatland: increasing saturation as an approach to improving clinical success. *Journal of Medicinal Chemistry*, **52**, 6752–6756.

64 Koehn, F.E. and Carter, G.T. (2005) The evolving role of natural products in drug discovery. *Nature Reviews. Drug Discovery*, **4**, 206–220.

65 Zhang, M.Q. and Wilkinson, B. (2007) Drug discovery beyond the 'rule-of-five'. *Current Opinion in Biotechnology*, **18**, 478–488.

66 Arya, P., Joseph, R., Gan, Z., and Rakic, B. (2005) Exploring new chemical space by stereocontrolled diversity-oriented synthesis. *Chemistry and Biology*, **12**, 163–180.

67 Schreiber, S.L. (2000) Target-oriented and diversity-oriented organic synthesis in drug discovery. *Science*, **287**, 1964–1969.

68 Tan, D.S. (2005) Diversity-oriented synthesis: exploring the intersections between chemistry and biology. *Nature Chemical Biology*, **1**, 74–84.

69 Driggers, E.M., Hale, S.P., Lee, J., and Terrett, N.K. (2008) The exploration of macrocycles for drug discovery:

an underexploited structural class. *Nature Reviews. Drug Discovery*, 7, 608–624.

70 Baber, J.C. and Feher, M. (2004) Predicting synthetic accessibility: application in drug discovery and development. *Mini Reviews in Medicinal Chemistry*, **4**, 681–692.

71 Ertl, P. and Schuffenhauer, A. (2009) Estimation of synthetic accessibility score of drug-like molecules based on molecular complexity and fragment contributions. *Journal of Cheminformatics*, **1**, 8.

72 Miller, J.L. (2006) Recent developments in focused library design: targeting gene-families. *Current Topics in Medicinal Chemistry*, **6**, 19–29.

73 Gregori-Puigjane, E. and Mestres, J. (2008) Coverage and bias in chemical library design. *Current Opinion in Chemical Biology*, **12**, 359–365.

74 Morphy, R. (2006) The influence of target family and functional activity on the physicochemical properties of pre-clinical compounds. *Journal of Medicinal Chemistry*, **49**, 2969–2978.

75 Vieth, M. and Sutherland, J.J. (2006) Dependence of molecular properties on proteomic family for marketed oral drugs. *Journal of Medicinal Chemistry*, **49**, 3451–3453.

76 Balakin, K.V., Tkachenko, S.E., Lang, S.A., Okun, I., Ivashchenko, A.A., and Savchuk, N.P. (2002) Property-based design of GPCR-targeted library. *Journal of Chemical Information and Computer Sciences*, **42**, 1332–1342.

77 Rognan, D. (2007) Chemogenomic approaches to rational drug design. *British Journal of Pharmacology*, **152**, 38–52.

78 Schneider, P., Tanrikulu, Y., and Schneider, G. (2009) Self-organizing maps in drug discovery: compound library design, scaffold-hopping, repurposing. *Current Medicinal Chemistry*, **16**, 258–266.

79 Lavrador, K., Murphy, B., Saunders, J., Struthers, S., Wang, X., and Williams, J. (2004) A screening library for peptide activated G-protein coupled receptors. 1. The test set. *Journal of Medicinal Chemistry*, **47**, 6864–6874.

80 Lamb, M.L., Bradley, E.K., Beaton, G., Bondy, S.S., Castellino, A.J., Gibbons, P.A., Suto, M.J., and Grootenhuis, P.D. (2004) Design of a gene family screening library targeting G-protein coupled receptors. *Journal of Molecular Graphics and Modelling*, **23**, 15–21.

81 Mason, J.S., Morize, I., Menard, P.R., Cheney, D.L., Hulme, C., and Labaudiniere, R.F. (1999) New 4-point pharmacophore method for molecular similarity and diversity applications: overview of the method and applications, including a novel approach to the design of combinatorial libraries containing privileged substructures. *Journal of Medicinal Chemistry*, **42**, 3251–3264.

82 Sun, D., Chuaqui, C., Deng, Z., Bowes, S., Chin, D., Singh, J., Cullen, P., Hankins, G., Lee, W.C., Donnelly, J., Friedman, J., and Josiah, S. (2006) A kinase-focused compound collection: compilation and screening strategy. *Chemical Biology and Drug Design*, **67**, 385–394.

83 Decornez, H., Gulyas-Forro, A., Papp, A., Szabo, M., Sarmay, G., Hajdu, I., Cseh, S., Dorman, G., and Kitchen, D.B. (2009) Design, selection, and evaluation of a general kinase-focused library. *ChemMedChem*, **4**, 1273–1278.

84 Evans, B.E., Rittle, K.E., Bock, M.G., DiPardo, R.M., Freidinger, R.M., Whitter, W.L., Lundell, G.F., Veber, D.F., Anderson, P.S., Chang, R.S. *et al.* (1988) Methods for drug discovery: development of potent, selective, orally effective cholecystokinin antagonists. *Journal of Medicinal Chemistry*, **31**, 2235–2246.

85 DeSimone, R.W., Currie, K.S., Mitchell, S.A., Darrow, J.W., and Pippin, D.A. (2004) Privileged structures: applications in drug discovery. *Combinatorial Chemistry and High Throughput Screening*, 7, 473–494.

86 Lewell, X.Q., Judd, D.B., Watson, S.P., and Hann, M.M. (1998) RECAP: retrosynthetic combinatorial analysis procedure: a powerful new technique for identifying privileged molecular fragments with useful applications in combinatorial chemistry. *Journal of*

Chemical Information and Computer Sciences, **38**, 511–522.

87 Vieth, M., Erickson, J., Wang, J., Webster, Y., Mader, M., Higgs, R., and Watson, I. (2009) Kinase inhibitor data modeling and *de novo* inhibitor design with fragment approaches. *Journal of Medicinal Chemistry*, **52**, 6456–6466.

88 Crisman, T.J., Bender, A., Milik, M., Jenkins, J.L., Scheiber, J., Sukuru, S.C., Fejzo, J., Hommel, U., Davies, J.W., and Glick, M. (2008) "Virtual fragment linking": an approach to identify potent binders from low affinity fragment hits. *Journal of Medicinal Chemistry*, **51**, 2481–2491.

89 Akritopoulou-Zanze, I. and Hajduk, P.J. (2009) Kinase-targeted libraries: the design and synthesis of novel, potent, and selective kinase inhibitors. *Drug Discovery Today*, **14** 291–297.

90 Schnur, D.M., Hermsmeier, M.A., and Tebben, A.J. (2006) Are target-family-privileged substructures truly privileged? *Journal of Medicinal Chemistry*, **49**, 2000–2009.

91 Jacoby, E., Schuffenhauer, A., Popov, M., Azzaoui, K., Havill, B., Schopfer, U., Engeloch, C., Stanek, J., Acklin, P., Rigollier, P., Stoll, F., Koch, G., Meier, P., Orain, D., Giger, R., Hinrichs, J., Malagu, K., Zimmermann, J., and Roth, H.J. (2005) Key aspects of the Novartis compound collection enhancement project for the compilation of a comprehensive chemogenomics drug discovery screening collection. *Current Topics in Medicinal Chemistry*, **5**, 397–411.

92 Lowrie, J.F., Delisle, R.K., Hobbs, D.W., and Diller, D.J. (2004) The different strategies for designing GPCR and kinase targeted libraries. *Combinatorial Chemistry and High Throughput Screening*, **7**, 495–510.

93 Aronov, A.M. and Bemis, G.W. (2004) A minimalist approach to fragment-based ligand design using common rings and linkers: application to kinase inhibitors. *Proteins*, **57**, 36–50.

94 Kubinyi, H. and Müller, G. (2005) Chemogenomics in drug discovery: a medicinal chemistry perspective, in *Methods and Principles in Medicinal Chemistry* (eds R. Mannhold, H., Kubinyi, and G. Folkers) Wiley-VCH Verlag GmbH, Weinheim.

95 Harris, C.J. and Stevens, A.P. (2006) Chemogenomics: structuring the drug discovery process to gene families. *Drug Discovery Today*, **11**, 880–888.

96 Schuffenhauer, A., Floersheim, P., Acklin, P., and Jacoby, E. (2003) Similarity metrics for ligands reflecting the similarity of the target proteins. *Journal of Chemical Information and Computer Sciences*, **43**, 391–405.

97 Surgand, J.S., Rodrigo, J., Kellenberger, E., and Rognan, D. (2006) A chemogenomic analysis of the transmembrane binding cavity of human G-protein-coupled receptors. *Proteins*, **62**, 509–538.

98 Deng, Z., Chuaqui, C., and Singh, J. (2004) Structural interaction fingerprint (SIFt): a novel method for analyzing three-dimensional protein–ligand binding interactions. *Journal of Medicinal Chemistry*, **47**, 337–344.

99 Frimurer, T.M., Ulven, T., Elling, C.E., Gerlach, L.O., Kostenis, E., and Hogberg, T. (2005) A physicogenetic method to assign ligand-binding relationships between 7TM receptors. *Bioorganic and Medicinal Chemistry Letters*, **15**, 3707–3712.

100 Martin, R.E., Green, L.G., Guba, W., Kratochwil, N., and Christ, A. (2007) Discovery of the first nonpeptidic, small-molecule, highly selective somatostatin receptor subtype 5 antagonists: a chemogenomics approach. *Journal of Medicinal Chemistry*, **50**, 6291–6294.

101 Crossley, R. (2004) The design of screening libraries targeted at G-protein coupled receptors. *Current Topics in Medicinal Chemistry*, **4**, 581–588.

102 Klabunde, T., Giegerich, C., and Evers, A. (2009) Sequence-derived three-dimensional pharmacophore models for G-protein-coupled receptors and their application in virtual screening. *Journal of Medicinal Chemistry*, **52**, 2923–2932.

103 Keiser, M.J., Roth, B.L., Armbruster, B.N., Ernsberger, P., Irwin, J.J., and Shoichet, B.K. (2007) Relating protein pharmacology by ligand chemistry. *Nature Biotechnology*, **25**, 197–206.

104 Vieth, M., Sutherland, J.J., Robertson, D.H., and Campbell, R.M. (2005) Kinomics: characterizing the therapeutically validated kinase space. *Drug Discovery Today*, **10**, 839–846.

105 Gozalbes, R., Rolland, C., Nicolaï, E., Paugam, M.-F., Coussy, L., Horvath, D., Barbosa, F., Mao, B., Revah, F., and Froloff, N. (2005) QSAR strategy and experimental validation for the development of a GPCR focused library. *QSAR & Combinatorial Science*, **24**, 508–516.

106 Boehm, M., Wu, T.Y., Claussen, H., and Lemmen, C. (2008) Similarity searching and scaffold hopping in synthetically accessible combinatorial chemistry spaces. *Journal of Medicinal Chemistry*, **51**, 2468–2480.

107 Rarey, M. and Stahl, M. (2001) Similarity searching in large combinatorial chemistry spaces. *Journal of Computer-Aided Molecular Design*, **15**, 497–520.

108 Lessel, U., Wellenzohn, B., Lilienthal, M., and Claussen, H. (2009) Searching fragment spaces with feature trees. *Journal of Chemical Information and Modeling*, **49**, 270–279.

109 Yu, N. and Bakken, G.A. (2009) Efficient exploration of large combinatorial chemistry spaces by monomer-based similarity searching. *Journal of Chemical Information and Modeling*, **49**, 745–755.

110 Degen, J., Wegscheid-Gerlach, C., Zaliani, A., and Rarey, M. (2008) On the art of compiling and using 'drug-like' chemical fragment spaces. *ChemMedChem*, **3**, 1503–1507.

111 Mauser, H. and Stahl, M. (2007) Chemical fragment spaces for *de novo* design. *Journal of Chemical Information and Modeling*, **47**, 318–324.

112 Schurer, S.C., Tyagi, P., and Muskal, S.M. (2005) Prospective exploration of synthetically feasible, medicinally relevant chemical space. *Journal of Chemical Information and Modeling*, **45**, 239–248.

113 Zhou, J.Z., Shi, S., Na, J., Peng, Z., and Thacher, T. (2009) Combinatorial library-based design with Basis Products. *Journal of Computer-Aided Molecular Design*, **23** (10), 725–736.

114 van Hoorn, W.P. and Bell, A.S. (2009) Searching chemical space with the Bayesian Idea Generator. *Journal of Chemical Information and Modeling*, **49**, 2211–2220.

115 Ghosh, S., Nie, A., An, J., and Huang, Z. (2006) Structure-based virtual screening of chemical libraries for drug discovery. *Current Opinion in Chemical Biology*, **10**, 194–202.

116 Degen, J. and Rarey, M. (2006) FlexNovo: structure-based searching in large fragment spaces. *ChemMedChem*, **1**, 854–868.

117 Oprea, T.I. and Tropsha, A. (2006) Target, chemical and bioactivity databases: integration is key. *Drug Discovery Today: Technologies*, **3**, 357–365.

118 Irwin, J.J. and Shoichet, B.K. (2005) ZINC: a free database of commercially available compounds for virtual screening. *Journal of Chemical Information and Modeling*, **45**, 177–182.

119 Chen, J.H., Linstead, E., Swamidass, S.J., Wang, D., and Baldi, P. (2007) ChemDB update: full-text search and virtual chemical space. *Bioinformatics*, **23**, 2348–2351.

120 Xie, X.Q. and Chen, J.Z. (2008) Data mining a small molecule drug screening representative subset from NIH PubChem. *Journal of Chemical Information and Modeling*, **48**, 465–475.

121 Chen, B., Wild, D., and Guha, R. (2009) PubChem as a source of polypharmacology. *Journal of Chemical Information and Modeling*, **49**, 2044–2055.

122 Seiler, K.P., George, G.A., Happ, M.P., Bodycombe, N.E., Carrinski, H.A., Norton, S., Brudz, S., Sullivan, J.P., Muhlich, J., Serrano, M., Ferraiolo, P., Tolliday, N.J., Schreiber, S.L., and Clemons, P.A. (2008) ChemBank: a small-molecule screening and cheminformatics resource database. *Nucleic Acids Research*, **36**, D351–D359.

123 Wishart, D.S., Knox, C., Guo, A.C., Shrivastava, S., Hassanali, M., Stothard, P., Chang, Z., and Woolsey, J. (2006) DrugBank: a comprehensive resource for *in silico* drug discovery and

exploration. *Nucleic Acids Research*, **34**, D668–D672.

124 Olah, M., Mracec, M., Ostopovici, L., Rad, R., Bora, A., Hadaruga, N., Olah, I., Banda, M., Simon, Z., Mracec, M., and Oprea, T.I. (2005) WOMBAT: World of Molecular Bioactivity, in *Chemoinformatics in Drug Discovery* (ed. T.I. Oprea), Wiley-VCH Verlag GmbH, Weinheim, pp. 221–239.

125 Banville, D.L. (2006) Mining chemical structural information from the drug literature. *Drug Discovery Today*, **11**, 35–42.

126 Rhodes, J., Boyer, S., Kreulen, J., Chen, Y., and Ordonez, P. (2007) Mining patents using molecular similarity search. Proceedings of the Pacific Symposium on Biocomputing, pp. 304–315.

127 Barnard, J.M. and Wright, P.M. (2009) Towards in-house searching of Markush structures from patents. *World Patent Information*, **31**, 97–103.

128 Fliri, A., Moysan, E., Benichou, P., and Nolte, M. (2009) Methods for processing generic chemical structure representations. Patent WO09051741.

2
Preparing and Filtering Compound Databases for Virtual and Experimental Screening

Maxwell D. Cummings, Éric Arnoult, Christophe Buyck, Gary Tresadern, Ann M. Vos, and Jörg K. Wegner

2.1
Introduction

In drug discovery research, the term screening is used to describe a process in which members of what can be a very large set of molecules are evaluated for a specific biochemical activity, most commonly enzyme inhibition or receptor antagonism or agonism. High-throughput screening (HTS) involves the testing of tens of thousands to a million or more small molecules, seeking new starting points for medicinal chemistry-based drug discovery. Increasingly, computer-based virtual screening is used to prioritize the set of molecules that will be tested experimentally, by using one or more scoring functions to predict the desired biochemical activity. In this context, virtual screening methods are also used to explore virtual combinatorial libraries and catalogs of purchasable compounds to selectively guide the synthesis or purchase of additional compounds to enrich screening collections.

The term virtual screening spans a range of techniques; here, we use it to refer to 3D methods like pharmacophore-based searching, automated docking, and shape-based matching. These methods screen on the basis of matching a set of pharmacophoric points, complementary to a specified region of a target protein or overall shape matching (often with chemical features mapped to the query shape), respectively. What these computational approaches have in common is that they all are essentially methods for mining databases of molecules. A common resource for all these virtual experiments is the collection or database of small molecules to be mined.

Database preparation is an important aspect of virtual screening. Molecules must be represented by one or more chemically sensible states and must be formatted appropriately for the virtual screening tool to be used. Relevant considerations include storage format(s), 2D–3D conversion or 3D structure generation, stereochemistry, charge, tautomers, protonation, and conformers. The impact of different database preparation protocols has not been thoroughly evaluated. Limited information in this area indicates that database preparation does impact final screening

Virtual Screening. Edited by C. Sotriffer

ISBN: 978-3-527-32636-5

outcome (discussed below), but an ultimate best practice, if such is possible, remains to be detailed.

Database "filtering" most typically refers to methods for "cleaning up" a virtual compound database, by removing undesirable (e.g., reactive functional groups, high molecular weight (MW)) compounds; the same approaches can be used to preselect a database subset enriched in desired properties. Here, we briefly summarize several aspects of database management and discuss and expand upon material presented in our previous survey of this topic [1]. Then we briefly review a few recent papers as well as some relevant technological developments that were not considered in our previous survey. Finally, we focus on various types of property- and target-based filtering, as these approaches are an integral aspect of building, maintaining, and using a large screening collection.

2.2 Ligand Databases

Ligand preparation and database maintenance can be divided into several subtopics. Ligands need to be represented as chemical data structures. Some ligands may require multiple structures, with comprehensive representation requiring treatment of chirality and/or tautomerization and/or protonation state(s). Dependent on the intended use of the database, each structure may further require elucidation of one or more 3D conformers. Each of the resultant representations may then be annotated with various types of information, for example, conformational energy, MW, purchase or synthesis source, and amount of physical compound available. This body of information must then be stored as completely and as compactly as possible. In this section, we explore and comment on some of these aspects of virtual ligand preparation.

2.2.1 Chemical Data Structures

Chemical file formats provide different levels of accuracy, and this translates to different levels of reproducibility when structures are built from files. Translation errors of chemical structures can occur when moving between programs if the two programs are not communicating at the same level of data accuracy. SMILES [2] is widely used to store chemical structures. In principle, SMILES can encode the full set of structural information. In practice, unfortunately, different SMILES readers/writers exist and this can lead to inconsistencies in chemical structures (Figure 2.1). The MDL SD [3] and Sybyl mol2 (http://tripos.com/tripos_resources/fileroot/pdfs/mol2_format2.pdf) formats can include 2D and 3D information, in contrast to SMILES that contains the topological arrangement of atoms but no atom type, 2D or 3D coordinate information. (Based on SMILES, 2D coordinates can be created with structure diagram algorithms (e.g., Ref. [4]), and 3D coordinates built with conformer generation algorithms (discussed below).) The OEChem/OpenBabel

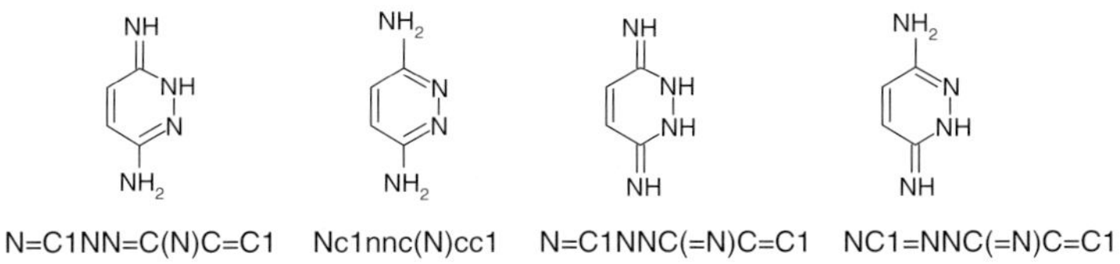

Figure 2.1 Tautomers and SMILES. Each tautomer is represented by a different SMILES string. This type of difference can lead to inconsistencies between programs.

toolkit (http://www.eyesopen.com/products/toolkits/oechem.html) [5] provides a rich set of atom types spanning most other chemical formats, but limitations can arise upon translation to other formats. Since not all programs interface with OEChem/OpenBabel directly, perfect molecule conversion is not guaranteed. A practical approach is to use MDL SD or Sybyl mol2 formats for any data exchange, with some risk of incorrect atom typing. The most verbose data format is the Chemical Markup Language (CML) [6], but this standard is not (yet) widely distributed within commercial software packages.

In principle, canonical SMILES strings can be used to identify duplicate compounds, but in practice canonicalization differs between programs (the theoretical canonicalization algorithms are often not documented and can vary in details). The use of canonical SMILES to select and remove duplicate molecules is only recommended when consistently using one program or set of programs known to abide by the same canonicalization scheme. For more consistent, documented, and standardized duplicate removal, the IUPAC International Chemical Identifier (InChI, InChIKey) (http://www.iupac.org/inchi/release101.html) (http://www.iupac.org/inchi/release102.html) is recommended. The InChI is a text identifier for chemical substances, developed with the goal of providing an open source and freely available standard for encoding molecular structure (Table 2.1). The goal of the InChIKey is to provide one molecule identifier for different tautomeric and protomeric forms, for example, InChIKey = GPMMYQITJVUZAT-UHFFFAOYSA-N, which can be split into a molecule skeleton GPMMYQITJVUZAT, an isomerism layer UHFFFAOYSA, and the charge (in this case "N" for neutral). One advantage of the InChI/InChIKey is that this identifier can be indexed by search engines (e.g., Google and ChemSpider) and can be freely used by publishers. In contrast, this is

Table 2.1 Comparison of SMILES and InChIKeys.

SMILES	InChIKeyStd skeleton	InChIKeyStd isomerism	InChIKeyStd charge
C1=CC(=O)CCC1(=O)	GPMMYQITJVUZAT	UHFFFAOYSA	N
c1cc(−O)ccc1(−O)	QIGBRXMKCJKVMJ	UHFFFAOYSA	N
C1C(=O)C=CC(=O)C1	GPMMYQITJVUZAT	UHFFFAOYSA	N

The InChIKey addresses some tautomerization challenges in chemical encoding, but may create different keys based on the aromaticity encoding of the underlying input structure. It is recommended to use a chemical expert system prior to the InChIKey calculation (which was not done here) to avoid such issues.

often not possible or practical for SMILES, due to stemming (text mining) or the enumeration problems mentioned above.

Tautomerization (reviewed in detail in Ref. [7]) can lead to alternate SMILES strings for "the same" ligand (see also Figure 2.1), and inconsistencies in SMILES interpretation can thus lead to inconsistencies in tautomer representation. Several programs are able to enumerate canonical tautomers (e.g., Accelrys, CCG, OpenEye, and Schrodinger), and this is recommended for consistent processing of molecules. Commercial software suites typically provide utilities to produce one or more specific tautomeric and protonation states of molecules based on definition files or user specification. A few studies exploring the impact of tautomer and protonation state enumeration on automated docking results were reviewed in our earlier survey [1]. Several recent papers have explored these aspects of database management in virtual screening in some depth [7–10]. A new method of tautomer stability prediction and an extensive analysis of several small-molecule databases have also been presented [11].

2.2.2
3D Conformations

For 3D virtual screening applications, a database of one or more 3D conformers per entry is required. Many screening tools (e.g., automated flexible ligand docking) have integral conformational search engines, thus requiring only one conformer as input. Other approaches (e.g., rigid docking) require precalculated conformers. A virtual screening tool that generates conformers on the fly avoids the calculation and storage of a multiconformer database, but requires additional computation time for each execution. Alternatively, generating conformers as a separate process may allow more control and fine-tuning of this important step.

In the context of structure-based design, an important question is, when a ligand binding mode is known or can be reliably predicted, whether a given conformational search protocol generates a similar conformer. However, the usefulness of this as a general performance metric is questionable, and how to best evaluate conformer generation in the context of predicting ligand binding modes or bioactive conformations remains an open and actively studied question, with several alternative performance metrics described [12–18].

Comparison of the observed conformations of small molecules bound to proteins with those calculated with molecular mechanics-based conformational search tools has been studied. Bostrom *et al.* initially studied relatively small sets of molecules [19, 20], and this was later expanded upon by Perola and Charifson [21]. In these studies, the conformational energy penalty paid upon binding was observed to be surprisingly high for a significant fraction of the studied systems. These results clearly highlight the potential for error in selecting one or a few low-energy conformers as a representative set (un)likely to include the bioactive conformer for a given small molecule. Several more recent studies further validate this concern [14–17]. Many of these papers also describe comparison of various conformational search tools, and thus can be instructive in understanding how to generate conformer sets for small-molecule databases.

2.2.3
Data Storage

When preparing conformational ligand databases, we are interested in maximally leveraging the time required for database preparation and the space required for data storage. Since the data can typically be used for multiple target systems, each with different small-molecule requirements, it is most efficient to tag the compounds with a variety of information. This allows the incorporation of physicochemical properties as well as target- or therapeutic area-specific information (see later sections of this chapter), all of which can be used to select subsets of the compounds for specific purposes.

Since most compression algorithms are designed to remove redundant data, it is recommended to compress any text-based formats, for example, SD mol or Sybyl mol2, with gzip, a format supported by most programs. Some vendors use specific compression routines with, for example, vendor-specific binary formats. In general it is recommended to use the most commonly available format (e.g., SD) and a program with many output formats and scripting options (e.g., OEChem and OpenBabel) to store conformational databases, allowing maximal downstream flexibility for transforming the conformational data into software-specific formats for use with various programs. It would be most efficient if all vendors would agree on a common conformational database format, but this ideal state has not been reached. Table 2.2 shows an estimate of the disk size needed to store chemical structures in some of the most commonly used file formats. Whatever format is used to store the molecular data, the programs used for ligand preparation and virtual screening must have fast disk access.

2.2.4
Workflow Tools

Managing large compound collections requires a well-designed informatics infrastructure [22, 23]. The growth in size of small-molecule databases being studied has encouraged automation of molecular structure preparation and filtering. Increasingly, workflow tools such as Pipeline Pilot, (http://accelrys.com/products/scitegic/) Inforsense, (http://www.inforsense.com) and the open-source tools Knime (http://www.knime.org) and Taverna [24] are used for various aspects of molecular structure database management. These tools facilitate cheminformatic programming through

Table 2.2 Disk size needed to store 10 000 druglike compounds selected randomly from the World Drug Index.

	Disk size (KB)	3D information
SDF	19701	Yes
SMILES	703	No
InChI	1775	No

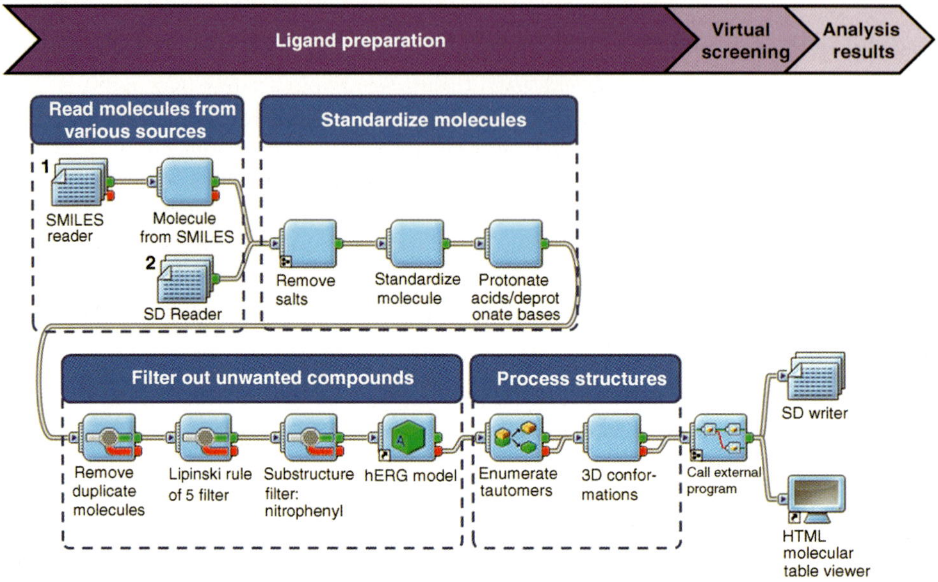

Figure 2.2 Example of a workflow for ligand preparation created using Pipeline Pilot.

a visual interface that allows the connection of data sources, applications, and services into workflows (pipelines). An example of a typical workflow is shown in Figure 2.2. More expert programmers can build custom workflows by incorporating additional programming and scripting languages such as Python and the cheminformatics libraries that were released publicly in the last decade: CDK [4], OELib (http://www.eyesopen.com/products/toolkits/oelib.html), and JOELib (http://www.ra.cs.uni-tuebingen.de/software/joelib/). Factors contributing to the widespread adoption of these cheminformatic tools are the high reusability and ready integration of the resulting workflows.

2.2.5
Past Reviews and Recent Papers

We recently reviewed aspects of database preparation in the context of automated docking-based virtual screening, giving an overview of the virtual screening process and highlighting some of the key issues involved [1]. Aspects of several papers describing docking-based virtual screens were surveyed to provide some perspective on current practices employed in the field. One study aimed specifically at exploring the effect of different database preparation schemes [25] was reviewed in some detail. Bologa *et al.* have also reviewed database preparation for virtual screening [26], providing a rich overview of relevant tools and approaches. These papers, together with an early study of artificial enrichment [27], can provide a broad introduction to some of the major issues of small-molecule database preparation for virtual screening, and can also serve as a resource for identifying relevant software tools and Internet resources.

Here we briefly review several additional papers that have been published since our previous article on the subject. We have not intended to exhaustively analyze all recent work; rather, we have noted a few additional papers (see also preceding paragraph) that would be helpful to those readers interested in building or managing compound collections for virtual and/or experimental screening.

McGaughey *et al.* at Merck have described virtual screening benchmarking studies, comparing the performance of 2D and 3D ligand similarity and protein structure-based docking methods with 11 protein targets [28]. This study is particularly important in that it was published somewhat later than several previous comprehensive docking comparisons (reviewed in Ref. [1]), and therefore provides an evolved perspective on some of the issues related to this type of work. The authors compare several proprietary software tools with various commercial products, and some detail is provided on specific database preparation requirements for the virtual screening methods used. This study uses two different small-molecule databases, one of which (derived from the MDDR database [29]) is available for public use.

Irwin, one of the developers of the ZINC [30] and DUD [31] databases, has commented on the state of screening libraries in a brief review [32], providing an overview of issues to be considered in building and maintaining a screening collection. Topics covered include chemical space, screening artifacts, fragment-based screening, natural products versus synthetic molecules, and clustering and compound acquisition, providing a succinct overview and citing many worthwhile references.

A detailed discussion of compound acquisition has been presented [33], with comparison of different commercial sources of chemical collections. Also included are useful discussions of methods for compound and library evaluation and comparison and practical aspects of actually purchasing compounds. This review also provides an extensive set of compound vendor Web sites.

Researchers from BMS have detailed the results of their efforts to enhance their HTS process [34]. Their papers discuss the subjectivity of the typical chemical structure triage process as it relates to HTS analysis, a topic worth some investigation by anyone involved in this type of selection process. With the aim of reducing subjectivity in this area, the authors systematically review their filters for physicochemical properties (this topic discussed in more detail below) and unwanted chemical moieties. Much of the work is aimed at understanding and detecting promiscuous compounds – those that initially appear to be hits in many screens (this topic discussed in more detail below). Importantly, the authors have made some of the related tools available for public use.

Brenk *et al.* at the University of Dundee have outlined the lessons learned from assembling screening libraries for neglected diseases in an academic setting [35]. This work offers an interesting perspective in that compound purchases were not made to augment an already large proprietary collection as is typically the case in industrial pharmaceutical research, but rather a new collection was being built for use in an academic drug discovery setting. A detailed description of the tools and processes involved in virtual compound analysis is provided, as are some experimental analyses for purity and solubility. These authors have also made some of the information tools derived from their work available for public use.

2.3 Considering Physicochemical Properties

2.3.1 Druglikeness

The physicochemical properties of small molecules can be applied to compound databases to selectively enrich the collection in molecules with desirable property profiles and to selectively deplete the collection of molecules with undesirable property profiles. In the late 1990s, a number of groups began reporting observed trends between calculated physicochemical properties and oral bioavailability. Oral bioavailability is a complex pharmacokinetic parameter that includes absorption and clearance components. In turn, absorption is itself dependent on solubility and permeability [36]. Chan and Stewart observed that intestinal permeability increased with lipophilicity but decreased with MW or H-bonding potential, and that clearance in bile increased with both MW and lipophilicity [37]. They recommended that new chemical entities should have a balance of such properties. Lipinski's rule of five mnemonic states that a compound with more than 5 H-bond donors (HBD), 10 H-bond acceptors (HBA), $MW > 500$, and $\mathrm{Clog}P > 5$ is more likely to manifest poor absorption or permeation [38]. Hits identified by HTS were more lipophilic and less soluble than the set of drugs used in the comparison study. The rules were presented with an emphasis on improving both compound collections and initial chemical leads for drug discovery projects. Refinements were suggested by Ghose *et al.*, who set more specific range limits for two of the rules: $160 \leq MW \leq 480$ and $-0.4 \leq \mathrm{Alog}P \leq 5.6$ [39].

Lipinski *et al.* noted that finding good starting points for medicinal chemistry-based drug discovery is key to overall project success as well as the quality of the final optimized compounds [38]. While some library design examples may have considered diversity, there was no overall understanding of the impact of the physicochemical properties of the compounds or their druglikeness [40], and these properties were not widely applied in the design of screening decks. Subsequently, more druglike considerations were applied [41]. As compound collections in pharmaceutical companies grew, Lipinski's rule of five was used to filter purchased compounds. Lipinski's rules were elaborated on by Veber *et al.*, who recommended using a number of rotatable bonds (NRB) filter, with $NRB > 7$ appearing to be detrimental for oral bioavailability [42]. In addition, from a review of modeling work, the role of polar surface area (PSA) was highlighted as a useful descriptor for passive absorption [43]. Finally, it has been shown that the physicochemical properties governing oral bioavailability are different for anions and cations at pH 6–7. PSA is the sole property criterion for anions, whereas for neutral and cationic species the rule of five is predictive [44, 45]. Acids were shown, on average, to have higher oral bioavailability [45]. Interesting retrospective studies have examined the druglikeness concept and its impact on medicinal chemistry [46], and have explored whether current approaches to descriptor calculation are an oversimplification [47].

2.3.2
Leadlikeness and Beyond

Following Lipinski's work on the rule of five [38], Teague *et al.* pointed out the disparity between the physicochemical properties of marketed drugs and the leads or chemical starting points from which they came [48]. Increasingly, it became clear that compound collections should contain molecules with sufficiently low MW and lipophilicity to allow physicochemical property space (i.e., "room") for lead optimization. Progressing from lead to drug was accompanied by a median increase in MW of 69 and a median increase in Clog$P$ of 0.43, among other properties studied. Filters of leadlikeness were defined: MW < 450, $-3.5 \leq \text{Clog}P \leq 4.5$, $-4 \leq \log D_{\text{pH 7.4}} \leq 4$, ≤ 5 rings, ≤ 10 nonterminal single bonds, ≤ 5 HBD, and ≤ 8 HBA [49]. More theoretical discussions of molecular complexity suggested that leads tend to be less complex than drugs [50]. Subsequent work in this area recommended even lower MW to allow coverage of a greater percentage of the total virtual chemical space. Tighter reduced complexity filters identify attractive molecules for high-concentration screening: MW < 350, NRB ≤ 6, heavy atoms ≤ 22, HBD ≤ 3, HBA ≤ 8, and Clog$P \leq 2.2$ [51]. These filters are similar to the so-called rule of three, MW < 300, Clog$P$ < 3, HBD < 3, and NRB < 3, proposed for fragment-based lead discovery [52]. A recent study has shown that aromatic ring count is a significant factor in compound developability [53].

2.4
Undesirables

An important task in drug discovery is to identify a ligand that is selective for a specific protein target and that does not participate in adverse drug interactions. It is also important to identify potential screening artifacts. Hence, there is a clear motivation to evaluate compound pharmacological promiscuity and propensity for artifactual behavior as early as possible in the drug discovery process. By identifying such problematic compounds, virtual database filtering can help reduce the number of such compounds that are ultimately screened.

The terms "frequent hitter," "promiscuous compound," "screening artifact," and "false positive" are often used synonymously and, at times, inconsistently. The term "promiscuous ligand" was first used in the context of drug discovery in 1987 [54], describing compounds of pharmacological interest that bind with high affinity to more than one receptor. In this definition, the term refers to a truly polypharmacological profile. More recently, in the screening field, the term "promiscuous molecule" has been used to refer to hits that appear nondruglike: they act noncompetitively, show little relation between structure and activity, and have poor selectivity [55]. These compounds show up reproducibly in a given primary screening assay, but later fail in more advanced assays. Their initial detection is an artifact of the screen and is not based on specific activity toward the protein target of interest. They differ from "false positives," a term used in HTS to describe compounds active in an initial test that fail confirmation in repeat or dose–response testing. Another term describing compounds that show up as hits in many different biological assays covering a wide range of targets is "frequent hitters" [56].

To avoid confusion, here we use the term "pharmacologically promiscuous compound" to refer to compounds that are truly active on several drug targets and the term "screening artifact" to describe compounds that are active in an assay for any reason other than specific activity toward the protein target of interest.

2.4.1
Screening Artifacts

When a compound interferes with an assay such that it leads to an apparently positive result, this is a screening artifact. There are various possible mechanisms of assay interference, and it is therefore important to understand the screening assay(s) and potential sources of interference [57].

Compounds may interfere directly with wavelengths used in colorimetric assay readouts (e.g., fluorescence, quenching, absorbance, and luminescence). Such compounds show similar activity profiles in other assays that rely on the same wavelengths and assay conditions. In some cases, very slight changes in the assay conditions can lead to distinctly different compound properties (e.g., halochromic pH indicator-like dyes used at pH close to their dissociation constant). Depending on the assay conditions, light-interfering compounds can also be a source of false negatives; in this case, the active compound can mask its own activity by, for example, fluorescence quenching. Substructure filters or other *in silico* models that can detect dye-like compounds are useful for flagging these cases.

Compounds that form aggregates in solution can be problematic. These hits, often with low micromolar activities, typically show steep dose–response curves [58]. The observed activity of these compounds does not originate from the molecule itself, but rather from the suspensions or aggregates formed by the molecules [59, 60]. One such colloidal particle can sequester up to 10 000 enzyme molecules [61]. It is believed that compounds showing this behavior represent a large fraction of the observed hits (up to 95%) in some screening campaigns [62]. Assay conditions have been proposed to reduce the effect of this class of false positives [63], and there are models aimed at predicting this behavior [64].

Another source of nonspecific behavior can be observed in cellular assays [65], when a compound does not interfere with the (overexpressed) investigated target but does interfere with a different cellular target, and this result ultimately cascades down to the same assay readout. An example is the measurement of the activity of an overexpressed GPCR by monitoring intracellular Ca^{2+} levels with Ca^{2+}-sensitive dyes [66, 67]. If the compound stimulates an endogenous wild-type receptor that also leads to Ca^{2+} mobilization, then this compound will show up (artifactually) as active in this type of assay. In most cases, this type of mechanism-based interference is unlikely to be predicted initially. It is possible to discriminate this kind of screening artifact by using "wild-type" (without the overexpressed target) control assays, and, based on data from such control assays, generate *in silico* models for subsequent computational filtering.

Toxic compounds are another source of screening artifacts in cellular assays. In many reporter gene assays, decrease of the signal is the desired readout. However, toxic compounds that lead to a decrease in cell number are a major source of false positives when the data are not normalized with respect to a toxicity parameter (e.g., cell mass determination). There are different manifestations of cellular toxicity, with some toxic compounds showing a rapid toxic effect (e.g., blocking cellular respiration), while other compounds may take several days to show their effect (e.g., blocking cell proliferation through kinase inhibition) [68, 69]. It is difficult to come up with generally applicable *in silico* models for toxicity filtering of databases, since the underlying toxicity mechanism(s) are variable. In most cases where cell toxicity leads to screening artifacts, control assays are used to weed out toxicity artifacts.

2.4.2
Pharmacologically Promiscuous Compounds

It is estimated that, on average, a drug molecule interacts (i.e., shows low micromolar affinity) with 6.3 target proteins [70]. While this is an average, it does seem like a big number. This estimate includes both known (literature documented) and predicted (not yet documented, but extrapolated from a validated set of *in silico* predictions) ligand–target pairs. Pharmacologically promiscuous compounds can be sorted broadly into two classes, those active on multiple similar targets and those active on various (apparently) unrelated targets.

Human kinases, comprising more than 500 distinct enzymes, are a large and well-explored target class. Kinase inhibitors often inhibit multiple kinases, and are a familiar example(s) of pharmacologically promiscuous compounds [71]. The vast majority of these enzymes use ATP as a substrate, and it is thus not surprising that ATP-competitive inhibitors often exhibit cross-reactivity within the set of kinases. When the protein target being investigated is not a kinase, it can be helpful to flag the known or suspected kinase inhibitors in the set of molecules being screened, since kinase inhibition in a cellular screen can be a source of screening artifacts if the inhibited kinases alter normal cell behavior. In addition to potential artifacts, it may also be of interest to monitor kinase activity during compound optimization. Substructure selection [72], Bayesian models [73], and/or pharmacophore searching [74] can all be used to aid in tracking potential kinase activity or promiscuity.

Prediction of compound promiscuity toward (apparently) unrelated target proteins is currently an active area of research. Interesting research has been published on linking proteins by the chemical similarity of their ligands, and unexpected links between proteins were found; testing of some of these compounds on their predicted targets confirmed their predicted polypharmacology [75–77]. Polypharmacology may lead to desirable clinical profiles, as is the case for antidepressants [78]. Of course, the inverse is also true – pharmacological promiscuity can lead to undesirable adverse events that can ultimately lead to the withdrawal of a compound from the market [79].

Some target proteins are promiscuous by nature. Metabolic cytochromes (CYPs) have evolved to process a variety of substrates [80]. Both lipophilicity and charge are contributors to CYP susceptibility, with increased lipophilicity generally leading to greater CYP affinity and the impact of charge being CYP specific [45]. The hERG channel is another renowned protein with fearsome promiscuity; high lipophilicity and the presence of a positive charge are important contributors to affinity for this protein. Further elucidation of hERG structure–activity relationships is an active field of research [81, 82].

In addition to the use of *in vitro* screens for the profiling of initial hits, there are also *in silico* profiling screens that are useful for this purpose [83]. Several groups have investigated substructural or physicochemical property correlations with promiscuous compound behavior. Most studies indicate that high lipophilicity leads to increased promiscuity [46, 83–86], and that the presence of a positive charge at neutral pH [46, 86] increases the chance of a polypharmacological profile.

In general, and perhaps not surprisingly, pharmacological promiscuity diminishes as compounds progress through preclinical and clinical development [83]. This observation is relevant to the fields of drug repositioning [87, 88] and selective optimization of side activities (SOSA) [89], techniques that focus on compounds that have survived the rigors of the initial stages of the drug development process and are therefore highly enriched in druggable properties. Exploring the polypharmacology of this relatively small set of well-studied compounds can lead to new uses for old drugs (drug repositioning), as well as yield excellent starting points for new discovery projects (SOSA). When a "hit" is detected in these contexts, it may be worthwhile to retrace the optimization route that yielded the molecule of interest and explore the new activity in less "mature" analogues from the identified chemical series.

2.5
Property-Based Filtering for Selected Targets

Removal of undesirable compounds, as discussed above, is clearly one important application for database filtering. However, just as many simple filters can be useful in identifying undesirable compounds, filtering can also select desirable molecules. Targeted selections for desirable compounds may be quite general (e.g., compiling a general-purpose screening deck for various targets) or very specific (e.g., targeting a specific enzyme). In the preceding sections, we have reviewed background material related to filtering for both desirable and undesirable compounds, largely focusing on physicochemical properties, and we have discussed selected aspects of undesirable compounds. In this final section, we review material related to filtering aimed at enriching a selection in desired compounds, covering three target areas:

antibacterials, central nervous system (CNS), and protein–protein interactions. Antibacterials are a particularly important class of molecules, and they exhibit distinct physicochemical characteristics. Penetration of the blood–brain barrier (BBB) presents a unique challenge for CNS drug discovery, and understanding how to target this characteristic is an active area of research. Protein–protein interactions have recently emerged as a distinct class of targets for drug discovery, and we are only just beginning to try to understand the unique requirements of small-molecule drug discovery in this arena.

2.5.1
Antibacterials

Antibacterial drug discovery remains of vital importance. Unfortunately, screens of antibacterial targets typically yield poor hit rates [90]. After many years of medicinal chemistry efforts, often based on the modification of known antibacterial scaffolds, it is increasingly difficult to deliver new chemical leads for optimization and drug development. One goal of antibacterial-targeted small-molecule library design is to facilitate the identification of novel chemical classes as drug discovery leads, for both new and established bacterial targets.

Antibacterials differ from other drugs in many respects [91]), and the Lipinski rules [38] need to be adapted for this drug class, especially for those derived from natural products (e.g., macrolides and glycopeptides; Table 2.3). Antibacterial drugs tend to have high molecular weights and "repellently" complex structures [91]. Many antibacterial drugs have to satisfy the requirements for both parenteral and oral administration, and they must also penetrate bacteria. According to Nikaido [92],

Table 2.3 Natural product-derived antibacterials versus "other" drugs.

Topic		Antibacterials	Other drugs (*Lipinski etc.*)
Target/Mode of Action		Multiple targets, multivalent, block target	Single target, selective, modulate target
Structure		Complex, multiple pharmacophores	Simple, single pharmacophore
Physicochemistry	M_W (g/mol)	>500	<500
	log MA (pH 7.5)	<3 (Parenteral) <5 (oral)	<5
	Rotatable bonds	>10	<10
	H-donors	>5 (Parenteral)	<5
	H-acceptors	>10	<10
	solubility (g/L)	>0.5–2	<1
Pharmacokinetics	Dose	Often high	Often low
	Protein binding (%)	Critical	Less critical

Empirical rules of thumb. Reprinted from Table 6 of Ref. [91] with permission.

porins prevent the entry of overly lipophilic molecules in Gram-negative bacteria. Bacterial penetration by antibacterial compounds seems to be at least partially defined by a molecular polarity window. Von Nussbaum *et al.* noted that parenteral antibacterials have to be polar (log MA < 3, where MA = membrane affinity) [91, 93], but at the same time bacterial penetration by overly polar molecules is limited by the bacterial membrane [94]. A "preferred polarity window" may apply. These observations are consistent with the more recent work of Leeson and Davis, wherein the authors demonstrate that antibacterial drugs have the highest mean molecular weight, lowest mean lipophilicity, highest O + N (O plus N atoms) and H-bond acceptor counts, and the largest number of rings of all drug classes [95].

O'Shea and Moser have concluded, similar to von Nussbaum, that most antibacterial drugs are substantially more polar than drugs from other therapeutic classes [91, 96]. Furthermore, it is important to distinguish Gram-negative and Gram-positive antibacterials. In their study of 147 antibacterial agents, the average Clog*P* value of antibacterial agents effective against Gram-negative organisms was −0.1, while the corresponding Clog*P* values for antibacterial agents active against Gram-positive organisms was +2.1 [96]. This difference reflects differences in Gram-negative and Gram-positive cell wall structures (lipid composition, charge distribution, and fluidity), which in turn affects permeability and drug efflux. According to the authors, the two major differences between antibacterials and other drugs are in MW and lipophilicity (Table 2.4).

Understanding the physicochemical features of antibacterial property space can enhance screening efforts aimed at identifying novel antibacterials in synthetic or semisynthetic chemical libraries. Relatively simple filtering, based on a set of physicochemical property rules, can help to optimize an antibacterial screening deck. A recent study suggests that natural products should be investigated to identify novel antibacterial hits [97]. In addition to increased overall structural complexity and diversity, natural products are more likely (than synthetic molecules) to fulfill the physicochemical property requirements of antibacterial compounds due to their greater density of polar functionalities.

Table 2.4 Comparison of average (mean) compound property values of three drug data sets representing general (CMC, excluding antibiotics) and antibacterial drugs.

Parameter	CMC data set	Antibacterials (only Gram-positive activity)	Antibacterials (Gram-negative activity)
MW	338	813	414
Clog*P*	2.7	2.1	−0.1
Clog$D_{7.4}$	1.6	−0.2	−2.8
PSA (Å^2)	70	243	165
rel PSA (%)	22	30	42
H-donor	1.6	7.1	5.1
H-acceptor	4.9	16.3	9.4

Reprinted from Table 1 of Ref. [96] with permission.

2.5.2
CNS

A fundamental of CNS drug discovery research is that compounds must cross the blood–brain barrier and, consequently, a modified (compare with other drugs) physicochemical property profile is required to describe CNS agents [49]. The BBB is composed of a network of capillaries lined with endothelial cells joined by complex tight junctions, protecting the brain from xenobiotics present in the peripheral circulation. Active transport uptake and efflux systems, and metabolic mechanisms, are numerous. Analysis of CNS-active and CNS-inactive drugs has shown that MW, PSA, Clog*P*, and log*D* are important descriptors for discriminating CNS activity. It was suggested that MW should ideally be <450 and $1 \leq \log D \leq 3$ [98]. Kelder *et al.* determined that drugs entering the CNS via passive transport across the BBB should not have PSA > 120 Å^2, with PSA < 60–70 preferred [99]. Qualitative rules suggested by Lipinski state that MW < 400, Clog*P* < 5, HBD <3, and HBA <7 are attributes of successful CNS drugs [100]. Other simple rules of thumb were proposed by Norinder and Haeberlein: if the sum of nitrogen and oxygen atoms (N + O) is <5, the molecule has a high chance of entering the brain; likewise, if [Clog*P* − (N + O)] > 0 [101]. Lipophilicity, represented by either Clog*P* or log*D*, is a common feature of BBB permeation models [102]. It has been shown that positively charged molecules at pH 7–8 tend to favor brain penetration [103], whereas a negatively charged group with $pK_a < 4$ is unfavorable for brain penetration [104]. A detailed summary of the qualitative rules describing BBB permeation is available [105]. There have been many attempts to construct quantitative models for BBB permeation, and this topic has been reviewed [102, 106].

Qualitative models are useful in approximating the requirements of the underlying mechanisms of CNS penetration. Quantitative models are typically built from smaller data sets, from which compounds known to cross the BBB by active transport are excluded. Thus, many quantitative models focus only on passive permeation. It has been suggested that a compound with sufficient intestinal uptake and little or no susceptibility to BBB efflux and metabolism should be BBB penetrant [107]. Avoidance of efflux mediated by permeability glycoprotein (P-gp) is a requirement for CNS activity [108]. Efforts are underway to model P-gp efflux, but it remains a challenging property to predict [109]. Plasma protein binding has also been shown to be detrimental to CNS penetration [110, 111], since only unbound drug is free to permeate the BBB. Thus, many factors affect small-molecule penetration of the BBB. While simple qualitative rule-based approaches are a gross oversimplification, they overlap to some extent with concepts of drug- and leadlikeness, and one can therefore expect that application of such models or filters in the earliest stages of drug discovery will, on average, pay dividends.

Typically, in targeting CNS-active compounds, a series of physicochemical property filters is applied to early discovery work such as *de novo* library design, virtual screening analysis, and the design of screening decks. These filters reflect a desire to identify good starting points for medicinal chemistry-based lead optimization (i.e., leadlike molecules), as well as a preference for molecules exhibiting properties similar to those of previously successful CNS compounds. The following characteristics are typically emphasized: $MW < 400$, $1 \leq ClogP \leq 4$, $HBD < 2$, $HBA < 9$, $NRB < 9$, and $PSA < 80$, with negatively charged species excluded. The leadlike and CNS-like origins of these filters are clear, given the discussion above, and are broadly consistent with a recent analysis [112]. The Clog*P* range is a compromise, somewhat lower than that of known CNS drugs since we anticipate an increase in Clog*P* during lead optimization.

Figure 2.3 shows the effect of applying these CNS leadlike filters to an in-house data set of 298 compounds. As the aim was to demonstrate how a conventional lead differs from a CNS lead, all compounds in the data set were compliant with the leadlike filters specified by Oprea *et al.* [49]. A univariate analysis was performed with all 2D descriptors available in the Molecular Operating Environment (MOE) program, and the most highly correlated individual descriptors (TPSA, vsa_pol, vsa_acc) were related to surface polarity.

Figure 2.3a shows the plot of log(BB) (log brain:blood ratio) versus calculated 2D PSA. The compounds compliant with the CNS leadlike filters are enriched with respect to higher log(BB) values. Classification of the same compound set into three groups, CNS + + ($\log(BB) > 0$), CNS+ ($-0.5 \leq \log(BB) \leq 0$), and CNS− ($\log(BB) < -0.5$), shows that the CNS leadlike filters achieve good separation of CNS + + penetrant and CNS− nonpenetrant compounds (Figure 2.3b). With classifier models, there are uncertainties around the cutoff boundaries, and in this case the CNS+ class was more difficult to predict. Approximately 75% (58/77) of the CNS + + compounds passed all the CNS leadlike filters, whereas only 33% (32/96) of the CNS− compounds were filter compliant. Thus, simple physicochemical property

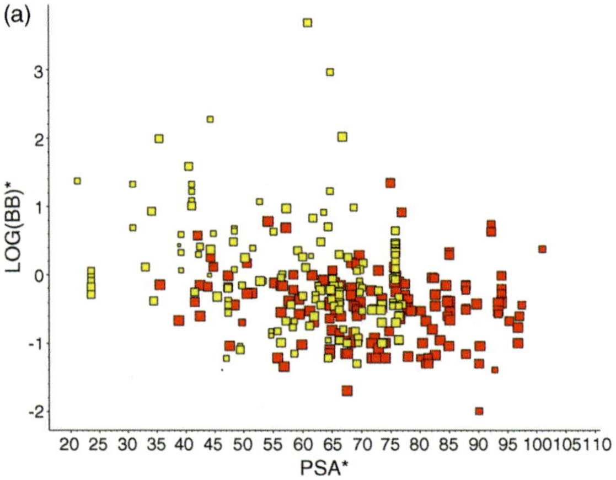

Figure 2.3 (a) Plot of log(BB) versus PSA for an in-house set of leadlike compounds. Data points are sized by MW; compounds that comply with the CNS leadlike filters (see text) are highlighted in gold. (b) Histogram for the same data set split according to CNS −, CNS +, and CNS + +; compounds that comply with the CNS leadlike filters (see text) are highlighted in gold.

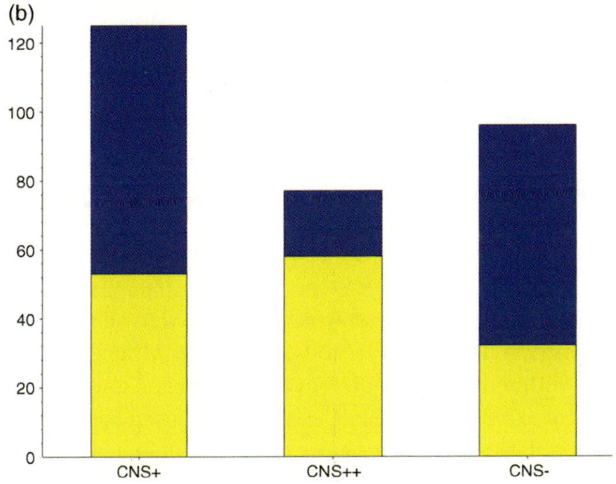

Figure 2.3 (*Continued*).

descriptors deliver enrichment of CNS-positive compounds. These results are satisfying, given the expected difficulty of such discrimination within a set of leadlike compounds.

2.5.3
Protein–Protein Interactions

Analysis of biomolecular interactions continues to increase our understanding of the complex metabolic pathways and molecular interaction networks on which biology and disease depend [113]. Interactions between proteins are a foundation of biology, and over the past two decades the perception of protein–protein interactions as a vast set of potential drug discovery targets spanning all disease areas has emerged ([114, 115] and reviews therein). Currently, it is generally accepted that protein–protein interactions are difficult targets for small-molecule drug discovery. Many factors have been put forward to explain this difficulty, including interface size, the relative (to enzyme active sites) flatness of protein–protein interfaces, absence of a site that has evolved to bind a small molecule, and lack of a known small-molecule "starting point" for a medicinal chemistry-based discovery effort. Since many industrial drug discovery efforts originate from screening, the simple fact that historical collections have been built from compounds targeting enzymes and receptors may explain the difficulty of small-molecule drug discovery for protein–protein interactions. In other words, current screening collections have not evolved to target protein–protein interactions.

The term "peptidomimetic" typically refers to mimicry of a few adjacent residues in a peptide sequence, and this type of molecular design approach is unlikely to be relevant to most protein–protein interfaces, since binding typically involves structural features derived either from one large secondary structural element or two or more disparate stretches of the protein sequence. Hamilton and colleagues coined the term proteomimetics to describe small molecules that mimic larger areas of a protein surface [116]; much of their work has focused on α-helix mimicry (reviewed in [117]). Helix mimicry has been successfully employed against the oncology-related p53-HDM2 protein–protein interaction (discussed in, for example, Ref. [118]), and the helix binding site in Bcl-2 family proteins has also proven susceptible to small-molecule discovery [119], with Abbott having advanced a compound to phase 2 clinical studies [120]. Many other protein–protein targets have been reviewed ([114, 115] and references therein).

Several groups have analyzed sets of inhibitors of protein–protein interactions and compared them to drugs or druglike molecules. In 2004, Pagliaro *et al.* analyzed 19 small molecules targeting 12 different protein–protein interactions, showing that more than half of the inhibitors exceeded Lipinski's criteria (discussed above) and providing a hint that suitable small molecules for many protein–protein targets may be absent from large compound collections [121]. In 2005, Fischer reviewed the field and also concluded that the majority of small-molecule inhibitors of protein–protein interactions fall outside the rule of five [122]. Wells and McClendon applied the ligand efficiency (LE) concept [123] to a set of small-molecule inhibitors of protein–protein interactions, concluding that a K_d of 10 nM translates to MW = 645 Da [115]. Most recently, Higueruelo *et al.* analyzed a larger set of 104 small molecules targeting 20 different protein–protein targets, comparing them to various drug discovery-related small-molecule collections [124]. Generally consistent with the earlier studies noted above, these authors also conclude that while the studied compounds do span a large range of physicochemical property values, they tend to be larger, more lipophilic, more rigid, and contain fewer hydrogen bonding centers than drugs or molecules in screening collections. These and other authors [122] note that these properties are characteristic of promiscuous compounds, and also caution that there is only limited profiling data available for these compounds. In addition to the observations on physicochemical properties, this set of compounds exhibits a higher occurrence of carboxylic acids, sulfonamides, aromatic rings, and nitro groups and a lower occurrence of ethers than the compared set of drugs.

2.6 Summary

Data format, tautomers, protonation states, 3D structure generation, and conformers are some of the aspects to be considered when managing compound collections for virtual, and experimental, screening. Issues such as generating and storing maximal information and ensuring compatibility between multiple software tools will also be influential. We have outlined some of the relevant issues and cited many references to studies that in some way shed light on one or more of these issues. End users want to remove undesirable compounds from their screening sets and design sets of compounds suitable for the target area in which they work. Analysis of antibacterials has led to the conclusion that the rule of five is not relevant to this therapeutic area.

Contrast this with research in CNS, where it is often desirable to work in an even more limited physicochemical descriptor space. Indeed, it has been shown that filters frequently applied to CNS library design and virtual screening can be considered a modified and more restrictive version of leadlike filters. Finally, protein–protein interactions as a target class are just emerging, and it seems premature to attempt general characterization of small molecule inhibitors of this class at this time.

References

1 Cummings, M.D., Gibbs, A.C., and DesJarlais, R.L. (2007) Processing of small molecule databases for automated docking. *Medicinal Chemistry*, **3**, 107–113.

2 Weininger, D. (1988) SMILES, a chemical language and information system. 1. Introduction to methodology and encoding rules. *Journal of Chemical Information and Computer Sciences*, **28**, 31–36.

3 *MDL chemical data file* (2010) Available from http://www.symyx.com/downloads/public/ctfile/ctfile.pdf.

4 Steinbeck, C., Han, Y., Kuhn, S., Horlacher, O., Luttmann, E., and Willighagen, E. (2003) The Chemistry Development Kit (CDK): an open-source Java library for chemo- and bioinformatics. *Journal of Chemical Information and Computer Sciences*, **43**, 493–500.

5 O'Boyle, N.M., Morley, C., and Hutchison, G.R. (2008) Pybel: a Python wrapper for the OpenBabel cheminformatics toolkit. *Chemistry Central Journal*, **2**, 5.

6 Murray-Rust, P. and Rzepa, H.S. (1999) Chemical markup, XML, and the Worldwide Web. 1. Basic principles. *Journal of Chemical Information and Computer Sciences*, **39**, 928–942.

7 Martin, Y.C. (2009) Let's not forget tautomers. *Journal of Computer-Aided Molecular Design*, **23**, 693–704.

8 Kalliokoski, T., Salo, H.S., Lahtela-Kakkonen, M., and Poso, A. (2009) The effect of ligand-based tautomer and protomer prediction on structure-based virtual screening. *Journal of Chemical Information and Modeling*, **49** (12), 2742–2748.

9 ten Brink, T. and Exner, T.E. (2009) Influence of protonation, tautomeric, and stereoisomeric states on protein–ligand docking results. *Journal of Chemical Information and Modeling*, **49**, 1535–1546.

10 Deng, W. and Verlinde, C.L. (2008) Evaluation of different virtual screening programs for docking in a charged binding pocket. *Journal of Chemical Information and Modeling*, **48**, 2010–2020.

11 Milletti, F., Storchi, L., Sforna, G., Cross, S., and Cruciani, G. (2009) Tautomer enumeration and stability prediction for virtual screening on large chemical databases. *Journal of Chemical Information and Modeling*, **49**, 68–75.

12 Hawkins, P.C., Warren, G.L., Skillman, A.G., and Nicholls, A. (2008) How to do an evaluation: pitfalls and traps. *Journal of Computer-Aided Molecular Design*, **22**, 179–190.

13 Jain, A.N. (2007) Surflex-Dock 2.1: robust performance from ligand energetic modeling, ring flexibility, and knowledge-based search. *Journal of Computer-Aided Molecular Design*, **21**, 281–306.

14 Kirchmair, J., Wolber, G., Laggner, C., and Langer, T. (2006) Comparative performance assessment of the conformational model generators omega and catalyst: a large-scale survey on the retrieval of protein-bound ligand conformations. *Journal of Chemical Information and Modeling*, **46**, 1848–1861.

15 Takagi, T., Amano, M., and Tomimoto, M. (2009) Novel method for the evaluation of 3D conformation generators. *Journal of Chemical Information and Modeling*, **49**, 1377–1388.

16 Agrafiotis, D.K., Gibbs, A.C., Zhu, F., Izrailev, S., and Martin, E. (2007) Conformational sampling of bioactive molecules: a comparative study. *Journal of Chemical Information and Modeling*, **47**, 1067–1086.

17 Chen, I.J. and Foloppe, N. (2008) Conformational sampling of druglike molecules with MOE and catalyst: implications for pharmacophore modeling and virtual screening. *Journal of Chemical Information and Modeling*, **48**, 1773–1791.

18 Matter, H. and Potter, T. (1999) Comparing 3D pharmacophore triplets and 2D fingerprints for selecting diverse compound subsets. *Journal of Chemical Information and Computer Sciences*, **39**, 1211–1225.

19 Bostrom, J. (2001) Reproducing the conformations of protein-bound ligands: a critical evaluation of several popular conformational searching tools. *Journal of Computer-Aided Molecular Design*, **15**, 1137–1152.

20 Bostrom, J., Norrby, P.O., and Liljefors, T. (1998) Conformational energy penalties of protein-bound ligands. *Journal of Computer-Aided Molecular Design*, **12**, 383–396.

21 Perola, E. and Charifson, P.S. (2004) Conformational analysis of drug-like molecules bound to proteins: an extensive study of ligand reorganization upon binding. *Journal of Medicinal Chemistry*, **47**, 2499–2510.

22 Chen, W.L. (2006) Chemoinformatics: past, present, and future. *Journal of Chemical Information and Modeling*, **46**, 2230–2255.

23 Engel, T. (2006) Basic overview of chemoinformatics. *Journal of Chemical Information and Modeling*, **46**, 2267–2277.

24 Hull, D., Wolstencroft, K., Stevens, R., Goble, C., Pocock, M.R., Li, P., and Oinn, T. (2006) Taverna: a tool for building and running workflows of services. *Nucleic Acids Research*, **34**, W729–W732.

25 Knox, A.J., Meegan, M.J., Carta, G., and Lloyd, D.G. (2005) Considerations in compound database preparation: "hidden" impact on virtual screening results. *Journal of Chemical Information and Modeling*, **45**, 1908–1919.

26 Bologa, C.G., Olah, M.M., and Oprea, T.I. (2006) Chemical database preparation for compound acquisition or virtual screening. *Methods in Molecular Biology*, **316**, 375–388.

27 Verdonk, M.L., Berdini, V., Hartshorn, M.J., Mooij, W.T., Murray, C.W., Taylor, R.D., and Watson, P. (2004) Virtual screening using protein–ligand docking: avoiding artificial enrichment. *Journal of Chemical Information and Computer Sciences*, **44**, 793–806.

28 McGaughey, G.B., Sheridan, R.P., Bayly, C.I., Culberson, J.C., Kreatsoulas, C., Lindsley, S., Maiorov, V., Truchon, J.F., and Cornell, W.D. (2007) Comparison of topological, shape, and docking methods in virtual screening. *Journal of Chemical Information and Modeling*, **47**, 1504–1519.

29 http://www.mdl.com/products/knowledge/drug_data_report/index.jsp.

30 Irwin, J.J. and Shoichet, B.K. (2005) ZINC: a free database of commercially available compounds for virtual screening. *Journal of Chemical Information and Modeling*, **45**, 177–182.

31 Huang, N., Shoichet, B.K., and Irwin, J.J. (2006) Benchmarking sets for molecular docking. *Journal of Medicinal Chemistry*, **49**, 6789–6801.

32 Irwin, J.J. (2006) How good is your screening library? *Current Opinion in Chemical Biology*, **10**, 352–356.

33 Richardson, R. (2006) Compound collections: acquisition, annotation, and access, in *Exploiting Chemical Diversity for Drug Discovery* (eds P.A. Bartlett and M. Entzeroth), Royal Society of Chemistry, Cambridge, UK, pp. 112–136.

34 Pearce, B.C., Sofia, M.J., Good, A.C., Drexler, D.M., and Stock, D.A. (2006) An empirical process for the design of high-throughput screening deck filters. *Journal of Chemical Information and Modeling*, **46**, 1060–1068.

35 Brenk, R., Schipani, A., James, D., Krasowski, A., Gilbert, I.H., Frearson, J., and Wyatt, P.G. (2008) Lessons learnt from assembling screening libraries for

drug discovery for neglected diseases. *ChemMedChem*, **3**, 435–444.
36 Martinez, M.N. and Amidon, G.L. (2002) A mechanistic approach to understanding the factors affecting drug absorption: a review of fundamentals. *Journal of Clinical Pharmacology*, **42**, 620–643.
37 Chan, O.H. and Stewart, B.H. (1996) Physicochemical and drug delivery considerations for oral drug bioavailability. *Drug Discovery Today*, **1**, 461–473.
38 Lipinski, C.A., Lombardo, F., Dominy, B.W., and Feeney, P.J. (1997) Experimental and computational approaches to estimate solubility and permeability in drug discovery and development settings. *Advanced Drug Delivery Reviews*, **23**, 3–25.
39 Ghose, A.K., Viswanadhan, V.N., and Wendoloski, J.J. (1999) A knowledge-based approach in designing combinatorial or medicinal chemistry libraries for drug discovery. 1. A qualitative and quantitative characterization of known drug databases. *Journal of Combinatorial Chemistry*, **1**, 55–68.
40 Alper, J. (1994) Drug discovery on the assembly line. *Science*, **264**, 1399–1401.
41 Fecik, R.A., Frank, K.E., Gentry, E.J., Menon, S.R., Mitscher, L.A., and Telikepalli, H. (1998) The search for orally active medications through combinatorial chemistry. *Medicinal Research Reviews*, **18**, 149–185.
42 Veber, D.F., Johnson, S.R., Cheng, H.Y., Smith, B.R., Ward, K.W., and Kopple, K.D. (2002) Molecular properties that influence the oral bioavailability of drug candidates. *Journal of Medicinal Chemistry*, **45**, 2615–2623.
43 Clark, D.E. and Pickett, S.D. (2000) Computational methods for the prediction of 'drug-likeness'. *Drug Discovery Today*, **5**, 49–58.
44 Martin, Y.C. (2005) A bioavailability score. *Journal of Medicinal Chemistry*, **48**, 3164–3170.
45 Gleeson, M.P. (2008) Generation of a set of simple, interpretable ADMET rules of thumb. *Journal of Medicinal Chemistry*, **51**, 817–834.
46 Leeson, P.D. and Springthorpe, B. (2007) The influence of drug-like concepts on decision-making in medicinal chemistry. *Nature Reviews. Drug Discovery*, **6**, 881–890.
47 Vistoli, G., Pedretti, A., and Testa, B. (2008) Assessing drug-likeness: what are we missing? *Drug Discovery Today*, **13**, 285–294.
48 Teague, S.J., Davis, A.M., Leeson, P.D., and Oprea, T. (1999) The design of leadlike combinatorial libraries. *Angewandte Chemie, International Edition*, **38**, 3743–3748.
49 Oprea, T.I., Davis, A.M., Teague, S.J., and Leeson, P.D. (2001) Is there a difference between leads and drugs? A historical perspective. *Journal of Chemical Information and Computer Sciences*, **41**, 1308–1315.
50 Hann, M.M., Leach, A.R., and Harper, G. (2001) Molecular complexity and its impact on the probability of finding leads for drug discovery. *Journal of Chemical Information and Computer Sciences*, **41**, 856–864.
51 Hann, M.M. and Oprea, T.I. (2004) Pursuing the leadlikeness concept in pharmaceutical research. *Current Opinion in Chemical Biology*, **8**, 255–263.
52 Congreve, M., Carr, R., Murray, C., and Jhoti, H. (2003) A 'rule of three' for fragment-based lead discovery? *Drug Discovery Today*, **8**, 876–877.
53 Ritchie, T.J. and Macdonald, S.J. (2009) The impact of aromatic ring count on compound developability: Are too many aromatic rings a liability in drug design? *Drug Discovery Today*, **14**, 1011–1020.
54 Lehmann, F.P.A. (1987) Stereoselectivity and affinity in molecular pharmacology. Part 12. A quantitative stereo-structure activity relationship analysis of the binding of promiscuous chiral ligands to different receptors. *Quantitative Structure–Activity Relationships*, **6**, 57–65.
55 McGovern, S.L., Caselli, E., Grigorieff, N., and Shoichet, B.K. (2002) A common mechanism underlying promiscuous inhibitors from

virtual and high-throughput screening. *Journal of Medicinal Chemistry*, **45**, 1712–1722.

56 Roche, O., Schneider, P., Zuegge, J., Guba, W., Kansy, M., Alanine, A., Bleicher, K., Danel, F., Gutknecht, E.-M., Rogers-Evans, M., Neidhart, W., Stalder, H., Dillon, M., Sjoegren, E., Fotouhi, N., Gillespie, P., Goodnow, R., Harris, W., Jones, P., Taniguchi, M., Tsujii, S., von Saal, W., Zimmermann, G., and Schneider, G. (2002) Development of a virtual screening method for identification of "frequent hitters" in compound libraries. *Journal of Medicinal Chemistry*, **45**, 137–142.

57 Hueser, J., Lohrmann, E., Kalthof, B., Burkhardt, N., Brueggemeier, U., and Bechem, M. (2006) High-throughput screening for targeted lead discovery. *Methods and Principles in Medicinal Chemistry*, **35**, 15–36.

58 Shoichet, B.K. (2006) Interpreting steep dose–response curves in early inhibitor discovery. *Journal of Medicinal Chemistry*, **49**, 7274–7277.

59 Coan, K.E., Maltby, D.A., Burlingame, A.L., and Shoichet, B.K. (2009) Promiscuous aggregate-based inhibitors promote enzyme unfolding. *Journal of Medicinal Chemistry*, **52**, 2067–2075.

60 Feng, B.Y., Shelat, A., Doman, T.N., Guy, R.K., and Shoichet, B.K. (2005) High-throughput assays for promiscuous inhibitors. *Nature Chemical Biology*, **1**, 146–148.

61 Coan, K.E. and Shoichet, B.K. (2008) Stoichiometry and physical chemistry of promiscuous aggregate-based inhibitors. *Journal of the American Chemical Society*, **130**, 9606–9612.

62 Feng, B.Y., Simeonov, A., Jadhav, A., Babaoglu, K., Inglese, J., Shoichet, B.K., and Austin, C.P. (2007) A high-throughput screen for aggregation-based inhibition in a large compound library. *Journal of Medicinal Chemistry*, **50**, 2385–2390.

63 Coan, K.E. and Shoichet, B.K. (2007) Stability and equilibria of promiscuous aggregates in high protein milieus. *Molecular Biosystems*, **3**, 208–213.

64 Seidler, J., McGovern, S.L., Doman, T.N., and Shoichet, B.K. (2003) Identification and prediction of promiscuous aggregating inhibitors among known drugs. *Journal of Medicinal Chemistry*, **46**, 4477–4486.

65 Caldwell, J.S. and Janes, J. (2006) High-throughput screening and data analysis. *Methods and Principles in Medicinal Chemistry*, **35**, 297–322.

66 Heilker, R., Wolff, M., Tautermann, C.S., and Bieler, M. (2009) G-protein-coupled receptor-focused drug discovery using a target class platform approach. *Drug Discovery Today*, **14**, 231–240.

67 Thomsen, W., Frazer, J., and Unett, D. (2005) Functional assays for screening GPCR targets. *Current Opinion in Biotechnology*, **16**, 655–665.

68 Schoonen, W.G., Westerink, W.M., and Horbach, G.J. (2009) High-throughput screening for analysis of *in vitro* toxicity. *EXS*, **99**, 401–452.

69 Xu, J.J., Diaz, D., and O'Brien, P.J. (2004) Applications of cytotoxicity assays and pre-lethal mechanistic assays for assessment of human hepatotoxicity potential. *Chemico-Biological Interactions*, **150**, 115–128.

70 Mestres, J., Gregori-Puigjane, E., Valverde, S., and Sole, R.V. (2008) Data completeness: the Achilles heel of drug-target networks. *Nature Biotechnology*, **26**, 983–984.

71 Manning, G., Whyte, D.B., Martinez, R., Hunter, T., and Sudarsanam, S. (2002) The protein kinase complement of the human genome. *Science*, **298**, 1912–1934.

72 Perola, E. (2006) Minimizing false positives in kinase virtual screens. *Proteins*, **64**, 422–435.

73 Xia, X., Maliski, E.G., Gallant, P., and Rogers, D. (2004) Classification of kinase inhibitors using a Bayesian model. *Journal of Medicinal Chemistry*, **47**, 4463–4470.

74 Aronov, A.M. and Murcko, M.A. (2004) Toward a pharmacophore for kinase frequent hitters. *Journal of Medicinal Chemistry*, **47**, 5616–5619.

75 Keiser, M.J., Roth, B.L., Armbruster, B.N., Ernsberger, P., Irwin, J.J., and Shoichet, B.K. (2007) Relating

protein pharmacology by ligand chemistry. *Nature Biotechnology*, **25**, 197–206.

76 Cleves, A.E. and Jain, A.N. (2006) Robust ligand-based modeling of the biological targets of known drugs. *Journal of Medicinal Chemistry*, **49**, 2921–2938.

77 Keiser, M.J., Setola, V., Irwin, J.J., Laggner, C., Abbas, A.I., Hufeisen, S.J., Jensen, N.H., Kuijer, M.B., Matos, R.C., Tran, T.B., Whaley, R., Glennon, R.A., Hert, J., Thomas, K.L., Edwards, D.D., Shoichet, B.K., and Roth, B.L. (2009) Predicting new molecular targets for known drugs. *Nature*, **462**, 175–181.

78 Roth, B.L., Sheffler, D.J., and Kroeze, W.K. (2004) Magic shotguns versus magic bullets: selectively non-selective drugs for mood disorders and schizophrenia. *Nature Reviews. Drug Discovery*, **3**, 353–359.

79 Fermini, B. and Fossa, A.A. (2003) The impact of drug-induced QT interval prolongation on drug discovery and development. *Nature Reviews. Drug Discovery*, **2**, 439–447.

80 Zhou, S.-F. (2008) Drugs behave as substrates, inhibitors and inducers of human cytochrome P450 3A4. *Current Drug Metabolism*, **9**, 310–322.

81 Diller, D.J. (2009) In *silico* hERG modeling: challenges and progress. *Current Computer-Aided Drug Design*, **5**, 106–121.

82 Zhu, T., Guo, J.-l., Wang, Y., Jiang, Z.-z., Shang, J., and Zhang, L.-y. (2008) Application of computational model approaches in predicting the metabolism properties of compounds. *Yaoxue Jinzhan*, **32**, 385–390.

83 Azzaoui, K., Hamon, J., Faller, B., Whitebread, S., Jacoby, E., Bender, A., Jenkins, J.L., and Urban, L. (2007) Modeling promiscuity based on *in vitro* safety pharmacology profiling data. *ChemMedChem*, **2**, 874–880.

84 Hopkins, A.L., Mason, J.S., and Overington, J.P. (2006) Can we rationally design promiscuous drugs? *Current Opinion in Structural Biology*, **16**, 127–136.

85 Whitlock, G.A., Fish, P.V., Fray, M.J., Stobie, A., and Wakenhut, F. (2008) Pyridyl-phenyl ether monoamine reuptake inhibitors: impact of lipophilicity on dual SNRI pharmacology and off-target promiscuity. *Bioorganic & Medicinal Chemistry Letters*, **18**, 2896–2899.

86 Peters, J.-U., Schnider, P., Mattei, P., and Kansy, M. (2009) Pharmacological promiscuity: dependence on compound properties and target specificity in a set of recent Roche compounds. *ChemMedChem*, **4**, 680–686.

87 Ashburn, T.T. and Thor, K.B. (2004) Drug repositioning: identifying and developing new uses for existing drugs. *Nature Reviews. Drug Discovery*, **3**, 673–683.

88 Graul, A.I., Revel, L., Barrionuevo, M., Cruces, E., Rosa, E., Verges, C., Lupone, B., Diaz, N., and Castaner, R. (2009) The year's new drugs & biologics: 2008. *Drug News Perspectives*, **22**, 7–29.

89 Ravichandran, V., Jain, P.K., and Agrawal, R.K. (2007) Discovery of a new drug from old drug: an overview on selective optimization of side activities. *Journal of Pharmaceutical Research*, **6**, 178–184.

90 Payne, D.J., Gwynn, M.N., Holmes, D.J., and Pompliano, D.L. (2007) Drugs for bad bugs: confronting the challenges of antibacterial discovery. *Nature Reviews. Drug Discovery*, **6**, 29–40.

91 von Nussbaum, F., Brands, M., Hinzen, B., Weigand, S., and Habich, D. (2006) Antibacterial natural products in medicinal chemistry: exodus or revival? *Angewandte Chemie, International Edition*, **45**, 5072–5129.

92 Nikaido, H. (2003) Molecular basis of bacterial outer membrane permeability revisited. *Microbiology and Molecular Biology Reviews*, **67**, 593–656.

93 Hartmann, T. and Schmitt, J. (2004) Lipophilicity – beyond octanol/water: a short comparison of modern technologies. *Drug Discovery Today*, **1**, 431–439.

94 Nikaido, H. (2001) Preventing drug access to targets: cell surface permeability barriers and active efflux in bacteria. *Seminars in Cell & Developmental Biology*, **12**, 215–223.

95 Leeson, P.D. and Davis, A.M. (2004) Time-related differences in the physical property profiles of oral drugs. *Journal of Medicinal Chemistry*, **47**, 6338–6348.

96 O'Shea, R. and Moser, H.E. (2008) Physicochemical properties of antibacterial compounds: implications for drug discovery. *Journal of Medicinal Chemistry*, **51**, 2871–2878.

97 Clardy, J., Fischbach, M.A., and Walsh, C.T. (2006) New antibiotics from bacterial natural products. *Nature Biotechnology*, **24**, 1541–1550.

98 van de Waterbeemd, H., Camenisch, G., Folkers, G., Chretien, J.R., and Raevsky, O.A. (1998) Estimation of blood–brain barrier crossing of drugs using molecular size and shape, and H-bonding descriptors. *Journal of Drug Targeting*, **6**, 151–165.

99 Kelder, J., Grootenhuis, P.D., Bayada, D.M., Delbressine, L.P., and Ploemen, J.P. (1999) Polar molecular surface as a dominating determinant for oral absorption and brain penetration of drugs. *Pharmaceutical Research*, **16**, 1514–1519.

100 Raub, T.J. (2004) Early preclinical evaluation in support of hit identification and lead optimization for brain exposure. AAPS Workshop: Optimization of Drug-Like Properties During Lead Optimization, Parsippany, NJ.

101 Norinder, U. and Haeberlein, M. (2002) Computational approaches to the prediction of the blood–brain distribution. *Advanced Drug Delivery Reviews*, **54**, 291–313.

102 Hou, T., Wang, J., Zhang, W., Wang, W., and Xu, X. (2006) Recent advances in computational prediction of drug absorption and permeability in drug discovery. *Current Medicinal Chemistry*, **13**, 2653–2667.

103 Lobell, M., Molnar, L., and Keseru, G.M. (2003) Recent advances in the prediction of blood–brain partitioning from molecular structure. *Journal of Pharmaceutical Sciences*, **92**, 360–370.

104 Fischer, H., Gottschlich, R., and Seelig, A. (1998) Blood–brain barrier permeation: molecular parameters governing passive diffusion. *The Journal of Membrane Biology*, **165**, 201–211.

105 Pajouhesh, H. and Lenz, G.R. (2005) Medicinal chemical properties of successful central nervous system drugs. *NeuroRx*, **2**, 541–553.

106 Clark, D.E. (2005) Computational prediction of blood–brain barrier permeation. *Annual Reports in Medicinal Chemistry*, **40**, 403–415.

107 Fagerholm, U. (2007) The highly permeable blood–brain barrier: an evaluation of current opinions about brain uptake capacity. *Drug Discovery Today*, **12**, 1076–1082.

108 Mahar Doan, K.M., Humphreys, J.E., Webster, L.O., Wring, S.A., Shampine, L.J., Serabjit-Singh, C.J., Adkison, K.K., and Polli, J.W. (2002) Passive permeability and P-glycoprotein-mediated efflux differentiate central nervous system (CNS) and non-CNS marketed drugs. *The Journal of Pharmacology and Experimental Therapeutics*, **303**, 1029–1037.

109 Ha, S.N., Hochman, J., and Sheridan, R.P. (2007) Mini review on molecular modeling of P-glycoprotein (Pgp). *Current Topics in Medicinal Chemistry*, **7**, 1525–1529.

110 Maurer, T.S., Debartolo, D.B., Tess, D.A., and Scott, D.O. (2005) Relationship between exposure and nonspecific binding of thirty-three central nervous system drugs in mice. *Drug Metabolism and Disposition: The Biological Fate of Chemicals*, **33**, 175–181.

111 Di, L., Kerns, E.H., and Carter, G.T. (2008) Strategies to assess blood–brain barrier penetration. *Expert Opinion on Drug Discovery*, **3**, 677–687.

112 Hitchcock, S.A. and Pennington, L.D. (2006) Structure–brain exposure relationships. *Journal of Medicinal Chemistry*, **49**, 7559–7583.

113 Yamada, T. and Bork, P. (2009) Evolution of biomolecular networks: lessons from metabolic and protein interactions. *Nature Reviews. Molecular Cell Biology*, **10**, 791–803.

114 Arkin, M.R. and Wells, J.A. (2004) Small-molecule inhibitors of protein–protein

interactions: progressing towards the dream. *Nature Reviews. Drug Discovery*, **3**, 301–317.

115 Wells, J.A. and McClendon, C.L. (2007) Reaching for high-hanging fruit in drug discovery at protein–protein interfaces. *Nature*, **450**, 1001–1009.

116 Örner, B.P., Ernst, J.T., and Hamilton, A.D. (2001) Toward proteomimetics: terphenyl derivatives as structural and functional mimics of extended regions of an alpha-helix. *Journal of the American Chemical Society*, **123**, 5382–5383.

117 Saraogi, I. and Hamilton, A.D. (2008) alpha-Helix mimetics as inhibitors of protein–protein interactions. *Biochemical Society Transactions*, **36**, 1414–1417.

118 Cummings, M.D., Schubert, C., Parks, D.J., Calvo, R.R., LaFrance, L.V., Lattanze, J., Milkiewicz, K.L., and Lu, T. (2006) Substituted 1,4-benzodiazepine-2,5-diones as alpha-helix mimetic antagonists of the HDM2-p53 protein–protein interaction. *Chemical Biology & Drug Design*, **67**, 201–205.

119 Oltersdorf, T., Elmore, S.W., Shoemaker, A.R., Armstrong, R.C., Augeri, D.J., Belli, B.A., Bruncko, M., Deckwerth, T.L., Dinges, J., Hajduk, P.J., Joseph, M.K., Kitada, S., Korsmeyer, S.J., Kunzer, A.R., Letai, A., Li, C., Mitten, M.J., Nettesheim, D.G., Ng, S., Nimmer, P.M., O'Connor, J.M., Oleksijew, A., Petros, A.M., Reed, J.C., Shen, W., Tahir, S.K., Thompson, C.B., Tomaselli, K.J., Wang, B., Wendt, M.D., Zhang, H., Fesik, S.W., and Rosenberg, S.H. (2005) An inhibitor of Bcl-2 family proteins induces regression of solid tumours. *Nature*, **435** 677–681.

120 Zeitlin, B.D., Zeitlin, I.J., and Nor, J.E. (2008) Expanding circle of inhibition: small-molecule inhibitors of Bcl-2 as anticancer cell and antiangiogenic agents. *Journal of Clinical Oncology*, **26**, 4180–4188.

121 Pagliaro, L., Felding, J., Audouze, K., Nielsen, S.J., Terry, R.B., Krog-Jensen, C., and Butcher, S. (2004) Emerging classes of protein–protein interaction inhibitors and new tools for their development. *Current Opinion in Chemical Biology*, **8**, 442–449.

122 Fischer, P.M. (2005) Protein–protein interactions in drug discovery. *Drug Design Reviews*, **2**, 179–207.

123 Hopkins, A.L., Groom, C.R., and Alex, A. (2004) Ligand efficiency: a useful metric for lead selection. *Drug Discovery Today*, **9**, 430–431.

124 Higueruelo, A.P., Schreyer, A., Bickerton, G.R., Pitt, W.R., Groom, C.R., and Blundell, T.L. (2009) Atomic interactions and profile of small molecules disrupting protein–protein interfaces: the TIMBAL database. *Chemical Biology & Drug Design*, **74**, 457–467.

3
Ligand-Based Virtual Screening

Herbert Koeppen, Jan Kriegl, Uta Lessel, Christofer S. Tautermann, and Bernd Wellenzohn

3.1
Introduction

Virtual screening is a computational approach for the knowledge-based identification of compounds with a defined biological activity. In contrast to high-throughput screening (HTS), the compounds do not need to exist physically. For this reason, virtual screening can search extremely large parts of the chemical space, which is a key advantage compared to HTS. The big challenge, however, is the need for a high-throughput assessment of the biological activity of each compound within the screened chemical space.

Virtual screening can start either from the 3D structure of a target (target-based virtual screening) or from at least one known ligand of this target (ligand-based virtual screening). If both target and ligand structures are known, the whole information can be used in a combined approach. Since the first published virtual screening applications more than 10 years ago [1, 2], many researchers both in academic groups and in the pharmaceutical industry have gained experience in virtual screening and thousands of publications illustrate the progress in methods as well as the successful application of virtual screening in the search for bioactive compounds. A number of recent reviews can be found in Refs [3–10].

The focus of this chapter is ligand-based virtual screening. The underlying principle is the assumption that similar molecules should exhibit similar binding properties with respect to a given target [11]. Molecular similarities are based on descriptors and similarity measures. Section 3.2 introduces the calculation of descriptors. Some selected descriptors are discussed in detail. The choice of descriptors does not mean an assessment; however, it is driven by the experience of the authors.

To conduct a ligand-based virtual screening, at least one active query molecule and a search database are required. Section 3.3 discusses the preparation of search databases and the choice of the queries.

Virtual Screening. Edited by C. Sotriffer

ISBN: 978-3-527-32636-5

Section 3.4 discusses the most common ligand-based virtual screening techniques where similarity searches are the most straightforward approach. The extension of standard similarity searches to huge virtual spaces requires special techniques, which will be discussed separately. These chemical spaces can result from virtual combinatorial libraries and virtual screening in such libraries is a rather new but promising field. In cases where a wealth of data (active and inactive ligands) for a target is available, machine learning approaches enter the field of virtual screening. Models can be trained to predict the activity of molecules in a search database.

Finally, Section 3.5 summarizes the status of ligand-based virtual screening from the perspective of a practitioner in an industrial research environment.

3.2
Descriptors

The similarity between two objects, be it persons or molecules, can be described by the degree of overlap between characteristic features of these objects. Characteristic features of human beings are, for example, the color of the hair, the weight, or the body size if the visual appearance is the focus of interest. However, if candidates applying for an open position are to be ranked, other features such as educational career or the experience in a particular profession are more important. In other words, the sensible choice of the features to be compared depends on the goal of the comparison.

Basically the same is true for comparing molecules. Again, the similarity of molecules is based on a comparison of their key features. These key features are in most cases directly derived from the molecular structure and translated into descriptors, being a set of real numbers or vectors. It is worth to mention that descriptors can also be derived from experimental properties of molecules. Examples of this type are so-called bioprints that consist of experimentally determined affinities of a set of compounds to a panel of biological targets [12]. Their calculated counterpart is the Flexsim-X descriptor that is derived from the docking scores against a panel of 3D target structures [13].

A wealth of methods for the calculation of molecular descriptors is published and a comprehensive discussion would go beyond the scope of this chapter. The interested reader is referred to recent reviews [7, 14]. The choice of the appropriate descriptor(s) is crucial for the similarity calculation and the whole virtual screening process. For example, some descriptors are better suited for recognizing similar chemical classes, while other descriptors describe the physicochemical behavior of the molecules. However, it is very important to keep in mind that in medicinal chemistry, similarity of molecules means similar behavior at a particular biological target. For example, thiorphan and retro-thiorphan (Figure 3.1) differ only in the amide group and have similar biological activity at thermolysin and the NEP24.11 receptor, respectively. Thus, these molecules could be considered to be similar. In contrast, the biological activity of the thiorphan/retro-thiorphan pair against the angiotensin-converting enzyme (ACE) differs considerably, that is, regarding ACE, the two molecules are

	Thermolysin	NEP 24.11	ACE
Thiorphan 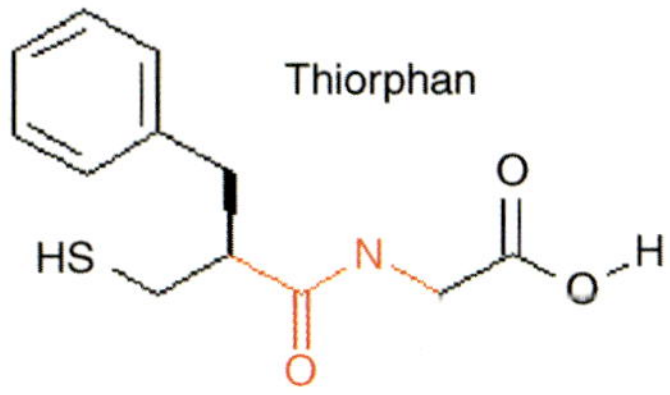	$K_i = 1.8\ \mu M$	$K_i = 0.0019\ \mu M$	$K_i = 0.14\ \mu M$
Retro-thiorphan 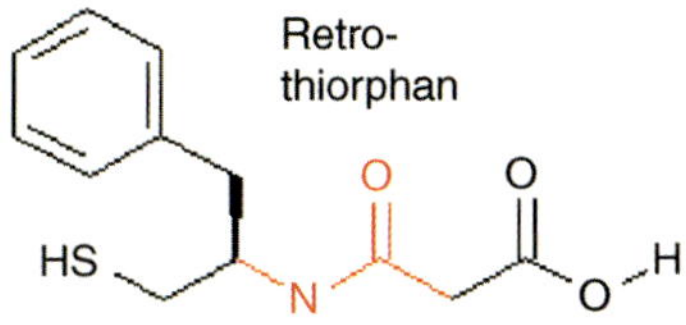	$K_i = 2.3\ \mu M$	$K_i = 0.0023\ \mu M$	$K_i > 10\ \mu M$

Figure 3.1 Thiorphan and retro-thiorphan show similar biological activity against thermolysin and NEP 24.11, but their activities are significantly different against ACE. The example demonstrates that molecular similarity depends on the structure of the target protein [15].

dissimilar. Since the way the structural similarity translates into biological similarity depends on the particular target, we need many different descriptors in order to handle this diversity in an adequate way [16].

Descriptors are often classified according to their dimension [17]. Descriptors such as the molecular weight or the number of heavy atoms are 1D descriptors because only the 1D information (sum formula) about the molecule is needed to calculate the descriptor value. Such 1D descriptors are more often used as rough filters for preprocessing the search database than for measuring similarities in virtual screening campaigns. On the basis of the chemical structure (2D representation), many different descriptors can be derived. The most straightforward virtual screening applications based on 2D descriptors are substructure searches. A substructure search is a virtual screen for all molecules that contain a defined molecular fragment, that is, a certain substructure. Of course, such a search will not lead to new scaffolds, but will allow to find analogues and possible variations in the decoration of known molecule classes. The exploration of HTS hits by searching for analogues in vendor databases is an example for this approach. Apart from this direct application for virtual screening purposes, substructure searches are often used for the elimination of reactive or toxic species in molecule databases.

Many numerical values such as the number of aromatic rings or rotatable bonds or the calculated log$P$ can be derived from the chemical structure. Like 1D descriptors, these numerical descriptors are often used for fast filtering of databases, for example, to sort out molecules with an unwanted lipophilicity. Since they are independent for the molecule conformation, 2D descriptors are usually well suited for similarity searches as well as for machine learning purposes.

Pearlman and Smith [18] developed the so-called BCUT descriptors that condense compound-specific atomic and molecular properties relevant to intermolecular interactions into a set of numbers. They are calculated from a matrix representation of the molecules with diagonal elements containing atomic properties like atomic charges, polarizabilities, and hydrogen bonding capabilities. The off-diagonal elements are derived from either the 2D connection table (e.g., bond types) or from the calculated 3D conformations (e.g., atomic distances). The highest and lowest eigenvalues of the different matrices provide more than 60 BCUT descriptors per molecule that can be used to define low-dimensional chemistry (property) spaces. In these spaces, diversity analyses and similarity searches can be performed.

Various methods exist to capture the relative location of pharmacophoric elements of molecules based on the 2D structure. They are mostly based on the connectivity and on the functional groups of a molecule. One such method is the feature trees originally described by Rarey and Dixon [19]. The feature trees reduce all rings and all functional groups to single nodes. Each node contains information about steric and intermolecular interaction features of the corresponding part in the molecule, for example, the volume, the number of hydrogen bond donors and acceptors, and the like. The nodes are connected in a way that the overall topology of the molecule is retained. If two fragments are connected in the molecule, the corresponding two nodes of the feature tree are also connected. Hence, the feature tree is a very generic representation of the molecule (see Figure 3.2) and can be considered as a 2D pharmacophore model. Rarey and Dixon also developed very efficient algorithms, thereby making similarity searches even in a million compounds a matter of minutes on standard workstations. Furthermore, the feature trees are well suited for searching very large combinatorial libraries (see below). Several successful applications of similarity searches by means of feature trees were reported [20].

In addition to calculated properties based on the molecular structure, the use of 2D fingerprints is very common in virtual screening applications [21–23]. A molecular fingerprint is a binary bit string representing characteristic properties of a molecular structure. An example is a structural fingerprint where each bit represents the

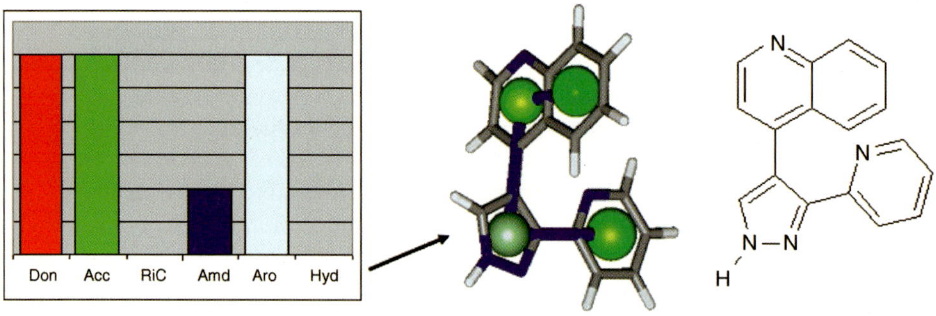

Figure 3.2 The figure shows a molecule overlapped with its feature tree (center). Each node in the feature tree contains the information of the corresponding part of the molecule. The feature profile of the pyrazole node is shown in the box on the left. This node contains hydrogen bond donor (Don), hydrogen bond acceptor (Acc), aromatic (Aro), and amid (Amd) like features. RiC and Hyd are ring closure and hydrophobic features. The importance of the features in an individual node indicated by the different bar heights is part of the comparison of feature tree nodes.

presence (TRUE) or absence (FALSE) of a specific fragment, most often a specific functional group or a substructure. Keyed fingerprints like MACCS keys or the BCI fingerprints have a predefined fragment dictionary and report the absence or presence of these fragments in the compound. Obviously, the result of a virtual screening campaign with keyed fingerprints highly depends on the list of structural fragments in the dictionary.

The often used Daylight fingerprint (Daylight Chemical Information Systems, Inc., 120 Vantis, Suite 550, Aliso Viejo, CA 92656, USA. Available at http://www.daylight.com/dayhtml/doc/theory/, March 20, 2010) is a so-called hashed fingerprint. Unlike keyed fingerprints with predefined fragments, the bits for a hashed fingerprint are generated by the following process: All linear substructures up to a length n in the molecule (with n often in the range of 7–8) are exhaustively enumerated starting with single atoms. Each substructure is assigned a numeric value depending on atom and bond properties. Each value serves as the seed for a pseudorandom number generator. The resulting integer is converted into the position of a "1" (TRUE) bit in a fixed-length fingerprint. Hashed fingerprints do not need a predefined fragment dictionary and are therefore not biased in a particular way. On the other hand, the above-described process may generate identical fingerprints for different structures. The probability of such a case decreases with increasing length of the fingerprint.

Fingerprints may also be generated by encoding the properties of circular structures of increasing diameter around each atom in a molecule [24]. An often used implementation of such an algorithm is the extended-connectivity fingerprints (ECFPs) [25]. Each atom collects information from its neighboring atom "shells" in terms of their atom types, charges, and bond properties. FCFPs (function-class fingerprints) are a variant thereof where the atoms are mapped onto generalized atom types as, for example, hydrogen bond donors or acceptors.

The CATS descriptor is a size- and conformation-independent topological pharmacophore fingerprint. To calculate the CATS descriptor, the atoms are assigned five generalized atom types (hydrogen bond donors, hydrogen bond acceptors, positively charged group, negatively charged group, and lipophilic group) and the distances are expressed as the number of bonds along the shortest path connecting each atom pair. For each molecule, the distances between all generalized atom-type pairs are counted and the histograms of the counts represent a simplified but exhaustive pharmacophore fingerprint [26].

The concept of fingerprints can be extended to 3D fingerprints by capturing the spatial arrangement of pharmacophoric features within a fingerprint. Such pharmacophoric features are hydrogen bond donors and acceptors, negative and positive charges, as well as hydrophobic and aromatic moieties. The 3D fingerprints store the information about pairs, triplets, or quartets of the pharmacophoric features for multiple 3D conformations. The distance ranges and the type of the pharmacophoric combinations are binned. Three-dimensional pharmacophoric features describe a molecule in a more abstract manner that it is independent of the chemical class it belongs to. Similarity searches using pharmacophore fingerprints may therefore result in hits with structural scaffolds that are clearly different from the query. This is advantageous if a "chemotype or scaffold hopping" is the goal of virtual screening (see Section 3.4.1.2). However, 3D descriptors depend on the molecular conformation. Both the conformational sampling and the often unknown bioactive conformation of a ligand might lead to deficiencies in the virtual screening process. Predictions of the protein-bound conformation of a ligand without experimental 3D information by X-ray or NMR are difficult since in the majority of cases, the bioactive conformation of a ligand does not correspond to the global energy minimum in the unbound state [27, 28]. Nevertheless, there are reports that the impact of the bioactive conformation on the enrichment of active compounds is low [29–31], and that similarity searches with 3D descriptors can be performed based on an energetically favored conformation of the reference ligand.

Besides the use of pharmacophore fingerprints, 3D pharmacophore searches are among the most prominent 3D virtual screening techniques. Here distances between pharmacophoric features of the reference structures are compared with the respective distances in the structures of the search database. Again, these distances are conformation dependent and may be precomputed for a number of low-energy conformers in the search database to speed up the virtual screening process. This important approach is discussed in detail in a separate chapter of this book.

A further important option for ligand-based virtual screening is to perform shape comparisons that have a pronounced scaffold hopping potential. An often used method of this kind is ROCS [31] (OpenEye Scientific Software, 9 Bisbee Court Suite D, Santa Fe, NM 87508, USA. Available at http://www.eyesopen.com, March 20, 2009). ROCS employs continuous functions that are derived from atom-centered Gaussians to calculate the volume overlap between two 3D structures. The use of Gaussians drastically speeds up the computational process, and ROCS is able to search even databases with millions of compounds for molecules that can adopt shapes similar to the reference compound. As in the case of 3D pharmacophore searches, the low-energy conformations must be precomputed for the search database.

At this point we want to emphasize that all sorts of descriptors can generally be used for all virtual screening applications. However, for each search strategy, there are preferred descriptors and their choice also depends on the query, the search database, and the applied method. Machine learning approaches are usually conducted employing 2D descriptors due to the uncertainty that might be introduced by the conformation dependency of 3D descriptors. For similarity searches, the choice of the descriptors is crucial and depends on the envisioned outcome of the virtual screening run (finding close analogues versus novel chemical classes). This is illustrated by the example of three different descriptors.

The similarity assessment of compounds by the Daylight fingerprints reflects the structural topology of the molecules. If the scaffold of an active compound provides a major contribution to its affinity, close analogues based on Daylight fingerprints also have high chances to be active. Pharmacophore-based descriptors focus on the essential target–ligand interaction features of the active compounds. Hence, the corresponding analogues can belong to different structural classes and nevertheless show affinity if the crucial part of the interacting features is similar in the query compounds and the virtual hits. BCUT values belong to a class of even more abstract descriptors. Usually the similarity of compounds in the BCUT space is not very obvious when looking at the structures with a chemist's eyes. In our experience, the performance of these abstract descriptors with respect to the enrichment of active compounds in virtual screening is often only moderate. However, their application may lead to very interesting bioactive molecules with completely new scaffolds [32].

3.3
Search Databases and Queries

As mentioned in Section 3.1, a ligand-based virtual screening crucially depends on the knowledge of active query molecules, which can either stem from literature or in-house efforts. In some cases, a wealth of information is available, but not all known active compounds are equally suitable queries for virtual screening. The proper choice of the query and the preparation of both the query and the search database will be discussed in the following section.

3.3.1
Selection of Reference Ligands

In principle, any ligand known to be active at the target can be used as a reference molecule to search for additional ligands. Even if only one reference ligand is sufficient to perform similarity searches, it is recommended to include as much information as possible in the search. Therefore, it is worth to think about searches based on several ligands if available. In such a situation, the reference ligands can be aligned and 3D pharmacophore model can be used for virtual screening. This procedure, however, is only applicable if the ligands show a common binding mode and in many cases it is not obvious how the reference ligands should be aligned, especially if they are structurally diverse. Nevertheless, in these cases too, it is helpful to make use of several reference ligands by performing independent similarity searches for each of the ligands and merging the results. Methods to combine results from several similarity searches as well as the use of machine learning techniques in case of larger numbers of active and inactive compounds will be discussed later (see below).

There is still a lack of studies regarding the impact of the affinity of the reference compounds on the success of virtual screening. Ligands with high affinity are a good choice to start with, but there is no evidence from literature that weaker queries (in the micromolar range) cannot lead to enrichments.

The physicochemical properties are a further aspect of both reference ligand and descriptor selection. If reference ligands have properties in an undesired range (e.g., high lipophilicity), ligand-based virtual screening will often yield compounds with similar undesired properties. This is more pronounced if atom- or fragment-based descriptors are used in contrast to shape- or pharmacophore-based descriptors. The shape or the pharmacophoric pattern describes a structure on a more abstract level and gives room for more variations of the underlying chemical scaffold within the virtual screening hits. These descriptors are therefore preferable in such cases.

However, if the target prefers lipophilic molecules over hydrophilic ones, even a perfect match of shape between query and hits does not lead to interesting biological activities if the compounds are not lipophilic enough or do not fulfill other crucial requirements of the active site. Only more insight into the properties of the binding site or the structure–activity relationships (SARs) of the ligands may help to decide how to proceed best in such cases.

3.3.2
Preparation of the Search Database

The database to be searched has to be prepared according to the requirements of the selected descriptors and virtual screening methods, respectively. Depending on the descriptors and on the virtual screening method, the protonation state of the compounds may be important and has to be determined. Different tautomers of the compounds are usually considered as different molecules and are not included automatically. As different tautomers can show different descriptors, for example, the pharmacophoric properties of 4-pyridone and 4-hydroxy-pyridine, it might be worth to repeat a similarity search with other tautomeric forms of a query. Alternatively, different tautomers of the compounds in the database can be included in the searches. If 3D descriptors are used for similarity searches, different conformers of the compounds must also be taken into account. In many cases, the programs offered for the descriptor calculation include tools for the preparation of the molecules to be treated. The preparation of the structures as well as the descriptor calculation can be performed on the fly, but in particular if the preparation step is computationally expensive, the molecules are prepared in advance and stored in files or databases. Useful hints for the best preparation of search databases can often be taken from the manuals of the software for descriptor calculation and molecule comparison. Some general aspects for preparing search databases with respect to druglikeness are summarized by Bologa *et al.* [33].

It is common to use a cascade of filtering steps that reduces the size of the database to be searched. Fast substructure filters, for example, to eliminate unwanted functional groups, are applied first. These pre-processing filters not only reduce the size of the database and speed up the virtual screening process. They also improve the quality of the resulting hit list since compounds with unwanted properties are eliminated early. More time-consuming operations like docking into the 3D target structure are typically applied late in the process when only a small number of structures is left for detailed investigations. An example of such a screening cascade is described in the work of Perez-Pineiro *et al.* [34].

3.4
Virtual Screening Techniques

In this chapter, we discuss various methods that are applied for virtual screening. The simplest case is a similarity search where a single active query molecule and an enumerated search database are required. More complex are similarity searches in combinatorial spaces where the enumeration of all search database molecules is not possible due to their sheer number. This case requires special search algorithms and molecule descriptors. Finally, for machine learning approaches, the knowledge of many active and inactive molecules is required in order to train models to categorize the actives and the inactives in the search database.

3.4.1 Similarity Searches

Similarity searches can be performed on a small information basis that makes them suitable for the detection of actives in early project phases. The minimum information that is needed is a single active compound. In most cases, the aim is to detect new chemotypes, but of course similarity searches can also be used for the exploration of a hit class. The outcome can be controlled to a certain degree by the choice of the descriptors.

3.4.1.1 Similarity Measures

There is no unique way for the quantification of the similarity between objects. As this is an important topic for many scientific disciplines, a lot of different similarity coefficients have been developed that were reviewed by Willett *et al.* [35].

There are direct similarity measures like Tanimoto, Dice, and Cosine coefficients as well as distance similarity measures (e.g., Euclidean distance or the Hamming distance). The value of distance similarity measures is 0 for identical objects, whereas direct similarity measures show their maximum values for identical molecules. The so-called monotonic coefficients like Hamming and Euclidean distances or Tanimoto and Dice coefficients generate identical rankings despite their different numeric values. The most widespread similarity coefficient for fingerprints is the Tanimoto coefficient. For other tasks, Euclidean distances are frequently used. Direct similarity measures such as the Tanimoto coefficient depend on the number of fingerprint bits set because they take into account the presence of common features, whereas Hamming and Euclidean distances consider the difference of attributes. Therefore, small molecules with usually a smaller number of bits set tend to show lower similarity values using the former coefficients and can reveal higher numerical similarities using Hamming or Euclidean distances [36]. This is illustrated in Figure 3.3.

3.4.1.2 Practice of Similarity Searches

After the selection of an active query ligand and a search database, it has to be decided which descriptor(s) and which similarity measure shall be employed. The result of a similarity search is a list of compounds (so-called nearest neighbors) that is ranked according to the similarity of the reference compound and the searched structures. The list can be limited to a certain number of nearest neighbors to the reference compound or to compounds with a similarity above a certain threshold. There is no general rule to determine this threshold, especially since there is no similarity value that clearly discriminates between active and inactive compounds. The number

Molecule 1	Molecule 1	Tanimoto	Hamming
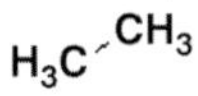	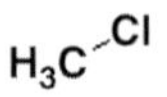	0.286	10
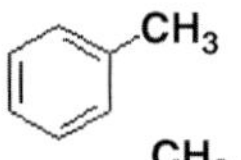	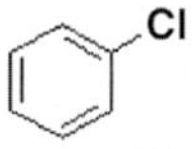	0.413	27
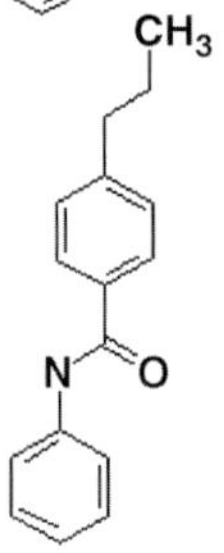	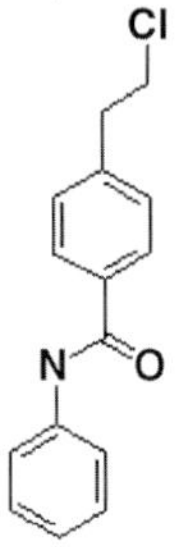	0.851	20
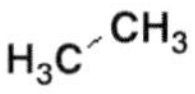	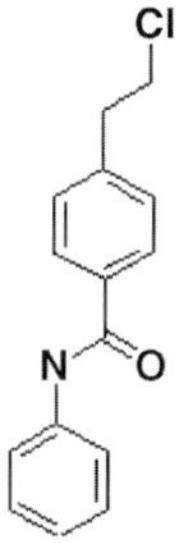	0.055	120

Figure 3.3 The similarity coefficients shown have been calculated based on Daylight fingerprints with a fixed length of 1024 bits. The first three pairs of molecules with increasing molecular weight differ only by the substitution of a methyl group with the chlorine. Although the Hamming distances (similarity range from 0 to 1024) indicate high similarity for all three pairs, the similarity according to the Tanimoto coefficient (similarity range from 1 to 0) increases with the molecular weight. The last example shows a pair of molecules with low similarity.

of compounds that are eventually selected is rather determined by pragmatic reasons like the budget for compound acquisition or the available test capacity.

If the virtual screening process is successful, the bioactive compounds will be "enriched" in the upper part of this ranked list. Enriched means that there are more active compounds in this part of the list than that one would expect based on the average content of bioactive compounds in the searched database. This enrichment can be determined only in retrospective studies where both the active and the inactive compounds in the database are known. The enrichment factor is typically used in such studies as a quality criterion for a particular virtual screening approach. Since the enrichment factor depends on the chosen subset of the ranked list, it is common to calculate enrichment curves where the cumulated number of hits is plotted against the ranked list of compounds in the search database. In recent years, more and more researchers prefer other types of enrichment plots (e.g., ROC curves). The interested reader is referred to the literature [37]. However, in a prospective virtual screening campaign, it should be kept in mind that a low number of experimentally confirmed virtual screening hits can be either the result of a successful virtual screening (substantial enrichment, i.e., the average number of actives in the database is even lower) or the poor result of a virtual screening run without enrichment (the average number of actives in the database is equal or even higher than that in the virtual screening list).

Very often the aim of a virtual screening campaign is the detection of a bioactive compound of a novel chemical class that shows bioactivity at the same target as the query compound(s) (scaffold hopping) in order to gain intellectual property or to open up new ways out of pharmacokinetic liabilities to name only two reasons. Thus, methods that are capable of identifying related chemical classes instead of only chemically related compounds are desired. The above-mentioned 2D fingerprint methods, although being very successful for similarity searches, are not always optimally designed for scaffold hopping. Reducing the chemical structure to a more general scheme that only represents the important chemical features of a molecule results in a more appropriate description for scaffold hopping. The above-mentioned feature trees are an example of such a descriptor. The potential of reduced graphs in identifying similarities between compounds belonging to different chemotypes is demonstrated in a number of publications (see, for example, Refs [38–40]).

3.4.1.3 **Selection of Descriptors**

Although models are usually built on the basis of a whole bunch of descriptors in machine learning techniques, in most cases simple similarity searches first rank the compounds according to single descriptors (for the combination of results with different descriptors, see below). To support the selection of the most appropriate descriptors, many studies have been published assessing the performance of different descriptors or descriptor combinations in similarity searches. Selected publications can be found in the reference list [16, 30, 41–47]. Most of them discuss the behavior of descriptors on individual test data sets in retrospective studies. They often focus on the comparison of 2D versus 3D descriptors and/or on the potential to detect new chemotypes. A detailed discussion of all these studies is beyond the scope of this contribution, but some general observations are presented.

Two-dimensional descriptors are performing well in similarity searches. Three-dimensional descriptors do not generally outperform 2D descriptors, maybe due to an insufficient sampling of the conformational space. As already mentioned, there is no globally best descriptor for ligand-based virtual screening. The results with different descriptors are only partly overlapping (that is, they detect different actives) and so it is recommended to use several descriptors in a virtual screening campaign and to combine the results (see below).

The simplest way to compare the performance of different descriptors is to perform a retrospective study and to count the numbers of true actives found in different virtual screening hit lists of predefined size and compare them with the hit rate in the search database (enrichment). Enrichment factors, however, are not sufficient to assess the scaffold hopping potential of a descriptor or a search method.

In this case, the ranks of the first representatives of each class or average ranks of the class members have to be taken into account.

Altogether the performance of descriptors depends on the target, the reference ligands, and the search database. Performance assessments of descriptors or virtual screening methods should therefore be considered with care. Phenomena like "artificial enrichment" [48] and the so-called analogue bias [44] can lead to overoptimistic estimates of virtual screening performance. An artificial enrichment is the differentiation between actives and inactives in a data set where they are different in obvious parameters, for example, the molecular weight. Analogue bias often occurs in data sets from drug discovery projects in which certain scaffolds are overrepresented.

3.4.1.4 **Data Fusion**

The combination of virtual screening results with several reference ligands and/or several search methods is called "data fusion." Whittle *et al.* [49, 50] refer to the combination of similarity searches for one reference ligand with different descriptors as similarity fusion, whereas the combination of the results for a set of reference ligands with one method is called group fusion. Many reports on different methods and results of data fusion approaches can be found in the literature [41, 46, 51–53].

Data fusion can be performed in a number of ways. Most often used are the MIN, MAX, and SUM rules. According to these rules, the minimum or maximum score value or the sum of the scores is taken from a list of different similarity values for a compound that result from different virtual screening runs. It was also recommended to consider only the ranks of the compound in the corresponding nearest-neighbor lists [51]. Hert *et al.* [41] observed the superiority of the SUM rule when fusion is performed on ranks, whereas the MAX rule gives better results if the fusion is performed on scores, which is in line with earlier results from Schuffenhauer *et al.* [52]. Whittle *et al.* [50] observed a superiority of the MAX rule over the SUM rule for group fusion.

Most researchers agree that data fusion is insensitive to the presence of a poorly performing method. This leads to a more consistent level of search performance compared to individual methods, because the performance of individual methods varies from target to target in an unpredictable manner.

In essence, the chance to find active compounds is higher if they are detected by more than one descriptor. On the other hand, by concentrating only on compounds that are detected by several methods, a lot of valid actives will be missed. Therefore, the authors prefer to simply merge the nearest-neighbor lists of different virtual screening methods and reference structures, respectively.

3.4.2 **Similarity Searches in Very Large Chemical Spaces**

Virtual screening is often used to complement internal screening sets in a target-specific manner with interesting compounds from external vendors that offer in the order of 10–20 million compounds. But even if all these millions of compounds were searched, only a small part of the whole chemical universe with an estimated size of up to 10^{180} molecules [54] would be taken into account. Virtual screening allows the screening of large parts of this virtual space because the compounds do not need to exist physically. But still the conventional virtual screening techniques require the molecules in the searched chemical space to be enumerated at least temporarily, which limits the number of compounds that can be handled. Recently, nonenumerating virtual screening methods have been developed to overcome this problem.

One such approach is the use of fragment spaces. A fragment space is a set of small compounds (fragments) with one or more attachment points (linkers) and a set of rules laying down how to combine these fragments. Even a small set of fragments and connection rules can span a huge virtual library due to the so-called combinatorial explosion. The rules contain the information that linkers are compatible in terms of chemical reactions. Therefore, the definition of the connection rules and the fragments is critical in determining the chemical feasibility of the resulting molecules. Very often retro-synthetic rules like RECAP [55] are applied on existing compounds to get suitable fragments. The recombination of these fragments applying the same rules should lead to synthetically accessible molecules. A different approach is the use of protocols from combinatorial chemistry. A combinatorial library usually consists of a core and several "R"-groups that represent the possible decoration of the core. By using the core and the R-groups as fragments and the corresponding connection rules, all possible combinations of the core with the R-groups are mapped. Such combinatorial libraries can span huge chemical spaces. A fragment space of 82 synthesis protocols from the literature was recently published (BioSolveIT GmbH, An der Ziegelei 79, 53757 Sankt Augustin, Germany. Available at http://www.biosolveit.de/datasets/, March 20, 2010). Böhm *et al.* described the formation of a virtual library of 3×10^{13} compounds, consisting of 358 combinatorial libraries [56].

Several methods are suited for navigation within such huge chemical spaces [56–59]. An extension of the above-mentioned feature tree descriptor makes it possible to search large virtual combinatorial libraries without enumeration [38]. The so-called feature tree fragment space (FTree-FS) method uses dynamic programming techniques and allows the detection of the molecule with the highest similarity to the query that can be found in the fragment space. The efficiency of searches in fragment spaces versus searches in product spaces can be easily shown. A fragment space of three sets of reagents with 100 reagents per set (i.e., 300 reagents) will yield 100^3 products. In a conventional similarity search, all products must be enumerated and searched, while in the fragment space only 300 fragments have to be compared. Nevertheless, the FTree-FS searches do not simply compare fragments but rather generate the most similar products on the fly. The selection and the matching of the fragments are guided by locally maximizing the similarity to the query molecule using the dynamic programming algorithm. The nature of the feature tree descriptor and the search algorithm ensure that the most similar molecule is detected by the search. Recently, successful applications of the FTree-FS software for detection of new biologically active molecules were reported [20].

Several other search techniques in very large virtual spaces are available, in particular optimization by means of evolutionary algorithms (genetic algorithms and evolution strategies) or simulated annealing. They are broadly applicable and can use all different types of scoring functions such as the similarity of compounds to a reference structure. A full enumeration of the search space is avoided with these algorithms. Instead of starting from a random selection of "parent" structures, new molecules with an improved score are generated in a stepwise manner. The iterative algorithm restricts the sampling of the search space to those parts where the optimization of the score is most likely. For example, Schneider *et al.* [60] used an evolution strategy to optimize a score in a large fragment-based chemical space. The score was derived from a 2D pharmacophore similarity to a reference compound. Starting from a randomly selected parent generation, the score could be improved in several successive optimization cycles. Some of the designed molecules showed a bioactivity comparable to the reference compound. Scoring functions can contain additional constraints like a range of allowed physicochemical parameters. It is also possible to constrain the solutions to a matrix format that optimizes the score of a whole combinatorial library instead of single molecules.

It is the authors' experience that the combination of virtual screening and combinatorial chemistry has proven to be very effective. The combinatorial synthesis of the virtual hits is fast and robust. Moreover, it generates small targeted libraries instead of singletons. Since the SARs in a project can be steep and nonadditive, such targeted libraries are preferred in order to explore the potential of a scaffold. Furthermore, after the detection of an active compound in the targeted library, follow-up libraries are fast and easily accessible. The authors use the FTree-FS software to virtually screen the in-house virtual libraries and subsequently perform a 3D postprocessing by means of shape or pharmacophore filtering.

3.4.3
Machine Learning in Virtual Screening

Besides searching for similar compounds that are supposed to have a similar affinity toward a target, one can also utilize sets of compounds with known activities to train models that aim to separate active from inactive molecules. This can be done by means of machine learning methods.

Machine learning methods have the distinct advantage over plain similarity searches in that the information of many active and inactive molecules is utilized for model generation. These methods were originally developed by computer scientists to distinguish, for instance, handwritten characters [61, 62] and are nowadays widely applied in pharmaceutical industry [63]. Both the active and inactive molecules are represented by molecular descriptors or fingerprints (see above), and the classification or regression models are built from these so-called training sets to relate compound structural information to the biological activity of interest. By also taking into account the information on inactive compounds, machine learning methods have the advantage of harvesting SARs that are already present in the set of known molecules. To reduce hit lists to a size that can be managed during follow-up activities, one can also consider predicted property profiles. Most pharmaceutical companies test their compounds for off-target or ADMET properties on a routine basis. Large data sets comprising compounds with more or less favorable profiles have been compiled. Again, machine learning methods can be used to generate predictive models from those data. For a survey on endpoints that have been addressed, we refer to recent reviews [64–66].

Machine learning techniques can be subdivided into so-called unsupervised and supervised methods.

3.4.3.1 Unsupervised Methods

Starting from a data set in which compounds are encoded as molecular descriptors and one or more biological activities are given as either continuous or discrete values, unsupervised machine learning techniques such as self-organizing maps or principal component analysis (see below) utilize only the descriptor information to provide an overview of the data set [63, 67]. Generally, unsupervised methods may be seen as techniques to project high-dimensional descriptor data sets onto few dimensions (usually up to two or three dimensions). This projection reveals clusters of compounds that are closely related according to the input descriptors. It also allows, for instance, to detect sparsely populated regions of the data set. By mapping the biological activities onto the projection, one can identify regions with predominantly active or inactive compounds. Compounds from vendor databases or virtual molecules are mapped onto the projection. They can then be categorized according to the initial mapping. If new molecules are found close to regions with mostly active compounds, one assumes that they are active as well. If they are far off the active region, the molecules are predicted to be inactive.

One major advantage of unsupervised methods is that the number of adjustable parameters is usually low. Therefore, these methods are usually very robust since overfitting (see below) cannot happen. A clear disadvantage is the fact that the features that are actually important for activity are not necessarily important for the projection. This means that the actives do not need to cluster in the projection.

3.4.3.2 Supervised Methods

In contrast to unsupervised methods, supervised machine learning techniques also take into account the biological activity for model training. In general, a regression or classification function is trained that aims to minimize an error function while keeping the complexity of the underlying function as low as possible [63, 68].

For all supervised methods, a subset of the initial data set with inactive and active molecules must be selected for model training, while the remaining data are used to test the predictivity of the model. This is necessary because models that usually include many tunable parameters may adjust perfectly to the data set they have been trained on, but they may be unable to make useful predictions for previously unseen compounds. This effect is called overfitting. One has to be aware that model building is always a trade-off between increasing complexity of the model (thus, perfectly fitting the training data) and its general validity. Usually one accepts that some molecules of the training data set are predicted incorrectly by the final model if the model is able to perform quite well for other molecules outside the training data. There exist various ways to split the data set into training and test data, but in all cases a significant fraction of the available data is used for testing the model. This waste of information (large amount of data are not used for model building) led to cross-validation approaches. Here, several models are built, and for each single model, a certain training set and test set is defined. Often the test data are randomly taken as a certain fraction of the available molecules. All resulting models are combined in the end in order to give one so-called cross-validated model.

Although complex cross-validation schemes are applied, the final assessment of the model quality and predictivity can only be achieved when the model is applied to compounds that were not seen by the model before. This so-called model validation is often the direct application of the model to prospective virtual screening projects or to predicting ADMET properties and the model quality may only be assessed after biological testing of the predicted compounds.

To sum up, independent of the method applied, model building is a very delicate task and a lot of experience is required to reliably construct stable and predictive models. This is some drawback in comparison to similarity searches whose application also requires experience but is conceptionally simpler. However, in cases where a sufficient number of active and inactive compounds are available, machine learning techniques are valuable tools for virtual screening (see Section 3.4.3.4).

3.4.3.3 Selected Techniques

In the following, we will discuss very few important techniques for machine learning. There exists a wealth of methods [69] and we try to focus here on the ones primarily applied to virtual screening. The list, however, is not exhaustive and the interested reader is redirected to excellent machine learning literature in order to get the full picture where details of the applicability domain of models and error estimations are also discussed [69–72].

Principal Component Analysis (PCA) Principal component analysis (PCA) is the only unsupervised method that will be discussed here in detail. PCA is a linear projection method that is designed to preserve the variance in the data. This means that populated regions that are far apart in high-dimensional descriptor space will also end up far apart in the projection. Visually one can imagine that a high-dimensional ellipsoid is drawn that encloses all data apart from some outliers. The principal components then correspond to the longest axes of the ellipsoid comprising a linear combination of the original axes in feature space. Therefore, the new axes and thus the whole model can still be interpreted because they are composed of certain descriptors. As an example, one may imagine a principal axis mainly made of the molecular mass and the clog$P$ descriptors. The molecules along this axis are increasing in weight and lipophilicity. Figure 3.4 sketches the principle of PCA.

PCA is widely used for descriptor selection in order to identify correlations between descriptors, but there are also examples where PCA is directly used for virtual screening. In a recent work by Knox *et al.* [73], PCA was applied in a virtual screening run to identify ligands for the estrogen receptor by identifying the part of the chemical space where known estrogen receptor ligands lie.

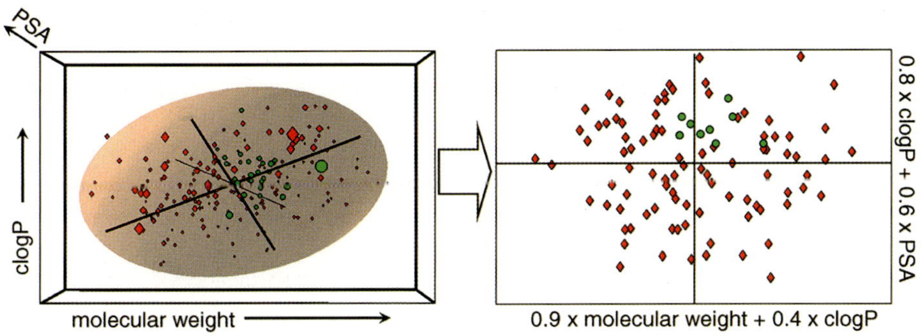

Figure 3.4 The principle of PCA is the linear projection of higher dimensional data (left) to few dimensions (right). Molecules clustering in higher dimensions (green dots represent active molecules) still cluster in the projection. In the example shown here, the molecules are described by their weight, their calculated log*P* (clog*P*), and their calculated polar surface area (PSA). The new axes in the PCA (right part of the figure) are linear combinations of the original axes.

Decision Trees A decision tree is a hierarchical data structure (a so-called tree) based on the divide and conquer strategy [74]. The method is also called recursive partitioning. A molecule enters the tree at its root and at each node a decision is made if the molecule is sorted to the left or to the right (usually every node has two children nodes). The decision may be based on the occurrence of a certain substructure or on the value of a certain descriptor. The decision procedure at each node is trained in a way that the tree is able to split the training data set optimally into active and inactive molecules. Thus, at each node the descriptor is sought that is able to split the entering molecules most satisfyingly. In the end the optimal tree has highly populated leaves that are filled with either only active or inactive molecules. To predict the activity of a new molecule, it enters the tree at its root and follows the corresponding decisions at each node until it ends up at a leaf that tells if the molecule is to be predicted active or inactive.

To overcome limitations of a single decision tree, especially overfitting, many trees resulting from training with different subsets of the training data set are combined to give a so-called random forest [75].

Support Vector Machines (SVM) A classifying support vector machine is a method that separates the active and inactive molecules of the training data set in a high-dimensional space. The input features of a molecule (descriptors) are transformed into a coordinate space of usually higher dimension. Then a hyperplane is determined that separates the active from the inactive molecules. This is done while maximizing the margin between both classes [62, 76]. Figure 3.5 depicts the underlying principle of SVMs. Many kinds of SVMs are described in the literature (see, for example, Ref. [77]. The main difference is in the way the input data are mapped on to a higher dimensional space. This transforming function is called "kernel." The user usually tests different predefined kernels for their performance on a specific virtual screening

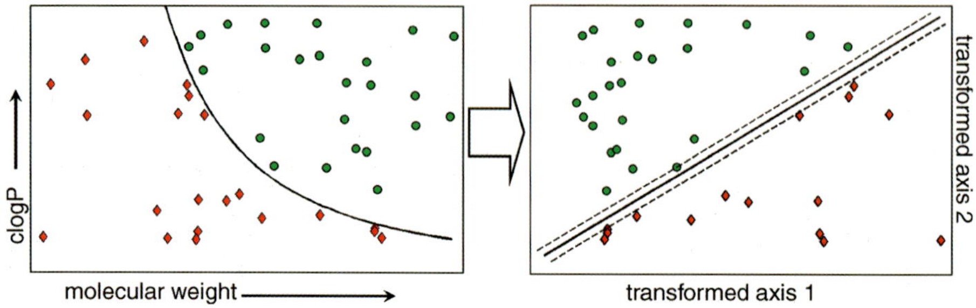

Figure 3.5 Schematic representation of the principle of SVMs in two dimensions. Data from two activity classes, which are not separable by a straight line (left), become transformed so that they are separable in the new coordinate space (right). The dashed lines indicate the margin, which is maximized by SVMs. In the example shown here, the molecules are described by their weight and their calculated log*P*. The axes of the new coordinate space are not interpretable.

problem. Since there is no way to predict the suitability of a kernel for a specific application, the user usually picks the kernel that gives best results in the cross-validation. Once the model is trained based on the known data, the virtual screening search is performed by taking the molecules from the search database and transforming their descriptors into their high-dimensional representation employing the kernel. The predicted activities of the molecules depend on which side of the hyperplane they come to lie.

3.4.3.4 **Machine Learning Applications for Virtual Screening**

Random forests and SVMs are currently the most commonly used machine learning methods in virtual screening. The recent publications [71, 78–80] compare state-of-the-art machine learning approaches in their virtual screening performance on many different data sets. In Ref. [71], a number of studies about virtual screening by machine learning from the literature have been summarized, showing that machine learning methods are well able to enrich active compounds in a data set. The studies of Refs [78, 79] are conducted in a way that several different machine learning methods are used for virtual screening on a set of five different biological targets. All current papers show that the performance of different methods strongly depends on the data set, but as a conclusion it is seen that SVMs and random forests always perform well in terms of the number of recovered actives and the enrichment [71, 78, 79, 81].

3.4.4 Validation of Methods and Prediction of Success

The outcome of virtual screening is very much method, target, and data set dependent. It would be very helpful for practitioners to be able to predict the chance for success of a prospective virtual screening. Building models with machine learning tools implies a model validation (see above). Together with a check whether the compounds in the search database belong to the applicability domain of the model, a cautious assessment of its performance can be achieved. But for similarity searches, this is still challenging and in recent years several groups published methods to tackle this problem.

Martin *et al.* [82] retrospectively analyzed the results of 115 HTS campaigns at Abbott and found that compounds with a Tanimoto coefficient >0.85 to a known active based on Daylight fingerprints had only a 30% chance to be active at the same target. Others, namely, Patterson *et al.* [83], Horvath and Jeandenans [84], and Papadatos *et al.* [85] published methods to quantify how far the structural similarity defined by a descriptor corresponds to the similarity in biological activity. Recently, methods were published [86, 87] to determine the likelihood that a compound exhibits a specific activity based on descriptor values of actives and inactives and the divergence of their probability distributions. Recovery rates of active compounds could be successfully predicted. However, all these methods mentioned above require the knowledge of a significant number of actives and inactives. In case of only a single known reference ligand, the authors are not aware of any possibility to predict the chance for success of a virtual screening run.

3.5 Conclusions

Virtual screening has attracted increasing attention during the last decade as a tool to computationally search for new chemotypes with a specified bioactivity. The role of virtual screening in the research process, however, depends on the availability of other lead identification techniques and on the timing of virtual screening within this process.

Research projects in pharmaceutical industry that are in an early phase need bioactive chemotypes as potential lead structures for optimization. Hits with a medium or even weak activity can serve as leads if the overall profile looks attractive. HTS of the in-house compound libraries is the most common source of these lead structures. If information about the 3D structure of the target and/or about bioactive ligand(s) is available, virtual screening can be used to add further active chemotypes either from the existing compounds, for example, from vendor catalogues, or from the virtual chemical space, for example, from virtual combinatorial libraries. Virtual screening can also be used to select a subset from the in-house screening collection if a full HTS is not possible due to cost or time limitations.

In contrast, biotech companies with only a small or even without an in-house screening pool depend on virtual screening techniques to access potentially active compounds from external sources. The same is true for academic groups that in most cases neither have access to an in-house compound library nor have access to HTS facilities.

Therefore, the role of virtual screening depends on the alternatives that are available regarding the access to new, bioactive chemotypes. In pharmaceutical industry, hits from virtual screening often compete with those from HTS in early projects. Virtual screening will add value only if novel and attractive chemotypes are found that favorably complement the hit set from HTS and provide new lead options.

In many early projects, only little is known about active ligands of the respective target. In these cases, similarity searches are the only option for ligand-based virtual screening. Based on the authors' experience, it is worth to try a similarity search even if the reference structure has a moderate activity in the micromolar range. The search for new chemotypes usually yields only low enrichments and in most cases only weakly active hits whose optimization potential has to be evaluated in a hit exploration campaign. In most cases, additional virtual screening and optimization cycles with support from medicinal chemistry are necessary to get novel lead structures. As part of the research process, virtual screening must meet the timelines of HTS and hit exploration in order to provide active compounds for the lead selection process.

Projects in a more progressed phase may need support from virtual screening if the chemotypes that are in optimization have liabilities such as serious pharmacokinetic or patent problems. A virtual screening in external databases or in virtual libraries can provide new chemotypes with favorable properties. In such projects, much information about active and inactive structures and SARs is available that can be used for virtual screening. However, even if the chance for a successful virtual screening may be better, in these advanced projects the expectations regarding affinity and additional compound properties like selectivity or solubility of compounds are typically high. Weak hits from virtual screening are compared with compounds in the high affinity range and often do not look attractive enough to the medicinal chemists. Even if a new chemotype does not show the liabilities of the existing compounds, further multiparameter optimization will be needed, which again may take years. Despite these challenges, virtual screening may help advanced projects, but it is important to keep these constraints in mind and to avoid unrealistic expectations.

References

1 Horvath, D. (1997) A virtual screening approach applied to the search for trypanothione reductase inhibitors. *Journal of Medicinal Chemistry*, **40** (15), 2412–2423.

2 Walters, W.P., Stahl, M.T., and Murcko, M.A. (1998) Virtual screening: an overview. *Drug Discovery Today*, **3** (4), 160–178.

3 Clark, D.E. (2008) What has virtual screening ever done for drug discovery? *Expert Opinion Drug Discovery*, **3** (8), 841–851.

4 Guido, R.V.C., Oliva, G., and Andricopulo, A.D. (2008) Virtual screening and its integration with modern drug design technologies. *Current Medicinal Chemistry*, **15** (1), 37–46.

5 Kontoyianni, M., Madhav, P., Suchanek, E., and Seibel, W. (2008) Theoretical and practical considerations in virtual screening: a beaten field? *Current Medicinal Chemistry*, **15** (2), 107–116.

6 Muegge, I. (2008) Synergies of virtual screening approaches. *Mini Reviews in Medicinal Chemistry*, **8** (9), 927–933.

7 Rester, U. (2008) From virtuality to reality – virtual screening in lead discovery and lead optimization: a medicinal chemistry perspective. *Current Opinion in*

Drug Discovery & Development, **1** (4), 559–568.

8 Seifert, M.H.J. and Lang, M. (2008) Essential factors for successful virtual screening. *Mini Reviews in Medicinal Chemistry*, **8** (1), 63–72.

9 Kirchmair, J., Distinto, S., Schuster, D., Spitzer, G., Langer, T., and Wolber, G. (2008) Enhancing drug discovery through *in silico* screening: strategies to increase true positives retrieval rates. *Current Medicinal Chemistry*, **15** (20), 2040–2053.

10 Koeppen, H. (2009) Virtual screening: what does it give us? *Current Opinion in Drug Discovery & Development*, **12** (3), 397–407.

11 Johnson, M.A. and Maggiora, G.M. (eds) (1990) *Concepts and Applications of Molecular Similarity*, John Wiley & Sons, Inc., New York.

12 Dixon, S.L. and Villar, H.O. (1998) Bioactive diversity and screening library selection via affinity fingerprinting. *Journal of Chemical Information and Computer Sciences*, **38** (6), 1192–1203.

13 Lessel, U.F. and Briem, H. (2000) Flexsim-X: a method for the detection of molecules with similar biological activity. *Journal of Chemical Information and Computer Sciences*, **40** (2), 246–253.

14 Mauser, H. and Guba, W. (2008) Recent developments in *de novo* design and scaffold hopping. *Current Opinion in Drug Discovery & Development*, **11** (3), 365–374.

15 Kubinyi, H. (2002) Chemical similarity and biological activities. *Journal of the Brazilian Chemical Society*, **13** (6), 717–726.

16 Sheridan, R.P. and Kearsley, S.K. (2002) Why do we need so many chemical similarity search methods? *Drug Discovery Today*, **7** (17), 903–911.

17 Bajorath, J. (2002) Integration of virtual and high-throughput screening. *Nature Reviews. Drug Discovery*, **1** (11), 882–894.

18 Pearlman, R.S. and Smith, K.M. (1998) Novel software tools for chemical diversity. *Perspectives in Drug Discovery and Design*, **9–11**, 339–353.

19 Rarey, M. and Dixon, J.S. (1998) Feature trees: a new molecular similarity measure based on tree matching. *Journal of Computer-Aided Molecular Design*, **12** (5), 471–490.

20 Lessel, U., Wellenzohn, B., Lilienthal, M., and Claussen, H. (2009) Searching fragment spaces with feature trees. *Journal of Chemical Information and Modeling*, **49** (2), 270–279.

21 Ewing, T., Baber, J.C., and Feher, M. (2006) Novel 2D fingerprints for ligand-based virtual screening. *Journal of Chemical Information and Modeling*, **46** (6), 2423–2431.

22 Flower, D.R. (1998) On the properties of bit string-based measures of chemical similarity. *Journal of Chemical Information and Computer Sciences*, **38** (3), 379–386.

23 Lounkine, E., Hu, Y., Batista, J., and Bajorath, J. (2009) Relevance of feature combinations for similarity searching using general or activity class-directed molecular fingerprints. *Journal of Chemical Information and Modeling*, **49** (3), 561–570.

24 Morgan, H.L. (1965) Generation of a unique machine description for chemical structures: a technique developed at chemical abstracts service. *Journal of Chemical Documentation*, **5** (2), 107–113.

25 Rogers, D., Brown, R.D., and Hahn, M. (2005) Using extended-connectivity fingerprints with Laplacian-modified Bayesian analysis in high-throughput screening follow-up. *Journal of Biomolecular Screening*, **10** (7), 682–686.

26 Schneider, G., Neidhart, W., Giller, T., and Schmid, G. (1999) "Scaffold-Hopping" by topological pharmacophore search: a contribution to virtual screening. *Angewandte Chemie, International Edition*, **38** (19), 2894–2896.

27 Perola, E. and Charifson, P.S. (2004) Conformational analysis of drug-like molecules bound to proteins: an extensive study of ligand reorganization upon binding. *Journal of Medicinal Chemistry*, **47** (10), 2499–2510.

28 Takagi, T., Amano, M., and Tomimoto, M. (2009) Novel method for the evaluation of 3D conformation generators. *Journal of Chemical Information and Modeling*, **49** (6), 1377–1388.

29 Renner, S., Schwab, C.H., Gasteiger, J., and Schneider, G. (2006) Impact of conformational flexibility on three-dimensional similarity searching using

correlation vectors. *Journal of Chemical Information and Modeling*, **46** (6), 2324–2332.

30 Zhang, Q. and Muegge, I. (2006) Scaffold hopping through virtual screening using 2D and 3D similarity descriptors: ranking, voting, and consensus scoring. *Journal of Medicinal Chemistry*, **49** (5), 1536–1548.

31 Hawkins, P.C.D., Skillman, A.G., and Nicholls, A. (2007) Comparison of shape-matching and docking as virtual screening tools. *Journal of Medicinal Chemistry*, **50** (1), 74–82.

32 Lessel, U. (2007) Ligand based virtual screening using BCUT descriptors. Abstracts of papers presented at 234th ACS National Meeting, Boston, MA, August 19–23, 2007.

33 Bologa, C.G., Olah, M.M., and Oprea, T.I. (2006) Chemical database preparation for compound acquisition or virtual screening. *Methods in Molecular Biology*, **316**, 375–388.

34 Perez-Pineiro, R., Burgos, A., Jones, D.C., Andrew, L.C., Rodriguez, H., Suarez, M., Fairlamb, A.H., and Wishart, D.S. (2009) Development of a novel virtual screening cascade protocol to identify potential trypanothione reductase inhibitors. *Journal of Medicinal Chemistry*, **52** (6), 1670–1680.

35 Willett, P., Barnard, J.M., and Downs, G.M. (1998) Chemical similarity searching. *Journal of Chemical Information and Computer Sciences*, **38** (6), 983–996.

36 Holliday, J.D., Salim, N., Whittle, M., and Willett, P. (2003) Analysis and display of the size dependence of chemical similarity coefficients. *Journal of Chemical Information and Computer Sciences*, **43** (3), 819–828.

37 Kirchmair, J., Markt, P., Distinto, S., Wolber, G., and Langer, T. (2008) Evaluation of the performance of 3D virtual screening protocols: RMSD comparisons, enrichment assessments, and decoy selection: what can we learn from earlier mistakes? *Journal of Computer-Aided Molecular Design*, **22** (3–4), 213–228.

38 Rarey, M. and Stahl, M. (2001) Similarity searching in large combinatorial chemistry spaces. *Journal of Computer-Aided Molecular Design*, **15** (6), 497–520.

39 Gillet, V.J., Willett, P., and Bradshaw, J. (2003) Similarity searching using reduced graphs. *Journal of Chemical Information and Computer Sciences*, **43** (2), 338–345.

40 Barker, E.J., Buttar, D., Cosgrove, D.A., Gardiner, E.J., Kitts, P., Willett, P., and Gillet, V.J. (2006) Scaffold hopping using clique detection applied to reduced graphs. *Journal of Chemical Information and Modeling*, **46** (2), 503–511.

41 Hert, J., Willett, P., Wilton, D.J., Acklin, P., Azzaoui, K., Jacoby, E., and Schuffenhauer, A. (2004) Comparison of fingerprint-based methods for virtual screening using multiple bioactive reference structures. *Journal of Chemical Information and Computer Sciences*, **44** (3), 1177–1185.

42 Renner, S. and Schneider, G. (2006) Scaffold-hopping potential of ligand-based similarity concepts. *ChemMedChem*, **1** (2), 181–185.

43 Hristozov, D.P., Oprea, T.I., and Gasteiger, J. (2007) Virtual screening applications: a study of ligand-based methods and different structure representations in four different scenarios. *Journal of Computer-Aided Molecular Design*, **21** (10–11), 617–640.

44 Good, A.C., Hermsmeier, M.A., and Hindle, S.A. (2004) Measuring CAMD technique performance: a virtual screening case study in the design of validation experiments. *Journal of Computer-Aided Molecular Design*, **18** (7–9), 529–536.

45 Bender, A., Mussa, H.Y., Glen, R.C., and Reiling, S. (2004) Similarity searching of chemical databases using atom environment descriptors (MOLPRINT 2D): evaluation of performance. *Journal of Chemical Information and Computer Sciences*, **44** (5), 1708–1718.

46 Bender, A., Jenkins, J.L., Scheiber, J., Sukuru, S.C.K., Glick, M., and Davies, J.W. (2009) How similar are similarity searching methods? A principal component analysis of molecular descriptor space. *Journal of Chemical Information and Modeling*, **49** (1), 108–119.

47 Brown, R.D. and Martin, Y.C. (1997) The information content of 2D and 3D structural descriptors relevant to ligand–receptor binding. *Journal of Chemical Information and Computer Sciences*, **37** (1), 1–9.

48 Verdonk, M.L., Berdini, V., Hartshorn, M.J., Mooij, W.T.M., Murray, C.W., Taylor, R.D., and Watson, P. (2004) Virtual screening using protein–ligand docking: avoiding artificial enrichment. *Journal of Chemical Information and Computer Sciences*, **44** (3), 793–806.

49 Whittle, M., Gillet, V.J., Willett, P., and Loesel, J. (2006) Analysis of data fusion methods in virtual screening: theoretical model. *Journal of Chemical Information and Modeling*, **46** (6), 2193–2205.

50 Whittle, M., Gillet, V.J., Willett, P., and Loesel, J. (2006) Analysis of data fusion methods in virtual screening: theoretical model. *Journal of Chemical Information and Modeling*, **46** (6), 2206–2219.

51 Ginn, C.M.R., Willett, P., and Bradshaw, J. (2000) Combination of molecular similarity measures using data fusion. *Perspectives in Drug Discovery and Design*, **20**, 1–16.

52 Schuffenhauer, A., Floersheim, P., Acklin, P., and Jacoby, E. (2003) Similarity metrics for ligands reflecting the similarity of the target proteins. *Journal of Chemical Information and Computer Sciences*, **43** (2), 391–405.

53 Baber, J.C., Shirley, W.A., Gao, Y., and Feher, M. (2006) The use of consensus scoring in ligand-based virtual screening. *Journal of Chemical Information and Modeling*, **46** (1), 277–288.

54 Gorse, A.-D. (2006) Diversity in medicinal chemistry space. *Current Topics in Medicinal Chemistry*, **6** (1), 3–18.

55 Lewell, X.Q., Judd, D., Watson, S., and Hann, M. (1998) RECAP-retrosynthetic combinatorial analysis procedure: a powerful new technique for identifying privileged molecular fragments with useful applications in combinatorial chemistry. *Journal of Chemical Information and Computer Sciences*, **38** (3), 511–522.

56 Boehm, M., Wu, T.-Y., Claussen, H., and Lemmen, C. (2008) Similarity searching and scaffold hopping in synthetically accessible combinatorial chemistry spaces. *Journal of Medicinal Chemistry*, **51** (8), 2468–2480.

57 Cramer, R.D., Jilek, R.J., Guessregen, S., Clark, S.J., Wendt, B., and Clark, R.D. (2004) "Lead hopping". Validation of topomer similarity as a superior predictor of similar biological activities. *Journal of Medicinal Chemistry*, **47** (27), 6777–6791.

58 Olender, R. and Rosenfeld, R. (2001) A fast algorithm for searching for molecules containing a pharmacophore in very large virtual combinatorial libraries. *Journal of Chemical Information and Computer Sciences*, **41** (3), 731–738.

59 Yu, N. and Bakken, G.A. (2009) Efficient exploration of large combinatorial chemistry spaces by monomer-based similarity searching. *Journal of Chemical Information and Modeling*, **49** (4), 745–755.

60 Schneider, G., Clement-Chomienne, O., Hilfiger, L., Schneider, P., Kirsch, S., Bohm, H.-J., and Neidhart, W. (2000) Virtual screening for bioactive molecules by evolutionary *de novo* design. *Angewandte Chemie, International Edition*, **39** (22), 4130–4133.

61 Hearst, M.A., Dumais, S.T., Osuna, E., Platt, J., and Schölkopf, B. (1998) SVMs: a practical consequence of learning theory. *IEEE Intelligent Systems*, **13**, 18–28.

62 Müller, K.-R., Mika, S., Rätsch, G., Tsuda, K., and Schölkopf, B. (2001) An introduction to kernel-based learning algorithms. *IEEE Transactions on Neural Networks*, **12** (2), 181–201.

63 Schneider, G. and Baringhaus, K-.H. (eds) (2008) *Molecular Design*, Wiley-VCH Verlag GmbH, Weinheim.

64 Fox, T. and Kriegl, J.M. (2006) Machine learning techniques for *in silico* modeling of drug metabolism. *Current Topics in Medicinal Chemistry*, **6** (15), 1579–1591.

65 Sakiyama, Y. (2009) The use of machine learning and nonlinear statistical tools for ADME prediction. *Expert Opinion on Drug Metabolism & Toxicology*, **5** (2), 49–169.

66 Hutter, M.C. (2009) In *silico* prediction of drug properties. *Current Medicinal Chemistry*, **16** (2), 189–202.

67 Ivanenkov, Y.A., Savchuk, N.P., Ekins, S., and Balakin, K.V. (2009) Computational mapping tools for drug discovery. *Drug Discovery Today*, **14** (15/16), 767–775.

68 Hastie, T., Tibshirami, R., and Friedman, J. (2001) *The Elements of Statistical Learning*, Springer, New York.

69 Alpaydin, E. (2004) *Introduction to Machine Learning*, MIT Press, Cambridge.

70 Hert, J., Willett, P., Wilton, D.J., Acklin, P., Azzaoui, K., Jacoby, E., and Schuffenhauer, A. (2006) New methods for ligand-based virtual screening: use of data fusion and machine learning to enhance the effectiveness of similarity searching. *Journal of Chemical Information and Modeling*, **46** (2), 462–470.

71 Ma, X.H., Jia, J., Zhu, F., Xue, Y., Li, Z.R., and Chen, Y.Z. (2009) Comparative analysis of machine learning methods in ligand-based virtual screening of large compound libraries. *Combinatorial Chemistry & High Throughput Screening*, **12** (4), 344–357.

72 Schwaighofer, A., Schroeter, T., Mika, S., and Blanchard, G. (2009) How wrong can we get? A review of machine learning approaches and error bars. *Combinatorial Chemistry & High Throughput Screening*, **12** (5), 453–468.

73 Knox, A.J.S., Meegan, M.J., and Lloyd, D.G. (2006) Estrogen receptors: molecular interactions, virtual screening and future prospects. *Current Topics in Medicinal Chemistry*, **6** (3), 217–243.

74 Rusinko, A., III, Farmen, M.W., Lambert, C.G., Brown, P.L., and Young, S.S. (1999) Analysis of a large structure/biological activity data set using recursive partitioning. *Journal of Chemical Information and Computer Sciences*, **39** (6), 1017–1026.

75 Svetnik, V., Liaw, A., Tong, C., Culberson, J.C., Sheridan, R.P., and Feuston, B.P. (2003) Random forest: a classification and regression tool for compound classification and QSAR modeling. *Journal of Chemical Information and Computer Sciences*, **43** (6), 1947–1958.

76 Cortes, C. and Vapnik, V.N. (1995) Support vector networks. *Machine Learning*, **20** (3), 273–297.

77 Schölkopf, B. and Smola, A.J. (2002) *Learning with Kernels*, MIT Press, London.

78 Plewczynski, D., Spieser, S.A.H., and Koch, U. (2006) Assessing different classification methods for virtual screening. *Journal of Chemical Information and Modeling*, **46** (3), 1098–1106.

79 Plewczynski, D., Spieser, S.A.H., and Koch, U. (2009) Performance of machine learning methods for ligand-based virtual screening. *Combinatorial Chemistry & High Throughput Screening*, **12** (4), 358–368.

80 Melville, J.L., Burke, E.K., and Hirst, J.D. (2009) Machine learning in virtual screening. *Combinatorial Chemistry & High Throughput Screening*, **12** (4), 332–343.

81 Briem, H. and Guenther, J. (2005) Classifying "kinase inhibitor-likeness" by using machine-learning methods. *ChemBioChem*, **6** (3), 558–566.

82 Martin, Y.C., Kofron, J.L., and Traphagen, L.M. (2002) Do structurally similar molecules have similar biological activity? *Journal of Medicinal Chemistry*, **45** (19), 4350–4358.

83 Patterson, D.E., Cramer, R.D., Ferguson, A.M., Clark, R.D., and Weinberger, L.E. (1996) Neighborhood behavior: a useful concept for validation of "molecular diversity" descriptors. *Journal of Medicinal Chemistry*, **39** (16), 3049–3059.

84 Horvath, D. and Jeandenans, C. (2003) Neighborhood behavior of *in silico* structural spaces with respect to *in vitro* activity spaces: a novel understanding of the molecular similarity principle in the context of multiple receptor binding profiles. *Journal of Chemical Information and Computer Sciences*, **43** (2), 680–690.

85 Papadatos, G., Cooper, A.W.J., Kadirkamanathan, V., Macdonald, S.J.F., McLay, I.M., Pickett, S.D., Pritchard, J.M., Willett, P., and Gillet, V.J. (2009) Analysis of neighborhood behavior in lead optimization and array design. *Journal of Chemical Information and Modeling*, **49** (2), 195–208.

86 Vogt, M. and Bajorath, J. (2007) Introduction of an information-theoretic method to predict recovery rates of active compounds for Bayesian *in silico* screening: theory and screening trials. *Journal of Chemical Information and Modeling*, **47** (2), 337–341.

87 Muchmore, S.W., Debe, D.A., Metz, J.T., Brown, S.P., Martin, Y.C., and Hajduk, P.J. (2008) Application of belief theory to similarity data fusion for use in analog searching and lead hopping. *Journal of Chemical Information and Modeling*, **48** (5), 941–948.

4
The Basis for Target-Based Virtual Screening: Protein Structures

Jason C. Cole, Oliver Korb, Tjelvar S.G. Olsson, and John Liebeschuetz

4.1
Introduction

When beginning a virtual high-throughput screening (vHTS) campaign against a given target, scientists have to make several decisions with regard to the starting material they will use. In particular, they have to choose one or more starting structural models to use in docking. Furthermore, said models have to be altered such that the setup of the protein is suitable for the underlying software being used for vHTS.

Consequently, this chapter is split into two main sections. The first tries to convey information about the pitfalls in protein crystal structures, in order to make an informed decision about structure selection. The second deals with the common issues one faces when trying to use one or more structures in the context of virtual screening.

4.2
Selecting a Protein Structure for Virtual Screening

This section focuses on how to select a structure for virtual screening. The discussion is specific to structures determined by X-ray crystallography. There are, of course, other structure elucidation methods (via NMR or via homology modeling). It should be noted, however, that structures determined by these methods are also subject to imprecision and inaccuracy. NMR yields multiple models, so the user has to select the one or more appropriate NMR conformations to use in vHTS. Use of homology models for docking-based vHTS should probably be done only as a last resort, as the side chain placement in the binding site in such models is likely to be less accurate than in the models generated using experimental information.

4.2.1
Why Are There Errors in Crystal Structures?

When presented with a structural file, one's initial temptation is to treat the contained coordinates as a direct 3D image of a protein structure; the reality, however, is that the

Virtual Screening. Edited by C. Sotriffer

ISBN: 978-3-527-32636-5

structural file represents an *atomic model* of the protein crystal structure. A modeler or medicinal chemist would be well advised to understand how this model was generated, at least at a superficial level, so as to understand possible underlying issues in a given structure. In this brief section, we will try to summarize the causes of error in the context of structural data.

To elucidate a crystal structure, a crystallographer collects a set of observed diffraction intensities for a crystal diffracting in an X-ray beam. The intensities alone, however, are insufficient to construct a model; the crystallographer needs to predict a set of unknowns called the reflection phases. These are initially estimated by various techniques to give a starting model. The starting model is then refined, and the refined model is used to recalculate the phases, allowing the calculation of an improved electron density map, which can be reinterpreted. The process is cyclical, but hopefully leads to an accurate interpretation of the reflection intensities.

Note that a pattern of X-ray intensities reflects the distribution of electrons in the underlying crystal. The atomic model is therefore an *interpretation* of this electronic distribution. One consequence of this is that elements can be misinterpreted in a model, as elements of a similar atomic number (such as carbon, nitrogen, and oxygen) can be used almost equally well to model regions of the electronic distribution. This problem is interlinked with the problem of structural "resolution" (see Section 4.5.2). A low resolution indicates that the underlying diffraction data will be harder to interpret as an atomic model due to a lack of information content in the diffraction pattern.

Figure 4.1 shows the effect of resolution on the electron density for histidine residues in three kinase protein structures of varying resolution. In the highly resolved structure, the density reveals the clear shape of a histidine; one can resolve atomic centers in the density. In the less well-resolved structures, the interpretation is more subjective. Even in the high-resolution structure, a flip around the exocyclic bond would still yield a model that fitted to the density reasonably well.

Crystallographic refinement programs utilize chemical knowledge and sequence information to assist in electron density interpretation. Threading algorithms map a 3D model of a protein sequence directly into the calculated electron density map. Crystallographic restraints are used during the refinement process to tie down bond lengths and angles in crystallographic models, but invariably some ambiguity exists, which can lead to misinterpretations of the electron density.

An additional problem with crystal structures that can give rise to a misleading model is the thermal motion and disorder within the crystalline lattice. Local regions of electron density can be poorly defined, even for structures with relatively good resolution if, for example, a protein residue is labile in the crystalline state. If undetected, a residue can be poorly modeled, misassigned, or omitted from the model. Even when detected and fully modeled, disorder implies flexibility, which may need specific handling in a docking study.

Errors occur if rigorous care is not taken, but another factor can also be at play. Gerd Vriend has pointed out (personal communication) that most protein structures included in the open literature are refined by research students who have little

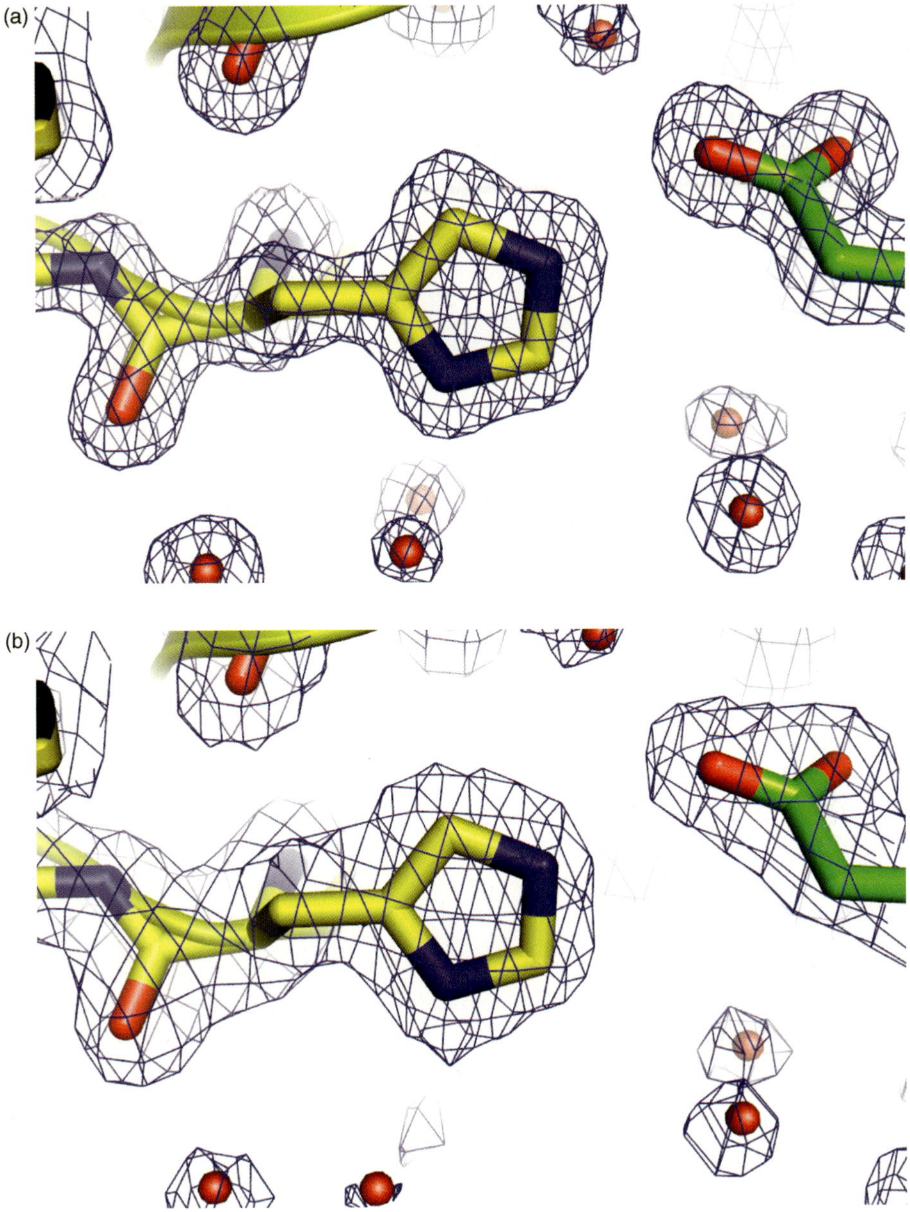

Figure 4.1 Variance of fit of a histidine with structural resolution. Three examples of histidine residues are shown superimposed on their electron density as generated from a $2mF_O$-DF_C map. (a) Histidine residue 268 (chain A) from PDB ID 2uv4 at 1.33 Å resolution. (b) Histidine residue 268 (chain A) from PDB ID 2uv6 at 2.0 Å resolution. (c) Histidine residue 179 (chain A) from PDB ID 2waj at 2.4 Å resolution.

(c)

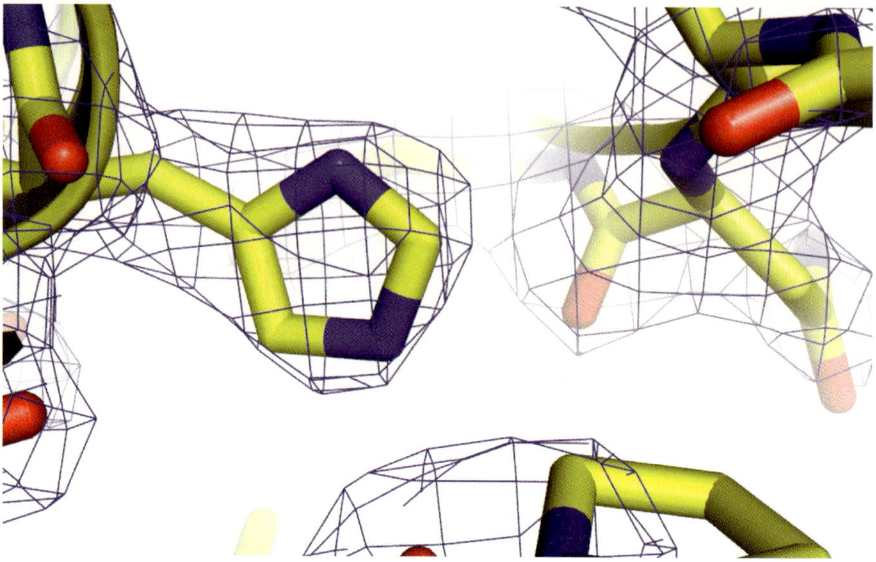

Figure 4.1 (*Continued*)

previous experience in protein crystallography. It is possible that this, combined with an eagerness to publish, and perhaps less than rigorous supervision, may result in errors creeping in to the public domain. Sometimes a given error is in a structural region that is of little interest to the original publishing authors, but critical for a third party using the model. An example here might be the difference of focus of a biologist interested in overall fold as compared to a medicinal chemist who may be interested in a very specific binding site.

Finally, inexperienced crystallographers have, in the past, tended to focus on global refinement metrics, such as the R-factor (see Section 4.5.1), to judge the relative merit of a model. Such metrics, however, only tell the user about the relative fit of the observed data to that calculated from the model; they say nothing about the chemical sense of the model used. Trusting such metrics is fraught with danger, as the metric is calculated using the data that were used to generate the model. Protein structure refinements require the inclusion of geometric restraints as there are often more parameters to refine than experimental observations. Consequently, the R-factor can reflect overfitting of a poor model rather than the merit of said model. Use of R-free [1] in recent years has improved the situation somewhat, as the experimental data set used to elucidate R-free is genuinely independent of the data used to refine the model.

All these issues are, from a modeling perspective, problematic, particularly when dealing with structures from the public domain. A modeler, however, can ameliorate such problems by effective communication with the crystallographer responsible for the structure and by careful evaluation when first dealing with a new structure.

4.2.2
Possible Problems That May Occur in a Crystal Structure

This section will give a brief summary of common problems in crystal structures. Two excellent reviews were recently published in this area by Davis *et al.* [2, 3] that deal with limitations of X-ray data with real case examples, some of which are highlighted below. Furthermore, there are online resources available for modelers to teach methods for structural validation [4].

4.2.2.1 Entirely Incorrect Models

Very occasionally a structure is deposited in the Protein Data Bank [5] (Rutgers University, The Protein Data Bank. Available at www.pdb.org and www.pdb.org) (PDB) that is completely wrong. Though these are mercifully rare, there have been some recent high-profile examples in the literature [6]. If you are unfortunate enough to end up performing a vHTS campaign against such a structure, then the results are unlikely to be of any value.

4.2.2.2 Sequencing Errors

A more common error in proteins occurs when a crystallographer erroneously assigns one or more residues of incorrect type, and consequently models the underlying electron density using an incorrect atomic model.

The worst assignment error is called a "frameshift" where the initial tracing of the protein into the sequence misses a particular residue in the electron density causing an offsetting in the assigned residue type (see Figure 4.2). Such errors rarely end up in the final model as they are usually detected and corrected during the refinement process. A more likely error is one where the initial sequence used for the tracing process contains errors, meaning that the density for an individual residue is fitted to the wrong residue type.

4.2.2.3 Misplaced Side Chains

By far the most common issue in a protein is that of a misplaced amino acid side chain. In particular, asparagines, glutamine, and histidine residues can be flipped from the correct orientation. This occurs due to the similar scattering nature of the δO and δN in asparagine residues and the εN and εO atoms in glutamine residues. Furthermore, it is easy for a crystallographer to flip a histidine as the electron density is delocalized around the ring. Davis *et al.* [2] reported in 2003 that as many as one in six asparagines,

True Sequence in density	KVILVAVHVASGYIEAEVI PAETG
Fitted Sequence in density	KVILVAV HVASGYIEAEVIPAETG

Figure 4.2 A schematic diagram of a tracing error in protein crystallography. Initially, on tracing the density, the residue in blue is missed by the tracing algorithm. Consequently, the residue subsequent to this is erroneously assigned as a histidine when it is, in fact, a valine. The errors propagate along the sequence until the tracing algorithm fits two residues into the observed density of one residue, when the sequences synchronize.

glutamines, and histidines are flipped in PDB structures. It is hoped that newer checking software such as Molprobity [7], PROCHECK [8], and WHAT_CHECK [9] will have significantly reduced this in newer structures since then, but still one would be well advised to treat these residues with particular caution.

4.2.2.4 **Structural Disorder**

Disordering of the crystal structure is not an error on the part of the crystallographer unless it goes undetected. That said, a disorder presents its own set of practical problems for setup in a virtual screen. Disorder reflects a situation where a part of the underlying molecule can be positioned in alternative locations. If detected, the modeler is effectively presented with two or more different models for the protein in question. The modeler then has to decide whether to dock into one or the other, or dock into both. Ensemble and flexible side chain docking methods are well suited to this problem, as they allow the user to model multiple conformations in a single docking run.

4.2.2.5 **Poorly Modeled Cofactors and Ligands**

For many years, cofactors and ligands were the molecular black sheep of the macromolecular crystallography world. The majority of interest from a structural perspective was directed at understanding the overall fold adopted by a given protein. Bound cofactors and ligands, consequently, did not receive the same attention as the protein backbone. The programs used to refine proteins contained libraries to constrain peptidic residues into geometrically reasonable conformations, but equivalents did not exist for cofactors and ligands. Consequently, ligands and cofactors could refine into unlikely geometries. In recent years, the increase in use of protein crystallography in structure-based drug design has led to a recognition that the protein–ligand interface is as important structurally as the overall fold, and consequently more attention is now paid to the binding sites of proteins in order to ensure that ligands are better treated. That said, a molecular modeler would be well advised to view ligands with due caution.

Evidence suggests that a large proportion of ligand structures in the Protein Data Bank have geometries that may be incorrect. Certainly, a number of authors have pointed out entries that contain ligands that are clearly wrong [2, 9, 10]. Some of these errors may be because of a mistake by the protein crystallographer, the application of an incorrect restraint perhaps; or a mistake in the chemistry that is modeled, perhaps through making a subtle error in stereochemistry.

There are two reasons other than direct human error for why poor ligand geometries may result. First, the resolution of diffraction patterns obtained from protein structures is such that it is usually impossible to refine to individual atom positions, unlike the case for small-molecule structures. So, a model structure has to be used that will force restraints to be applied between proximal atom positions, within the bounds decided by the force field associated with the refinement program. The force field parameters in general use for the refinement of amino acid residues (i.e., the restraints applied during crystallographic refinement of protein structures, the so called Engh–Huber parameters [11]) are well established and are generally considered reliable. This is not necessarily the case for the force field that is applied to the ligand. Many different chemical functionalities can potentially be expressed in a ligand structure. Each possible chemical substructure requires a number of specific bond length, bond angle, and torsion parameters that can be used to restrain the refinement to within known limits. Such a collection of parameters is known as a "ligand dictionary" by crystallographers. Such dictionaries take time and effort to build and, since there are a huge number of possible fragments that could be considered, most refinement packages only have the restraint parameters for the commonest substructures to be found in ligands. As a consequence, poor ligand geometry can result from a poor set of restraints.

The second source of error arises from insufficient exploration of alternative viable ligand conformations in the model building phase. The chemistry of the initial ligand model may be correct, but the conformation used leads, on refinement, to a ligand conformation that is high energy. Refinement is often applied as a minimization technique where the nearest local minimum from the initial model, in fit to electron density, is sought, and minima with better but significantly different ligand geometry to the initial model may be missed. Sometimes such poor ligand geometries are easy to spot by the knowledgeable chemist. So, for instance, the observance of twist boat and boat forms of cyclohexane and piperidine are reasonably common (see PDB ID 1hak [12], for example). This is usually an error and a chair form for these six-membered rings is almost invariably to be preferred. Crystallographers do not necessarily have the chemical knowledge to easily identify this type of error by eye. Quite frequently, this type of error may escape the attention of even experienced and chemically aware crystallographers. Sometimes such errors can be identified from seeing where the fit to the electron density may be imperfect. However, the geometrical errors can be so subtle that even this is not possible to spot. The only thing that can be done in such cases is that all reasonable ligand conformational models should be tried by the protein crystallographer during refinement and that the final ligand model be selected based on the best trade-off between fits to the electron density and the ligand strain.

The amount of nonstandard geometry or, in other words, the amount of strain that should be expected in a bound ligand is something of an open question. After all, one established mechanism of enzyme action is the creation of strain in the cognate substrate, thereby rendering it amenable to chemical reaction at physiological temperature [13, 14]. A good example of such an enzyme is neuraminidase, the target of the influenza medication Tamiflu. The chair form of the natural substrate is converted to a high-energy boat conformation that activates it to reaction [15]. Some estimates of allowable ligand strain in protein–ligand complexes have been as high as 9 kcal/mol [16]. However, an alternative viewpoint is emerging that suggests that much of this "strain" is artifactual and a consequence of poor ligand geometry is generated on refinement. It has been suggested that alternative low-energy conformations can be found that fit the structural data as well or better for many of these high-energy complexes [17, 18].

What then is the proportion of structures in the PDB that are likely to have poor ligand geometry? We have endeavored to answer this question by analyzing samples of ligand structures from the PDB and assessing their geometric quality against the geometric information available in the Cambridge Structural Database [19]. This is a comprehensive database of small-molecule organic and metallo-organic X-ray structures (~500 000 in 2009), curated and compiled since 1965 by the Cambridge Crystallographic Data Centre. The small-molecule structures derived via X-ray diffraction are usually refined without use of restraints at the final step and so give accurate molecular geometries. The tool Mogul [20], a component of the Cambridge Structural Database System, can be used to analyze all the geometric features of a model structure (bonds, angles, torsions, and ring geometries) against those same features embedded within similar substructures and found in the CSD. The number of structures available in the CSD means that usually the appropriate chemical environment for the query feature is reasonably well represented.

Samples of ligands submitted either pre-2000 or in 2006 were looked at. Ligands with significantly unusual torsion angles were first identified using the criterion that less than 5% of the CSD-derived torsion distribution be found within 10° of the questionable ligand torsion angles. These cases were then analyzed further to see if other unusual geometric features were observed. Significantly unusual geometry was identified in 60% of the structures in the samples submitted pre-2000 and in 45% of structures in the sample from 2006. Unusual geometry cannot *per se* be considered incorrect in a way that is liable to mislead the user of the model, without other factors being considered. *Bona fide* strain of the ligand by the protein may occur in some cases. In others the error may relate to a small part of the ligand and correction of the error would result in no different interpretation of the complex. An objective assessment was therefore made on a case-by-case basis. Consideration was given to the fit to electron density, where available, and in addition, the interaction of the ligand with the binding site was surveyed to identify interactions that might stabilize a strained ligand. When examples of truly strained ligands were identified and excluded, giving the benefit of the doubt to the deposited structures in cases of uncertainty, it was still found that at least 25% of the structures in the pre-2000 sample and 16% in the 2006 sample could be considered "wrong." In other words, for these structures, it is almost certain that an alternative low-strain ligand model of significantly different geometry could be constructed, which is likely to fit the electron density equally well or better than the model deposited. There is an apparent improvement in ligand quality in the more recently submitted structures. The present work is aimed at expanding this study and checking if this improvement is real or a statistical blip.

4.2.2.6 **Erroneous Solvent**

Solvent in a protein model should be analyzed carefully as mismodeled solvent can mask larger scale errors in a protein. Davis *et al.* [3] refer to an interesting case where a fatty acid molecule was initially mismodeled as a solvent chain within a binding site. However, more subtle errors can occur. Elements with a similar molecular weight to oxygen can be misinterpreted as a solvent molecule; for example, sodium ions can be misinterpreted as solvent in a binding site. Finally, on occasions, a structural disordering of a side chain in a binding site can be misinterpreted as one or more solvent molecules.

4.2.3
Structural Relevance

Although a structure may be reasonably error free, there can still be issues that would make using a given structural model of questionable use in a virtual HTS campaign. For example, a structure that is determined at a pH far from that *in vivo* will be protonated differently from the biologically active form and in extreme cases can have a significantly different conformation.

4.2.3.1 The Biologically Relevant Unit and Crystal Packing

Another aspect of crystallography that modelers need to be aware of is that only the coordinates of atoms that form part of the asymmetric unit will be included in the final output. This means that the coordinates present in the PDB file may not represent the biological unit or may represent multiple copies of the biological unit. This is illustrated in Figure 4.3, which shows the backbone of three different entries of HIV protease (PDB IDs 1hhp [21], 1hsg [22], and 3gga [23]). The biological unit of HIV protease is a homodimer, and as such the 1hhp structure that only contains one chain would need to be symmetry expanded to get the biological unit. Information on the transformations required to generate the biologically active unit is often present in the PDB header (Figure 4.4). If no information on the biologically active unit is present in the PDB header, one can make us of PQS (protein quaternary structure file server) to predict it [24].

A related issue is that of crystal packing, where the pose of the ligand or the conformation of the binding site, or both, is affected by neighboring symmetry-related molecules. Many interesting examples where this is particularly pertinent, for example, PDB ID 1qs4 [25] (Figure 4.5), are highlighted by Bergner *et al.* [26] who also describe how Relibase [27] can be used to identify such crystallographic packing effects.

One also needs to consider whether the structural model is in the appropriate mechanistic state. Some targets (e.g., nuclear hormone receptor), can exist either in active or in inactive state. One can wish to design either antagonists or agonists for such targets. The appropriate state for use in vHTS depends on the mode of action desired.

A common mechanism of regulating the state of a protein is via phosphorylation/dephosphorylation (by kinases and phosphatases, respectively). Serine and threonine residues are the most commonly phosphorylated residues. Tyrosine residues can also be phosphorylated as can histidines. Other mechanisms of controlling the state of proteins include sulfonation and methylation (by sulfotransferases and methyltransferases, respectively). Such posttranslational modifications to the protein are key to the behavior of the target in question and a vHTS study should target the state of interest. One should also be wary of engineered proteins, where one or more residues may have been mutated to alter the biological behavior of said protein.

Some deposited structures in the PDB, such as binding proteins, may only represent part of the story. The biologically relevant unit may, in fact, be an aggregate of more than one chemically distinct structural domain; the crystal structure in the PDB may represent only one of these domains. An example is the set of matrix metalloproteinases (MMP) structures. Some MMPs are bound to hemopoxin moi-

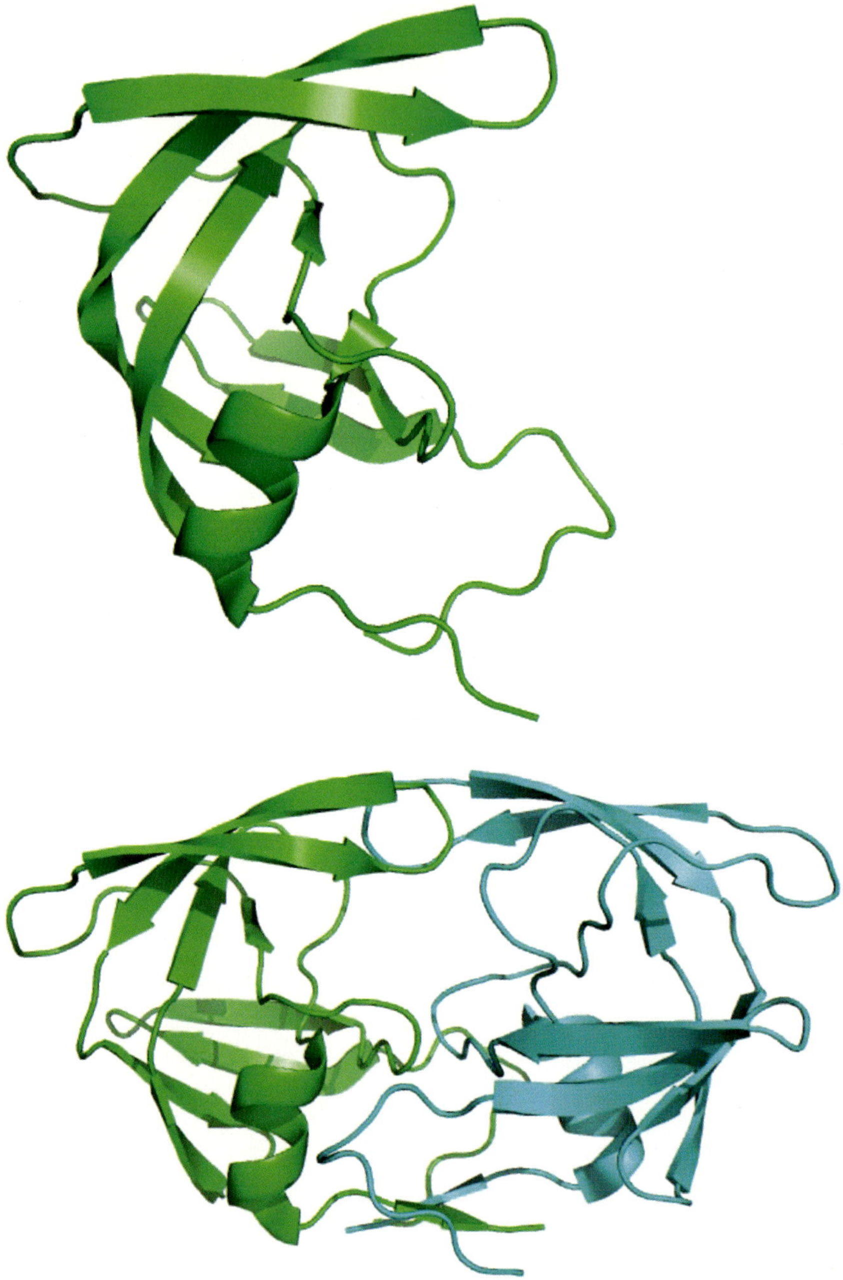

Figure 4.3 Symmetry and the biological unit of an HIV protease structure. (a) Backbone generated from coordinates in 1hhp only represent half of the biological unit. (b) Backbone generated from coordinates in 1hsg is equivalent to the biological unit. (c) Backbone generated from coordinates in 1gga contains three biological units.

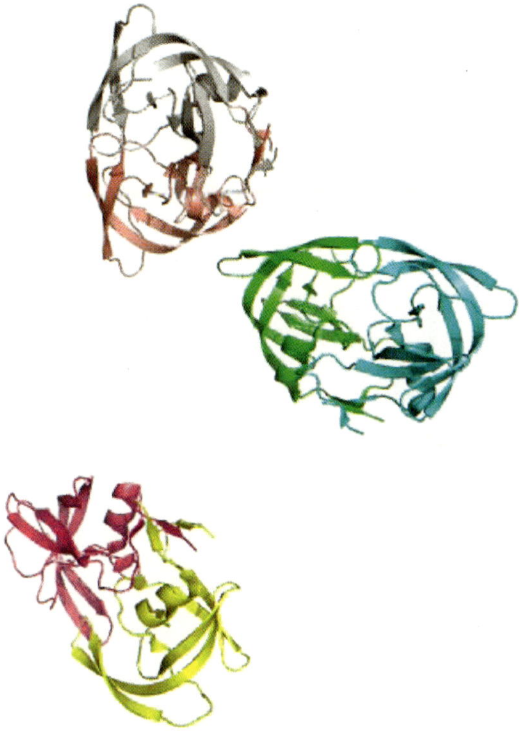

Figure 4.3 (*Continued*)

```
REMARK 300 BIOMOLECULE: 1
REMARK 300 THIS ENTRY CONTAINS THE CRYSTALLOGRAPHIC ASYMMETRIC UNIT
REMARK 300 WHICH CONSISTS OF 1 CHAIN(S). SEE REMARK 350 FOR
REMARK 300 INFORMATION ON GENERATING THE BIOLOGICAL MOLECULE(S).
REMARK 350
REMARK 350 GENERATING THE BIOMOLECULE
REMARK 350 COORDINATES FOR A COMPLETE MULTIMER REPRESENTING THE KNOWN
REMARK 350 BIOLOGICALLY SIGNIFICANT OLIGOMERIZATION STATE OF THE
REMARK 350 MOLECULE CAN BE GENERATED BY APPLYING BIOMT TRANSFORMATIONS
REMARK 350 GIVEN BELOW.  BOTH NON-CRYSTALLOGRAPHIC AND
REMARK 350 CRYSTALLOGRAPHIC OPERATIONS ARE GIVEN.
REMARK 350
REMARK 350 BIOMOLECULE: 1
REMARK 350 APPLY THE FOLLOWING TO CHAINS: A
REMARK 350   BIOMT1   1  1.000000  0.000000  0.000000        0.00000
REMARK 350   BIOMT2   1  0.000000  1.000000  0.000000        0.00000
REMARK 350   BIOMT3   1  0.000000  0.000000  1.000000        0.00000
REMARK 350   BIOMT1   2  0.000000  1.000000  0.000000        0.00000
REMARK 350   BIOMT2   2  1.000000  0.000000  0.000000        0.00000
REMARK 350   BIOMT3   2  0.000000  0.000000 -1.000000        0.00000
```

Figure 4.4 Extract of PDB header record for 1hpp.

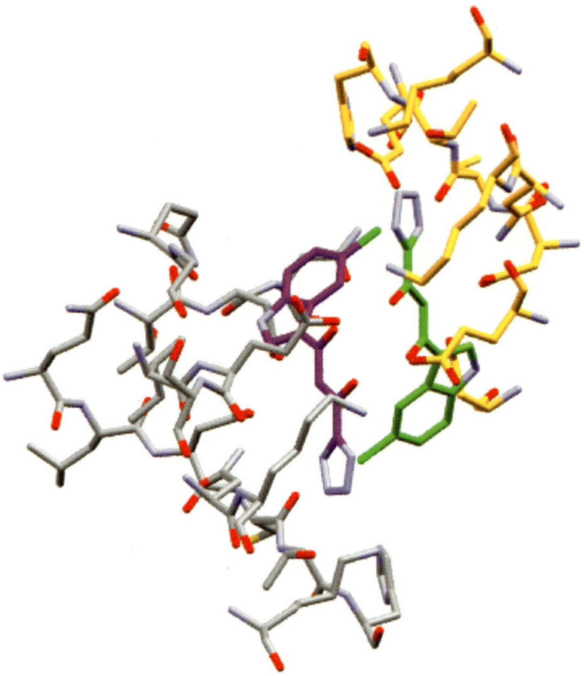

Figure 4.5 Example of how crystallographic packing effects can lead to ligand binding modes that are not biologically relevant. The yellow and green structure (PDB ID 1qs4: the catalytic core domain of HIV integrase) shows atom coordinates generated by expanding symmetry-related molecules.

eties in their active configuration, others are not. One needs to understand if a given structure actually represents the active form.

When selecting a structure for vHTS, one sometimes is presented with both "holo" and "apo" forms. An apo form is not biased by the presence of a ligand, and so may be regarded as the most suited option for vHTS. That said, an apo form may also be more closed than a system bound to a given ligand, so a docking program may miss *bona fide* binding modes due to steric clash that could, in reality, be alleviated by protein motion.

In summary, crystallographic symmetry brings up issues in terms of packing and the biological unit. In both cases, the modeler needs to make an informed decision on whether the model used is biologically relevant or not. Furthermore, it is important to understand the biochemistry underneath a protein when making a judgment as to its relevance for virtual screening.

4.2.4
Critical Evaluation of Models: Recognizing Issues in Structures

The original PDB file is a rich source of information for a modeler. Crystallographers do not intentionally include errors in structures; often, there will be known issues in the structure, which the crystallographer will have reported. Crystallographers include REMARK records in PDB files that can inform the reader of this.

```
REMARK 465 MISSING RESIDUES
REMARK 465 THE FOLLOWING RESIDUES WERE NOT LOCATED IN THE
REMARK 465 EXPERIMENT. (M=MODEL NUMBER; RES=RESIDUE NAME; C=CHAIN
REMARK 465 IDENTIFIER; SSSEQ=SEQUENCE NUMBER; I=INSERTION CODE.)
REMARK 465
REMARK 465   M RES C SSSEQI
REMARK 465     GLY A    289
REMARK 465     SER A    290
REMARK 465     SER A    291
...
REMARK 470
REMARK 470 MISSING ATOM
REMARK 470 THE FOLLOWING RESIDUES HAVE MISSING ATOMS (M=MODEL NUMBER;
REMARK 470 RES=RESIDUE NAME; C=CHAIN IDENTIFIER; SSEQ=SEQUENCE NUMBER;
REMARK 470 I=INSERTION CODE):
REMARK 470   M RES CSSEQI   ATOMS
REMARK 470     SER A 319     OG
REMARK 470     TYR A 320     CG    CD1   CD2   CE1   CE2   CZ    OH
REMARK 470     ARG A 341     CD    NE    CZ    NH1   NH2
REMARK 470     LYS A 345     CE    NZ
...
```

Figure 4.6 Remark records taken from PDB ID 2cdz showing information regarding missing atoms and missing residues.

Experimental details of crystallization are recorded in many header files, which can inform the would-be user of a structure of, for example, the pH at which the crystal was crystallized. This can aid in the interpretation of protonation states of residues around the binding site.

Often, one can find information about missing atoms and/or residues; for example, in the PDB file for entry 2cdz [28], we see remarks as shown in Figure 4.6. These have been automatically generated by the refinement program: the REMARK record indicates that some residues are missing in the structure, and that certain residues have side chain atoms that have been omitted. If these atoms are in proximity to the binding site, their omission could have an effect on docking.

If possible, the best way to critically analyze a structure is to go back to the original electron density map around the binding site region and view the residues placed in the calculated electron density. For newer public domain structures (where intensity data have been deposited in the PDB), the EDS server [29, 30] at Uppsala University can be used. This methodology was used recently to construct a test set of complexes for docking program evaluation [31]. Subsequent to publication, however, an undetected error was spotted in one entry, showing that checking the fit to electron density alone is not sufficient for validation. The entry in question was PDB ID 1jd0 [32]. In Figure 4.7, the acetazolamide ligand in entry 1jd0 is shown superimposed with the electron density generated by using a $2mF_o$-DF_c map (see Section 4.5.3) localized to show only the density around the ligand. This structure was elucidated at relatively high resolution (the resolution in the PDB file is cited as 1.5 Å). The map looks reasonably well defined. The chemistry of the ligand, however, is somewhat suspect. When the ligand is analyzed in Mogul [20], several issues are identified. The amide nitrogen subtends a C–N.am–C angle that is larger than would be expected. Similarly, the

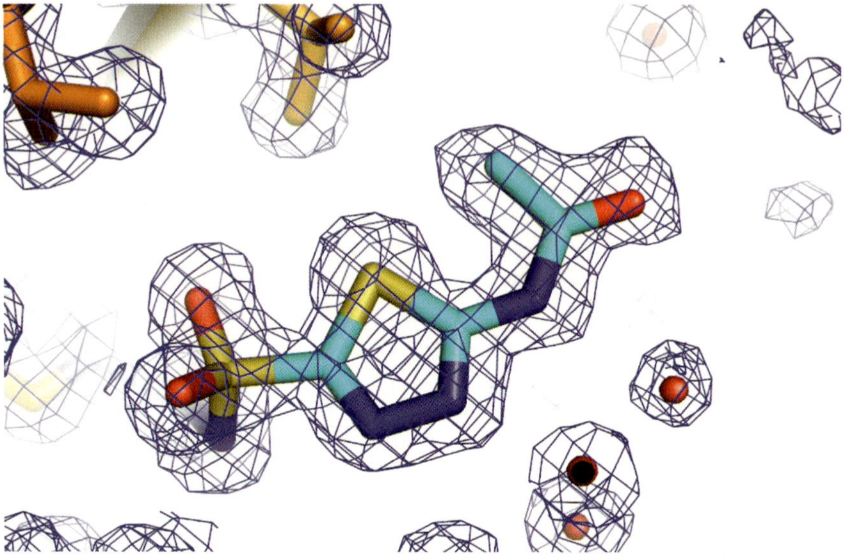

Figure 4.7 Good fit of electron density does not necessarily mean a correct atomic model. The image shows the atomic model of a ligand in entry 1jd0 overlayed with the electron density generated by using a $2mF_o$-DF_c map. The terminal amide group is incorrectly modeled, however, with the methyl group and oxygen switched in the electron density.

exocyclic C–C–N.am angle is also larger than suggested by Mogul. Mogul also recognizes that the amide occupies a *cis*-conformation. By flipping the amide torsion and adjusting the internal angles, a more chemically reasonable model is produced that fits the density equally well. Furthermore, switching the amide group in this way leads to a better stacking arrangement of GLN92 with the ligand amide group.

If looking at the electron density directly is impractical, then a critical evaluation of data in the PDB file can help. A single residue that is incorrectly assigned can sometimes be detected by looking at the temperature factors and occupancies of a given residue. If the occupancies for atoms in the residue have been set to zero or to low values, one should regard said residue with suspicion. Furthermore, very high or very low temperature factors can indicate problems with the overall modeling of a particular residue. Residues in such a form can reflect either incorrect assignment to the electron density (in which case the residue is not the amino acid specified) or a situation where there is a high degree of thermal motion or disorder in the structure, rendering resolution of atomic coordinates impossible.

One check that can be performed is to cross-validate the actual residue sequence as directly extracted from the atomic coordinates with independent references: entries in the PDB will habitually have a "SEQRES" field that lists the expected sequence. This, however, may have been generated from the atoms automatically. For public domain structures, one can cross-reference to independent sources of sequence data such as UniProt [33, 34]. Cross-referencing, however, only illuminates discrepancies; it does not tell the modeler the correct sequence.

Kleywegt, with coworkers, has published several papers on the subject of crystallographic validation [35, 36]. One interesting observation was that the error rate in structural studies seems to be positively correlated to journal impact factor, so "hotter" structures scientifically were more error prone. This, in all probability, reflects the urgency to publish a given structure.

Crystallographers use several global metrics to assess overall model quality. In recent years, validation tools have been developed to aid crystallographers in checking structures. Molprobity [7], WHAT_CHECK [9], and PROCHECK [8] will highlight specific errors, and will also allow the fixing of some errors automatically. As previously described, Mogul contains tools to validate conformations of ligands based on expected geometric preferences, as dictated by high-resolution crystal structures from the Cambridge Structural Database.

Residues that may be flipped (histidine, asparagine, and glutamine) in the region of the binding site should be closely scrutinized for reasons outlined above. Sometimes hydrogen bonding patterns can be used to identify flipped residues, but the right answer is not always certain. Indeed, in certain cases, the right answer may be that both models are equally likely. In such cases, one may wish to consider ensemble docking or a small degree of side chain flexibility to allow both models to be tested. Similarly, structural disordering can be treated either as multiple fixed conformations for flexible side chain docking or as a set of separate ensemble members.

For the modeler, another useful approach for detecting issues with a given structure is comparison with other similar structures around the binding site. Such an example where binding site superposition can be useful is seen in PDB ID 2bvr [37] (a thrombin protein–ligand complex). The structure was solved from very high resolution data (1.25 Å). In this structure, a sodium ion has been misassigned as a solvent molecule (HOH2340). Several characteristics signify that it is probably in error in this structure. HOH2340 has a temperature factor that is significantly lower than its local environment and forms relatively short contacts with the protein, and commensurate with metal–protein coordination. This can be seen easily using the Waterbase module in Relibase [27] (see Figure 4.8a). The coordination contacts around the solvent molecule occupy sites on a putative octahedron, suggesting that the solvent molecule is, in fact, a metal. Comparison with structures of a similar sequence via binding site superposition in Relibase (Figure 4.8b) further indicates that the site has been incorrectly assigned; many similar structures, such as PDB ID 3dhk [38], have a sodium ion at the same location.

4.3 Setting Up a Protein Model for vHTS

4.3.1 Binding Site Definition

Before docking can proceed, most docking programs require an approximate binding location to be defined. Most commercial software packages include tools for binding

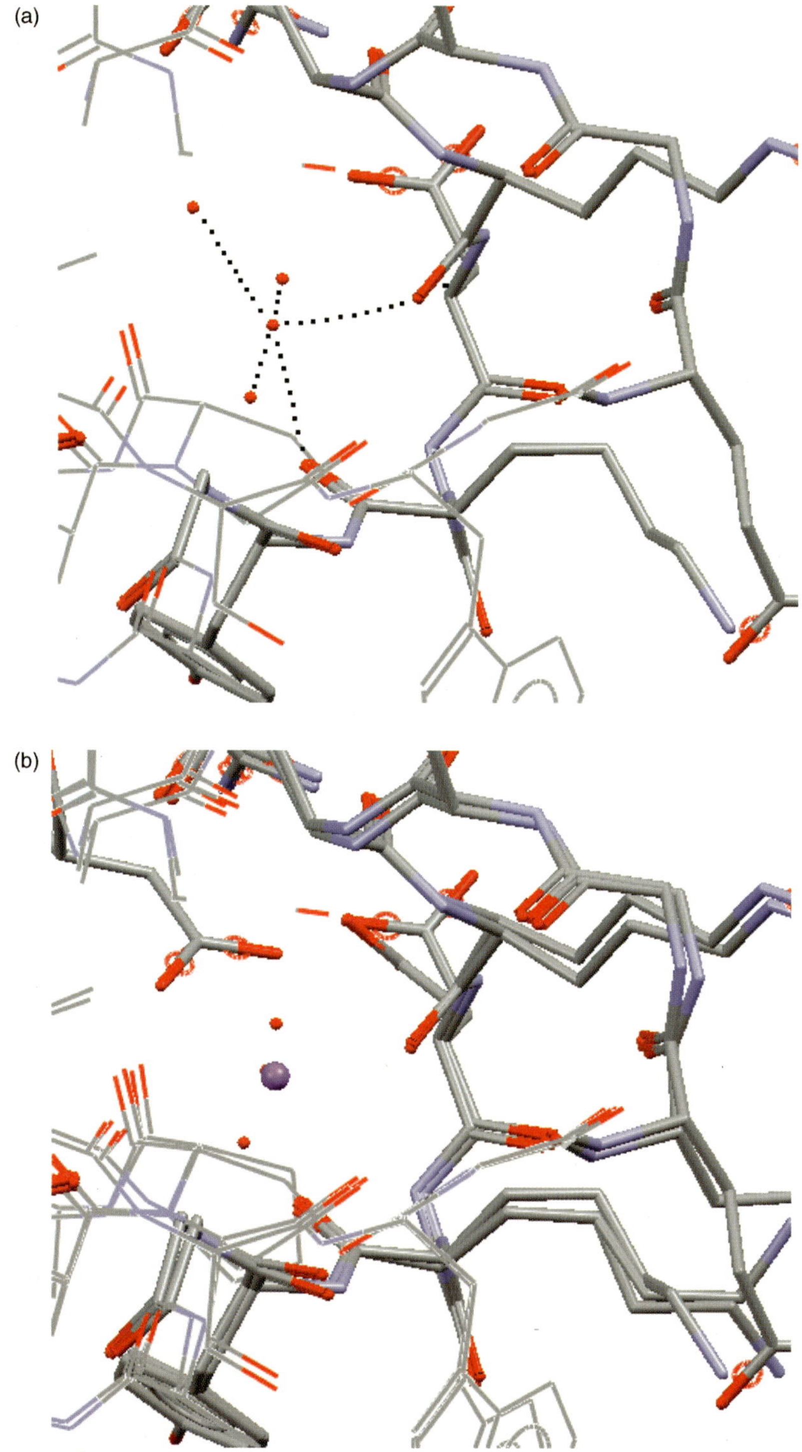
(a)
(b)

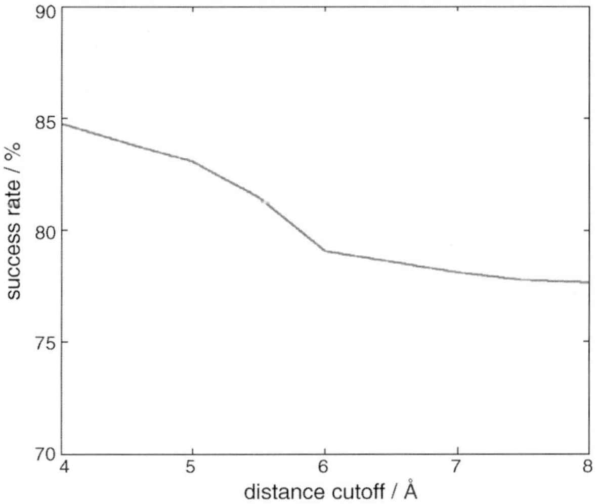

Figure 4.9 Docking success rate as a function of atoms included in the binding site. As the binding site gets larger, docking success falls due to the larger search space available for docking.

site detection using one of a number of published binding site detection algorithms. Current methods have been recently reviewed by Fuller et al. [39]. These algorithms give the user an idea of the location, extent, and shape of binding sites in a protein, but give little indication of the likelihood of a pocket being suitable for ligand binding [40]. Methods do exist for assessing pocket druggability (see, for example, Refs [39, 41]), but such methods are still at an early stage of development.

Once the binding region is selected, care should be taken with the actual definition of the binding site specified in the docking program of choice; the user needs to ensure that sufficient atoms are considered to allow unbiased docking of any possible ligand of a reasonable molecular size.

With the docking program GOLD [42, 43], for example, one can see quite large effects on docking success rates, depending upon atoms included in the binding site. By default, GOLD can be configured to do the binding site detection for the user automatically, but this mode can be switched off and the binding site can be specified manually. In Figure 4.9 we see the effect on pose prediction rates of specifying binding sites to contain protein atoms within a certain distance of the known bound ligand at a sequence of different distances. Success rates are shown for entries in the Astex Diverse Set [44].

High success rates are observed for short radii. The effect is, however, misleading: smaller spheres around the ligand reduce the search space and so focus

Figure 4.8 HOH2340 in 2bvr. (a) The atom is surrounded by five coordinating oxygen atoms at the points associated with an octahedral coordination sphere. (b) When the local environment is superimposed with a different high-resolution PDB ID (3dhk), we see an alternative atom type located at the same site, suggesting that the water in 2bvr has been misassigned.

docking very tightly on the region where the known ligand binds. Using a short radius in virtual screening may, inadvertently, discard ligands that use different binding modes.

4.3.2 Protonation

Standard pK_a values of the ionizable groups of the amino acids provide the simplest way of protonating a protein model at a given pH. For example, at pH 3.9 the carboxylic acid side chain of aspartate (pK_a of 3.9) will be 50% deprotonated, whereas at pH 4.9 and 5.9 it will be 90 and 99% deprotonated, respectively. This means that ionizable groups with pK_a values close to the pH of interest will be the most difficult to evaluate. As the pH environment of most proteins is around 7.4 (physiological pH), the imidazole side chains of histidine residues (pK_a of 6.0) are the ones likely to be the most difficult to evaluate. An issue that further complicates the protonation of proteins is the fact that the pK_a values of the amino acids are affected by their local environment. The imidazole group of histidine, for example, has been reported to have pK_a values ranging 7 units [45]. Many computational approaches have therefore been developed to estimate the pK_a values of ionizable groups of a protein from structural models. The methods are reviewed by Czodrowski *et al.* [46]. The methodologies include computationally expensive techniques such as the Poisson–Boltzmann equation [47] and the protein–dipole Langevin–dipole method [48], as well as fast empirical rule-based algorithms [49, 50]. It is possible to use any of these techniques to protonate the protein model before conducting a docking experiment. However, one should be aware that ligand binding alters the local environment of ionizable groups in the binding site, which can lead to changes in the protonation state of the protein [46]. An interesting recent development in the field is the introduction of a fast, empirical method of calculating pK_a values of ionizable groups in protein–ligand complexes [51]. However, as of yet there is no evidence that evaluating the protonation state of each protein–ligand complex would benefit protein–ligand docking. On the contrary, studies on the effect of protonation and tautomeric states of ligands have revealed docking to be relatively robust with regard to these types of structural variations [52, 53].

4.3.3 Treatment of Solvent in Docking

A perennial problem with docking is the treatment of bound solvent. In certain cases, a protein can contain a solvent molecule that is tightly bound to the protein. The modeler has to decide whether the water can be displaced on ligand binding. Thermodynamically, displacement of a solvent leads to a loss in binding enthalpy but an increase in configurational entropy [54]. The binding enthalpy is usually partially recovered by alternative interactions with the bound ligand. Hence, solvent can be displaced by a ligand when the recovered enthalpy, and the entropy gain, is sufficient to overcome the loss of the solvent–protein enthalpy. The problem is further complicated by ligand desolvation on binding, but in the case of a lone solvent molecule one could argue that the associated ligand desolvation is, in turn, compensated for by the solvent molecule solvation and so cancels out.

In most cases, solvent displacement is favored provided the ligand forms equivalent hydrogen bonds to the protein as the displaced water. There may, however, also be binding modes where a water molecule mediates an interaction between the protein and a ligand. Such binding modes need consideration in a virtual screen.

To tackle this problem, a docking software user has a number of possible paths. Tools such as GRID [55], HINT [56], or SuperStar [57, 58] can be useful for predicting how strongly bound a solvent molecule is at a given location using either force field-based or knowledge-based probes. In addition, there are empirical methods, such as Consolv [59] and WaterScore [60], that can be used for predicting whether a given water molecule is displaceable. Finally, one can use higher order methods such as double decoupling with replica exchange thermodynamic integration [61] to assess the free energy of binding of solvent molecules.

The user may wish to consider leaving strongly bound solvent molecules in place during docking. Weakly bound solvents may be removed. Alternatively, the user could choose to dock into both possible configurations for all ligands and pick the higher scoring poses for each ligand. In such an approach, the user may find it necessary to attempt to account for score attributable to solvent–protein contacts that would not be included in the water-bound docking score explicitly. Finally, some docking packages (e.g., GOLD [62]) allow explicit solvent modeling during docking in which case the problem can be automatically handled.

4.3.4
Use of Protein-Based Constraints in Docking

Many techniques for constraining docking have been developed for different docking programs; different docking programs will use different strategies to implement the constraints provided.

Constraints can be implemented as hard constraints or soft constraints. A hard constraint is strict, forcing all poses to obey the requirement specified. A soft constraint is implemented either as a penalty or as a reward function; dockings are penalized by some weighted score term if they do not conform to the desired constraint or rewarded if they do conform. This means the docking program can generate nonconformant poses, but these poses are down weighted in the score. Such constraints will often have harmonic or Gaussian-based penalty or reward functions, meaning that the scoring shift applied is less for poses that are close to being conformant with the constraint.

Broadly speaking, for the benefit of virtual screening, one can separate types of constraint into three categories (consult your docking program's documentation for details). Category 1 covers constraints that enforce specific interactions to the protein (see, for example, Ref. [63]). One specialization of this constraint is a covalent constraint: this allows a docking program to place ligands that are known to be covalently bound to the protein. Category 2 covers constraints that do not enforce direct interactions, but rather ensure that a specific region in space is occupied on docking. Category 3 covers constraints that enforce similarity to a known binding mode of a ligand (see, for example, Ref. [64]). In this category, there are scaffold-based constraints, where a known ligand scaffold is detected in each ligand and made to occupy the same site as an ideally placed scaffold. Alternatively, there are shape and interaction similarity constraints, motif-based constraints, and pharmacophore constraints. These constraints can be used to enforce similarity of binding mode without the need for equivalent substructures in a given ligand.

All three categories of constraint can prove useful in virtual screening as a means to incorporate known preconditions on the poses generated. For example, kinase inhibitors that target the ATP binding site bind to the adenine region of the binding site [65]. If such a condition is known for realistic binding modes, it can be useful to constrain docking to force solutions to contain the requisite interactions. The adenine binding region lends itself well to a motif constraint, where the docking algorithm is instructed to tolerate multiple possible binding motifs at the specified region.

Use of constraints is to be encouraged in virtual screening when the condition implied by the constraint is a known precondition for binding, but a user should consider that by constraining dockings one may preclude possible unknown modes of binding.

4.3.5
Protein Flexibility

Another important step is the selection of a single or even multiple protein structures to be used in the virtual screening campaign. The outcome of the screening may crucially depend on this selection. Like the ligand conformation, the protein conformation can change upon binding, which is also known as the *induced fit* effect [66]. Induced fit effects can be observed, for example, when comparing different holo structures of the same protein. *Protein kinase A* (PKA) will serve as an illustrative example for assessing the outcome of docking calculations when considering partial protein flexibility. Figure 4.10 illustrates changes in the binding site upon binding of ligand staurosporine (PDB ID 1stc [67]) and (*S*)-2-methyl-1-[(4-methyl-5-isoquinoline) sulfonyl]-homopiperazine (PDB ID 1q8u [68]). In the following sections, results for pose prediction and virtual screening will be discussed when applying a *rigid receptor, ensemble,* and a *flexible side chain docking* protocol. For the simplified virtual screening example, a single, arbitrarily chosen decoy molecule has been added as a third potential ligand that approximately matches the property distributions of the ligand in 1q8u. The *rigid receptor docking* protocol treats each protein structure independently, which means each ligand is docked into each structure and the average performance per protein structure is assessed. In the *ensemble docking* case, all results from the rigid docking protocol are used and for each ligand the best scoring function value obtained for the two protein structures is selected. Finally, the *flexible side chain* protocol resembles the rigid one, but the side chain of residue PHE327 is treated flexible.

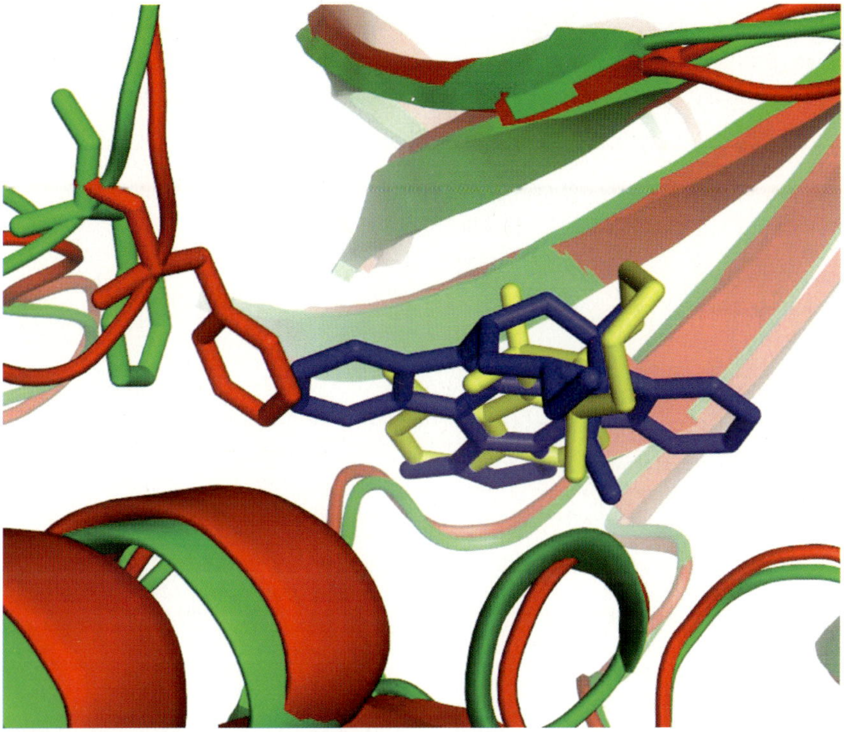

Figure 4.10 Superimposition of protein kinase A structures 1stc (green) and 1q8u (red) together with their cocrystallized ligands staurosporine (blue) and (*S*)-2-methyl-1-[(4-methyl-5-isoquinoline) sulfonyl]- homopiperazine (yellow). Ligand *staurosporine* shows a steric clash with the side chain of residue PHE327 in the nonnative protein structure 1q8u. The same side chain is also highlighted for the protein structure of PDB code 1stc.

4.3.5.1 **Pose Prediction**

The superimposition of the protein structures and the ligand binding modes shows a steric clash between ligand staurosporine and the side chain of PHE327 in protein conformation of 1q8u. Thus, using a rigid receptor hypothesis for this target is expected to result in a pose prediction failure when using only the protein conformation of PDB ID 1q8u that is confirmed by the cross-docking results presented in the upper part of Table 4.1. While the ligand of PDB ID 1q8u can be docked correctly into both protein structures, this is only the case for the protein conformation of PDB ID 1stc when docking ligand staurosporine. This results in an average pose prediction success rate of 50% for protein structure 1q8u and 100% for protein structure 1stc. In contrast, the ensemble docking protocol reaches a pose prediction success rate of 100% as the highest scoring function values for each ligand are observed for the conformation correctly predicted in their native protein structures. Also, when treating the side chain of residue PHE327 flexible, all ligand conformations can be predicted correctly in all protein conformations (see lower part of Table 4.1).

Table 4.1 *Protein kinase A* cross-docking results for rigid and flexible receptor docking (side chain of PHE327 flexible).

	Protein Structure	
Rigid receptor		
Ligand	**1q8u**	**1stc**
1q8u	**54.4** (0.5 Å)	50.6 (0.6 Å)
1stc	55.4 (3.0 Å)	**84.7** (0.2 Å)
Decoy	59.4	**61.0**
Flexible side chain		
1q8u	54.0 (0.6 Å)	51.0 (0.5 Å)
1stc	60.7 (0.6 Å)	83.0 (0.3 Å)
Decoy	58.8	61.7

For each docking experiment carried out with GOLD [43], the GoldScore value (higher is better) and the corresponding rmsd between the predicted and the experimentally observed ligand conformation are reported (except for the decoy molecule used in virtual screening). The ligand of PDB code 1q8u can be reproduced correctly in both receptor conformations (rmsd values given in brackets are below 1 Å), while the conformation of ligand staurosporine (PDB code 1stc) can only be predicted correctly in its native protein conformation (PDB code 1stc). Bold entries mark the scoring function values selected by the *ensemble docking* approach. When treating the side chain of residue PHE327 flexible (lower part), all ligand conformations can be predicted correctly.

4.3.5.2 **Virtual Screening**

The scoring function values obtained for the pose prediction experiments (see Table 4.1) can be used to derive virtual screening rankings as reported in Table 4.2. For this simplified virtual screening example, all protocols result in the same order, that is, ranking staurosporine best, then the decoy, and finally the ligand of PDB ID 1q8u, except when applying the rigid receptor protocol to protein structure 1q8u. The wrong pose of staurosporine when using the rigid receptor structure of 1q8u is also reflected in a bad scoring function value, which is nearly 30 scoring function units worse than the one obtained for its native protein structure 1stc. Although staurosporine is ranked better than the decoy when using the flexible side chain protocol for 1q8u, the difference in the scoring function value compared to the one in the native structure is still around 24 scoring function units, which can be attributed to overall less favorable interactions of staurosporine with the protein conformation of 1q8u. Thus, the best performing protocols in terms of maximizing the scoring function value difference between active ligands and the decoy molecule are the rigid receptor and flexible side chain docking protocol for protein structure 1stc as well as the ensemble docking protocol. Unfortunately, it is unlikely to know a priori that protein structure 1stc will show a better screening performance than 1q8u.

This simple example illustrates that the selection of the protein structure and also the explicit or implicit treatment of protein flexibility can have a large impact on docking results. Selecting a single receptor structure based on the assumption that all ligands bind to the same protein conformation can be misleading as observed for protein structure 1q8u. A priori it is usually unknown which single protein structure

Table 4.2 *Protein kinase A* virtual screening rankings obtained for the *rigid*, *ensemble*, and *flexible* docking protocols.

Protocol	Ranking
rigid 1q8u	DAA
rigid 1stc	ADA
rigid ensemble	ADA
flexible 1q8u	ADA
flexible 1stc	ADA

A, active; D, decoy.
Correctly predicted ligand conformations are colored green, while wrong ones are colored red. The optimum ranking is AAD.

will perform best in pose prediction and screening. As presented, the integration of side chain flexibility may improve results if limited conformational flexibility in the protein is sufficient. Nonetheless, there are two major problems associated with side chain flexibility. First, there are no guidelines for determining the selection of side chains that should be treated as flexible in the docking calculation except for expert knowledge of the target. Second, scoring side chain conformations is a difficult task as it also involves the scoring of intraprotein interactions. In this sense, an ensemble docking protocol seems to be more robust as it relies on scoring functions initially calibrated on rigid protein structures. In principle also, the large-scale protein movements as observed, for example, in p38 MAP kinase can be handled by this approach if a conformationally diverse set of protein structures is selected. However, it must be noted that the performance of this protocol also depends on the selection of the conformational ensemble as well as the scoring function used.

4.4 Summary

Protein structures are delightful to study, but equally enigmatic. This chapter highlights a number of specific features that need consideration when using protein structures in vHTS, but broadly these can be summarized into a small number of recommendations. These are as follows:

1) Understand the way in which the protein structure was elucidated and be sufficiently skeptical of what you see.
2) Understand the biochemistry of the system that you are dealing with, and consider if what you have is relevant to your problem.
3) Understand the dynamic nature of the system that you are dealing with, and consider if a single protein structure is sufficient.
4) If you are unsure of the structure, then do not be shy: talk to the primary source of the structure. Crystallographers are generally quite approachable; ultimately, they are keen to see use of the structures they provide.

5) Be careful when setting up the protein for vHTS to ensure that the model used is, as far as possible, correct.

4.5 Glossary of Crystallographic Terms

4.5.1 R-Factor

The R-factor of a crystal structure is a statistical measure of the deviation of the calculated intensity values (or more correctly the structure factors) from those observed in the diffraction pattern. R-free is the same measure, but calculated on a randomly selected cross-validation subset of reflections (typically 5–10% of the data set) that were omitted from the structural refinement.

4.5.2 Resolution

The resolution of a crystal structure reflects the degree to which a given crystal diffracted when analyzed. The resolution is quoted as a distance in Angstroms as it reflects the smallest d-spacing between diffraction planes. Lower angle reflections are separated by higher d-spacings, so a resolution with a larger value indicates that a crystal diffracted out to a lower 2θ angle. At the simplest level, one can draw a rough analogy to visible optics; a higher resolution lens allows viewing of more sharply defined image of a magnified object. Analogously, a higher resolution diffraction pattern allows generation of more easily interpretable electron density maps.

4.5.3 2mFo-DFc Map

A $2mF_o$-DF_c [69] map is a "σA weighted electron density map" used by crystallographers to illustrate the fit of the current model to the predicted electron density. The σA weighting here attempts to correct the map produced for missing atoms and poorly positioned atoms in the model. More information is available in Ref. [69] and references therein.

References

1 Brünger, A.T. (1997) Free R value: cross-validation in crystallography. *Methods in Enzymology*, **227**, 366–396.
2 Davis, A.M., Teague, S.J., and Kleywegt, G.J. (2003) Application and limitations of X-ray crystallographic data in structure-based ligand and drug design. *Angewante Chemie, International Edition*, **42** (24), 2718–2736.
3 Davis, A.M., St-Gallay, S.A., and Kleywegt, G.J. (2008) Limitations and lessons in the use of X-ray structural

information in drug design. *Drug Discovery Today*, **13** (19–20), 831–841.

4 Kleywegt, G.J. (2009) Practical Model Validation – EMBO Bioinformatics Course – Uppsala 2001, Uppsala University. Available at http://xray.bmc.uu.se/embo2001/modval/ and http://xray.bmc.uu.se/embo2001/modval/. Accessed January 29.

5 Berman, H.M., Westbrook, J., Feng, Z., Gilliland, G., Bhat, T.N., Weissig, H., Shindyalov, I.N., and P.E., Bourne. (2000) The Protein Data Bank. *Nucleic Acid Research*, **28**, 235–242.

6 Chang, G., Roth, C.B., Reyes, C.L., Pornillos, O., Chen, YJ., and Chen, A.P. (2006) Retraction. *Science*, **314** (5807), 1875.

7 Davis, I.W., Leaver-Fay, A., Chen, V.B., Block, J.N., Kapral, G.J., Wang, X., Murray, L.W., Arendall, W.B., III, Snoeyink, J., Richardson, J.S., and Richardson, D.C. (2007) MolProbity: all-atom contacts and structure validation for proteins and nucleic acids. *Nucleic Acids Research*, **35** (Web Server Issue), W375–W383.

8 Laskowski, R.A., MacArthur, M.W., Moss, D.S., and Thornton, J.M. (1993) PROCHECK: a program to check the stereochemical quality of protein structures. *Journal of Applied Crystallography*, **26**, 283–291.

9 Hooft, R.W.W., Vriend, G., Sander, C., and Abola, E.E. (1996) Errors in protein structures. *Nature*, **381**, 272–272.

10 Nissink, J.W.M., Murray, C., Hartshorn, M., Verdonk, V.L., Cole, J.C., and Taylor, R. (2002) A new test set for validating predictions of protein–ligand interaction. *Proteins*, **49**, 457–471.

11 Engh, R.A. and Huber, R. (1991) Accurate bond and angle parameters for X-ray protein structure refinement. *Acta Crystallographica A*, **47**, 392–400.

12 Kaneko, N., Ago, H., Matsuda, R., Inagaki, E., and Miyano, M. (1997) PDB ID 1hak. *Journal of Molecular Biology*, **274**, 16–20.

13 Grant, A.J. and Mulholland, I.M. (2007) Computational enzymology: insights into enzyme mechanism and catalysis from modelling, in *Challenges and Advances in Computational Chemistry and Physics: Molecular Materials with Specific Interactions: Modelling and Design*, Springer, The Netherlands.

14 Anderson, V.E. (2005) Quantifying energetic contributions to ground state stabilisation. *Archives of Biochemistry and Biophysics*, **433** (1), 27–33.

15 Taylor, N, and von Itzstein, M. (1994) Studies on ligand binding to Sialidase from influenza virus and the mechanism of catalysis. *Journal of Medicinal Chemistry*, **37** (5), 616–624.

16 Perola, E. and Charifson, P.S. (2004) Conformational analysis of drug-like molecules bound to proteins: an extensive study of ligand reorganisation upon binding. *Journal of Medicinal Chemistry*, **47**, 2499–2510.

17 Wlodek, S., Skillman, A.G., and Nicholls, A. (2006) Automated ligand placement and refinement with a combined force field and shape potential. *Acta Crystallographica D*, **62**, 741–749.

18 Warren, G. and Stahl, M. (2010) Methods for automated structure determination for ligands within a protein–ligand complex. MMS Technology Networks. Available at http//mmstechnologynetworksnet/posters/0266pdf and http://mms.technologynetworks.net/posters/0266.pdf.

19 Allen, F.H. (2002) The Cambridge structural database: a quarter of a million structures and rising. *Acta Crystallographica B*, **58**, 380–388.

20 Bruno, I.J., Cole, J.C., Kessler, M., Luo, J., Motherwell, W.D.S., Purkis, L.H., Smith, B.R., Taylor, R., Cooper, R.I., Harris, S.E., and Orpen, A.G. (2004) Retrieval of crystallographically-derived molecular geometry information. *Journal of Chemical Information and Computer Science*, **44**, 2133–2144.

21 Spinelli, S., Liu, Q.Z., Alzari, P.M., Hirel, P.H., and Poljak, R.J. (1991) PDB ID 1hhp. *Biochimie*, **73**, 1391–1396.

22 Chen, Z., Li, Y., Chen, E., Hall, D.L., Darke, P.L., Culberson, C., Shafer, J.A., and Kuo, L.C. (1994) PDB ID 1hsg. *Journal of Molecular Biology*, **264**, 26344–26348.

23 Degoey, D.A., Grampovnik, D.J., Flentge, CA., Flosi, W.J., Chen, H.J., Yeung, C.M., Randolph, J.T., Klein, L.L., Dekhtyar, T.,

Colletti, L., Marsh, K.C., Stoll, V., Mamo, M., Morfitt, D.C., Nguyen, B., Schmidt, J.M., Swanson, S.J., Mo, H., Kati, W.M., Molla, A., and Kempf, D.J. (2009) PDB ID 3gga. *Journal of Medicinal Chemistry*, **52**, 2571–2586.

24 Henrick, K. and Thornton, J.M. (1998) PQS: a protein quaternary structure file server. *Trends in Biochemical Sciences*, **23**, 358–361.

25 Goldgur, Y., Craigie, R., Cohen, G.H., Fujiwara, T., Yoshinaga, T., Fujishita, T., Sugimoto, H., Endo, T., Murai, H., and Davies, D.R. (1999) PDB ID 1qs4. *Proceedings of the National Academy of Sciences of the United States of America*, **96**, 13040–13043.

26 Bergner, A., Günther, J., Hendlich, M., Klebe, G., and Verdonk, M. (2001) Use of relibase for retrieving complex three-dimensional interaction patterns including crystallographic packing effects. *Biopolymers (Nucleic Acid Science)*, **61**, 99–110.

27 Hendlich, M., Bergner, A., Günther, J., and Klebe, G. (2003) Relibase: design and development of a database for comprehensive analysis of protein–ligand interactions. *Journal of Molecular Biology*, **326**, 607–620.

28 Eswaran, J., Lee, WH., Debreczeni, JE., Filippakopoulos, P., Turnbull, A., Fedorov, O., Deacon, SW., Peterson, JR., and Knapp, S. (2007) PDB ID 2cdz. *Structure*, **15** (2), 201.

29 Kleywegt, G.J., Harris, M.R., Zou, J.Y., Taylor, T.C., Wählby, A., and Jones, T.A. (2004) The Uppsala electron-density server. *Acta Crystallographica D*, **60** (12), 2240–2249.

30 Kleywegt, G.J. (2004) The Uppsala Electron-Density Server. Available at http://eds.bmc.uu.se/eds/ and http://eds.bmc.uu.se/eds/. Accessed January 1.

31 Hartshorn, M.J., Verdonk, M.L., Chessari, G., Brewerton, S.C., Mooij, W.TM., Mortenson, P.N., and Murray, C.W. (2007) Diverse, high-quality test set for the validation of protein–ligand docking performance. *Journal of Medicinal Chemistry*, **50**, 726–741.

32 Whittington, D.A., Waheed, A., Ulmasov, B., Shah, G.N., Grubb, J.H., Sly, W.S., and Christianson, D.W. (2001) PDB ID 1jd0. *Proceedings of the National Academy of Sciences of the United States of America*, **98**, 9545.

33 The Uniprot Consortium (2009) The Universal Protein Resource (UniProt). Available at http://www.uniprot.org and http://www.uniprot.org. Accessed January 1.

34 Jain, E., Bairoch, A., Duvaud, S., Phan, I., Redaschi, N., Suzek, B.E., Martin, M., McGarvey, P., and Gasteiger, E. (2009) Infrastructure for the life sciences: design and implementation of the UniProt Website. *BMC Bioinformatics*, **10**, 136.

35 Read, R.J. and Kleywegt, GJ. (2009) Case-controlled structure validation. *Acta Crystallographic D*, **65** (Part 2), 140–147.

36 Kleywegt, G. (2009) On vital aid: the why, what and how of validation. *Acta Crystallographica Section D*, **65** (2), 134–139.

37 Neumann, T., Junker, HD., Keil, O., Burkert, K., Ottleben, H., Gamer, J., Sekul, R., Deppe, H., Feurer, A., Tomandl, D., and Metz, G. (2005) PDB ID 2bvr. *Letters in Drug Design and Discovery*, **2**, 590.

38 Baum, B., Hangauer, D., Heine, A., and Klebe, G., PDB ID 3dhk.

39 Fuller, J.C., Burgoyne, N.J., and Jackson, R.M. (2009) Predicting druggable binding sites at the protein–protein interface. *Drug Discovery Today*, **14** (3/4), 155–161.

40 Hajduk, P.J., Huth, J.R., and Tse, C. (2005) Predicting protein druggability. *Drug Discovery Today*, **10** (23–24), 1675–1682.

41 Cheng, A.C., Coleman, G.R., Smyth, K.T., Cao, Q., Soulard, P., Caffrey, D.R., Salzberg, A.C., and Huang, E.S. (2007) Structure-based maximal affinity model predicts small-molecule druggability. *Nature Biotechnology*, **25** (1), 71–75.

42 Cole, J.C., Nissink, J.W.M., and Taylor, R. (2005) Protein–ligand docking and virtual screening with GOLD, in *Virtual Screening in Drug Discovery* (eds B. Shoichet and J. Alvarez), Taylor & Francis CRC Press, Boca Raton.

43 Jones, G., Willett, P., Glen, R.C., Leach, A.R., and Taylor, R. (1997) Development and validation of a genetic algorithm for flexible docking. *Journal of Molecular Biology*, **267**, 727–748.

44 Hartshorn, M.J., Verdonk, M.L., Chessari, G., Brewerton, S.C., Mooij, W.T.M., Mortenson, P.N., and Murray, C.W. (2007) Diverse, high-quality test set for the validation of protein–ligand docking performance. *Journal of Medicinal Chemistry*, **50** (4), 726–741.

45 Edgcomb, S.P. and Murphy, K.P. (2002) Variability in the pK_a of histidine side-chains correlates with burial within proteins. *Proteins: Structure, Function, and Genetics*, **49**, 1–6.

46 Czodrowski, P., Sotriffer, C.A., and Klebe, G. (2007) Protonation changes upon ligand binding to trypsin and thrombin: structural interpretation based on pK_a calculations and ITC experiments. *Journal of Molecular Biology*, **367**, 1347–1356.

47 Bashford, D. and Karplus, M. (1990) pK_a's of ionizable groups in proteins: atomic detail from a continuum electrostatic model. *Biochemistry*, **29** (44), 10219–10225.

48 Warshel, A. (1981) Calculations of enzymatic reactions: calculations of pK_a, proton transfer reactions, and general acid catalysis reactions in enzymes. *Biochemistry*, **20**, 3167–3177.

49 Wisz, M.S. and Hellinga, H.W. (2003) An empirical model for electrostatic interactions in proteins incorporating multiple geometry-dependent dielectric constants. *Proteins*, **51**, 360–377.

50 Li, H., Robertson, A., and Jensen, J. (2005) Very fast empirical prediction and rationalization of protein pK_a values. *Proteins: Structure, Function, and Bioinformatics*, **61**, 704–721.

51 Bas, D.C., Rogers, D.M., and Jensen, J.H. (2008) Very fast prediction and rationalization of pK_a values for protein–ligand complexes. *Proteins: Structure, Function, and Bioinformatics*, **73**, 765–783.

52 Todorov, N.P., Monthoux, P.H., and Alberts, I.L. (2006) The influence of variations of ligand protonation and tautomerism on protein–ligand recognition and binding energy landscape. *Journal of Chemical Information and Modeling*, **46**, 1134–1142.

53 ten Brink, T. and Exner, T.E. (2009) Influence of protonation, tautomeric, and stereoisomeric states on protein–ligand docking results. *Journal of Chemical Information and Modeling*, **49**, 1535–1546.

54 Ladbury, J.E. (1996) Just add water! The effect of water on the specificity of protein–ligand binding sites and its potential application to drug design. *Chemistry & Biology*, **3** (12), 973–980.

55 Goodford, PJ. (1985) A computational procedure for determining energetically favorable binding sites on biologically important macromolecules. *Journal of Medicinal Chemistry*, **28** (7), 849–857.

56 Spyrakis, F., Cozzini, P., Bertoli, C., Marabotti, A., Kellogg, G.E., and Mozzarelli, A. (2007) Energetics of the protein–DNA–water interaction. *BMC Structural Biology*, **7**, 4.

57 Verdonk, M.L., Cole, J.C., and Taylor, R. (1999) SuperStar: A knowledge-based approach for identifying interaction sites in proteins. *Journal of Molecular Biology*, **289**, 1093–1108.

58 Verdonk, M.L., Cole, J.C., Watson, P., Gillet, V., and Willett, P. (2001) SuperStar: Improved knowledge-based interaction fields for protein binding sites. *Journal of Molecular Biology*, **307**, 841–859.

59 Raymer, M.L., Shanschagrin, P.C., Punch, W.F., Venkataraman, S., Goodman, E.D., and Kuhn, L.A. (1997) Predicting conserved water-mediated and polar ligand interactions in proteins using a K-nearest-neighbors genetic algorithm. *Journal of Molecular Biology*, **265**, 445–464.

60 García-Sosa, A.T., Mancera, R.L., and Dean, P.M. (2003) WaterScore: a novel method for distinguishing between bound and displaceable water molecules in the crystal structure of the binding site of protein–ligand complexes. *Journal of Molecular Modelling*, **9**, 172–182.

61 Barillari, C., Taylor, J., Viner, R., and Essex, J.W. (2007) Classification of water molecules in protein binding sites. *Journal of the American Chemical Society*, **129** (9), 2577–2587.

62 Verdonk, M.L., Chessari, G., Cole, JC., Hartshorn, M.J., Murray, C.W., Nissink, J.W.M., Taylor, R.D., and Taylor, R. (2005) Modeling water molecules in protein–ligand docking using GOLD.

Journal of Medicinal Chemistry, **48**, 6504–6515.

63 Cole, J. (2003) Onward development of GOLD: selective dockings using known protein properties, in *EuroQSAR2002 Designing Drugs and Crop Protectants: Processes, Problems and Solutions* (eds M. Ford, D., Livingstone, J., Dearden, and H. Van de Waterbeemd), Blackwell, 140–143.

64 Fradera, X., Knegtel, R.M.A., and Mestres, J. (2000) Similarity-driven docking. *Proteins*, **40** (4), 623–626.

65 Liu, Y. and Gray, N.S. (2006) Rational design of inhibitors that bind to inactive kinase conformations. *Nature Chemical Biology*, **2**, 358–364.

66 Koshland, D.E. (1973) Protein shape and biological control. *Scientific American*, **229** (4), 52–64.

67 Prade, L., Engh, R.A., Girod, A., Kinzel, V., Huber, R., and Bossemeyer, D. (1997) PDB ID 1stc.

68 Breitenlechner, C., Gassel, M., Hidaka, H., Kinzel, V., Huber, R., Engh, R.A., and Bossemeyer, D. (2003) PDB ID 1q8u.

69 Read, R.J. (1986) Improved Fourier coefficients for maps using phases from partial structures with errors. *Acta Crystallographica A*, **42** (3), 140–149.

5
Pharmacophore Models for Virtual Screening

Patrick Markt, Daniela Schuster, and Thierry Langer

5.1
Introduction

Although the first definition of the pharmacophore as a concept for drug discovery has been attributed to Paul Ehrlich, recently van Drie [1] claimed that it was Kier who introduced it in a series of papers in the late 1960s and early 1970s [2–4] when describing common molecular features of ligands for important central nervous system receptors, followed by Höltje in 1974 [5]. The present definition of the pharmacophore concept was introduced by Wermuth *et al.* [6]: *A pharmacophore is the ensemble of steric and electronic features that is necessary to ensure the optimal supramolecular interactions with a specific biological target and to trigger or block its biological response.*

In early pharmacophore-based studies, computational models of pharmacophores were mainly deduced manually, assisted through the use of simple interactive molecular graphics visualization programs. Later on, the diversity and steadily growing complexity of molecular structures that characterize drug discovery led to the development of sophisticated computer programs for the determination, manipulation, and use of pharmacophore models. A considerable number of books, book sections, and reviews on the pharmacophore approach have been published [7–14], the most recent comprehensive one being by Leach *et al.* [15].

Today, 3D pharmacophore modeling is a well-established *in silico* technique providing several benefits for early drug design. First, pharmacophore models visualize chemical features that are supposed to be important for protein–ligand interactions and therefore for biological activity. Second, pharmacophore-based screening allows retrieval of ligands with structurally diverse bioisosteric scaffolds that would not have been discovered by systematic derivatization of existing compounds.

Pharmacophore-based screening is a virtual screening (VS) method used to automatically evaluate millions of compounds by computer programs [16]. A variety of applications for VS exist. It can be applied to obtain novel lead structures from corporate or commercial databases in early drug discovery, to search virtual

Virtual Screening. Edited by C. Sotriffer

ISBN: 978-3-527-32636-5

combinatorial databases for synthesizable structures in the lead optimization phase of drug development, or to predict new biological activities or side effects for existing drugs. Using VS before wet lab screening has proven to give significantly higher enrichments of active molecules than performing high-throughput screening (HTS). For instance, a study was published by Doman *et al.* [17] that described the comparison of HTS and VS performance based on molecular docking both aiming at the discovery of protein tyrosine phosphatase 1b (PTP1b) inhibitors. The HTS campaign resulted in a true positive hit rate of 0.02%, whereas a selection of 365 compounds by VS yielded 34.8% PTP1b inhibitors.

5.2 Compilation of Compounds

5.2.1 Chemical Structure Generation

2D structures of compounds used for pharmacophore modeling can be built using chemistry software such as ChemBioDraw Ultra [18] or the compound builder of molecular modeling suites such as DiscoveryStudio [19], MOE [20], and Maestro [21]. After structure generation, the correctness of chemical properties, for example, atomic valences, bond orders, aromaticity definitions, stereochemistry, charges, and protonation states at physiological pH, has to be checked before compounds can be applied for VS studies [9].

5.2.2 Conformational Analysis

Since 3D pharmacophore modeling is aiming at the discovery of biologically active compounds, the 3D structures of molecules used for pharmacophore modeling should represent the compound's conformer bound to the protein. These so-called bioactive conformations can be retrieved from crystal structures of protein–ligand complexes. However, only a limited number of cocrystallized ligands are available. Moreover, some crystallographers usually focus more on providing a precise representation of the overall protein structure than on accurately modeling the structure of the bound low molecular ligand into the experimentally derived electron density. On that account, the ligand structure of protein–ligand complexes is not always accurately resolved. Thus, computational programs are needed to predict the 3D structure of the bioactive conformer. Several studies have shown that the bioactive conformer is not necessarily related to the global energy minimum conformer and therefore cannot be obtained by simply calculating the conformer with the lowest strain energy. However, a set of diverse low-energy conformers has proven to be a good representation for the bioactive conformer [22–24]. Therefore, the generation of a conformational model for each compound consisting of low-energy conformers is a pivotal step in pharmacophore modeling.

For analysis of conformational space and generation of low-energy 3D structures, several conformer generators are available. Examples for popular software are OMEGA [25], ROTATE [26], and DS CATALYST CONFIRM [27].

5.3 Pharmacophore Model Generation

5.3.1 State of the Art

Several programs for pharmacophore modeling are widely used mainly because of their availability in commercial software packages, such as DS CATALYST [27, 28], GALAHAD [29], GASP [30], LIGANDSCOUT [31, 32], PHASE [21, 33], and the pharmacophore module of MOE [20]. In addition, many other pharmacophore elucidation algorithms have been described, especially in the last few years [34–42], probably as a reaction to the more and more disappointing performance of docking- and scoring-based VS approaches.

Basically, there are two approaches to generate pharmacophore models, depending upon the availability of information about the target's three-dimensional structure.

5.3.2 Structure-Based Methods

A structure-based pharmacophore modeling approach uses the information about protein–ligand interactions obtained from an experimentally derived 3D structure to generate a model. Structure-based methods in pharmacophore modeling have gained significant interest in the past 5 years since the number of protein–ligand crystal structures has grown constantly. They aim to be complementary to docking procedures, including the same level of information, but less demanding with respect to computational requirements and therefore much more efficient.

Traditional structure-based 3D pharmacophore models are directly derived from protein–ligand complexes using heuristics (e.g., LIGANDSCOUT) [31, 43] or from force field energy calculations, as in the grid-based pharmacophore model (GBPM) [44] approach or in FLAP [45]. The last two approaches utilize the widely validated program GRID by Goodford [46] for calculation of interaction energy hot spots.

In addition, several new approaches have been described, including the application of pharmacophore fingerprints for lead identification, for example, as implemented in the methods FLIP [47] and SIFt (structural interaction fingerprint) [48]. Such SIFts are 1D binary representations of the interaction patterns derived from a 3D protein–inhibitor complex. The fingerprint representation of the interaction patterns is compact and allows rapid clustering and analysis of massive numbers of complexes. For a group of structures binding to the same target protein, the receptor site is defined as the list of residues comprising the union of all residues involved in ligand binding over the entire library of structures. By default, seven different types of interactions occurring at each binding residue are extracted and classified. The resulting binary fingerprint can be extended to include the so-called p-SIFts (profile-based structural interaction fingerprints) [49]. This type of fingerprints use interaction profiles that provide a sensitive mean to compare and contrast multiple inhibitors binding to a drug target. Thus, a p-SIFt represents the degree to which interactions are conserved across a set of protein–ligand complexes.

5.3.3 Ligand-Based Methods

If no crystal structure of a protein–ligand complex is available, a pharmacophore model can also be derived from known ligands. In this case, either common chemical features of the so-called training set of active compounds are identified and translated into a model or a single compound serves as a template for pharmacophore elucidation.

Apart from commercial software such as DS CATALYST, GALAHAD, GASP, LIGANDSCOUT, MOE, and PHASE, which all offer algorithms for ligand-based pharmacophore elucidation, several new approaches have been described in literature. Among these, the approach by Young and coworkers [35] seems rather promising. Fingerprints of 3D features and a modification of Gibbs sampling to align a set of known flexible ligands, where all compounds are active, are used to discern possible pharmacophores. A clique detection method is used to map the features back onto the binding conformations. The basic algorithm is relatively fast and can easily deal with up to 100 compounds and tens of thousands of conformations, as shown in test sets of D2 and D4 ligands [35]. In a recent review, Schneider and coworkers [50] describe the application of alignment-free pharmacophore pattern using a correlation vector approach for several purposes in bioactive compound selection, similarity searching, and virtual library design. The concept of fuzzy 3D pharmacophores has been successfully exemplified in a study aimed at the discovery of novel ligands for RNA targets [51]. Translating the approach of fuzzy pharmacophores for the calculation of 2D fingerprints has been proposed by Horvath and coworkers [52] introducing a novel molecular description, the topological (2D) fuzzy pharmacophore triplets: 2D-FPT. This method uses the number of interposed bonds as a measure of separation between the atoms representing pharmacophore types (hydrophobic, aromatic, hydrogen-bond donor and acceptor, cation, and anion). It was recently used for establishing quantitative structure–activity relationships on a set of thermolysin inhibitors [53].

Feature trees as described by Rarey and Dixon [54] differ from most other descriptors in structure. The node-labeled tree structure is more closely related to the molecular than linear structures and implies, however, more complex comparison algorithms. The descriptor combines conformation independence with alignment dependence that makes it somehow unique. Alignment dependence is often seen as a disadvantage due to the more time-consuming comparison and the potential bias resulting from heuristic alignment schemes. Both arguments do not hold in the case of feature trees, since the optimal alignment can be computed within milliseconds by employing dynamic programming techniques.

5.3.4 Limitations of Ligand-Based Methods

In ligand-based pharmacophore generation procedures, there is always uncertainty about the binding mode and the selection of meaningful training sets for common-feature pharmacophore model generation or the choice of single ligands as templates for pharmacophore-based similarity screening. For example, training set ligands that are too flexible and therefore give rise to a large number of possible pharmacophores or active compounds that do not represent a popular binding mode can result in the generation of a common-feature model causing a low enrichment of active molecules in a virtual screen. Thus, an experienced computational chemist is needed to select a suitable training set. However, some developmental algorithms try to solve the training set selection problem in a fully automated way. One possibility is a pharmacophoric space-based clustering of compounds [1]. Such an automatic division of active ligands into groups of compounds with similar pharmacophoric pattern would allow easy generation of selective pharmacophore models. Furthermore, it would save time compared to a trial and error training set selection strategy.

5.4 Validation of Pharmacophore Models

As mentioned above, pharmacophore-based screening is a well-established *in silico* method for lead discovery in the early phase of drug design. In this phase, several compounds containing structurally diverse scaffolds are biologically evaluated to obtain structures that are subjected to medicinal chemistry optimization in the following drug design phases. To be of use for lead discovery, a good pharmacophore model should be able to enrich as many biologically active molecules from a structurally diverse molecule database as possible and to discard most of the inactive compounds. Several metrics exist that quantify this enrichment of actives on the basis of the results of pharmacophore-based screening of validation databases [9].

5.4.1 Chemical Databases for Validation

To evaluate the enrichment of a pharmacophore model, a proper set of active and inactive molecules has to be screened virtually. The generation of such validation databases is a difficult task. Ideally, a validation database should contain structurally diverse active compounds and inactive molecules that are structurally related to their

1) Wolber, G. (2009) Pharmacophore space-based clustering method implemented in LigandScout 3.0., personal communication.

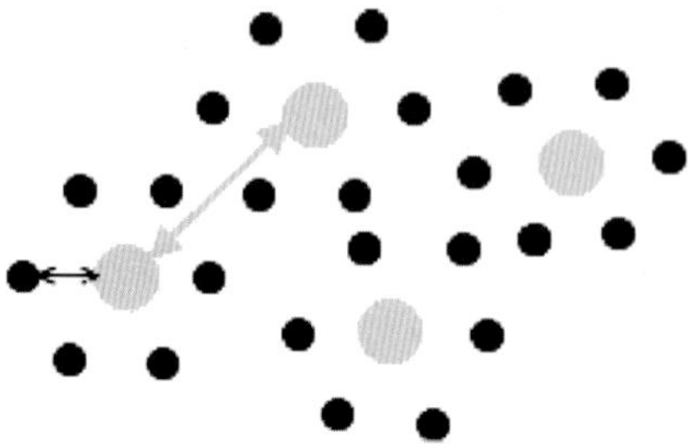

Figure 5.1 Chemical embedding of active molecules in an ideal validation database. A distribution of structurally diverse active compounds (gray) among inactive molecules (black) structurally related to actives but distant to other inactive compounds avoids artificial enrichments in model validation.

active analogues but structurally distant to their inactive neighbor molecules (Figure 5.1) [55].

With such a distribution of active molecules among inactive compounds, artificial enrichments can be eliminated. Artificial enrichments can be accomplished by a validation database consisting of inactive molecules structurally completely different from active molecules. When a model is screened against such an inappropriate validation database, the hit list will always contain a high ratio of active molecules since it would be more difficult for the model to match the chemical scaffold of any inactive molecule than to fit to the structure of another active compound [56]. Furthermore, a training set including active molecules comprising only one chemical scaffold can cause the so-called "analogue bias." In other words, the pharmacophore model will not be applicable to scaffold hopping but will produce high enrichments since it discards all compounds different from the single scaffold from which it has been derived [55, 57]. The artificial enrichment and analogue bias both contribute to inaccurate predictions of the discriminatory power of VS applications including pharmacophore modeling [55].

Except for the problem of appropriate chemical embedding of active molecules, the generation of proper validation databases can also be complicated by the lack of experimentally verified and publicly available active molecules for the target protein of interest. In the past, most databases containing data of experimentally determined molecules have been commercially available only (e.g., the Derwent World Drug Index [58], the WOMBAT database [59], and the MDDR database [60]). However, recently, the ChEMBL database [61], successor of the StarLite database, has been thrown open for public use. The database contains 2D structures of 622 824 bioactive, drug-like, and small molecules (version 02). In addition, physicochemical properties and data on biological testing (e.g., assays, binding constants, etc.) are included. The data of this exhaustive database of druglike compounds was extracted from literature.

Obtaining structural data of biologically tested inactive molecules is even more challenging. A limited number of inactive molecules have been published in literature. Thus, some computational chemistry groups used compounds structurally similar to actives but experimentally not tested for biological activity as putative inactive molecules or the so-called "decoys." A prominent validation database generated using decoy molecules is the Directory of Useful Decoys (DUD) [62]. To build this directory, 2950 active molecules for 40 proteins were derived from literature. For each of the 2950 actives, 36 decoys were added to the database. For this purpose, a total of 95 316 decoys were obtained from a set of drug-like commercially available compounds [62]. However, Irwin [63] reported several benchmark biases (e.g., analogue bias) discovered in the DUD database. Moreover, this fact cannot be denied that some of the commercial compounds used as decoys have biological activity for the corresponding target protein.

Recently, the Maximum Unbiased Validation data set (MUV) data set was published [55]. This publicly available validation database addresses both problems of the DUD. Its inactive molecules have been biologically tested on the target protein and the ideal distribution of actives avoids biases of enrichment assessments. For MUV generation, sets of active and inactive molecules were obtained from the PubChem database [64]. The PubChem offers publicly accessible data of primary HTS screenings and secondary low-throughput screenings serving as confirmation of HTS data. Biological data for more than 900 proteins are available for download at the PubChem homepage. However, the MUV contains only 18 target proteins due to lack of data matching the stringent filter criteria applied for compound selection. Each of these 18 MUV targets are represented by 30 active molecules selected from confirmatory screening data containing EC_{50} values and 15 000 inactive molecules obtained from HTS data [55]. The MUV is a promising validation database for VS methods. It contains well-distributed sets of active and inactive molecules, all molecules are experimentally tested, and each data set includes the same number of active and inactive molecules. On the other hand, the selection of only 18 target proteins may limit the scope of application for VS validation.

5.4.2 Enrichment Assessment

Once a proper validation database has been generated, the enrichment of actives caused by a pharmacophore model can be predicted by different methods. It can be either expressed as a single value or as a graph providing an overview of the enrichment for all possible hit list cutoffs. All enrichment-assessing methods are based on the following assumption:

In the case of a virtual screen where a pharmacophore model selects n compounds from a database comprising N molecules, a low percentage of selected compounds will possess biological activity (Figure 5.2). In terms of enrichment assessment, such compounds are named true positives (TP). The larger part of the pharmacophore-based hit list will consist of molecules that match the model features but are not biologically active. These compounds are falsely recognized as positives and thus named false positives (FP). Database molecules that are not retrieved by the pharmacophore model and do not show biological activity are true negatives (TN). Finally, database molecules will also exist that are not matched by the model although they are able to cause a biological response (false negatives) [9].

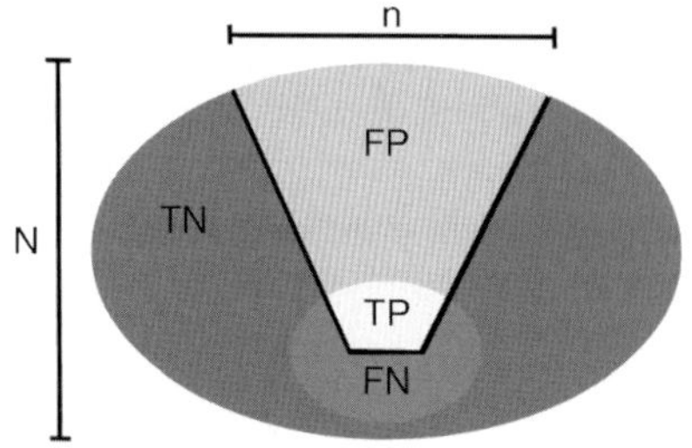

Figure 5.2 Schematic of a pharmacophore-based selection of n molecules from a database comprising N entries. The FP and TP database fraction represents the compounds obtained by a virtual screen.

5.4.3 Enrichment Metrics

Enrichment metrics are frequently derived from two basic values, the sensitivity (Se) and the specificity (Sp). Se or true positive rate is the ratio of the number of selected active molecules and the number of all biological active database molecules (5.1) [9, 65].

$$\mathrm{Se} = \frac{\text{selected actives}}{\text{all actives}} = \frac{\mathrm{TP}}{\mathrm{TP}+\mathrm{FN}} \tag{5.1}$$

Sp or false positive rate describes the ability of a pharmacophore model to discard inactive compounds. It is defined as the ratio of inactive molecules not selected by the model and all inactive molecules (5.2) [65].

$$\mathrm{Sp} = \frac{\text{discarded inactives}}{\text{all inactives}} = \frac{\mathrm{TN}}{\mathrm{TN}+\mathrm{FP}} \tag{5.2}$$

An outline of well-known enrichment metrics is provided in Table 5.1.

The Accuracy (Acc) is used to correctly determine the amount of database molecules classified by the pharmacophore model [66–68]. Another metric for calculating the correctness of compound classification by a model is the balanced labeling performance l_{bal}. For this metric, a value of 1 means that all active and inactive molecules have been correctly identified [69, 70]. If the biological activity of some database molecules has not been measured, the analysis of efficiency (AE) can be used for enrichment assessment. In the AE equation, the term U_s/U_t describes the ratio of compounds with unknown activity selected by the model and all molecules with missing activity data [71]. In contrast to the metrics mentioned above, Ford's M contains an adjustable weight ω. If $\omega = A/N = 1/2$ and $U_s = 0$, Acc, l_{bal}, AE, and Ford's M are equal [9, 72]. Further metrics for assessing VS success are the discrimination ratio (DR), the information content (I), and the "Matthews" correlation coefficient (C) [73–76]. Using C for enrichment assessment, a perfect pharmacophore model that selects only active compounds and discards all inactive molecules would obtain a value of 1. In particular created for determining the

Table 5.1 Definitions of several well-known enrichment metrics.

Enrichment metric	Equation	References
Accuracy	$\mathrm{Acc} = \frac{\mathrm{TP}+\mathrm{TN}}{N} = \frac{A}{N} \cdot \mathrm{Se} + \left(1-\frac{A}{N}\right) \cdot \mathrm{Sp}$	[66–68]
Balanced labeling performance	$l_{\mathrm{bal}} = \frac{1}{2} \cdot \mathrm{Se} + \frac{1}{2} \times \mathrm{Sp}$	[69, 70]
Analysis of efficiency	$\mathrm{AE} = \frac{1}{2} \cdot (\mathrm{Se} + \mathrm{Sp}) \cdot \left(1-\frac{\mathrm{U_s}}{\mathrm{U_{total}}}\right)$	[71]
Ford's M	$M = \omega \cdot \mathrm{Se} + (1-\omega) \cdot \mathrm{Sp}$	[9, 72]
Discrimination ratio	$\mathrm{DR} = \frac{\mathrm{TP}/A}{\mathrm{TN}/(N-A)} = \frac{\mathrm{Se}}{\mathrm{Sp}}$	[73]
Information content	$I = \mathrm{TP} \times \log\left(\frac{\mathrm{TP}}{\mathrm{FP}}\right) + \mathrm{FN} \cdot \log\left(\frac{\mathrm{FN}}{\mathrm{TN}}\right)$	[74]
Matthews correlation coefficient	$C = \frac{\mathrm{TP}\times\mathrm{TN}-\mathrm{FN}\times\mathrm{FP}}{((\mathrm{TN}+\mathrm{FN})\times(\mathrm{TN}+\mathrm{FP})\times(\mathrm{TP}+\mathrm{FN})\times(\mathrm{TP}+\mathrm{FP}))^{1/2}}$	[75, 76]
Goodness of hit list	$\mathrm{GH} = \left(\frac{3}{4}\mathrm{Ya} + \frac{1}{4}\mathrm{Se}\right) \times \mathrm{Sp}$	[7]
Yield of actives	$Ya = \frac{TP}{n}$	[7, 9, 66]
Enrichment factor	$\mathrm{EF} = \frac{\mathrm{TP}/n}{A/N}$	[9, 66, 77, 78]

discriminatory power of pharmacophore models, the Goodness of Hit List (GH) is not only based on Se and Sp but also includes a term named yields of actives (Ya). Ya is a popular metric, although it does not include information about the consistence of the molecule database and simply describes the ratio of active molecules among all compounds selected by the model. Since the definition of GH contains a higher weight for Ya than for Se, GH favors discarding inactive molecules over retrieving as much active database compounds as possible [7, 9, 66].

The enrichment factor (EF) represents another frequently used enrichment metric. The EF shows how many times more active molecules are retrieved by the pharmacophore model than by a random selection of the same number of compounds [9, 66, 77, 78]. Thus, an EF value of 1 corresponds to a model performing equal to random and EF value >1 is obtained for model-based compound selections containing more actives than random. The EF is an easy to read metric displaying the enrichment improvement compared to random. However, if the EF is used for enrichment assessment, the computational chemist should keep in mind that it suffers from two significant drawbacks. First, the EF highly depends on the ratio of active molecules in the database. Therefore, EF values obtained for pharmacophore models that have been validated by screening validation databases with different ratios of actives cannot be used for comparing VS performance. Only EF values determined by screening the same validation database will allow an exact comparison of pharmacophore model efficiency [65, 79]. Second, the EF does not possess a weight that favors active molecules ranked at the top of the hit list by a model-to-compound alignment score. This so-called "early recognition" problem in VS is important if all compounds of the hit list cannot be biologically evaluated [79]. In this case, the EF cannot discriminate between a hit list where all actives have the best alignment scores and a hit list with top-ranked inactive compounds and only low-ranked active molecules.

5.4.4
Receiver Operating Characteristic Curve Analysis

Enrichment metrics provide a single value that allows comparison of the discriminatory power of different pharmacophore models. This is a fast and convenient way of selecting the best performing pharmacophore model. However, if not all molecules from the pharmacophore-based hit list can be subjected to biological evaluation, a specific number of top-ranked hit list compounds have to be selected. To determine the hit list cutoff that leads to a compound selection with the optimal ratio of actives to inactive molecules, a validation method is needed that gives an easy to read enrichment overview for all possible thresholds. For this purpose, the receiver operating characteristic (ROC) curve analysis can be used. The ROC curve method is based on a hit list ranked by model-to-compound alignment scores and starts with the top-scored compounds. For all possible score thresholds, the Se and Sp values are calculated by determining the number of active and inactive molecules. Subsequently, all Se values are plotted as a function of 1-Sp (Figure 5.3) [65].

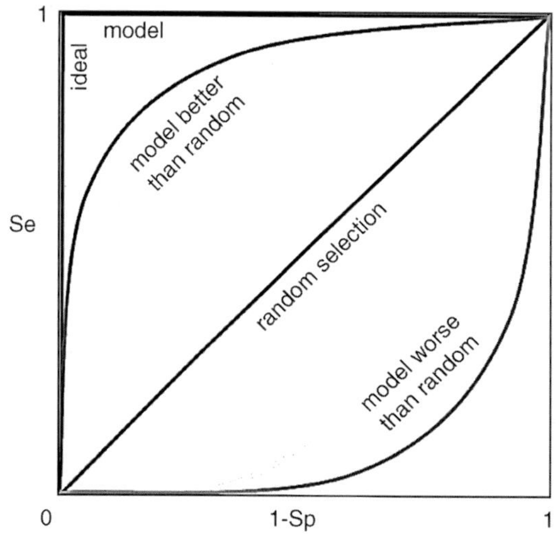

Figure 5.3 ROC curves. A random selection results in a curve that asymptotically tends toward the Se = 1-Sp line. An ideal pharmacophore-based virtual screen causes a straight vertical line between the origin and the upper left corner until all actives are selected. Afterward, scoring of remaining inactive molecules results in the continuation of the curve to the upper right corner. An ROC curve between the ideal and the random curve represents a model performing better than random, whereas curves located in the area below the Se = 1-Sp line indicate a discriminatory power of the model lower than a random selection.

Since in pharmacophore-based VS only a part of the database molecules matches the model and therefore obtains an alignment score, a limited number of Se and 1-Sp values can be calculated and plotted. Thus, a selective model would result in an ROC curve that starts at the origin and finishes before it reaches the upper right corner where all active and inactive molecules are scored. However, to simplify the explanation of the ROC curve method, we suggest that the model would retrieve and score all database molecules, either because all database molecules are very similar or because partial matching of model features is allowed. In this case, an ideal pharmacophore model will score all actives higher than inactive database molecules. The corresponding ROC curve will start at the origin and go straight to the upper left corner where all active molecules are scored by the model. Afterward, only inactive compounds are available and the ROC curve will continue as a horizontal line to the upper right corner until all database molecules are scored. If no pharmacophore model is used for screening and the compounds are randomly selected, the ROC curve will tend toward the diagonal between the origin and the upper right corner asymptotically. A pharmacophore model that enriches more actives than a random selection will give an ROC curve located between the Se = 1-Sp diagonal (random) and the ideal ROC curve, whereas the ROC curve for a model performing worse than random will be situated below the Se = 1-Sp line [65].

As mentioned above, the ROC curve gives an intuitive overview of the VS performance allowing the selection of hit list cutoffs by simply looking at the slope of the curve. An ROC curve with a steep slope at the beginning shows a high enrichment of actives among the top-ranked hit list compounds. If the slope decreases, a cutoff can be made for the number of top-ranked compounds. Another advantage of the ROC curve method is the easy comparability between the selectivity of two models. As long as the ROC curves of two models do not cross each other, the model causing the curve with the steeper slope has the better overall screening performance. Finally, since the ROC curve method does not depend on the ratio of actives in the molecule database used for enrichment assessment, it also allows a comparison of two pharmacophore models validated by screening different databases [65, 80].

5.4.5
Area Under the ROC Curve

If tens or hundreds of models have to be validated, a simple metric providing a value can be more comfortable for enrichment comparison than the visual analysis of tens or hundreds of ROC curves. For this purpose, a metric also derived from the area under the ROC curve (AUC) exists. The AUC value can be obtained by simply adding the areas of rectangles formed by Se and 1-Sp for the ith active molecule (5.3) [65].

$$\mathrm{AUC} = \sum_i [(\mathrm{Se}_{i+1})(\mathrm{Sp}_i\text{-}\mathrm{Sp}_{i+1})] \tag{5.3}$$

A pharmacophore model can obtain an AUC value between 0 (ranking all inactive molecules first) and 1 (ranking all actives first). An AUC value of 0.5 refers to a random selection. Thus, an AUC value of >0.5 has to be determined for a pharmacophore model useful for VS [65]. If the pharmacophore model does not score all database molecules because its features match only a subset of the compounds, as it is the common case in VS practice, the AUC for a specific fraction of top-ranked molecules can be determined. For example, the AUC for the top-ranked 25% of false positives can be measured and divided by 0.25 to obtain the AUC25 value that is also limited by 0 and 1 (Figure 5.4) [81].

Active molecules ranked top in the hit list contribute more to the AUC than other actives do. Thus, to some extent, a higher AUC value means a higher early recognition of active molecules. However, if the ROC curves cross each other, there are some cases where the early recognition ability of two different models cannot be determined using the AUC (Figure 5.5) [80, 82].

On that account, the ROC curve is more useful than the AUC if the best model for addressing the early recognition problem has to be selected.

To sum up, a variety of enrichment metrics for evaluating VS methods are available. Among these enrichment metrics, the EF and the AUC value, as well as visualizations of ROC curves, represent popular methods for assessing the enrichment of active molecules by pharmacophore models [83–85]. The two disadvantages of many of these enrichment metrics are the lack of information about early enrichment of active molecules and the missing comparability between validation

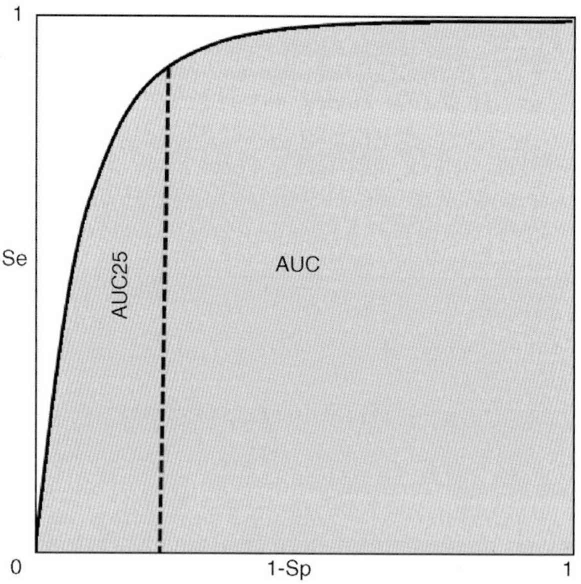

Figure 5.4 The AUC value represents the area under the ROC curve and is limited by 0 and 1. Since pharmacophore-based screening mostly results in the selection of a limited number of database molecules that are subjected to alignment scoring, the AUC, not for all database molecules but for a top-ranked fraction of false positives, such as the AUC25, can serve as enrichment metric.

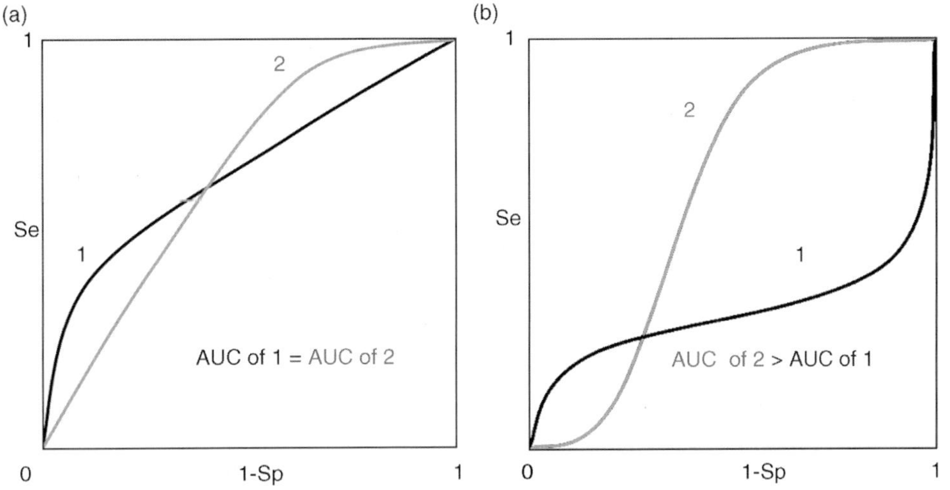

Figure 5.5 Comparison of AUC values obtained for two pharmacophore models. The AUC can give a clue which model has the better early recognition of active molecules. However, if ROC curve 1 that has a steep slope at the beginning is cutting across ROC curve 2, which starts with a small slope, the AUC of curve 1 does not necessarily have to be larger than the AUC of curve 2. In fact, the AUC of curve 1 can also be equal to (a) or smaller (b) than the AUC of curve 2.

results gained by screening molecule databases with different ratio of actives. The ROC curve does not suffer from these two drawbacks and thus represents an interesting and easy to interpret validation method [65, 80].

5.5 Pharmacophore-Based Screening

As mentioned above, DS CATALYST, GALAHAD, GASP, LIGANDSCOUT, MOE, and PHASE represent popular pharmacophore modeling algorithms applied for lead discovery. Although their pharmacophore-based screening algorithms may differ in detail, the common rationale of all these screening tools is the use of a pharmacophore model as query for a virtual screen of databases consisting of 3D structures of small molecules [86]. The single database molecules are usually represented by a set of conformers that are ideally closely related to the molecule conformer responsible for the biological interaction with the target protein. If the database is virtually screened, all conformers that match a user-specified number of model features are stored in a hit list [9]. Depending on the selectivity of the pharmacophore-based model, such a virtual screen of chemical databases consisting of millions of small molecules can result in tens to thousands of hits [15]. For the latter case, especially for academic research where usually only a limited number of molecules can be subjected to biological testing, an additional filter criterion is needed. For this purpose, pharmacophore-based screening algorithms allow calculation of a score determining the quality of the match between the pharmacophore model and each molecule of the VS hit list [9]. The following sections describe the generation of this alignment score and the pharmacophore-based screening algorithms of DS CATALYST, GALAHAD, GASP, LIGANDSCOUT, MOE, and PHASE.

5.5.1
DS CATALYST

First, DS CATALYST performs a fast filtering of database conformers including, for example, feature type and interfeature distance matches between pharmacophore model and the geometries of the database conformers. To be considered as a possible pharmacophore–molecule match, either all chemical features of the model or a user-specified number of model features have to be mapped by the conformer of the database molecule. Second, if all pharmacophore–molecule matches are determined, the distances between the conformer and the model are minimized. For this fitting step of the pharmacophore-based screening, DS CATALYST offers three options. The "Rigid" and "Flexible" fitting options use the Kabsch algorithm [87] for minimizing the distance between model features and chemical functions of the molecule conformer. "Flexible" fitting generates new and energetically optimized conformers before starting Kabsch distance minimization, whereas only existing conformers are used for Kabsch calculations if the "Rigid" option is selected. The third fitting option, "None," does not perform any distance minimization [27].

After distance minimization, the so-called fit value that is DS CATALYSTs score for measuring the quality of the pharmacophore–molecule mapping, is calculated. For each pharmacophore model feature f, the product of the user-specified weight of the feature weight(f) and the accuracy of its mapping on the corresponding chemical group of the conformer SSE(f) is calculated (5.4). SSE(f) is needed to take the so-called location constraint c of the model feature into consideration for fit value calculations. The location constraint is a sphere around the model feature that represents the space where a chemical group has to be located to be mapped by the feature. SSE(f) is expressed as the square of the ratio between the displacement of the matching chemical function of the conformer from the center of the model feature $D(c)$ and the radius of the model feature's tolerance sphere $T(c)$ (5.5). This product is determined for each model feature. The sum of all products represents the "Fit value" for the pharmacophore–molecule mapping [27].

$$\text{Fit} = \sum_{f} \text{weight}\ (f)^{*}[1 - \text{SSE}\ (f)] \tag{5.4}$$

$$\text{SSE}\ (f) = (D(c)/T(c))^2 \tag{5.5}$$

5.5.2
UNITY (GALAHAD/GASP)

Pharmacophore models derived by the GALAHAD or GASP algorithm can be screened against a 3D compound database applying UNITY [88], the database search module of the molecular modeling suite SYBYL [89]. By default, UNITY 3D database screening performs a prefiltering of database compounds discarding all molecules that do not match Lipinski's rule of five. The remaining compounds are subjected to a conformationally flexible 3D alignment based on the directed tweak algorithm [90]. For each compound, this algorithm generates low-energy conformers that possess the shortest distance to the model features. Thus, no conformational model for database compounds is needed and the VS is accelerated by avoiding the fitting of large numbers of compound conformers [91].

UNITY allows partial matching of pharmacophore features. Therefore, similar to DS CATALYST, not all features of the model have to be mapped by the database compound in order to be stored as hit. The success of pharmacophore feature alignment is expressed as QFIT. This score is based on the sum of (1 – (distance between compound atoms and center of the feature)^2) for all model features and used to determine the best conformer mapping for each compound. In accordance with DS CATALYSTs fit value, a high QFIT score corresponds to a good alignment between pharmacophore model and compound conformer [91].

5.5.3
LIGANDSCOUT

The recently developed pharmacophore-based alignment algorithm of LIGANDSCOUT differs significantly from established methods in translating the 3D conformer into a set of pharmacophore points instead of directly using atom positions to align the compound to the model. This novel concept allows an intuitive comparison of molecules in terms of bioisosterism and expands the range of possible applications for this algorithm. Thus, the algorithm can be used not only for pharmacophore-based VS but also for common-feature pharmacophore elucidation and 3D-QSAR studies [92].

The first step in VS applying this algorithm is the generation of 3D pharmacophoric points identified for the database conformer. Subsequently, the algorithm creates for each feature type a set of interfeature distances. The distance sets created for the pharmacophore model and for the conformers' pharmacophoric points are then compared in a pairwise manner. In order to find the optimal pair assignment, the so-called Hungarian matching algorithm is executed. Finally, the feature distances between model and conformer are minimized using the Kabsch alignment algorithm [87, 92]. For scoring the alignment quality, four different scores are available. The pharmacophore fit score calculates the number of matching pharmacophore features and the root mean square distance (RMSD) for pharmacophore alignment. The overlap of atom van der Waals spheres is determined by the atom sphere overlap score, whereas an overlap of Gaussian function representations of molecular volume is measured to obtain the Gaussian shape similarity score. Finally, a combo score of the first two scores is available as pharmacophore fit and atom overlap score [32].

5.5.4 MOE

For an efficient screening, MOE database search starts with prefiltering steps including the discard of conformers that do not match feature types and interfeature distances of the pharmacophore model. After this fast filtering of database molecules, the fitting between the model features and the chemical functions of the conformer starts. For this purpose, MOE performs a rigid body superimposition between conformer and model features. In other words, only translational and strain-free rotational movement is allowed for model fitting. Similar to DS CATALYST, only conformers of database molecules are retrieved that fall within the tolerance radii of a user-specified number of pharmacophore model features [20].

For scoring of mapping quality, MOE simply uses the RMSD calculated for the model–conformer superposition. Thus, contrary to DS CATALYST, a low score corresponds to a good alignment between model features and conformer features [20].

5.5.5 PHASE

Virtual database screening using PHASE pharmacophore models is executed in two steps called "finding" and "fetching." The finding step represents a prefiltering of database conformers for the following fetching step. During finding, PHASE searches for database conformers with geometries containing chemical functions with distances from each other as observed for the pharmacophore model. If the chemical functions of the database conformers are able to match the feature types and the corresponding distances between the model features, the conformer is stored and subjected to the following fetching step. As known for other pharmacophore-based screening algorithms, the user can specify if all the model features have to be mapped by the conformer or if a partial matching is possible, storing also hits that map a smaller number of model features [21].

Fetching is the fitting step of PHASE pharmacophore-based screening algorithm. It minimizes distances between chemical groups of the conformer and the features of the model and calculates the so-called fitness Score. This score consists of a term for the quality of pharmacophore–compound alignment, as well as terms for measuring the spatial deviation of matching vector features and matching conformer from their original locations. Finally, if partial matching is chosen, a penalty term for a conformer that does not map all features of the pharmacophore model is added to the fitness score [21].

To summarize, all six pharmacophore modeling tools – DS CATALYST, GALAHAD, GASP, LIGANDSCOUT, MOE, and PHASE – use a VS algorithm that performs a prefiltering of database conformers (e.g., calculating feature type and distance similarity of the conformer to the pharmacophore model) followed by a computationally more expensive conformer-to-model alignment. In contrast to other screening algorithms, the alignment step of the VS procedure of DS CATALYST is an independent option and can be switched off. Without the alignment option, DS CATALYST allows fast filtering of large small-molecule databases. However, the lack of conformer-to-model fitting produces a larger hit list containing lots of molecules that would not fall within the tolerance radii of the model features if an alignment would be performed. Thus, a DS CATALYST hit list filtered by the optional alignment and ranked by the fit value was the basis of several published VS studies aiming at the discovery of novel, biologically active ligands [85, 93–96].

5.6 Postprocessing of Pharmacophore-Based Screening Hits

As mentioned above, with respect to model selectivity and database size, hit lists of pharmacophore-based screenings can comprise tens to thousands of small molecules and can be prioritized and filtered by conformer-to-model alignment scores. For further filtering of hit lists, postprocessing methods using criteria for lead- and druglikeness, as well as structural diversity analysis, are available.

5.6.1 Lead- and Druglikeness

Hann *et al.* [97] defined criteria for leadlikeness of compounds as follows: a molecular weight equal to or smaller than 460, a clog P between -4 and 4.2, a log S_w equal to or larger than -5, a number of rotatable bonds equal to or smaller than 10, a number of rings equal to or smaller than 4, a number of hydrogen bond donors equal to or smaller than 5, and a number of hydrogen bond acceptors equal to or smaller than 9.

The most famous filter for druglikeness is Lipinski's rule of five [98]. According to Lipinski, a compound is most likely to have good absorption and permeability if it has equal to or less than 5 hydrogen bond donors, equal to or less than 10 hydrogen bond acceptors, a molecular weight equal to or less than 500, and a clog P equal to or less than 5.

Using scientific informatics software such as Pipeline Pilot [99] or script languages such as Perl [100] and Python [101], hit lists can be filtered with respect to these lead- and druglikeness criteria.

5.6.2 Structural Similarity Analysis

However, not only lead- and drug-likeness criteria are of importance for compound selection. If the compounds meet these criteria but are only derivatives of one single scaffold that is structurally closely related to already known biologically active molecules, the VS results will not be of interest for further drug development. Therefore, clustering of compounds with respect to their structural similarity to each other and to known ligands plays an important role in hit list postprocessing. For example, graph representations of molecules can be used as descriptor for analysis of

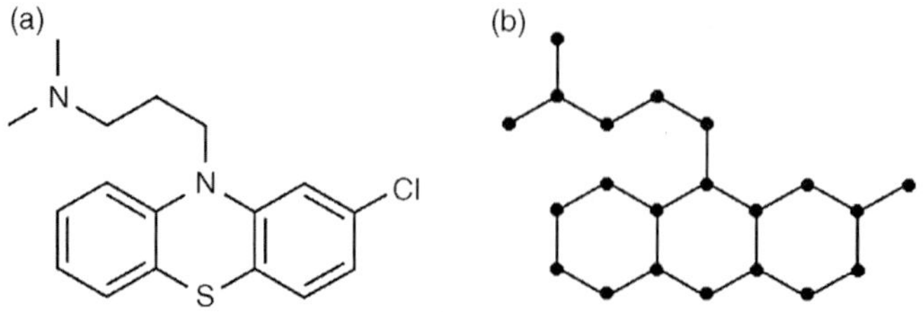

Figure 5.6 Chemical structure (a) and graph representation (b) of the antipsychotic drug chlorpromazine.

structural similarity [102, 103]. These representations only contain information about the connectivity properties of molecules. Atoms are displayed as vertices and bonds as lines. No information about the atom type is provided (Figure 5.6) [102]. If such graph representations are clustered, each cluster contains a set of compounds with a unique chemical scaffold giving medicinal chemists an overview of structural diversity of VS hits.

If structural similarity analysis of hit lists should also consider atomic properties, for example, atom and bond types or charges, 2D fingerprints can serve as descriptor [85]. For example, SciTegic's extended connectivity fingerprints (ECFP) identify either a single atom or a chemical fragment as a feature. The size of features depends on a user-specified number of neighbor atoms considered for feature analysis. Each of these features is encoded as a bit and all bits together represent the ECFPs of the molecule [99]. The similarity between ECFPs of molecules can be calculated by a metric such as the Tanimoto coefficient [104].

The above-mentioned filters are useful tools for compound selection. However, visual inspection of hit list compounds is still necessary since compounds with reactive or toxic functional groups or difficult to synthesize or chemically optimized molecules should be avoided. Thus, the experience of a medicinal chemist will always be needed for identifying the most promising hits of a virtual screen.

5.7 Pharmacophore-Based Parallel Screening

VS campaigns usually aim at the discovery of biological active molecules for a protein target of interest. One or more pharmacophore models are created representing essential ligand binding features and are subsequently screened against a chemical database. Although this might be an adequate approach for lead discovery, there are some drug design problems that can be solved only if the compound's activity for several pharmacologically important proteins is known. In other words, the VS approach should not only retrieve biologically active ligands but also all proteins where the ligand is predicted to be active. Such a parallel screen of several proteins against sets of pharmacophore models results in a list of putative target proteins for each single compound of the database [105]. The concept of the so-called parallel screening and its future developments can be applied to solve the following screening problems:

i. **Identification of putative side effects**: Compounds of interest are screened against *in silico* models representing target proteins known for causing side effects (e.g., the hERG potassium channel) [106].
ii. **Identification of putative biological activities**: Especially in the case of natural product research, there is frequently a set of compounds with unknown biological activities available. These compounds have been extracted from plants with pharmacological activity (e.g., traditionally used medical plants) without knowing their mechanism of action and which of the compounds are responsible for biological activity. Therefore, parallel screening can be used to identify the correct biological target protein and the compounds that are important for drug research. Such an identification of target proteins is called "target fishing" [80, 105, 107].

5.8 Application Examples for Synthetic Compound Screening

The application of pharmacophore-based screening of chemical databases has led to the discovery of several synthetic leads for promising drug targets. The following two application examples represent a typical structure-based and ligand-based pharmacophore modeling study, respectively.

5.8.1 17β-Hydroxysteroid Dehydrogenase 1 Inhibitors

17β-Hydroxysteroid dehydrogenase 1 (17β-HSD1) is pivotal for the biosynthesis of sex hormones. It participates both in the generation of testosterone and in the conversion of estrone into the biologically more potent estrogen estradiol. Due to the enzyme's important role in estradiol biosynthesis, inhibitors of 17β-HSD1 could lead to the development of promising drugs against breast cancer in premenopausal women. Most 17β-HSD1 inhibitors possess a steroidal scaffold suffering from the drawbacks of low target protein specificity and possible biotransformation into bioactive metabolites that could interfere with steroid hormone metabolism [94]. Thus, novel nonsteroidal inhibitors are needed to develop a selective and safe drug against breast cancer. In order to identify such inhibitors, a structure-based pharmacophore modeling study was performed by Schuster *et al.* [94]

First, the Protein Data Bank (PDB) [108], a publicly accessible source of experimentally determined protein structures, was searched for 17β-HSD1–inhibitor complexes. The two complexes with the PDB entry codes 1equ and 1i5r were selected for structure-based pharmacophore modeling. For this purpose, the pharmacophore elucidation software LIGANDSCOUT was applied. The structure-based pharmacophore generation algorithm of LIGANDSCOUT automatically analyzed all possible protein–ligand interactions of 1equ and 1i5r and derived a model for each PDB entry (Figure 5.7).

In accordance with protein–ligand interactions described in literature for small 17β-HSD1 inhibitors, the 1i5r model was refined by deleting hydrogen bond features and by incorporating hydrophobic features. Subsequently, the modified 1i5r model and the

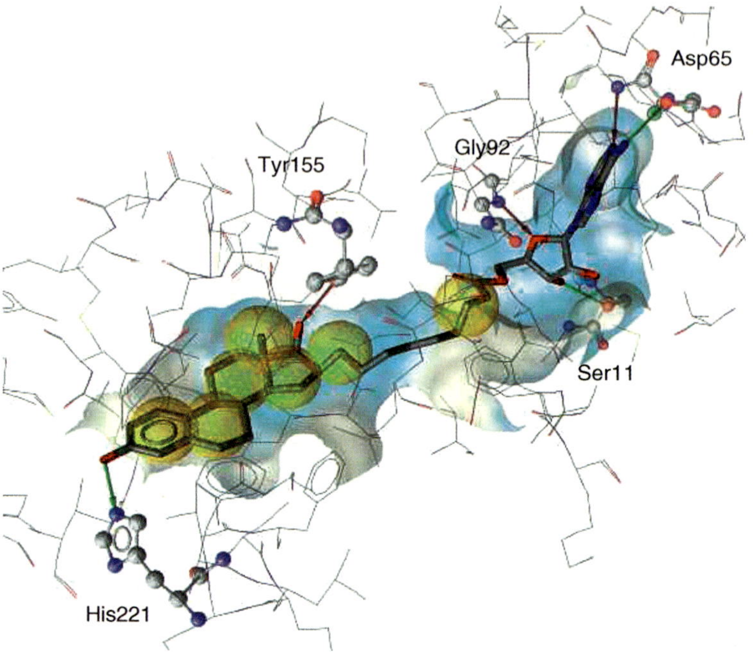

Figure 5.7 Depiction of the LIGANDSCOUT model generated for PDB entry 1i5r. Red arrows show hydrogen bond acceptors, green arrows display hydrogen bond donors, and yellow spheres represent hydrophobic interactions. The ligand binding pocket surface is shown by its aggregated lipophilicity/hydrophobicity.

1equ model were subjected to model validation. In order to determine their discriminatory power, each model was virtually screened against a set of known 17β-HSD1 inhibitors derived from literature and a set of decoys originating from the Derwent World Drug Index database [58], which consists of marketed and developmental drugs. On the basis of validation results, the modified 1i5r model was selected for VS of a commercial database and the compound collection of the National Cancer Institute. The pharmacophore-based screening hits were further analyzed by docking them into the 17β-HSD1 ligand binding pocket. Scores determined for fitting of the VS hits to the pharmacophore model and for docking to the binding site served as criteria to select compounds for biological testing. This workflow resulted in the identification of two steroidal and two nonsteroidal inhibitors with IC_{50} values below 50 μM. The most potent inhibitor showed an IC_{50} value of 5.7 μM and contained a nonsteroidal scaffold that represents an interesting starting point for further drug development (Figure 5.8) [94].

5.8.2
Cannabinoid Receptor 2 (CB_2) Ligands

Experimentally determined 3D structures of protein–ligand complexes are not always available. For example, the 3D structure of the promising drug target CB_2

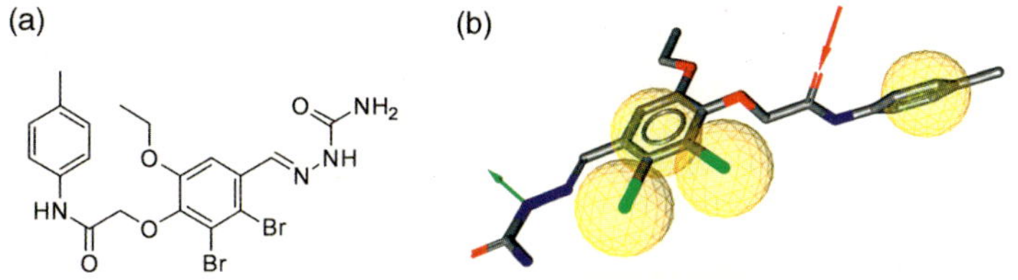

Figure 5.8 Structure of a novel nonsteroidal 17β-HSD1 inhibitor ($K_i = 5.7\,\mu M$) identified by pharmacophore-based screening (a) and fitted to the modified 1i5r model (b).

belonging to the family of G-protein-coupled receptors has not been identified. Agonists of CB_2 are known to reduce inflammation and neuropathic pain and could lead to the development of a novel generation of analgesics for chronic pain that do not possess the disadvantage of psychoactive side effects. In addition, inverse agonists of CB_2 are suggested to be of benefit in the therapy of bone loss. On that account, CB_2 represents the classical case of an interesting drug target for which novel ligands can be discovered virtually using a ligand-based approach only [109].

Thus, Markt *et al.* [109] created a ligand-based model for CB_2 ligands and applied it for a virtual screen of commercial chemical databases. For ligand-based pharmacophore modeling, the HipHop algorithm of DS CATALYST was used. This algorithm aligned five CB_2 agonists selected as training set and analyzed their common pharmacophoric features (Figure 5.9).

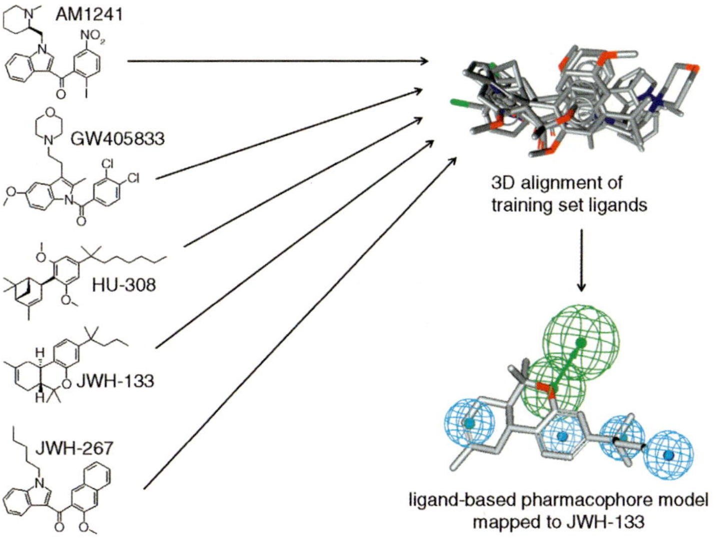

Figure 5.9 Generation of models for CB_2 ligands. The HipHop algorithm of DS CATALYST performed a 3D alignment of the five training set compounds AM1241, GW405 833, HU-308, JWH-133, and JWH-267 and identified common pharmacophoric patterns. This resulted in the creation of DS CATALYST pharmacophore models for CB_2 ligands. Chemical features of DS CATALYST models are color-coded as follows: hydrogen bond acceptors are shown as vectorized green spheres and hydrophobic interactions are represented by blue spheres.

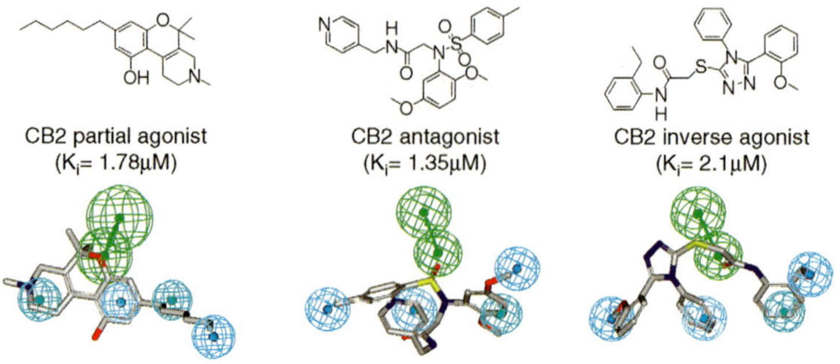

Figure 5.10 Pharmacophore-based screening resulted in three novel CB_2 ligands showing low micromolar binding affinities.

Models resulting from this common-feature analysis were validated by screening them against a set of CB_2 ligands from literature and decoys from the Derwent World Drug Index. The best EF values based on validation results were obtained for two models that were used as queries for a virtual screen of more than 900 000 commercially available compounds. Subsequently, the VS hits were filtered by their physicochemical properties. The filter criteria were derived from the properties of known CB_2 ligands from literature. Only compounds that did not differ significantly from the physicochemical property distribution of CB_2 ligands were stored. Afterward, a structural similarity analysis of the compounds based on 2D fingerprints was performed and only structurally diverse compounds were kept. Finally, the remaining VS hits were visually inspected in order to discard chemically reactive or toxic compounds. Using this workflow, 14 compounds were selected and biologically evaluated. Seven of these compounds showed a $K_i \leq 25\,\mu M$. Figure 5.10 shows the three most potent ligands: a CB_2 partial agonist ($K_i = 1.78\,\mu M$), a CB_2 antagonist ($K_i = 1.35\,\mu M$), and a CB_2 inverse agonist ($K_i = 2.1\,\mu M$) [109].

5.8.3
Further Application Examples

Apart from the structure-based discovery of novel 17β-HSD1 inhibitors and the ligand-based identification of CB_2 ligands, pharmacophore-based screening has provided a multitude of leads for drug development in the last few years. An outline of recent pharmacophore modeling studies resulting in the discovery of biologically active ligands is given in Table 5.2.

5.9
Application Examples for Natural Product Screening

The use of pharmacophore-based screening in the field of natural product drug discovery is one of the most recent application areas of pharmacophore models. It has been made possible by the introduction of several natural product databases for VS in

Table 5.2 Overview of recent pharmacophore-based screening studies aiming at the identification of synthetic leads for drug discovery.

Target protein	Therapeutic area	VS software	VS hits	References
5-Lipoxygenase	Inflammatory diseases	DS CATALYST	Two inhibitors ($IC_{50} = 14$ and 35 μM)	[110]
Angiotensin-converting enzyme	Hypertension	DS CATALYST	Four inhibitors showed moderate to high hypotensive activity *in vivo*	[111]
Aromatase	Breast cancer	DS CATALYST	Four inhibitors ($IC_{50} = 0.3$, 0.7, 9.8, and 15.5 μM, respectively)	[112]
β-Secretase	Alzheimer's disease	DS CATALYST	Inhibitor ($IC_{50} = 18.3$ μM)	[83]
Cancer cells	Cancer	DS CATALYST	Cytostatic compound ($IC_{50} < 2$ μM)	[113]
Carbonic anhydrase IX	Cancer	MOE	Inhibitor ($K_i = 0.3$ μM)	[114]
CB_1	Obesity	DS CATALYST	Antagonist ($K_i = 53$ nM)	[115]
CB_2	Inflammatory pain	FLAME	Agonist ($EC_{50} = 63$ nM)	[116]
c-Myc-Max heterodimer formation	Cancer	UNITY (GALAHAD)	Three inhibitors ($IC_{50} = 16.7$, 23, and 35 μM, respectively)	[117]
Complement component 3a receptor 1	Induction of immunity	DS CATALYST	Agonist ($EC_{50} = 310$ nM)	[118, 119]
Cruzain (cysteine protease of *Trypanosoma cruzi*)	Chargas disease	DS CATALYST	One inhibitor showed low micromolar activity	[120]
Disheveled PDZ domain	Cancer	UNITY (LIGANDSCOUT)	15 inhibitors (K_D between 8.6 and 78.8 μM)	[121]
Glycogen synthase kinase-3	Alzheimer's disease, cancer, chronic inflammation, and type-2 diabetes	DS CATALYST	Three inhibitors ($IC_{50} = 1.6$, 4.0, and 5.6 μM, respectively)	[122]
Heat shock protein 90	Cancer	DS CATALYST	Five inhibitors ($IC_{50} = 2.1$, 7.0, 25.3, 27.0 and 31.3 μM, respectively)	[123]
HIV-1 IN–LEDGF/p75 interaction	HIV infection	DS CATALYST (LIGANDSCOUT)	Inhibitor ($IC_{50} = 35$ μM)	[124]

(Continued)

Table 5.2 (*Continued*)

Target protein	Therapeutic area	VS software	VS hits	References
HIV-1 protease	HIV infection	MOE	Inhibitor ($IC_{50} = 18\,\mu M$)	[125]
Influenza neuraminidase	Flu	DS CATALYST	Three inhibitors ($IC_{50} = 1.8$, 7.3, and 12.5 μM, respectively)	[126]
Leukotriene A4 hydrolase	Inflammatory diseases	DS CATALYST	Inhibitor ($IC_{50} = 8\,nM$)	[127]
Lysophosphatidic acid 3 receptor	Gynecological and reproductive diseases	MOE	Antagonist ($IC_{50} = 24\,nM$)	[128]
N-Methyl-D-aspartate receptor NR2B subunit	Stroke	DS CATALYST	Antagonist ($IC_{50} = 769\,nM$)	[129]
Spleen tyrosine kinase	Allergic rhinitis, anaphylaxis, and asthma	DS CATALYST	Six inhibitors showed good *in vitro* potency	[130]
Thrombospondin-1	Angiogenesis-related diseases, cancer	DS CATALYST	Three inhibitors ($IC_{50} = 1.3$, 8.2, and $<50\,\mu M$, respectively)	[131]
Tubulin	Cancer	DS CATALYST	Inhibitor ($IC_{50} = 187\,nM$)	[132]

If the VS software was not used for model generation, the pharmacophore elucidation algorithm is mentioned in brackets.

the last few years. Today, a variety of commercial natural product libraries for VS purpose are available from vendors such as AnalytiCon (about 25 000 structures) [133, 134], InterBioScreen (more than 40 000 structures) [135], and VitasM (about 25 000 structures) [136]. Furthermore, several natural product databases exist, which were derived from literature. For example, Rollinger *et al.* [137] published the Natural Product Database (NPD, about 150 000 structures) comprising natural compounds obtained from literature and the DIOS database (about 10 000 structures) containing compounds extracted from medicinal plants with anti-inflammatory activity mentioned in the *De Materia Medica* of the ancient Greek physician Pedanius Dioscorides. Fakhrudin *et al.* [138] generated the Chinese Herbal Medicine database (CHM, about 10 000 structures) consisting of compounds from natural products reported in traditional Chinese medicine literature.

By pharmacophore-based screening of these natural product databases, several ligands with biological activity in the micro- and nanomolar range have been identified. The following sections report some of these successful natural product VS studies. Structures of the biologically most potent natural products identified by these VS campaigns are shown in Figure 5.11.

5.9.1
Cyclooxygenase (COX) Inhibitors

Since COX-1 and COX-2 play an important role in inflammation processes, inhibitors of these enzymes are known to lead to excellent anti-inflammatory drugs. The salicylic acid extracted from *Salix* species is a well-known anti-inflammatory compound from natural origin and has led to the development of the famous and frequently used drug acetylsalicylic acid. This shows that natural products have a great potential as COX inhibitors. Thus, Rollinger *et al.* [139] used a pharmacophore-based workflow for identifying novel ligands. They virtually screened the DIOS database and retrieved several compounds originating from the genus *Morus*. On the basis of these results, compounds from the methanol extract of the root bark of Morus were biologically evaluated. This resulted in the discovery of moderate COX inhibitors. For example, sanggenon E (**1**, Figure 5.11) gave an IC_{50} value of 10.8 μM for COX-1 inhibition [139].

5.9.2
Sigma-1 (σ_1) Receptor Ligands

Located in the endoplasmic reticulum of cells, the σ_1 receptor acts as a chaperone. The receptor is involved in a multitude of pathogenesis processes making σ_1 receptor ligands interesting drugs for the therapy of cocaine addiction, pain, depression, cancer, Alzheimer's disease, HIV infection, and other diseases [140]. Laggner *et al.* [141] created a ligand-based pharmacophore model to identify novel σ_1 receptor ligands. The model was screened against the Derwent World Drug Index. Except for synthetic molecules, this database also includes hormones and natural products from sources such as plants, marine organism, or microbial organisms. The most

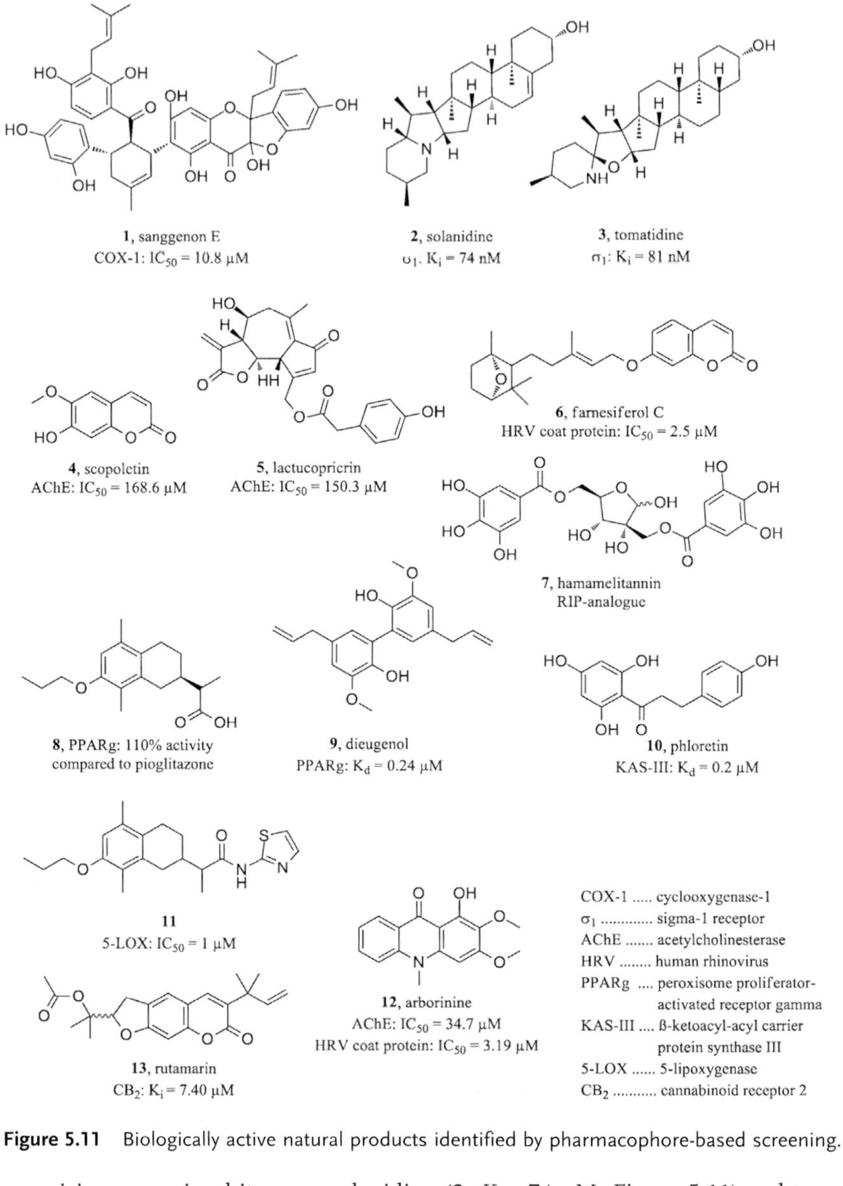

Figure 5.11 Biologically active natural products identified by pharmacophore-based screening.

promising screening hits were solanidine (**2**, $K_i = 74$ nM, Figure 5.11) and tomatidine (**3**, $K_i = 81$ nM, Figure 5.11) [141].

5.9.3 Acetylcholinesterase Inhibitors

Acetylcholinesterase (AChE) is responsible for acetylcholine degradation in the synaptic cleft. Therefore, inhibitors of AChE are increasing cholinergic neurotransmission. At present, AChE inhibitors are clinically used as drugs against Alzheimer's disease. A structure-based pharmacophore modeling study aiming at the discovery of natural AChE inhibitors has been published. In this study, a pharmacophore model was derived from the structure of an AChE–galanthamine complex. The resulting model was screened against the NPD. The coumarin scopoletin (**4**) was identified as a weak AChE inhibitor (IC_{50} = 168.6 μM, Figure 5.11) [142].

In a follow-up study, the same structure-based model was screened against a small database consisting of 47 compounds extracted from the roots of *Cichorium intybus* L. Biological testing of the hits resulted in two active sesquiterpene lactones, the most potent being lactucopicrin (**5**, IC_{50} = 150.3 μM, Figure 5.11) [143].

5.9.4 Human Rhinovirus Coat Protein Inhibitors

The coat protein of the human rhinovirus (HRV) is a promising drug target. HRV coat protein inhibitors could be useful as drugs against this virus that causes the common cold. To identify such inhibitors from natural sources, Rollinger *et al.* [144] developed a structure-based pharmacophore model and used it as query for a virtual screen of the DIOS database. Farnesiferol C (**6**), a sesquiterpene from the resin of the plant asafoetida, was identified as HRV coat protein inhibitor (IC_{50} = 2.5 μM, Figure 5.11) [144].

5.9.5 Quorum-Sensing Inhibitors

Staphylococci are responsible for most of the nosocomial infections. Since these bacteria are resistant to several antibiotics, there is an urgent need for novel drugs against Staphylococci infections. Quorum-sensing inhibitors that block the cell-to-cell communication between Staphylococci and thereby inhibit their virulence could represent an alternative to antibiotics. A pharmacophore-based screening retrieved hamamelitannin (**7**, Figure 5.11) from the bark and leaves of *Hamamelis virginiana*. *In vivo* evaluation of hamamelitannin showed that it was able to prevent device-associated Staphylococci infections [145].

5.9.6 Peroxisome Proliferator-Activated Receptor γ Ligands

The transcription factor peroxisome proliferator-activated receptor (PPAR) plays an important role in glucose and lipid metabolism. Three subtypes of PPAR exist: PPAR-α, PPAR-γ, and PPAR-δ. All subtypes are promising drug targets in the field of metabolic disorders. Fibrates are PPAR-α agonists currently applied as drugs against dyslipidemia, whereas a group of PPAR-γ agonists ("glitazones") has been approved by the FDA for the therapy of type-2 diabetes. In addition, PPAR-γ antagonists are investigated for their use as anti-obesity drugs [85]. Thus, PPAR-γ ligands are of interest for drug research in the area of the metabolic syndrome.

In order to discover natural product-based PPAR-γ agonists, Tanrikulu *et al.* [146] generated a pharmacophore model based on the alignment of bioactive conformations of three PPAR-γ agonists. A virtual screen of the NATx database of AnalytiCon and a subsequent *in vitro* testing of the hits resulted in compound **8** with 110% activity compared to the selective PPAR-γ agonist pioglitazone ($EC_{50} = 0.27\,\mu M$, Figure 5.11) [146].

Another pharmacophore-based screening study led to the identification of dieugenol (**9**, $K_i = 0.24\,\mu M$, Figure 5.11) and related neolignans as PPAR-γ partial agonist. In this study, a structure-based model was applied for a virtual screen of the DIOS and CHM database. Docking studies following the biological evaluation of the compounds rationalized the binding mode of **9** indicating the possibility that two molecules of this ligand could simultaneously bind to the PPAR-γ pocket [138].

5.9.7
β-Ketoacyl-Acyl Carrier Protein Synthase III Inhibitors

β-Ketoacyl-Acyl carrier protein synthase III (KAS III) is involved in the biosynthesis of fatty acids necessary for bacterial cell wall formation. In order to find natural lead structures for the development of novel antimicrobial drugs, a pharmacophore-based screening of about 900 natural products was carried out using a structure-based model for *Escherichia coli* KAS III. Four compounds were selected, of which two were identified as KAS III inhibitors in biological assays [147]. The structure of the most potent inhibitor (**10**, $K_d = 0.2\,\mu M$) is shown in Figure 5.11.

5.9.8
5-Lipoxygenase Inhibitors

Inhibitors of 5-lipoxygenase (5-LOX), which is responsible for the conversion of arachidonic acid into leucotrienic acid in the arachidonic acid cascade, are used as drugs for the treatment of asthma. Franke *et al.* [148] reported a pharmacophore-based screening aiming to discover new chemical scaffolds for these inhibitors. For this purpose, they applied a ligand-based method that uses the pharmacophoric features of a known active molecule as query for a similarity screening. In total, 43 active ligands were used as templates for screening the natural product databases MEGx [133] and NATx [134] from the AnalytiCon compound collection. The two hit compounds performing best in biological evaluation served as template molecules for a second VS run. By this stepwise workflow, one novel scaffold for 5-LOX inhibitors showing an IC_{50} value of 1 μM was obtained (**11**, Figure 5.11) [148].

5.9.9
11β-Hydroxysteroid Dehydrogenase Type 1 Inhibitors

Rollinger *et al.* used a previously experimentally validated pharmacophore model for 11β-hydroxysteroid dehydrogenase type 1 (11β-HSD1) to screen the DIOS database [95]. On the basis of the reported plant constituents in the hit list, triterpenoids from *Eriobotrya japonica* and related compounds were selected for biochemical evaluation [149]. This led to the discovery of ursolic acid and some of its derivatives as selective 11β-HSD1 inhibitors.

5.9.10
Pharmacophore-Based Parallel Screening of Natural Products

Especially in the area of natural product research where a fraction of compounds is extracted from a medicinal plant known from literature, the biological target proteins responsible for the biological effect are unknown. Thus, as mentioned above, a parallel screen of these compounds against several pharmacophore models representing different protein targets can be applied to predict possible biological targets.

One example for such a target fishing approach is the study by Rollinger *et al.* [150]. They investigated the biological activities of 16 secondary metabolites extracted from the plant *Ruta graveolens* L. by virtually screening them against 2208 pharmacophore models generated for 280 target proteins. The parallel screen predicted several targets of which three were selected for biological studies: AChE, HRV, and CB_2. Subsequently, the 16 metabolites were subjected to biological assays for these three targets. As a result of this biological testing, 6,7,8-trimethoxycoumarin and arborinine were identified as AChE and HRV coat protein inhibitors. Furthermore, isoplatydesmine (and norgraveoline) acted as AChE inhibitors, whereas daphnoretin methyl ether, methyl 3-(6-hydroxy-7-methoxybenzofuran-5-yl)propanoate, and (*S*)-ribalinine inhibited HRV coat protein. Finally, rutamarin showed activity for CB_2 [150]. Of all these compounds, arborinine (**12**, AChE: $IC_{50} = 34.7\,\mu M$ and HRV coat protein: $IC_{50} = 3.2\,\mu M$, Figure 5.11) and rutamarin (**13**, CB_2: $K_i = 7.4\,\mu M$, Figure 5.11) showed the highest *in vitro* potency. The study showed that the concept of *in silico* target fishing can support the research of pharmacognosists.

5.10
Conclusions

Over the past few years, pharmacophore-based screening has become a common technique for lead discovery in drug design. The basic concept of mapping a set of essential chemical features on functional groups of screening compounds does not only allow the identification of a variety of biologically active chemical scaffolds as novel leads. In fact, 3D pharmacophore models also hold great potential as visualization tools. A rotatable 3D depiction of important pharmacophoric features mapped on a protein–ligand complex provides an intuitive insight into the interaction patterns and thus facilitates interdisciplinary communication in the multidisciplinary drug discovery process. Furthermore, the rise of structure-based pharmacophore models challenges molecular docking techniques as the gold standard of structure-based VS. At least in terms of computational costs, structure-based pharmacophore models represent a promising alternative to docking. Due to low computational costs, parallel screening has evolved as a novel application of pharmacophore models. Until now, parallel screening has proven to be valuable for identifying target proteins of isolated natural products. Future developments in parallel screening have the potential to provide us with the selectivity needed for an efficient prediction of adverse drug reactions and off-target effects.

References

1 van Drie, J.H. (2007) Monty Kier and the origin of the pharmacophore concept. *Internet Electronic Journal of Molecular Design*, **6**, 271–279.

2 Kier, L.B. (1967) Molecular orbital calculation of preferred conformations of acetylcholine, muscarine, and muscarone. *Molecular Pharmacology*, **3**, 487–494.

3 Kier, L.B. (1970) Receptor mapping using molecular orbital theory, in *Fundamental Concepts in Drug–Receptor Interactions* (eds J.F. Danielli, J.F. Moran and D.J. Triggle), Academic Press, New York.

4 Kier, L.B. (1971) *Molecular Orbital Theory in Drug Research*, Academic Press, New York, pp. 164–169.

5 Höltje, H.D. (1974) Molecular orbital calculations for the structure of the muscarine–pharmacophore. *Archiv der Pharmazie (Weinheim)*, **307**, 969–972.

6 Wermuth, C.G. (1998) Glossary of terms used in medicinal chemistry (IUPAC recommendations 1998). *Pure and Applied Chemistry*, **70**, 1129–1143.

7 Guener, O.F. and Henry, D.R. (2000) *Pharmacophore: Perception Development and Use in Drug Design*, vol. 1, IUL Biotechnology Series (ed. O.F. Guener), IUL, La Jolla, CA, pp. 193–212.

8 Mason, J.S., Good, A.C., and Martin, E.J. (2001) 3-D pharmacophores in drug discovery. *Current Pharmaceutical Design*, **7**, 567–597.

9 Langer, T. and Hoffmann, R.D. (2006) Pharmacophores and pharmacophore searches, in *Methods and Principles in Medicinal Chemistry*, vol. **32** (eds R. Mannhold, H. Kubinyi, and G. Folkers), Wiley-VCH Verlag GmbH, Weinheim.

10 van Drie, J.H. (2003) Pharmacophore discovery: lessons learned. *Current Pharmaceutical Design*, **9**, 1649–1664.

11 Langer, T. and Wolber, G. (2004) Lead optimization. Pharmacophore definition and 3D searches. *Drug Discovery Today. Technologies*, **1**, 203–207.

12 Langer, T. and Hoffmann, R.D. (2006) Pharmacophore modelling: applications in drug discovery. *Expert Opinion on Drug Discovery*, **1**, 261–267.

13 Martin, Y.C. (2007) *Computer-Assisted Drug Design*, vol. 4, Comprehensive medicinal chemistry II (eds J.B. Taylor, D.J. Triggle and J.S. Mason), Elsevier, Oxford, pp. 119–147 and 515–536.

14 Laggner, C., Wolber, G., Kirchmair, J., Schuster, D., and Langer, T. (2008) Pharmacophore-based virtual screening in drug discovery, in *Chemoinformatics: An Approach to Virtual Screening* (eds A. Varnek and A. Tropsha), Royal Society of Chemistry, Cambridge, UK, pp. 76–119.

15 Leach, A.R., Gillet, V.J., Lewis, R.A., and Taylor, R. (2010) Three-dimensional pharmacophore methods in drug discovery. *Journal of Medicinal Chemistry*, **53**, 539–558.

16 Walters, W.P., Stahl, M.T., and Murcko, M.A. (1998) Virtual screening: an overview. *Drug Discovery Today*, **3**, 160–178.

17 Doman, T.N., McGovern, S.L., Witherbee, B.J., Kasten, T.P., Kurumbail, R., Stallings, W.C., Connolly, D.T., and Shoichet, B.K. (2002) Molecular docking and high-throughput screening for novel inhibitors of protein tyrosine phosphatase-1b. *Journal of Medicinal Chemistry*, **45**, 2213–2221.

18 CambridgeSoft (2009) ChemBioDraw Ultra, CambridgeSoft, Cambridge, MA 02140, USA.

19 Accelrys (2009) Discovery Studio, San Diego, CA.

20 CCG (2008) MOE, Montreal, Quebec, Canada.

21 Schrödinger LLC (2008) PHASE, New York, NY.

22 Kirchmair, J., Wolber, G., Laggner, C., and Langer, T. (2006) Comparative performance assessment of the conformational model generators Omega and Catalyst: a large-scale survey on the retrieval of protein-bound ligand conformations. *Journal of Chemical Information and Modeling*, **46**, 1848–1861.

23 Bostroem, J. (2001) Reproducing the conformations of protein-bound ligands: a critical evaluation of several popular conformational searching tools. *Journal of Computer-Aided Molecular Design*, **15**, 1137–1152.

24 Kirchmair, J., Laggner, C., Wolber, G., and Langer, T. (2005) Comparative analysis of protein-bound ligand conformations with respect to Catalyst's conformational space subsampling algorithms. *Journal of Chemical Information and Modeling*, **45**, 422–430.

25 Openeye Scientific Software Inc (2007) Omega, Santa Fe, NM, USA.

26 Molecular Networks (2010) ROTATE, Erlangen, Germany.

27 Accelrys (2009) DS Catalyst, San Diego, CA.

28 Barnum, D., Greene, J., Smellie, A., and Sprague, P. (1996) Identification of common functional configurations among molecules. *Journal of Chemical Information and Computer Sciences*, **36**, 563–571.

29 Richmond, N.J., Abrams, C.A., Wolohan, P.R., Abrahamian, E., Willett, P., and Clark, R.D. (2006) GALAHAD: 1. pharmacophore identification by hypermolecular alignment of ligands in 3D. *Journal of Computer-Aided Molecular Design*, **20**, 567–587.

30 Jones, G., Willett, P., and Glen, R.C. (1995) A genetic algorithm for flexible molecular overlay and pharmacophore elucidation. *Journal of Computer-Aided Molecular Design*, **9**, 532–549.

31 Wolber, G. and Langer, T. (2005) LigandScout: 3D pharmacophores derived from protein-bound ligands and their use as virtual screening filters. *Journal of Chemical Information and Modeling*, **45**, 160–169.

32 Wolber, G., Seidel, T., Bendix, F., Ibis, G., Dornhofer, A.A., Biely, M., Adaktylos, P., and Kosara, R. (2010) *LigandScout*, Inte: Ligand GmbH, Vienna, Austria.

33 Dixon, S.L., Smondyrev, A.M., Knoll, E.H., Rao, S.N., Shaw, D.E., and Friesner, R.A. (2006) PHASE: a new engine for pharmacophore perception, 3D QSAR model development, and 3D database screening: 1. Methodology and preliminary results. *Journal of Computer-Aided Molecular Design*, **20**, 647–671.

34 Cho, S.J. and Sun, Y. (2006) FLAME: a program to flexibly align molecules. *Journal of Chemical Information and Modeling*, **46**, 298–306.

35 Feng, J., Sanil, A., and Young, S.S. (2006) PharmID: pharmacophore identification using Gibbs sampling. *Journal of Chemical Information and Modeling*, **46**, 1352–1359.

36 Zhu, F. and Agrafiotis, D.K. (2007) Recursive distance partitioning algorithm for common pharmacophore identification. *Journal of Chemical Information and Modeling*, **47**, 1619–1625.

37 Marialke, J., Körner, R., Tietze, S., and Apostolakis, J. (2007) Graph-based molecular alignment (GMA). *Journal of Chemical Information and Modeling*, **47**, 591–601.

38 Todorov, N.P., Alberts, I.L., de Esch, I.J., and Dean, P.M. (2007) QUASI: a novel method for simultaneous superposition of multiple flexible ligands and virtual screening using partial similarity. *Journal of Chemical Information and Modeling*, **47**, 1007–1020.

39 Schneidman-Duhovny, D., Dror, O., Inbar, Y., Nussinov, R., and Wolfson, H.J. (2008) Deterministic pharmacophore detection via multiple flexible alignment of drug-like molecules. *Journal of Computational Biology*, **15**, 737–754.

40 Taminau, J., Thijs, G., and De Winter, H. (2008) Pharao: pharmacophore alignment and optimization. *Journal of Molecular Graphics and Modelling*, **27**, 161–169.

41 Anghelescu, A.V., DeLisle, R.K., Lowrie, J.F., Klon, A.E., Xie, X., and Diller, D.J. (2008) Technique for generating three-dimensional alignments of multiple ligands from one-dimensional alignments. *Journal of Chemical Information and Modeling*, **48**, 1041–1054.

42 Podolyan, Y. and Karypis, G. (2009) Common pharmacophore identification using frequent clique detection algorithm. *Journal of Chemical Information and Modeling*, **49**, 13–21.

43 Venkatachalam, C.M., Kirchoff, P., and Waldman, M. (2000) Receptor-based pharmacophore perception and modeling, in *Pharmacophore Perception, Development and Use in Drug Design* (ed O.F. Guener), IUL Biotechnology Series, IUL, La Jolla, CA, pp. 339–350.

44 Ortuso, F., Langer, T., and Alcaro, S. (2006) GBPM: GRID-based pharmacophore model: concept and application studies to protein–protein recognition. *Bioinformatics*, **22**, 1449–1455.

45 Baroni, M., Cruciani, G., Sciabola, S., Perruccio, F., and Mason, J.S. (2007) A common reference framework for analyzing/comparing proteins and ligands. Fingerprints for ligands and proteins (FLAP): theory and application. *Journal of Chemical Information and Modeling*, **47**, 279–294.

46 Goodford, P.J. (1985) A computational procedure for determining energetically favorable binding sites on biologically important macromolecules. *Journal of Medicinal Chemistry*, **28**, 849–857.

47 Karnachi, P. and Kulkarni, A. (2006) Application of pharmacophore fingerprints to structure-based design and data mining, in *Pharmacophores and Pharmacophore Searches* (eds T. Langer and R.D. Hoffmann), Wiley-VCH Verlag GmbH, Weinheim, pp. 193–206.

48 Deng, Z., Chuaqui, C., and Singh, J. (2004) Structural interaction fingerprint (SIFt): a novel method for analyzing three-dimensional protein–ligand binding interactions. *Journal of Medicinal Chemistry*, **47**, 337–344.

49 Chuaqui, C., Deng, Z., and Singh, J. (2005) Interaction profiles of protein kinase–inhibitor complexes and their application to virtual screening. *Journal of Medicinal Chemistry*, **48**, 121–133.

50 Renner, S., Fechner, U., and Schneider, G. (2006) Alignment-free pharmacophore patterns: a correlation-vector approach, in *Pharmacophores and Pharmacophore Searches* (eds T. Langer and R.D. Hoffmann), Wiley-VCH Verlag GmbH, Weinheim, pp. 49–80.

51 Tanrikulu, Y., Nietert, M., Scheffer, U., Proschak, E., Grabowski, K., Schneider, P., Weidlich, M., Karas, M., Göbel, M., and Schneider, G. (2007) Scaffold hopping by "fuzzy" pharmacophores and its application to RNA targets. *ChemBioChem*, **8**, 1932–1936.

52 Bonachéra, F., Parent, B., Barbosa, F., Froloff, N., and Horvath, D. (2006) Fuzzy tricentric pharmacophore fingerprints. 1. Topological fuzzy pharmacophore triplets and adapted molecular similarity scoring schemes. *Journal of Chemical Information and Modeling*, **46**, 2457–2477.

53 Bonachéra, F. and Horvath, D. (2008) Fuzzy tricentric pharmacophore fingerprints. 2. Application of topological fuzzy pharmacophore triplets in quantitative structure–activity relationships. *Journal of Chemical Information and Modeling*, **48**, 409–425.

54 Rarey, M. and Dixon, J.S. (1998) Feature trees: a new molecular similarity measure based on tree matching. *Journal of Computer-Aided Molecular Design*, **12**, 471–490.

55 Rohrer, S.G. and Baumann, K. (2009) Maximum unbiased validation (MUV) data sets for virtual screening based on PubChem bioactivity data. *Journal of Chemical Information and Modeling*, **49**, 169–184.

56 Verdonk, M.L., Berdini, V., Hartshorn, M.J., Mooij, W.T., Murray, C.W., Taylor, R.D., and Watson, P. (2004) Virtual screening using protein–ligand docking: avoiding artificial enrichment. *Journal of Chemical Information and Computer Sciences*, **44**, 793–806.

57 Good, A.C. and Oprea, T.I. (2008) Optimization of CAMD techniques 3. Virtual screening enrichment studies: a help or hindrance in tool selection. *Journal of Computer-Aided Molecular Design*, **22**, 169–178.

58 Thomson Scientific (2005) *Derwent World Drug Index*, Derwent Publications Ltd, London, UK.

59 Olah, M., Mracec, M., Ostopovici, L., Rad, R., Bora, A., Hadaruga, N., Olah, I., Banda, M., Simon, Z., and Opera, T.I. (2004) WOMBAT: world of molecular bioactivity, in *Cheminformatics in Drug Discovery* (ed T.I. Oprea), Wiley-VCH Verlag GmbH, New York, pp. 223–239.

60 AKos Consulting and Solutions GmbH (2010) MDDR: MDL Drug Data Report. AKos Consulting and Solutions GmbH, Steinen, Germany.

61 ChEMBL Group (2010) ChEMBL Database, EMBL-EBI, Cambridge, UK.

62 Huang, N., Shoichet, B.K., and Irwin, J.J. (2006) Benchmarking sets for molecular docking. *Journal of Medicinal Chemistry*, **49**, 6789–6801.

63 Irwin, J.J. (2008) Community benchmarks for virtual screening. *Journal of Computer-Aided Molecular Design*, **22**, 193–199.

64 Bolton, E.E., Wang, Y., Thiessen, P.A., and Bryant, S.H. (2008) PubChem: integrated platform of small molecules and biological activities. *Annual Reports in Computational Chemistry*, **4**, 217–241.

65 Triballeau, N., Acher, F., Brabet, I., Pin, J.P., and Bertrand, H.O. (2005) Virtual screening workflow development guided by the "receiver operating characteristic" curve approach. Application to high-throughput docking on metabotropic glutamate receptor subtype 4. *Journal of Medicinal Chemistry*, **48**, 2534–2547.

66 Jacobsson, M., Liden, P., Stjernschantz, E., Bostroem, H., and Norinder, U. (2003) Improving structure-based virtual screening by multivariate analysis of scoring data. *Journal of Medicinal Chemistry*, **46**, 5781–5789.

67 Shepherd, A.J., Gorse, D., and Thornton, J.M. (1999) Prediction of the location and type of b-turns in proteins using neural networks. *Protein Science*, **8**, 1045–1055.

68 Gao, H., Williams, C., Labute, P., and Bajorath, J. (1999) Binary quantitative structure–activity relationship (QSAR) analysis of estrogen receptor ligands. *Journal of Chemical Information and Computer Sciences*, **39**, 164–168.

69 Guha, R. and Jurs Peter, C. (2005) Determining the validity of a QSAR model: a classification approach. *Journal of Chemical Information and Modeling*, **45**, 65–73.

70 Weston, J., Perez-Cruz, F., Bousquet, O., Chapelle, O., Elisseeff, A., and Schoelkopf, B. (2003) Feature selection and transduction for prediction of molecular bioactivity for drug design. *Bioinformatics*, **19**, 764–771.

71 Martineau, E., Aman, A.M., and Kong, X. (2004) *Accelrysworld* Accelrys, Inc., San Diego, CA.

72 Ford, M.G. (2003) 2nd International Symposium on Computational Methods in Toxicology and Pharmacology Integrating Internet Resources, Thessaloniki, Greece.

73 Bradley, E.K., Miller, J.L., Saiah, E., and Grootenhuis, P.D.J. (2003) Informative library design as an efficient strategy to identify and optimize leads: application to cyclin-dependent kinase 2 antagonists. *Journal of Medicinal Chemistry*, **46**, 4360–4364.

74 Bradley, E.K., Beroza, P., Penzotti, J.E., Grootenhuis, P.D.J., Spellmeyer, D.C., and Miller, J.L. (2000) A rapid computational method for lead evolution: description and application to α1-adrenergic antagonists. *Journal of Medicinal Chemistry*, **43**, 2770–2774.

75 Matthews, B.W. (1975) Comparison of the predicted and observed secondary structure of T4 phage lysozyme. *Biochimica et Biophysica Acta*, **405**, 442–451.

76 Frimurer, T.M., Bywater, R., Nrum, L., Lauritsen, L.N., and Brunak, S. (2000) Improving the odds in discriminating "drug-like" from "non drug-like" compounds. *Journal of Chemical Information and Computer Sciences*, **40**, 1315–1324.

77 Hecker, E.A., Duraiswami, C., Andrea, T.A., and Diller, D.J. (2002) Use of catalyst pharmacophore models for screening of large combinatorial libraries. *Journal of Chemical Information and Computer Sciences*, **42**, 1204–1211.

78 Diller, D.J. and Li, R. (2003) Kinases, homology models, and high throughput

docking. *Journal of Medicinal Chemistry*, **46**, 4638–4647.

79 Truchon, J.F. and Bayly, C.I. (2007) Evaluating virtual screening methods: good and bad metrics for the "early recognition" problem. *Journal of Chemical Information and Modeling*, **47**, 488–508.

80 Markt, P., Schuster, D., Kirchmair, J., Laggner, C., and Langer, T. (2007) Pharmacophore modeling and parallel screening for PPAR ligands. *Journal of Computer-Aided Molecular Design*, **21**, 575–590.

81 Szilagyi, A. and Skolnick, J. (2006) Efficient prediction of nucleic acid binding function from low-resolution protein structures. *Journal of Molecular Biology*, **358**, 922–933.

82 Sheridan, R.P., Singh, S.B., Fluder, E.M., and Kearsley, S.K. (2001) Protocols for bridging the peptide to nonpeptide gap in topological similarity searches. *Journal of Chemical Information and Computer Sciences*, **41**, 1395–1406.

83 Huang, W., Yu, H., Sheng, R., Li, J., and Hu, Y. (2008) Identification of pharmacophore model, synthesis and biological evaluation of *N*-phenyl-1-arylamide and *N*-phenylbenzenesulfonamide derivatives as BACE 1 inhibitors. *Bioorganic & Medicinal Chemistry*, **16**, 10190–10197.

84 Dror, O., Schneidman-Duhovny, D., Inbar, Y., Nussinov, R., and Wolfson, H.J. (2009) Novel approach for efficient pharmacophore-based virtual screening: method and applications. *Journal of Chemical Information and Modeling*, **49**, 2333–2343.

85 Markt, P., Petersen, R.K., Flindt, E.N., Kristiansen, K., Kirchmair, J., Spitzer, G., Distinto, S., Schuster, D., Wolber, G., Laggner, C., and Langer, T. (2008) Discovery of novel PPAR ligands by a virtual screening approach based on pharmacophore modeling, 3D shape, and electrostatic similarity screening. *Journal of Medicinal Chemistry*, **51**, 6303–6317.

86 Wolber, G., Seidel, T., Bendix, F., and Langer, T. (2008) Molecule–pharmacophore superpositioning and pattern matching in computational drug design. *Drug Discovery Today*, **13**, 23–29.

87 Kabsch, W. (1978) A discussion of the solution for the best rotation to relate two sets of vectors. *Acta Crystallographica*, **A34**, 827–828.

88 Tripos (2010) UNITY, St. Louis, MO.

89 Tripos (2009) SYBYL, Tripos: St. Louis, MO.

90 Hurst, T. (1994) Flexible 3D searching: the directed tweak technique. *Journal of Chemical Information and Computer Sciences*, **34**, 190–196.

91 Tripos (2009) UNITY, Tripos: St. Louis, MO.

92 Wolber, G., Dornhofer, A.A., and Langer, T. (2006) Efficient overlay of small organic molecules using 3D pharmacophores. *Journal of Computer-Aided Molecular Design*, **20**, 773–788.

93 Markt, P., McGoohan, C., Walker, B., Kirchmair, J., Feldmann, C., De Martino, G., Spitzer, G., Distinto, S., Schuster, D., Wolber, G., Laggner, C., and Langer, T. (2008) Discovery of novel cathepsin S inhibitors by pharmacophore-based virtual high-throughput screening. *Journal of Chemical Information and Modeling*, **48**, 1693–1705.

94 Schuster, D., Nashev, L.G., Kirchmair, J., Laggner, C., Wolber, G., Langer, T., and Odermatt, A. (2008) Discovery of nonsteroidal 17beta-hydroxysteroid dehydrogenase 1 inhibitors by pharmacophore-based screening of virtual compound libraries. *Journal of Medicinal Chemistry*, **51**, 4188–4199.

95 Schuster, D., Maurer, E.M., Laggner, C., Nashev, L.G., Wilckens, T., Langer, T., and Odermatt, A. (2006) The discovery of new 11beta-hydroxysteroid dehydrogenase type 1 inhibitors by common feature pharmacophore modeling and virtual screening. *Journal of Medicinal Chemistry*, **49**, 3454–3466.

96 Brogi, S., Kladi, M., Vagias, C., Papazafiri, P., Roussis, V., and Tafi, A. (2009) Pharmacophore modeling for qualitative prediction of antiestrogenic activity. *Journal of Chemical Information and Modeling*, **49**, 2489–2497.

97 Hann, M.M. and Oprea, T.I. (2004) Pursuing the leadliness concept in

pharmaceutical research. *Current Opinion in Chemical Biology*, **8**, 255–263.
98 Lipinski, C.A., Lombardo, F., Dominy, B.W., and Feeney, P.J. (1997) Experimental and computational approaches to estimate solubility and permeability in drug discovery and development settings. *Advanced Drug Delivery Reviews*, **23**, 3–25.
99 Scitegic (2008) Pipeline Pilot, San Diego, CA, USA.
100 Wall, L. (2009) Perl, Perl.org: USA.
101 van Rossum, G. (2009) Python, Python Software Foundation, The Netherlands.
102 Bemis, G.W. and Murcko, M.A. (1996) The properties of known drugs. 1. Molecular frameworks. *Journal of Medicinal Chemistry*, **39**, 2887–2893.
103 Tiikkainen, P., Markt, P., Wolber, G., Kirchmair, J., Distinto, S., Poso, A., and Kallioniemi, O. (2009) Critical comparison of virtual screening methods against the MUV data set. *Journal of Chemical Information and Modeling*, **49**, 2168–2178.
104 Willett, P. and Winterman, V.A. (1986) Comparison of some measures for the determination of inter-molecular structural similarity. *Quantitative Structure–Activity Relationships*, **5**, 18–25.
105 Steindl, T.M., Schuster, D., Laggner, C., and Langer, T. (2006) Parallel screening: a novel concept in pharmacophore modeling and virtual screening. *Journal of Chemical Information and Modeling*, **46**, 2146–2157.
106 Bender, A., Scheiber, J., Glick, M., Davies, J.W., Azzaoui, K., Hamon, J., Urban, L., Whitebread, S., and Jenkins, J.L. (2007) Analysis of pharmacology data and the prediction of adverse drug reactions and off-target effects from chemical structure. *ChemMedChem*, **2**, 861–873.
107 Prathipati, P., Ma, N.L., Manjunatha, U.H., and Bender, A. (2009) Fishing the target of antitubercular compounds: *in silico* target deconvolution model development and validation. *Journal of Proteome Research*, **8**, 2788–2798.
108 Berman, H.M., Westbrook, J., Feng, Z., Gilliland, G., Bhat, T.N., Weissig, H., Shindyalov, I.N., and Bourne, P.E. (2000) The Protein Data Bank. *Nucleic Acids Research*, **28**, 235–242.
109 Markt, P., Feldmann, C., Rollinger, J.M., Raduner, S., Schuster, D., Kirchmair, J., Distinto, S., Spitzer, G.M., Wolber, G., Laggner, C., Altmann, K.H., Langer, T., and Gertsch, J. (2009) Discovery of novel CB2 receptor ligands by a pharmacophore-based virtual screening workflow. *Journal of Medicinal Chemistry*, **52**, 369–378.
110 Aparoy, P., Kumar Reddy, K., Kalangi, S.K., Chandramohan Reddy, T., and Reddanna, P. (2010) Pharmacophore modeling and virtual screening for designing potential 5-lipoxygenase inhibitors. *Bioorganic & Medicinal Chemistry Letters*, **20**, 1013–1018.
111 Ismail, M.A.H., Aboul-Enein, M.N., Abouzid, K.A.M., El Ella, D.A.A., and Ismail, N.S.M. (2009) ACE inhibitors hypothesis generation for selective design, synthesis and biological evaluation of 3-mercapto-2-methyl-propanoyl-pyrrolidine-3-imine derivatives as antihypertensive agents. *Bioorganic & Medicinal Chemistry*, **17**, 3739–3746.
112 Neves, M.A.C., Dinis, T.C.P., Colombo, G., and Sá e Melo, M.L. (2009) An efficient steroid pharmacophore-based strategy to identify new aromatase inhibitors. *European Journal of Medicinal Chemistry*, **44**, 4121–4127.
113 Deng, J., Taheri, L., Grande, F., Aiello, F., Garofalo, A., and Neamati, N. (2008) Discovery of novel anticancer compounds based on a quinoxalinehydrazine pharmacophore. *ChemMedChem*, **3**, 1677–1686.
114 Thiry, A., Ledecq, M., Cecchi, A., Frederick, R., Dongé, J.-M., Supuran, C.T., Wouters, J., and Masereel, B. (2009) Ligand-based and structure-based virtual screening to identify carbonic anhydrase IX inhibitors. *Bioorganic & Medicinal Chemistry*, **17**, 553–557.
115 Wang, H., Duffy, R.A., Boykow, G.C., Chackalamannil, S., and Madison, V.S. (2008) Identification of novel cannabinoid CB1 receptor antagonists by using virtual screening with a

pharmacophore model. *Journal of Medicinal Chemistry*, **51**, 2439–2446.

116 Cheng, Y., Albrecht, B.K., Brown, J., Buchanan, J.L., Buckner, W.H., DiMauro, E.F., Emkey, R., Fremeau, R.T.J., Harmange, J.C., Hoffman, B.J., Huang, L., Huang, M., Lee, J.H., Lin, F.F., Martin, M.W., Nguyen, H.Q., Patel, V.F., Tomlinson, S.A., White, R.D., Xia, X., and Hitchcock, S.A. (2008) Discovery and optimization of a novel series of *N*-arylamide oxadiazoles as potent, highly selective and orally bioavailable cannabinoid receptor 2 (CB2) agonists. *Journal of Medicinal Chemistry*, **51**, 5019–5034.

117 Mustata, G., Follis, A.V., Hammoudeh, D.I., Metallo, S.J., Wang, H., Prochownik, E.V., Lazo, J.S., and Bahar, I. (2009) Discovery of novel Myc-Max heterodimer disruptors with a three-dimensional pharmacophore model. *Journal of Medicinal Chemistry*, **52**, 1247–1250.

118 Klabunde, T., Giegerich, C., and Evers, A. (2009) Sequence-derived three-dimensional pharmacophore models for G-protein-coupled receptors and their application in virtual screening. *Journal of Medicinal Chemistry*, **52**, 2923–2932.

119 Legler, D.F., Loetscher, M., Jones, S.A., Dahinden, C.A., Arock, M., and Moser, B. (1996) Expression of high- and low-affinity receptors for C3a on the human mast cell line, HMC-1. *European Journal of Immunology*, **26**, 753–758.

120 Malvezzi, A., de Rezende, L., and -do Amaral, A.F. (2009) Pharmacopohore model of cruzain inhibitors. *QSAR & Combinatorial Science*, **28**, 781–784.

121 Shan, J. and Zheng, J.J. (2009) Optimizing Dvl PDZ domain inhibitor by exploring chemical space. *Journal of Computer-Aided Molecular Design*, **23**, 37–47.

122 Kim, H.-J., Choo, H., Cho, Y.S., No, K.T., and Pae, A.N. (2008) Novel GSK-3β inhibitors from sequential virtual screening. *Bioorganic & Medicinal Chemistry*, **16**, 636–643.

123 Sanam, R., Tanje, S., Gundla, R., Vadivelan, S., Machiraju, P.K., Dayam, R., Narasu, L., Jagarlapudi, S., and Neamati, N. (2010) Combined pharmacophore and structure-guided studies to identify diverse HSP90 inhibitors. *Journal of Molecular Graphics and Modelling*, **28**, 472–477.

124 De Luca, L., Barreca, M.L., Ferro, S., Christ, F., Iraci, N., Gitto, R., Monforte, A.M., Debyser, Z., and Chimirri, A. (2009) Pharmacophore-based discovery of small-molecule inhibitors of protein–protein interactions between HIV-1 integrase and cellular cofactor LEDGF/p75. *ChemMedChem*, **4**, 1311–1316.

125 Damm, K.L., Ung, P.M.U., Quintero, J.J., Gestwicki, J.E., and Carlson, H.A. (2008) A poke in the eye: inhibiting HIV-1 protease through its flap-recognition pocket. *Biopolymers*, **89**, 643–652.

126 Hammad, A.M.A. and Taha, M.O. (2009) Pharmacophore modeling, quantitative structure–activity relationship analysis, and shape-complemented *in silico* screening allow access to novel influenza neuraminidase inhibitors. *Journal of Chemical Information and Modeling*, **49**, 978–996.

127 Grice, C.A., Tays, K.L., Savall, B.M., Wei, J., Butler, C.R., Axe, F.U., Bembenek, S.D., Fourie, A.M., Dunford, P.J., Lundeen, K., Coles, F., Xue, X., Riley, J.P., Williams, K.N., Karlsson, L., and Edwards, J.P. (2008) Identification of a potent, selective, and orally active leukotriene A_4 hydrolase inhibitor with anti-inflammatory activity. *Journal of Medicinal Chemistry*, **51**, 4150–4169.

128 Fells, J.I., Tsukahara, R., Fujiwara, Y., Liu, J., Perygin, D.H., Osborne, D.A., Tigyi, G., and Parrill, A.L. (2008) Identification of non-lipid LPA_3 antagonists by virtual screening. *Bioorganic & Medicinal Chemistry*, **16**, 6207–6217.

129 Gitto, R., De Luca, L., Ferro, S., Occhiuto, F., Samperi, S., De Sarro, G., Russo, E., Ciranna, L., Costa, L., and Chimirri, A. (2008) Computational studies to discover a new NR2B/NMDA receptor antagonist and evaluation of pharmacological profile. *ChemMedChem*, **3**, 1539–1548.

130 Xie, H.-Z., Li, L.-L., Ren, J.-X., Zou, J., Yang, L., Wei, Y.-Q., and Yang, S.-Y. (2009) Pharmacophore modeling study based on known spleen tyrosine kinase inhibitors

together with virtual screening for identifying novel inhibitors. *Bioorganic & Medicinal Chemistry Letters*, **19**, 1944–1949.

131 Colombo, G., Margosio, B., Ragona, L., Neves, M., Bonifacio, S., Annis, D.S., Stravalaci, M., Tomaselli, S., Giavazzi, R., Rusnati, M., Presta, M., Zetta, L., Mosher, D.F., Ribatti, D., Gobbi, M., and Taraboletti, G. (2010) Non-peptidic thrombospondin-1 mimics as fibroblast growth factor-2 inhibitors. *The Journal of Biological Chemistry*, **285**, 8733–8742.

132 Chiang, Y.K., Kuo, C.C., Wu, Y.S., Chen, C.T., Coumar, M.S., Wu, J.S., Hsieh, H.P., Chang, C.Y., Jseng, H.Y., Wu, M.H., Leou, J.S., Song, J.S., Chang, J.Y., Lyu, P.C., Chao, Y.S., and Wu, S.Y. (2009) Generation of ligand-based pharmacophore model and virtual screening for identification of novel tubulin inhibitors with potent anticancer activity. *Journal of Medicinal Chemistry*, **52**, 4221–4233.

133 AnalytiCon Discovery GmbH (2010) MEGx Compound Collection, Potsdam, Germany.

134 AnalytiCon Discovery GmbH (2010) NATx Compound Collection, Potsdam, Germany.

135 InterBioScreen Ltd (2010) Natural Compound Library, Moscow, Russia.

136 VitasM Laboratory Ltd (2010) VitasM Tulip Library, Moscow, Russia.

137 Rollinger, J.M., Haupt, S., Stuppner, H., and Langer, T. (2004) Combining ethnopharmacology and virtual screening for lead structure discovery: COX-inhibitors as application example. *Journal of Chemical Information and Computer Sciences*, **44**, 480–488.

138 Fakhrudin, N., Ladurner, A., Atanasov, A.G., Heiss, E.H., Baumgartner, L., Markt, P., Schuster, D., Ellmerer, E.P., Wolber, G., Rollinger, J.M., Stuppner, H., and Dirsch, V.M. (2010) Computer-aided discovery, validation, and mechanistic characterization of novel neolignan activators of peroxisome proliferator-activated receptor γ. *Molecular Pharmacology*, **77**, 559–566.

139 Rollinger, J.M., Bodensieck, A., Seger, C., Ellmerer, E.P., Bauer, R., and Langer, T. (2005) Discovering COX-inhibiting constituents of Morus root bark: activity-guided versus computer-aided methods. *Planta Medica*, **71**, 399–405.

140 Maurice, T. and Su, T.P. (2009) The pharmacology of sigma-1 receptors. *Pharmacology & Therapeutics*, **124**, 195–206.

141 Laggner, C., Schieferer, C., Fiechtner, B., Poles, G., Hoffmann, R.D., Glossmann, H., Langer, T., and Moebius, F.F. (2005) Discovery of high-affinity ligands of sigma1 receptor, ERG2, and emopamil binding protein by pharmacophore modeling and virtual screening. *Journal of Medicinal Chemistry*, **48**, 4754–4764.

142 Rollinger, J.M., Hornick, A., Langer, T., Stuppner, H., and Prast, H. (2004) Acetylcholinesterase inhibitory activity of scopolin and scopoletin discovered by virtual screening of natural products. *Journal of Medicinal Chemistry*, **47**, 6248–6254.

143 Rollinger, J.M., Mocka, P., Zidorn, C., Ellmerer, E.P., Langer, T., and Stuppner, H. (2005) Application of the in combo screening approach for the discovery of non-alkaloid acetylcholinesterase inhibitors from *Cichorium intybus*. *Current Drug Discovery Technologies*, **2**, 185–193.

144 Rollinger, J.M., Steindl, T.M., Schuster, D., Kirchmair, J., Anrain, K., Ellmerer, E.P., Langer, T., Stuppner, H., Wutzler, P., and Schmidtke, M. (2008) Structure-based virtual screening for the discovery of natural inhibitors for human rhinovirus coat protein. *Journal of Medicinal Chemistry*, **51**, 842–851.

145 Kiran, M.D., Adikesavan, N.V., Cirioni, O., Giacometti, A., Silvestri, C., Scalise, G., Ghiselli, R., Saba, V., Orlando, F., Shoham, M., and Balaban, N. (2008) Discovery of a quorum-sensing inhibitor of drug-resistant staphylococcal infections by structure-based virtual screening. *Molecular Pharmacology*, **73**, 1578–1586.

146 Tanrikulu, Y., Rau, O., Schwarz, O., Proschak, E., Siems, K., Müller-Kuhrt, L., Schubert-Zsilavecz, M., and Schneider, G. (2009) Structure-based pharmacophore screening for natural-

product-derived PPARγ agonists. *ChemBioChem*, **10**, 75–78.

147 Lee, J.Y., Jeong, K.W., Lee, J.U., Kang, D.I., and Kim, Y. (2009) Novel *E. coli* beta-ketoacyl-acyl carrier protein synthase III inhibitors as targeted antibiotics. *Bioorganic & Medicinal Chemistry*, **17**, 1506–1513.

148 Franke, L., Schwarz, O., Müller-Kuhrt, L., Hoernig, C., Fischer, L., George, S., Tanrikulu, Y., Schneider, P., Werz, O., Steinhilber, D., and Schneider, G. (2007) Identification of natural-product-derived inhibitors of 5-lipoxygenase activity by ligand-based virtual screening. *Journal of Medicinal Chemistry*, **50**, 2640–2646.

149 Rollinger, J.M., Kratschmar, D.V., Schuster, D., Pfisterer, P.H., Gumy, C., Aubry, E.M., Brandstötter, S., Stuppner, H., Wolber, G., and Odermatt, A. (2010) 11Beta-hydroxysteroid dehydrogenase 1 inhibiting constituents from *Eriobotrya japonica* revealed by bioactivity-guided isolation and computational approaches. *Bioorganic & Medicinal Chemistry*, **18**, 1507–1515.

150 Rollinger, J.M., Schuster, D., Danzl, B., Schwaiger, S., Markt, P., Schmidtke, M., Gertsch, J., Raduner, S., Wolber, G., Langer, T., and Stuppner, H. (2009) In *silico* target fishing for rationalized ligand discovery exemplified on constituents of *Ruta graveolens*. *Planta Medica*, **75**, 195–204.

6
Docking Methods for Virtual Screening: Principles and Recent Advances

Didier Rognan

Writing a chapter on ligand docking is both easy and difficult. There are a great number of reviews (225) and application papers (>2800), and hence collecting these data and compiling them into one chapter is time consuming. This compilation is however comparatively easier to accomplish than attempting to write anew on this topic. Accordingly, this chapter will be divided into two parts. The first part recalls the basic principles of ligand docking for newcomers to the field. The most frequently used methods will be briefly described and discussed. For an exhaustive survey of algorithmic details, the reader is recommended to refer to recent reviews [1–11]. The second part illustrates the most remarkable advances of the past 2 years as well as the novel docking algorithms that have not been previously described by current reviews. These methodological advances will be discussed in the light of their applicability to virtual screening (VS). Whether a docking algorithm has to be applied to docking a single ligand or a large collection of compounds forces the user to adopt quite different strategies, notably with respect to protein flexibility and ligand setup. Therefore, computer-intensive docking methods notably based on molecular dynamics (MD) [12, 13] or normal mode analysis (NMA) [14] will not be reviewed here.

6.1
Principles of Molecular Docking

Given a small molecular weight compound and a target (usually a protein) of interest, docking is the computational answer to two basic questions: (1) What is the protein-bound conformation of the ligand? (2) What is the relative orientation of the ligand with respect to the target? This information is described by the proposed binding mode (pose) of the ligand for this particular target, illustrated by the Cartesian coordinates of the protein-bound ligand. To answer both questions, any molecular docking engine consists of two parts: a conformational search algorithm to sample all degrees of freedom (translational, rotational, and conformational) of the ligand, and a scoring function to rank putative poses for a compound and/or compounds from a large library.

Virtual Screening. Edited by C. Sotriffer

ISBN: 978-3-527-32636-5

6.1.1
Sampling Degrees of Freedom of the Ligand

There are basically three ways to handle ligand flexibility during docking: generation of conformers prior to docking, incremental ligand buildup, and stochastic methods. They will notably differ in their adaptability to the local protein environment, transferability to multiple docking engines, and speed.

6.1.1.1 Generation of Multiconformer Ligand Libraries

In the pioneering work of Kuntz and coworkers on the first standalone docking program (Dock), the ligand was considered rigid [15]. Ligand flexibility could thus be addressed only by preparing a set of suitable conformers for all ligands to be docked (so-called flexibases) [16]. There are now numerous programs to generate a set of three-dimensional (3D) conformers for small molecular weight ligands (e.g., Caesar [17], Catalyst (Accelrys Software Inc., San Diego, CA), and Omega (OpenEye Scientific Software, Santa Fe, NM)) that have been shown in benchmark studies to reproduce relatively well protein-bound ligand conformations [18, 19]. Once flexibases have been prepared, they can be easily transferred to most docking codes, which is a true advantage of this strategy.

The docking is completely rigid and consists in matching ligand with active site features. Since shape recognition is an essential component of protein–ligand interactions, many tools (e.g., Dock [15] and Fred [20]) look for shape complementarity between the ligand and an inverse image of the binding site, usually represented by a set of overlapping spheres. However, if the true protein-bound ligand conformation is not featured by a set of prepared conformers, there are few chances that even a final protein–ligand energy refinement will correct the erroneous pose. Moreover, for docking notably very large compound libraries, a significant amount of disk space (>100 GB) has to be reserved for the flexibase if standard file formats (sd, mol2) are chosen for data storage. Compressed binary formats as the OpenEye's oeb file format (OpenEye Scientific Software, Santa Fe, NM) are of special interest to address this issue.

6.1.1.2 Incremental Construction

Many docking programs (e.g., FlexX [21], Surflex [22], and Dock [23]) build up the ligand on the fly by first splitting the compound into its basic fragments, then docking a reference fragment (or base fragment) by geometric matching, and finally incrementally reconstructing the full ligand by adding fragments stepwise until the full molecule has been built. In order to speed up the process, only the most favorable values of a specific dihedral angle are browsed in a lookup table (e.g., the MIMUMBA conformer library [24]), the selected pose being the one that scored the best by a scoring function. An advantage of this method with respect to multiconformational databases is that the bound conformation of the ligand is generated in the presence of the target. However, if the bound conformer exhibits at least one unexpected torsional angle, incremental buildup techniques are unlikely to find a correct solution. Moreover, since many compounds share identical base fragments (e.g., heterocycles), there is a waste of time in repeating the same docking operation on simple fragments. It should be mentioned, however, that combinatorial docking algorithms [25] can take advantage of the fact that compounds share the same base fragment. Generating first all possible docking poses of all fragments and looking whether they have already been docked significantly speed up the process by storing a set of solutions for each fragment (e.g., in eHiTS [26]). Linkers must then be added to connect these fragments together, the full molecule being refined in a last step within the active site.

6.1.1.3 Stochastic Methods

The last category of conformational search methods samples ligand's conformation on the fly but does not necessarily give the same answer by repeating the docking. Two main computational methods are therefore used: Monte Carlo (MC) and Genetic algorithms (GAs). MC methods (e.g., in ICM [27] and Glide [28]) vary one parameter at a time (e.g., torsional angle and global rotation/translation of the ligand) and estimate the energy of newly generated poses. If that energy, whatever the scoring function used (empirical, knowledge-based potential of mean force, or force field), is lower than the previous one, it is kept. If not, a selection process (e.g., Metropolis criterion) will ensure the probability of a defined pose according to its Boltzmann weight factor $\exp(-E/kT)$. MC is often coupled to simulated annealing (e.g., in GlamDock [29]) that consists in progressively decreasing the temperature to trap the protein–ligand complex in a low energy minimum. During the initial docking steps, the temperature is set to higher values, thus enabling to cross energy barriers on the potential energy surface and efficiently browse conformational space. By cooling down the system during the docking, the conformational freedom of the ligand is continuously decreased until a minimum is reached.

The second popular category of stochastic methods uses GAs (e.g., in Gold [30] and AutoDock [31]). Most GAs are inspired from Darwin's theory of evolution. A population of individuals or chromosomes is set up first. A chromosome is here a ligand pose characterized by its properties (e.g., dihedral angle values and global rotation/translation vectors) encoded in genes. A population of chromosomes is left to evolve by genetic operations (mutation of one gene, crossing-over) and the fittest parents are allowed to create a new generation until a termination criterion is reached (e.g., rmsd of best ranked poses within a certain threshold).

Like MC methods, GAs may encounter a local energy minimum in which the best pose remains trapped. One cannot guarantee that the global minimum of the potential energy surface has been reached notably if this hypersurface is very rough as it is frequently the case for protein–ligand complexes. To cross local minima, tabu searches (e.g., in Pro_Leads [32]) can be combined to MC or GA in which a tabu list of already visited low-energy poses is stored and frequently updated to prevent the conformational sampling for premature convergence.

Alternatively, barrier heights can be erased in a method called stochastic tunneling (e.g., in FlexScreen [33]) that allows poses to tunnel through the potential energy surface.

6.1.2
Scoring Ligand Poses

There is a wide variety of different techniques available for predicting binding free energies from 3D structures of a protein–ligand complex [11, 34, 35]. These techniques differ significantly in accuracy and speed. If one wants to predict the binding free energy difference between a ligand and a reference molecule, very accurate but time-consuming techniques (free energy perturbation and thermodynamic integration) can be used [34]. If the aim is to compare free energies of hundreds or thousands of protein–ligand complexes (e.g., generated by virtual screening), much faster but thus less accurate scoring functions have to be used. Scoring functions can be mainly grouped into three categories [11, 35, 36]: empirical scoring functions, knowledge-based potential of mean force, and force field-based functions. In a virtual screening, scoring functions are used for two purposes: (i) during the docking process, they serve as fitness function in optimizing placement of the ligand; (ii) when the docking is completed, it is used to rank each ligand of the database for which a docking solution has been found. Different scoring functions are frequently used for these two purposes in recent updates of most docking tools.

6.1.2.1 Empirical Scoring Functions

Empirical scoring functions use several terms describing properties known to be important in ligand binding to construct a master equation for predicting binding affinity. Multilinear regression is used to optimize the coefficients to weight the computed terms using a training set of protein–ligand complexes for which both the binding affinity and an experimentally determined high-resolution 3D structure is known. These terms generally describe polar interactions such as hydrogen bonds and ionic interactions, apolar interactions such as lipophilic and aromatic interactions, loss of ligand flexibility (entropy), and eventually also desolvation effects. One major disadvantage of the empirical scoring functions is the need of a training set to derive the weight factors of the individual energy terms. One can therefore expect an empirical scoring function to perform well only for proteins similar to that used in the training set [36].

6.1.2.2 Knowledge-Based Potential of Mean Force

A major disadvantage of empirical scoring functions lies in the fact that it is unclear to what extent they can be applied to protein–ligand complexes that were not represented in the training set used for deriving the master equation. Furthermore, empirical scoring functions dissect the protein–ligand binding free energy into all its physically meaningful contributions and tries to evaluate them explicitly. Desolvation and entropy terms are, however, difficult to quantify. A more recently developed approach avoiding these disadvantages uses knowledge-based scoring functions with potentials of mean force. A potential of mean force simply encodes structural information gathered from protein–ligand X-ray coordinates into Helmholtz free interaction energies of protein–ligand atom pairs. It is assumed that the more often a protein atom of type i and ligand atom of type j are found at a certain distance r_{ij}, the more favorable is this interaction. Each interaction type between a protein atom of type i and a ligand atom type j at a distance r_{ij} is then assigned a protein–ligand interaction free energy $A(r)$ depending on its frequency.

$$A(r) = -k_{\mathrm{B}} T \ln g_{ij}(r)$$

where k_{B} is the Boltzmann constant, T is the absolute temperature, and $g_{ij}(r)$ is the atom pair distribution function for a protein–ligand atom pair ij. The distribution function is calculated from the occurrence of that pair ij at a certain distance r in a database of protein–ligand complexes (usually the PDB). The score is defined as the sum over all interatomic interactions of the protein–ligand complex. Advantages of this approach are that no fitting to experimentally determined binding free energies of the complexes in the training set is needed, and that solvation and entropic terms are treated implicitly.

6.1.2.3 **Force Fields**

Force field-based scoring functions are based on the nonbonded terms of a classical molecular mechanics force field (e.g., AMBER and CHARMM). A Lennard-Jones potential describes van der Waals interactions, whereas the Coulomb energy describes the electrostatic components of the interactions. The nonbonded interaction energy takes the following form:

$$E = \sum_{i=1}^{\mathrm{lig}} \sum_{j=1}^{\mathrm{rec}} \left[\frac{Aij}{r^{12}} - \frac{B_{ij}}{r^{6}} + 332 \frac{q_i q_j}{D r_{ij}} \right]$$

where A_{ij} and B_{ij} are respectively van der Waals repulsion and attraction parameters between two atoms i and j at a distance r_{ij}; q_i and q_j are the point charges on atoms i and j, respectively; D is the dielectric function; and 332 is a factor that converts the electrostatic energy into kilocalories per mole. The main drawback of force field calculations is the omission of the entropic component of the binding free energy. Therefore, attention should be paid not to overestimate the larger and most polar molecules that usually get the highest enthalpy interaction scores.

6.1.2.4 **Critical Evaluation of Scoring Functions**

Several independent studies agree to conclude that many fast scoring functions can indeed distinguish near-native poses (rmsd lower than 2.0 Å from the X-ray pose) from decoys for about 70% of high-resolution protein–ligand X-ray structures [36, 37]. However, when docking is applied to a large database, the corresponding scoring function should be robust enough to rank putative hits by increasing binding free energy values. Unfortunately, an accurate prediction of absolute binding free energies is still impossible whatever be the method: the treatment of solvation or the charge model [36–38]. Predicting binding free energy changes is possible provided that a customized scoring function is applied to a series of congeneric ligands. However, for a database containing a large diversity of compounds and for targets that have not been traditionally used for calibrating scoring functions, the obtained accuracy is usually limited (about 7 kJ/mol or 1.5 pK unit) [36].

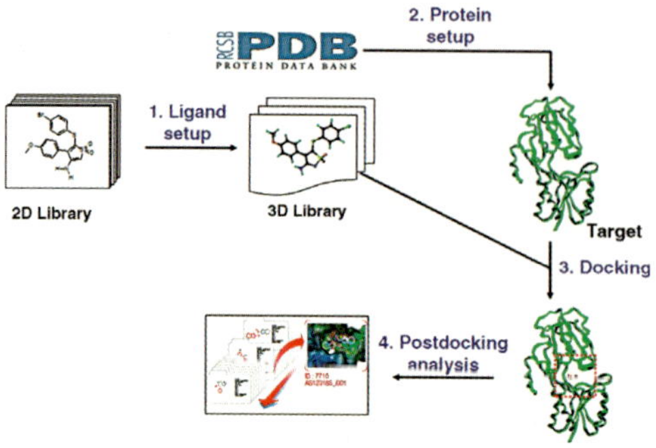

Figure 6.1 Typical docking flowchart.

6.2
Docking-Based Virtual Screening Flowchart

A typical docking flowchart is made of four invariant steps whose importance is critical to the outcome of the virtual screening (Figure 6.1).

Beginners usually have the impression that the docking step itself is crucial and may focus on this aspect only (e.g., conformational sampling method and free energy estimation of docking poses), which obviously is very dangerous. The four steps are of equal importance and will equally influence the quality of the results, notably for virtual screening applications where a compromise has to be found between quality and automation of input files. Docking is not only a matter of structural and computational biology but also of chemistry.

6.2.1
Ligand Setup

The very first step is to set up atomic coordinates and atom types/bond orders for ligands to dock (cf. also Chapter 2 of this book). Considering that atom types are correct, docking is still extremely sensitive to any parameter that may influence molecular interactions: protonation state, tautomeric state, and stereoisomeric state [39–41], notably when the user relies on empirical scoring functions to rank docking poses. Even the input file format (SMILES, SD, and MOL2) matters notably for equivalent atoms (e.g., oxygen atoms of a deprotonated carboxylic acid). The MOL2 file format is the gold standard for docking since it is compatible with most docking codes and addresses quite satisfactorily critical issues (treatment of symmetrical groups and variety of atom types). It is generally recommended to generate a reliable 3D conformation (e.g., using CORINA (Molecular Networks GmbH, 91052 Erlangen, Germany)) from a SMILES string or an SD file and quickly refine it with standard molecular mechanics energy minimization protocols [42]. Several automated ligand preparation flowcharts are now available in most docking programs (e.g., GLIDE (Schrodinger Inc., Portland, OR) and GOLD (Cambridge Crystallographic Data Centre, Cambridge, UK)) or chemoinformatic toolkits (CHEMAXON, FILTER (OpenEye Scientific

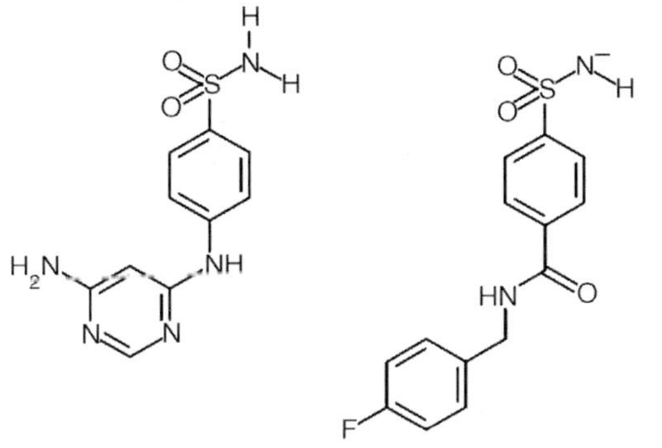

Figure 6.2 Influence of the binding site environment on the ionization state of arylsulfonamides. When bound to cdk2, the arylsulfonamide is neutral. Upon binding to carbonic anhydrase II, the arylsulfonamide is polarized by the metal ion present in the binding site and deprotonated.

Software, Santa Fe, NM), and PIPELINE PILOT (Accelrys Software Inc., San Diego, CA)). They should always be used with caution since they are based on predefined rules that usually miss the local influence of binding site atoms (Figure 6.2).

When applied to virtual screening, ligand setup also implies the choice of a collection of compounds (or more) to screen. In most of the cases, either screening decks (industrial environment) or commercially available compound collections (academic settings) are chosen. For prospective screening, there is generally no reason to favor one particular screening collection over another one. As most of them are easily accessible [43, 44], the best possible approach for an academic user is to start from a unified and filtered data set [45–47]. Of course, corporate and focused libraries may also be used. The former are particularly interesting for screening targets belonging to deeply investigated families (e.g., kinases and GPCRs) that usually contain a high percentage of true positives. Whatever the database selected, it is generally advisable to downsize the collection of molecules that will be submitted to 3D docking. A typical error from beginners is to screen the largest possible database, with the hope to optimize hit rate, chemotype enrichment, and binding modes. Such an approach only optimizes the noise to signal ratio for the simple reason that docking generates many false positives (about 90–95% in a VS) and to a lesser extent false negatives. Besides some important filters (chemical reactivity, druglikeness, etc.), it is generally advisable to first filter out those molecules that do not fulfill the simple 2D and/or 3D pharmacophoric features.

6.2.2 Protein Setup

Protein setup (cf. also Chapter 4 of this book) is technically easier since one has generally to care only about one macromolecule. It is advisable to start from a high-resolution X-ray structure [48], although homology models with a strong experimental support may also be used [49–51]. When several X-ray structures for the protein of interest are available, it is better to start from an holostructure (protein in complex with a ligand) than from an apostructure (ligand-free structure) [48]. When several holostructures are available, one should select at least one cocrystallized with a ligand in the binding site of interest. If a multiple choice still exists, it is advised to select an ensemble of structures reflecting the conformational flexibility of the binding site.

In any case, hydrogen atoms need to be added to the X-ray structure and a special care should be given to polar hydrogens (in serine, threonine, and tyrosine) in order to optimize the hydrogen bonding network at the binding site vicinity. A tautomeric state for histidine residues should be defined likewise, notably by taking into account how they interact with known ligands in existing crystal structures. Finally, the protein can be refined by a standard molecular mechanics protocol in order to remove putative clashes.

It is generally recommended to focus docking to a protein cavity of interest (catalytic site, inhibitor, or allosteric site) to limit the 3D space to sample. Usually, this information is inferred from known protein–ligand X-ray/NMR structures or existing site-directed mutagenesis studies. However, more and more apoprotein structures are solved nowadays by structural genomics consortia [52]. For many of these structures still expecting a functional annotation, there is no a priori information with regard to the protein region to scan for docking potential low molecular weight inhibitors. It might thus be necessary to scan the entire surface of the protein for potential cavities before docking [53]. When compared to local docking focusing on a predefined binding pocket, blind docking is generally less accurate because of the larger conformational space to scan. In addition, docking times are obviously significantly longer when a blind docking protocol is used, which thus limits the size of compound libraries to screen in a VS experiment.

6.2.3 Docking

From the pioneering work of Kuntz *et al.* [15], over 60 docking programs based on very different physicochemical approximations have been reported [11].

Since any docking tool needs to combine a docking engine with a fast scoring function, the recent literature is full of benchmarks addressing three possible issues: (i) the capability of a docking algorithm to reproduce the X-ray pose of selected small molecular weight ligands [54–57], (ii) the propensity of fast scoring functions to recognize near-native poses among a set of decoys and to predict absolute binding free energies [36, 37], and (iii) the discrimination of known binders from randomly chosen molecules in virtual screening experiments [54–56, 58]. However, analyzing all these data for a comparative analysis of available docking tools is very difficult. First, many tools are not available. Second, independent studies assessing the relative performance of docking algorithms/scoring functions are still rare and focus on the usage of few methods. Third, the quality judgment may vary depending on the examined properties (quality of the top-ranked pose, quality of all plausible poses, binding free energy prediction, and virtual screening utility). Fourth, most docking programs assume approximation levels that can vary considerably [59] and lead, for example, to very inhomogeneous docking paces ranging from few seconds to few hours. Finally, many docking programs have been calibrated and validated on small protein–ligand data sets. Hence, detailed benchmarks (>100 PDB-ligand complexes) are only reported for few docking tools. The most exhaustive validation studies on different data sets agree to conclude that the accuracy of a docking tool is largely target dependent [54–58] and should be examined on a case-by-case basis. The most robust programs generate near-native poses in about 75–80% of the cases [54–56], provided that several solutions are stored. A major problem is that the scoring function does not always (only in about 40–50% of the cases) predict the correct solution as the most probable one, which considerably complicates the analysis of docking results. Numerous reasons explain this limited accuracy [55]. Some are easy to correct (e.g., incorrect atom types for either the ligand or the protein), some are more difficult (e.g., resolution of the protein 3D structure, flexibility of the ligand, and accuracy of the scoring function), and some are really tricky to overcome (protein flexibility and the role of bound water). Trends observed in docking accuracy are also true considering virtual screening efficacy that is the ability to discriminate true binders from inactives and/or randomly chosen compounds [54, 55, 57, 58]. However, predicting that docking program will be the most suited for a research project is still unrealistic. If known ligands are available, the best possible option is to try a systematic combination of docking/scoring parameters and select for productive screening the one that best segregates true actives from true inactives. If no or very few ligands are available, some guides may be followed to choose the tool that seems the most appropriate to the physicochemical properties of the protein cavity [55].

6.2.4
Postdocking Analysis

The easiest way to mine docking results is to rank the top pose of database compounds by decreasing energy score. Unfortunately, this approach is absolutely to avoid for the simple reason that scoring function remains the Achilles' heel of docking programs. From this observation, two sources of improvement are possible: (i) design more accurate scoring functions [38], and (ii) design smarter strategies to postprocess docking outputs.

The reader is referred to Chapter 7 of this book dealing with scoring functions in detail. Many computational chemists actually favor the second option. The accuracy of scoring functions has leveled off several years ago, for the simple reason that some unknown parameters (e.g., role of bound water and protein flexibility) remain extremely difficult to predict whatever the physical principles used to derive a scoring function. Acknowledging that scoring functions are far from being perfect, a viable strategy to retrieve true positives from a virtual screen is first to detect false positives. Many strategies are possible. The simplest consists in rescoring poses with additional scoring functions; hoping that a consensus scoring [60, 61] will better identify true hits (top ranked by several scoring functions) from decoys. Comparing hit rates between simple and consensus scoring should however be realized on hit lists of comparative size [62]. However, customizing a consensus scoring scheme requires first the knowledge of several and chemically diverse true hits. Such data are not always available. Therefore, for poorly investigated targets, other strategies have to be designed. Topological filters can be used to filter out poses exhibiting steric or electrostatic mismatches between the ligand and its target [63]. Poses can also be minimized by a third party software [64, 65], clustered [66, 67], and analyzed by machine learning methods [68, 69]. In any case, the postprocessing treatment should be simple enough to be reproducible for a wide array of targets. An alternative strategy is to look at enrichment among true hits in precomputed substructures/scaffolds [70]. This presents the advantage to focus more on scaffolds and how docking scores are distributed among them and less on individual molecules. Therefore, false negatives may be recovered if they share a common scaffold with true positives.

Pharmacophoric constraints can be used to limit the chemical space to search. These constraints can be two dimensional (presence/absence of pharmacophoric features regardless of their relative location) or three dimensional (set of features and distances). There are two different conceptual ways of introducing pharmacophoric constraints in docking. Either constraints can be directly read in the docking algorithm in order to filter out unsuitable compounds [71] or constraints can be used as postfilters to prioritize poses fulfilling a pharmacophore query [72]. Both strategies may lead to significantly different results as to whether the docking is constrained by the pharmacophore or not. The first approach presents the advantage of unifying pharmacophore filtering and docking in a single computational step and does not require customizing a compound library before the docking step. It however restricts the choice of the docking software as pharmacophore filtering has to be implemented as an option (e.g., in FlexX-Pharm [71]). The last approach is softer as it only constrains the analysis and not the docking, but is independent of the docking code that is used. However, it does not mean that a compound library should not be customized first. In fact, it is strongly acknowledged to first set up a collection of compounds compatible with a simple 2D pharmacophore(s) describing the corresponding activity class, then dock, and finally analyze the docking poses under pharmacophoric constraints. All docking studies, notably applied to VS, agree that enrichment in true actives strongly depends on how ligand-based (pharmacophore) and receptor-based (docking) information is efficiently coupled [46, 73], irrespective to whether the pharmacophore filtering step is realized before or after docking [72].

Last but not the least, selected hits should be browsed in 3D target space for the ultimate selection: no algorithm yet outperforms the brain of an experienced modeler for such a task!

6.3
Recent Advances in Docking-Based VS Methods

6.3.1
Novel Docking Algorithms

In ASEDock [74], the ligand binding site is described as a concave portion of the protein surface and represented as a collection of alpha spheres. An alpha sphere is a sphere contacting n atoms at its boundaries (usually $n=4$), but containing no internal atoms. A so-called ASE model is defined by combining alpha spheres (allowed regions) with exclusion volumes (forbidden regions). Ligand docking is simply done by finding the optimal alignment of ligand atoms (from a predefined conformer library) to the ASE model using a simple Gaussian overlap scoring function. The last step is a full protein–ligand structure refinement with the MMFF94x force field. On a benchmark of 59 high-resolution protein–ligand complexes, ASEDock was able to find a pose within 2 Å rmsd from the X-ray solution in 98% of test cases. The code is interfaced with Moe (Chemical Computing Group, Montreal, QC, Canada) and was used to find inhibitors of the ribulose 1,5-bisphosphate carboxylase/oxygenase [75].

ADDock [76] is a recently described novel algorithm for placing flexible ligands into a rigid receptor. Terminal hydrogen atoms are iteratively selected as anchors for docking the entire ligand whose structure is rebuilt from a connection list describing each node of a graph-describing ligand. No global translational moves are considered; only global rotational moves by varying the value of four quaternions and dihedral angle values are optimized by a GA. Each pose is scored by a modified version of the PLP scoring function [77]. On a test set of 92 PDB protein–ligand complexes, ADDock was able to self-dock the native ligand in its PDB cavity with an accuracy of 91.3% (rmsd < 2.0 Å). In virtual screening mode, a simple receptor–ligand steric interaction energy could discriminate actives from decoys for three unrelated targets [76].

Several adaptations of known stochastic optimization methods to the problem of molecular docking have been described recently. FlexScreen [33] uses a stochastic tunneling optimization method for finding the absolute minimum of the free energy of a protein–ligand complex. Stochastic tunneling allows a classical force field optimizer to tunnel through the potential energy surface by flattening the hypersurface if an energy barrier of a certain height is met. It is expected to avoid usual flaws of many stochastic optimization methods (e.g., simulated annealing) that can remain trapped in a local energy minimum. Interestingly, FlexScreen handles both ligand and receptor flexibility (a few side chains) using small but continuous variations of dihedral angles. When applied to the Astex/CCDC data set of 83 high-resolution protein–ligand PDB structures, 80% of the ligands were docked within 2 Å rmsd from the X-ray pose [78].

In ISE-dock [79], an iterative stochastic elimination (ISE) algorithm was implemented in AutoDock 3.05 [31]. While the classical Lamarckian GA implemented in AutoDock is used to sample ligand's degrees of freedom, the ISE algorithm iteratively eliminates values for each degree of freedom that are statistically predominant in the worst solutions but not in the best solutions, as scored by the native AutoDock scoring function. The ISE approach enables to scan a large combination of solutions and to prune them relatively quickly. The method was shown to provide slightly better results than the native AutoDock in two independent benchmark studies. A small limitation of ISE-Dock is its relative slowness (about 7 min. per ligand) that precludes for the screening of large data sets, although massive computing environments are now accessible to most computational chemists.

Artificial intelligence algorithms have also been embedded in docking codes, notably ant colony optimization (ACO) and particle swarm optimization (PSO) [80, 81]. Both algorithms try to reproduce the behavior of self-organized systems. ACO is particularly well suited to optimize paths to a goal (best possible pose) by depositing artificial pheromones (variable weights) through the path. It has been implemented in the PLANTS program [82] with success rates comparable to state-of-the-art algorithms, but presents the noticeable advantage to converge more often than other algorithms to a near-native pose (unpublished in-house data). In PSO optimization, a group (swarm) of individuals (particles) explore the conformational space with an adjustable velocity, each particle keeping in memory the best solution encountered. PSO algorithms as implemented in SODOCK [80] or PSO@AUTODOCK [81] have been found to propose more reliable docking poses for highly flexible ligands than GA or MC optimizers that could readily get trapped in local minima.

6.3.2 Fragment Docking

Screening low molecular weight compounds (fragments) by biophysical methods (NMR, X-ray, and surface plasmon resonance) has gained considerable importance in the last decade [83]. Hence, fragment space is several orders of magnitude smaller than druglike or leadlike chemical space. The chemical diversity encoded in a few thousands fragments is far above than that seen in one million druglike compounds, and explains why fragment screening very often can rescue traditional high-throughput screening (HTS) in hit finding. Docking a fragment in a binding site is however considered difficult since it has to reflect a few weak interactions resulting in different binding poses that are equally considered by standard scoring functions [84]. In two elegant papers, Shoichet's group however demonstrates that fragment docking to polar cavities (β-lactamases) results in true hits whose predicted poses could be confirmed by cocrystallization [85, 86]. Interestingly, the specificity and affinity of fragments for a particular target increases with their molecular weight in a hit follow-up optimization step [86].

Another way to prioritize fragments was proposed by Fukunishi *et al.* [87] in the fragment screening by replica generation (FSRG) method. Instead of docking a library of fragments, the method first generates a set of replicas for each fragment by attaching six side chains to a diversity point and then generates higher molecular weight compounds that are supposed to be easier to dock. Analogues are classically docked and initial scaffolds are ordered according to the ranks of their corresponding replicas. Interestingly, polar interactions (Coulombic and hydrogen bonding) were ignored when ranking replicas and only shape complementarity guides scaffold ranking. The FSRG method was shown to be able to recover true active scaffolds from inhibitors of six different target proteins [87].

6.3.3 Postdocking Refinement

6.3.3.1 Rescoring with Rigorous Scoring Functions

A logical work-around to the inaccuracy of fast scoring functions is the use of more rigorous binding free energy estimation methods for either prioritizing virtual hits for experimental validation or optimizing them into leads. Most accurate methods (thermodynamic integration and free energy perturbation) [88] are limited to a few ligands with minor structural changes. Faster approaches like the linear interaction energy (LIE) method, estimating free energies from free and protein-bound ligand MD trajectories, have been occasionally used but are still hard to generalize as VS rescoring scheme [89]. Most popular rescoring methods use a combination of molecular mechanics (MM), continuum solvent model like Poisson–Boltzmann (PB) or Generalized Born (GB) approximations, and solvent-accessible surface area-dependent nonpolar solvation term (SA). MM-PB(GB)SA methods have been claimed to be fast enough to be applied to a few hundred compounds and able to rescue known deficiencies of fast scoring functions in estimating ligand desolvation and conformer focusing (change from free to bound conformation and loss of conformational entropy upon binding) [90]. Conclusions about the benefit of MM-PB (GB)SA rescoring of docking poses are still contradictory, at least target dependent [91]. While some studies show a true benefit in enriching hit lists in true hits [92–95], others are disappointing and do not detect significant improvements with respect to simple protein–ligand MM energy refinements [96, 97]. MM-GBSA rescoring with binding site minimization was shown on toy cavities (small buried cavities for fragment-like compounds dominated by a single intermolecular interaction) [98] to not only rescue docking false negatives (allowing bigger ligands to dock by cavity refinement) but also to produce novel false positives notably among top-ranked molecules. It presents the danger to significantly decrease hit rates if a very tiny percentage of top-ranked compounds are tested experimentally. Two reasons were invoked for this intriguing observation: inadequate ligand parametrization, and difficulties in treating electrostatic interactions when significant conformational changes are occurring at the protein cavity.

6.3.3.2 **Topological Scoring by Protein–Ligand Interaction Fingerprint (IFP)**

An IFP is a bit string registering how a ligand interacts with predefined active site residues [99]. For each active site residue or atom, a bit is set on or off whether or not a specific interaction (H-bond, ionic interaction, apolar contacts, aromatic interactions, and metal complexation) is detected. Poses may thus be ranked according to the IFP similarity to a known template (Figure 6.3). Contrary to what may be expected, IFP scoring does not prioritize virtual hits with high 2D similarity to a reference and is suitable for simple hit ranking [100–102], scaffold posing [84], and scaffold hopping [103].

Along the same idea, Renner *et al.* introduced the concept of scoring docking poses by searching for maximum common binding modes (MCBM) [104] with the assumption that true binding poses of similar ligands should be closer to each other than to poses of inactive compounds. The approach was validated in four different data sets and shows that MCBM scoring is superior to any individual scoring function. Instead of registering the presence/absence of protein–ligand interactions, the relative positions of interacting atom pairs can be encoded according to predefined distance ranges with the same advantage over classical energy-based scoring functions [105].

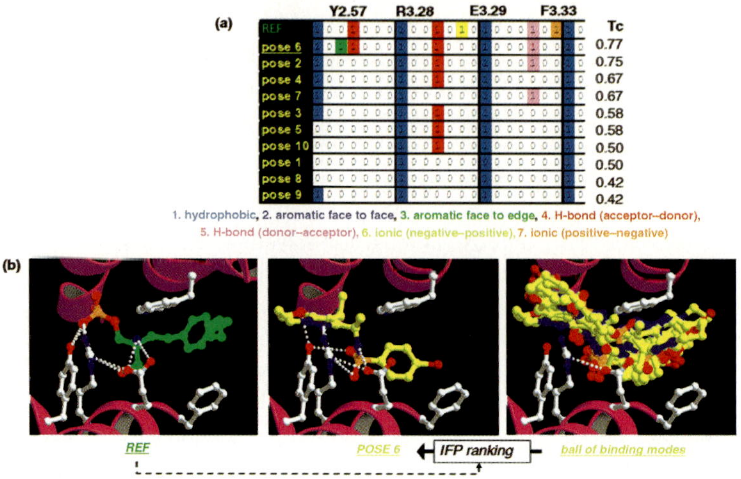

Figure 6.3 Converting a reference protein–ligand complex (REF) (a) into an interaction fingerprint (IFP) registering seven possible interactions with binding site residues. Docked poses (b) (right panel) are fingerprinted and the corresponding IFPs are compared to the reference IFP (REF) using a standard Tanimoto coefficient. The best pose (pose 6) exhibits the highest IFP similarity to the reference.

Extending the approach to a bioinformatics-guided docking protocol was recently proposed by Takaya *et al.* [106]. Ligand poses are scored by similarity to a knowledge-based ligand fingerprint gathered from a data set of target protein-oriented ligands (ligands of targets close to the one of interest) and optimized by a simulated annealing protocol.

6.3.4
Addressing Protein Flexibility

About 85% of proteins undergo conformational changes upon ligand binding, going from variation of a few rotameric states of key binding site residues [107] to larger domain rearrangements [108]. Moreover, cross-docking (docking a ligand to set of protein coordinates different from that of the cocrystal) to a single rigid target is known to be much less accurate than self-docking (docking a ligand to its native PDB structure) [109]. Besides deficiencies in predicting binding free energies, addressing protein flexibility is the most important issue in ligand docking (cf. also Chapters 8 and 9 of this book). The simplest way to encode protein flexibility is to fine-tune nonbonded energy potentials (soft docking) to tolerate some overlap between ligand and protein atoms. In a recent VS benchmark on 11 pharmaceutically interesting targets, soft docking enabled to dock more ligands than rigid docking, but at the cost of a lower specificity (inactives also dock better!) [33]. Soft docking is however limited to minor conformational changes of the target and will not be able to cope with backbone motions. Using multiple receptor conformations (MRCs) is therefore the most used approach to treat protein flexibility [2, 110]. There are two possible sources of receptor conformers, X-ray and/or NMR structures (high resolution but sometimes with a limited diversity), computed structures from molecular dynamics, Monte Carlo, or normal mode analysis. Motions may be limited to a few side chains by browsing rotamer libraries (e.g., in GOLD [111] and PLANTS [82]) with the danger of a strong dependency on the chosen library. Interestingly, selecting a few residues (3–5) for continuous dihedral rotation significantly enhances early enrichment factors in true hits but at the cost of increased computational times. Automating the selection of flexible residues for a target is proposed by docking known ligands and selecting the most clashing residues [33].

A cumbersome approach to MRC docking is to repeat the docking for all protein conformers, merge the results, and select the most appropriate pose whatever the protein conformer selected. Ensemble docking was recently shown to be able to rescue the poor suitability of single NMR structures or homology models for lead optimization by docking [112]. It is however computationally intensive. Therefore, most MRC approaches rely on conformational ensembles [110, 113] where interaction energies may be averaged from a unique grid to which all protein conformers have been matched (e.g., in DOCK [23] or AUTODOCK [31]), and FLEXE [114] uses a unified protein representation with a single set of invariant coordinates and various sets of coordinates for flexible moieties, but is limited to a few sets of coordinates and requires protein structures homogenization (unique number of common atoms and unique atom numbering). Finally, protein conformers may be encoded as an additional gene in a chromosome treated by a genetic algorithm (e.g., in FITTED) [115–117]. A frequent question in ensemble docking is which protein conformers to choose? Hence, different sets of protein conformers are likely to deliver different docking results. Conformers can be clustered according to rms deviations of key residues or molecular volumes of the binding site for generating a set of dissimilar representatives [118]. An automated protocol for selecting protein conformers for docking was recently proposed and consists in selecting the three entries maximizing the mean docking score for the top 1% database ligands [113]. Different approximations can be used for side chain and backbone atoms in hybrid methods as that proposed by May and Zacharias [119] in which side chain motions are described by precomputed rotameric states and backbone motions by elastic normal modes.

A good compromise between speed and accuracy was recently proposed by Bottegoni *et al.* as four-dimensional docking [120]. The fourth dimension in the docking is simply the target conformation. All conformers are simultaneously treated in a single docking run by switching, in a Monte Carlo sampling, between 3D grids storing interaction potentials of each conformer. When applied to 100 multiconformer PDB structures, 4D docking was nearly as accurate as ensemble docking (77% of successful dockings), although sparing 75% of cpu time dedicated to the ligand sampling phase.

FLIPDOCK [121] proposes a novel way of encoding both ligand and protein flexibility in docking. Molecular objects are recursively partitioned into independent nodes from a flexibility tree. Nodes are allowed to move with respect to each other through well-defined motions (shear, twist, screw, etc.), while normal modes are used to treat the node's internal flexibility. Side chain motions are considered classically by the use of rotamer libraries. Motion variables are encoded in a genetic algorithm and poses scored with the AutoDock 3.05 force field. In 400 cross-docking experiments, FLIPDock achieves a significantly higher successful docking rate than the original AutoDock engine.

6.3.5
Solvated or Dry?

Ligand binding is often mediated by key water molecules resulting in the impossibility to generate a good pose if these water molecules are systematically removed [117, 122]. At least, strongly bound waters (three H-bonds with the ligand and protein) should be considered with the danger to bias the VS toward hits sharing the same chemotype than that of the cocrystallized ligand. Many docking programs (FlexX [21], Gold [122], Fitted [115], and Dock [123]) now offer the possibility to switch "on" or "off" water molecules during the docking. Obtained results, as usual, are contradictory (cf. also Chapter 10 of this book). Some authors report a statistically improved docking accuracy with displaceable waters [117], while others note that for most of the targets, the docking is basically unaffected [122, 123]. Since the free energy change associated with the displacement of a water molecule is hard to compute, using displaceable waters clearly does not affect predicting binding free energies, whatever be the scoring function [124].

6.4
Future Trends in Docking

Structure-based (notably docking) and ligand-based (2D similarity searches, 3D shape, and pharmacophore searches) approaches have often been compared for their virtual screening accuracies [125–128]. Quite often, ligand-centric methods were shown to outperform structure-based virtual screening protocols, notably when sufficient knowledge is available on known ligands. Optimization of scoring protocols however show that peak performance in docking is rarely reached unless protein flexibility [2] and unconventional scoring functions are used to rank order docking poses [129]. Considerable breakthroughs have been noticed in the treatment of protein flexibility as well as in applying novel computational approaches to the global optimization of protein–ligand docking poses. Improving scoring functions is still extremely challenging. Fast scoring functions have reached their limit despite considerable efforts to vary the underlying physical principles and enlarge training data sets. Using more rigorous scoring functions often provides significant advantages, but at the cost of an extra computational burden, which limits their application to large ligand data sets. Fortunately, massive docking computing facilities have become available even for the academic community [130], and one can reasonably hope that this will force computational chemists not to increase the size of virtual libraries to screen but to fine-tune smarter docking/scoring protocols [131]. Taking the best out of docking-based virtual screening is more likely to be reached by designing integrated virtual screening workflows than for searching the ultimate scoring function. The rapid pace at which novel protein X-ray structures as well as chemogenomic data are generated will undoubtedly foster significant improvements in protein–ligand docking by an optimal use of known experimental data in docking protocols [106].

References

1 Tuccinardi, T. (2009) Docking-based virtual screening: recent developments. *Combinatorial Chemistry & High Throughput Screening*, **12**, 303–314.

2 Rao, C.B., Subramanian, J., and Sharma, S.D. (2009) Managing protein flexibility in docking and its applications. *Drug Discovery Today*, **14**, 394–400.

3 Dias, R. and de Azevedo, W.F., Jr. (2008) Molecular docking algorithms. *Current Drug Targets*, **9**, 1040–1047.

4 Kroemer, R.T. (2007) Structure-based drug design: docking and scoring. *Current Protein & Peptide Science*, **8**, 312–328.

5 Cavasotto, C.N. and Orry, A.J. (2007) Ligand docking and structure-based virtual screening in drug discovery. *Current Topics in Medicinal Chemistry*, **7**, 1006–1014.

6 Sousa, S.F., Fernandes, P.A., and Ramos, M.J. (2006) Protein–ligand docking: current status and future challenges. *Proteins*, **65**, 15–26.

7 Leach, A.R., Shoichet, B.K., and Peishoff, C.E. (2006) Prediction of protein–ligand interactions. Docking and scoring: successes and gaps. *Journal of Medicinal Chemistry*, **49**, 5851–5855.

8 Mohan, V., Gibbs, A.C., Cummings, M.D., Jaeger, E.P., and DesJarlais, R.L. (2005) Docking: successes and challenges. *Current Pharmaceutical Design*, **11**, 323–333.

9 Kitchen, D.B., Decornez, H., Furr, J.R., and Bajorath, J. (2004) Docking and scoring in virtual screening for drug discovery: methods and applications. *Nature Reviews. Drug Discovery*, **3**, 935–949.

10 Brooijmans, N. and Kuntz, I.D. (2003) Molecular recognition and docking algorithms. *Annual Review of Biophysics and Biomolecular Structure*, **32**, 335–373.

11 Moitessier, N., Englebienne, P., Lee, D., Lawandi, J., and Corbeil, C.R. (2008) Towards the development of universal, fast and highly accurate docking/scoring methods: a long way to go. *British Journal of Pharmacology*, **153** (Suppl. 1), S7–S26.

12 Davis, I.W. and Baker, D. (2009) RosettaLigand docking with full ligand and receptor flexibility. *Journal of Molecular Biology*, **385**, 381–392.

13 Taufer, M., Armen, R., Chen, J., Teller, P., and Brooks, C. (2009) Computational multiscale modeling in protein–ligand docking. *IEEE Engineering in Medicine and Biology Magazine*, **28**, 58–69.

14 Rueda, M., Bottegoni, G., and Abagyan, R. (2009) Consistent improvement of cross-docking results using binding site ensembles generated with elastic network normal modes. *Journal of Chemical Information and Modeling*, **49**, 716–725.

15 Kuntz, I.D., Blaney, J.M., Oatley, S.J., Langridge, R., and Ferrin, T.E. (1982) A geometric approach to macromolecule–ligand interactions. *Journal of Molecular Biology*, **161**, 269–288.

16 Kearsley, S.K., Underwood, D.J., Sheridan, R.P., and Miller, M.D. (1994) Flexibases: a way to enhance the use of molecular docking methods. *Journal of Computer-Aided Molecular Design*, **8**, 565–582.

17 Li, J., Ehlers, T., Sutter, J., Varma-O'brien, S., and Kirchmair, J. (2007) CAESAR: a new conformer generation algorithm based on recursive buildup and local rotational symmetry consideration. *Journal of Chemical Information and Modeling*, **47**, 1923–1932.

18 Bostrom, J. (2001) Reproducing the conformations of protein-bound ligands: a critical evaluation of several popular conformational searching tools. *Journal of Computer-Aided Molecular Design*, **15**, 1137–1152.

19 Kirchmair, J., Wolber, G., Laggner, C., and Langer, T. (2006) Comparative performance assessment of the conformational model generators omega and catalyst: a large-scale survey on the retrieval of protein-bound ligand conformations. *Journal of Chemical Information and Modeling*, **46**, 1848–1861.

20 McGann, M.R., Almond, H.R., Nicholls, A., Grant, J.A., and Brown, F.K. (2003) Gaussian docking functions. *Biopolymers*, **68**, 76–90.

21 Rarey, M., Kramer, B., Lengauer, T., and Klebe, G. (1996) A fast flexible docking method using an incremental construction algorithm. *Journal of Molecular Biology*, **261**, 470–489.

22 Jain, A.N. (2003) Surflex: fully automatic flexible molecular docking using a molecular similarity-based search engine. *Journal of Medicinal Chemistry*, **46**, 499–511.

23 Lang, P.T., Brozell, S.R., Mukherjee, S., Pettersen, E.F., Meng, E.C., Thomas, V., Rizzo, R.C., Case, D.A., James, T.L., and Kuntz, I.D. (2009) DOCK 6: combining techniques to model RNA–small molecule complexes. *RNA*, **15**, 1219–1230.

24 Klebe, G. and Mietzner, T. (1994) A fast and efficient method to generate biologically relevant conformations. *Journal of Computer-Aided Molecular Design*, **8**, 583–606.

25 Sun, Y., Ewing, T.J., Skillman, A.G., and Kuntz, I.D. (1998) CombiDOCK: structure-based combinatorial docking and library design. *Journal of Computer-Aided Molecular Design*, **12**, 597–604.

26 Zsoldos, Z., Reid, D., Simon, A., Sadjad, S.B., and Johnson, A.P. (2007) eHiTS: a new fast, exhaustive flexible ligand docking system. *Journal of Molecular Graphics & Modelling*, **26**, 198–212.

27 Totrov, M. and Abagyan, R. (1997) Flexible protein–ligand docking by global energy optimization in internal coordinates. *Proteins*, **29** (Suppl. 1), 215–220.

28 Friesner, R.A., Banks, J.L., Murphy, R.B., Halgren, T.A., Klicic, J.J., Mainz, D.T., Repasky, M.P., Knoll, E.H., Shelley, M., Perry, J.K., Shaw, D.E., Francis, P., and Shenkin, P.S. (2004) Glide: a new approach for rapid, accurate docking and scoring. 1. Method and assessment of docking accuracy. *Journal of Medicinal Chemistry*, **47**, 1739–1749.

29 Tietze, S. and Apostolakis, J. (2007) GlamDock: development and validation of a new docking tool on several thousand protein–ligand complexes. *Journal of Chemical Information and Modeling*, **47**, 1657–1672.

30 Jones, G., Willett, P., Glen, R.C., Leach, A.R., and Taylor, R. (1997) Development and validation of a genetic algorithm for flexible docking. *Journal of Molecular Biology*, **267**, 727–748.

31 Morris, G., Goodsell, D., Halliday, R., Huey, R., Hart, W., Belew, R., and Olson, A. (1998) Automated docking using a Lamarckian genetic algorithm and an empirical binding free energy solution. *Journal of Computational Chemistry*, **19**, 1639–1662.

32 Murray, C.W., Baxter, C.A., and Frenkel, A.D. (1999) The sensitivity of the results of molecular docking to induced fit effects: application to thrombin, thermolysin and neuraminidase. *Journal of Computer-Aided Molecular Design*, **13**, 547–562.

33 Kokh, D.B. and Wenzel, W. (2008) Flexible side chain models improve enrichment rates in *in silico* screening. *Journal of Medicinal Chemistry*, **51**, 5919–5931.

34 Jorgensen, W.L. (2009) Efficient drug lead discovery and optimization. *Accounts of Chemical Research*, **42**, 724–733.

35 Gohlke, H. and Klebe, G. (2002) Approaches to the description and prediction of the binding affinity of small-molecule ligands to macromolecular receptors. *Angewandte Chemie, International edition*, **41**, 2644–2676.

36 Ferrara, P., Gohlke, H., Price, D.J., Klebe, G., and Brooks, C.L., 3rd (2004) Assessing scoring functions for

protein–ligand interactions. *Journal of Medicinal Chemistry*, **47**, 3032–3047.

37 Wang, R., Lu, Y., and Wang, S. (2003) Comparative evaluation of 11 scoring functions for molecular docking. *Journal of Medicinal Chemistry*, **46**, 2287–2303.

38 Wang, R., Lu, Y., Fang, X., and Wang, S. (2004) An extensive test of 14 scoring functions using the PDBbind refined set of 800 protein–ligand complexes. *Journal of Chemical Information and Computer Science*, **44**, 2114–2125.

39 Feher, M. and Williams, C.I. (2009) Effect of input differences on the results of docking calculations. *Journal of Chemical Information and Modeling*, **49**, 1704–1714.

40 Knox, A.J., Meegan, M.J., Carta, G., and Lloyd, D.G. (2005) Considerations in compound database preparation: "hidden" impact on virtual screening results. *Journal of Chemical Information and Modeling*, **45**, 1908–1919.

41 Ten Brink, T. and Exner, T.E. (2009) Influence of protonation, tautomeric, and stereoisomeric states on protein–ligand docking results. *Journal of Chemical Information and Modeling*, **49**, 1535–1546.

42 Kirchmair, J., Markt, P., Distinto, S., Wolber, G., and Langer, T. (2008) Evaluation of the performance of 3D virtual screening protocols: RMSD comparisons, enrichment assessments, and decoy selection: what can we learn from earlier mistakes? *Journal of Computer-Aided Molecular Design*, **22**, 213–228.

43 Sirois, S., Hatzakis, G., Wei, D., Du, Q., and Chou, K.C. (2005) Assessment of chemical libraries for their druggability. *Computational Biology and Chemistry*, **29**, 55–67.

44 Baurin, N., Baker, R., Richardson, C., Chen, I., Foloppe, N., Potter, A., Jordan, A., Roughley, S., Parratt, M., Greaney, P., Morley, D., and Hubbard, R.E. (2004) Drug-like annotation and duplicate analysis of a 23-supplier chemical database totalling 2.7 million compounds. *Journal of Chemical Information and Computer Science*, **44**, 643–651.

45 Irwin, J.J. and Shoichet, B.K. (2005) ZINC: a free database of commercially available compounds for virtual screening. *Journal of Chemical Information and Modeling*, **45**, 177–182.

46 Kellenberger, E., Springael, J.Y., Parmentier, M., Hachet-Haas, M., Galzi, J.L., and Rognan, D. (2007) Identification of nonpeptide CCR5 receptor agonists by structure-based virtual screening. *Journal of Medicinal Chemistry*, **50**, 1294–1303.

47 Masciocchi, J., Frau, G., Fanton, M., Sturlese, M., Floris, M., Pireddu, L., Palla, P., Cedrati, F., Rodriguez-Tome, P., and Moro, S. (2009) MMsINC: a large-scale chemoinformatics database. *Nucleic Acids Research*, **37**, D284–D290.

48 McGovern, S.L. and Shoichet, B.K. (2003) Information decay in molecular docking screens against holo, apo, and modeled conformations of enzymes. *Journal of Medicinal Chemistry*, **46**, 2895–2907.

49 Bissantz, C., Bernard, P., Hibert, M., and Rognan, D. (2003) Protein-based virtual screening of chemical databases. II. Are homology models of G-protein coupled receptors suitable targets? *Proteins*, **50**, 5–25.

50 Oshiro, C., Bradley, E.K., Eksterowicz, J., Evensen, E., Lamb, M.L., Lanctot, J.K., Putta, S., Stanton, R., and Grootenhuis, P.D. (2004) Performance of 3D-database molecular docking studies into homology models. *Journal of Medicinal Chemistry*, **47**, 764–767.

51 Ferrara, P. and Jacoby, E. (2007) Evaluation of the utility of homology models in high throughput docking. *Journal of Molecular Modeling*, **13**, 897–905.

52 Dessailly, B.H., Nair, R., Jaroszewski, L., Fajardo, J.E., Kouranov, A., Lee, D., Fiser, A., Godzik, A., Rost, B., and Orengo, C. (2009) PSI-2: structural genomics to cover protein domain family space. *Structure*, **17**, 869–881.

53 Grosdidier, A., Zoete, V., and Michielin, O. (2009) Blind docking of 260 protein–ligand complexes with EADock 2.0. *Journal of Computational Chemistry*, **30**, 2021–2030.

54 Warren, G.L., Andrews, C.W., Capelli, A.M., Clarke, B., LaLonde, J., Lambert, M.H., Lindvall, M., Nevins, N., Semus, S.F., Senger, S., Tedesco, G., Wall, I.D.,

Woolven, J.M., Peishoff, C.E., and Head, M.S. (2006) A critical assessment of docking programs and scoring functions. *Journal of Medicinal Chemistry*, **49**, 5912–5931.

55 Kellenberger, E., Rodrigo, J., Muller, P., and Rognan, D. (2004) Comparative evaluation of eight docking tools for docking and virtual screening accuracy. *Proteins*, **57**, 225–242.

56 Kontoyianni, M., McClellan, L.M., and Sokol, G.S. (2004) Evaluation of docking performance: comparative data on docking algorithms. *Journal of Medicinal Chemistry*, **47**, 558–565.

57 Perola, E., Walters, W.P., and Charifson, P.S. (2004) A detailed comparison of current docking and scoring methods on systems of pharmaceutical relevance. *Proteins*, **56**, 235–249.

58 Cummings, M.D., DesJarlais, R.L., Gibbs, A.C., Mohan, V., and Jaeger, E.P. (2005) Comparison of automated docking programs as virtual screening tools. *Journal of Medicinal Chemistry*, **48**, 962–976.

59 Halperin, I., Ma, B., Wolfson, H., and Nussinov, R. (2002) Principles of docking: an overview of search algorithms and a guide to scoring functions. *Proteins*, **47**, 409–443.

60 Charifson, P.S., Corkery, J.J., Murcko, M.A., and Walters, W.P. (1999) Consensus scoring: a method for obtaining improved hit rates from docking databases of three-dimensional structures into proteins. *Journal of Medicinal Chemistry*, **42**, 5100–5109.

61 Bissantz, C., Folkers, G., and Rognan, D. (2000) Protein-based virtual screening of chemical databases. 1. Evaluation of different docking/scoring combinations. *Journal of Medicinal Chemistry*, **43**, 4759–4767.

62 Verdonk, M.L., Berdini, V., Hartshorn, M.J., Mooij, W.T., Murray, C.W., Taylor, R.D., and Watson, P. (2004) Virtual screening using protein–ligand docking: avoiding artificial enrichment. *Journal of Chemical Information and Computer Science*, **44**, 793–806.

63 Stahl, M. and Bohm, H.J. (2004) Development of filter functions for protein–ligand docking. *Journal of Molecular Graphics & Modelling*, **16**, 121–132.

64 Taylor, R.D., Jewsbury, P.J., and Essex, J.W. (2003) FDS: flexible ligand and receptor docking with a continuum solvent model and soft-core energy function. *Journal of Computational Chemistry*, **24**, 1637–1656.

65 Kalyanaraman, C., Bernacki, K., and Jacobson, M.P. (2005) Virtual screening against highly charged active sites: identifying substrates of alpha-beta barrel enzymes. *Biochemistry*, **44**, 2059–2071.

66 Paul, N. and Rognan, D. (2002) ConsDock: a new program for the consensus analysis of protein–ligand interactions. *Proteins*, **47**, 521–533.

67 Priestle, J.P. (2009) 3-D clustering: a tool for high throughput docking. *Journal of Molecular Modeling*, **15**, 551–560.

68 Klon, A.E., Glick, M., and Davies, J.W. (2004) Combination of a naive Bayes classifier with consensus scoring improves enrichment of high-throughput docking results. *Journal of Medicinal Chemistry*, **47**, 4356–4359.

69 Heuser, P. and Schomburg, D. (2007) Combination of scoring schemes for protein docking. *BMC Bioinformatics*, **8**, 279.

70 Nicolaou, C.A., Tamura, S.Y., Kelley, B.P., Bassett, S.I., and Nutt, R.F. (2002) Analysis of large screening data sets via adaptively grown phylogenetic-like trees. *Journal of Chemical Information and Computer Science*, **42**, 1069–1079.

71 Hindle, S.A., Rarey, M., Buning, C., and Lengaue, T. (2002) Flexible docking under pharmacophore type constraints. *Journal of Computer-Aided Molecular Design*, **16**, 129–149.

72 Muthas, D., Sabnis, Y.A., Lundborg, M., and Karlen, A. (2008) Is it possible to increase hit rates in structure-based virtual screening by pharmacophore filtering? An investigation of the advantages and pitfalls of post-filtering. *Journal of Molecular Graphics & Modelling*, **26**, 1237–1251.

73 Evers, A. and Klebe, G. (2004) Successful virtual screening for a submicromolar antagonist of the neurokinin-1 receptor

based on a ligand-supported homology model. *Journal of Medicinal Chemistry*, **47**, 5381–5392.

74 Goto, J., Kataoka, R., Muta, H., and Hirayama, N. (2008) ASEDock-docking based on alpha spheres and excluded volumes. *Journal of Chemical Information and Modeling*, **48**, 583–590.

75 Iwaki, T., Shiota, K., Al-Taweel, K., Kobayashi, D., Kobayashi, A., Suzuki, K., Yui, T., and Wadano, A. (2008) Inhibition of RuBisCO cloned from *Thermosynechococcus vulcanus* and expressed in *Escherichia coli* with compounds predicted by Molecular Operation Environment (MOE). *Journal of Bioscience and Bioengineering*, **105**, 26–33.

76 Lin, T.H. and Lin, G.L. (2008) An anchor-dependent molecular docking process for docking small flexible molecules into rigid protein receptors. *Journal of Chemical Information and Modeling*, **48**, 1638–1655.

77 Gehlhaar, D.K., Verkhivker, G.M., Rejto, P.A., Sherman, C.J., Fogel, D.R., Fogel, L.J., and Freer, S.T. (1995) Molecular recognition of the inhibitor AG-1343 by HIV-1 protease: conformationally flexible docking by evolutionary programming. *Chemistry & Biology*, **2**, 317–324.

78 Fischer, B., Basili, S., Merlitz, H., and Wenzel, W. (2007) Accuracy of binding mode prediction with a cascadic stochastic tunneling method. *Proteins*, **68**, 195–204.

79 Gorelik, B. and Goldblum, A. (2008) High quality binding modes in docking ligands to proteins. *Proteins*, **71**, 1373–1386.

80 Chen, H.M., Liu, B.F., Huang, H.L., Hwang, S.F., and Ho, S.Y. (2007) SODOCK: swarm optimization for highly flexible protein–ligand docking. *Journal of Computational Chemistry*, **28**, 612–623.

81 Namasivayam, V. and Gunther, R. (2007) pso@autodock: a fast flexible molecular docking program based on Swarm intelligence. *Chemical Biology & Drug Design*, **70**, 475–484.

82 Korb, O., Stutzle, T., and Exner, T.E. (2009) Empirical scoring functions for advanced protein–ligand docking with PLANTS. *Journal of Chemical Information and Modeling*, **49**, 84–96.

83 Congreve, M., Chessari, G., Tisi, D., and Woodhead, A.J. (2008) Recent developments in fragment-based drug discovery. *Journal of Medicinal Chemistry*, **51**, 3661 3680.

84 Marcou, G. and Rognan, D. (2007) Optimizing fragment and scaffold docking by use of molecular interaction fingerprints. *Journal of Chemical Information and Modeling*, **47**, 195–207.

85 Teotico, D.G., Babaoglu, K., Rocklin, G.J., Ferreira, R.S., Giannetti, A.M., and Shoichet, B.K. (2009) Docking for fragment inhibitors of AmpC beta-lactamase. *Proceedings of the National Academy of Science of the United States of America*, **106**, 7455–7460.

86 Chen, Y. and Shoichet, B.K. (2009) Molecular docking and ligand specificity in fragment-based inhibitor discovery. *Nature Chemical Biology*, **5**, 358–364.

87 Fukunishi, Y., Mashimo, T., Orita, M., Ohno, K., and Nakamura, H. (2009) *In silico* fragment screening by replica generation (FSRG) method for fragment-based drug design. *Journal of Chemical Information and Modeling*, **49**, 925–933.

88 Jorgensen, W.L. (2004) The many roles of computation in drug discovery. *Science*, **303**, 1813–1818.

89 Carlsson, J., Boukharta, L., and Aqvist, J. (2008) Combining docking, molecular dynamics and the linear interaction energy method to predict binding modes and affinities for non-nucleoside inhibitors to HIV-1 reverse transcriptase. *Journal of Medicinal Chemistry*, **51**, 2648–2656.

90 Tirado-Rives, J. and Jorgensen, W.L. (2006) Contribution of conformer focusing to the uncertainty in predicting free energies for protein–ligand binding. *Journal of Medicinal Chemistry*, **49**, 5880–5884.

91 Kuhn, B., Gerber, P., Schulz-Gasch, T., and Stahl, M. (2005) Validation and use of the MM-PBSA approach for drug discovery. *Journal of Medicinal Chemistry*, **48**, 4040–4048.

92 Lyne, P.D., Lamb, M.L., and Saeh, J.C. (2006) Accurate prediction of the relative

potencies of members of a series of kinase inhibitors using molecular docking and MM-GBSA scoring. *Journal of Medicinal Chemistry*, **49**, 4805–4808.

93 Zhou, Z., Bates, M., and Madura, J.D. (2006) Structure modeling, ligand binding, and binding affinity calculation (LR-MM-PBSA) of human heparanase for inhibition and drug design. *Proteins*, **65**, 580–592.

94 Xiong, Y., Li, Y., He, H., and Zhan, C.G. (2007) Theoretical calculation of the binding free energies for pyruvate dehydrogenase E1 binding with ligands. *Bioorganic & Medicinal Chemistry Letters*, **17**, 5186–5190.

95 Ferrari, A.M., Degliesposti, G., Sgobba, M., and Rastelli, G. (2007) Validation of an automated procedure for the prediction of relative free energies of binding on a set of aldose reductase inhibitors. *Bioorganic & Medicinal Chemistry*, **15**, 7865–7877.

96 Thompson, D.C., Humblet, C., and Joseph-McCarthy, D. (2008) Investigation of MM-PBSA rescoring of docking poses. *Journal of Chemical Information and Modeling*, **48**, 1081–1091.

97 Page, C.S. and Bates, P.A. (2006) Can MM-PBSA calculations predict the specificities of protein kinase inhibitors? *Journal of Computational Chemistry*, **27**, 1990–2007.

98 Graves, A.P., Shivakumar, D.M., Boyce, S.E., Jacobson, M.P., Case, D.A., and Shoichet, B.K. (2008) Rescoring docking hit lists for model cavity sites: predictions and experimental testing. *Journal of Molecular Biology*, **377**, 914–934.

99 Brewerton, S.C. (2008) The use of protein–ligand interaction fingerprints in docking. *Current Opinion in Drug Discovery & Development*, **11**, 356–364.

100 Deng, Z., Chuaqui, C., and Singh, J. (2004) Structural interaction fingerprint (SIFt): a novel method for analyzing three-dimensional protein–ligand binding interactions. *Journal of Medicinal Chemistry*, **47**, 337–344.

101 Kelly, M.D. and Mancera, R.L. (2004) Expanded interaction fingerprint method for analyzing ligand binding modes in docking and structure-based drug design. *Journal of Chemical Information and Computer Science*, **44**, 1942–1951.

102 Mpamhanga, C.P., Chen, B., McLay, I.M., and Willett, P. (2006) Knowledge-based interaction fingerprint scoring: a simple method for improving the effectiveness of fast scoring functions. *Journal of Chemical Information and Modeling*, **46**, 686–698.

103 Venhorst, J., Nunez, S., Terpstra, J.W., and Kruse, C.G. (2008) Assessment of scaffold hopping efficiency by use of molecular interaction fingerprints. *Journal of Medicinal Chemistry*, **51**, 3222–3229.

104 Renner, S., Derksen, S., Radestock, S., and Morchen, F. (2008) Maximum common binding modes (MCBM): consensus docking scoring using multiple ligand information and interaction fingerprints. *Journal of Chemical Information and Modeling*, **48**, 319–332.

105 Perez-Nueno, V.I., Rabal, O., Borrell, J.I., and Teixido, J. (2009) APIF: a new interaction fingerprint based on atom pairs and its application to virtual screening. *Journal of Chemical Information and Modeling*, **49**, 1245–1260.

106 Takaya, D., Takeda-Shitaka, M., Terashi, G., Kanou, K., Iwadate, M., and Umeyama, H. (2008) Bioinformatics based ligand-docking and *in-silico* screening. *Chemical & Pharmaceutical Bulletin*, **56**, 742–744.

107 Najmanovich, R., Kuttner, J., Sobolev, V., and Edelman, M. (2000) Side-chain flexibility in proteins upon ligand binding. *Proteins*, **39**, 261–268.

108 Moras, D. and Gronemeyer, H. (1998) The nuclear receptor ligand-binding domain: structure and function. *Current Opinion in Cell Biology*, **10**, 384–391.

109 Cavasotto, C.N. and Abagyan, R.A. (2004) Protein flexibility in ligand docking and virtual screening to protein kinases. *Journal of Molecular Biology*, **337**, 209–225.

110 Totrov, M. and Abagyan, R. (2008) Flexible ligand docking to multiple receptor conformations: a practical alternative. *Current Opinion in Structural Biology*, **18**, 178–184.

111 Verdonk, M.L., Cole, J.C., Hartshorn, M.J., Murray, C.W., and Taylor, R.D. (2003) Improved protein–ligand docking using GOLD. *Proteins*, **52**, 609–623.

112 Bolstad, E.S. and Anderson, A.C. (2008) In pursuit of virtual lead optimization: the role of the receptor structure and ensembles in accurate docking. *Proteins*, **73**, 566–580.

113 Rao, S., Sanschagrin, P.C., Greenwood, J.R., Repasky, M.P., Sherman, W., and Farid, R. (2008) Improving database enrichment through ensemble docking. *Journal of Computer-Aided Molecular Design*, **22**, 621–627.

114 Claussen, H., Buning, C., Rarey, M., and Lengauer, T. (2001) FlexE: efficient molecular docking considering protein structure variations. *Journal of Molecular Biology*, **308**, 377–395.

115 Corbeil, C.R., Englebienne, P., and Moitessier, N. (2007) Docking ligands into flexible and solvated macromolecules. 1. Development and validation of FITTED 1.0. *Journal of Chemical Information and Modeling*, **47**, 435–449.

116 Corbeil, C.R., Englebienne, P., Yannopoulos, C.G., Chan, L., Das, S.K., Bilimoria, D., L'Heureux, L., and Moitessier, N. (2008) Docking ligands into flexible and solvated macromolecules. 2. Development and application of fitted 1.5 to the virtual screening of potential HCV polymerase inhibitors. *Journal of Chemical Information and Modeling*, **48**, 902–909.

117 Corbeil, C.R. and Moitessier, N. (2009) Docking ligands into flexible and solvated macromolecules. 3. Impact of input ligand conformation, protein flexibility, and water molecules on the accuracy of docking programs. *Journal of Chemical Information and Modeling*, **49**, 997–1009.

118 Fradera, X., de la Cruz, X., Silva, C.H., Gelpi, J.L., Luque, F.J., and Orozco, M. (2002) Ligand-induced changes in the binding sites of proteins. *Bioinformatics*, **18**, 939–948.

119 May, A. and Zacharias, M. (2008) Protein–ligand docking accounting for receptor side chain and global flexibility in normal modes: evaluation on kinase inhibitor cross docking. *Journal of Medicinal Chemistry*, **51**, 3499–3506.

120 Bottegoni, G., Kufareva, I., Totrov, M., and Abagyan, R. (2009) Four-dimensional docking: a fast and accurate account of discrete receptor flexibility in ligand docking. *Journal of Medicinal Chemistry*, **52**, 397–406.

121 Zhao, Y. and Sanner, M.F. (2007) FLIPDock: docking flexible ligands into flexible receptors. *Proteins*, **68**, 726–737.

122 Verdonk, M.L., Chessari, G., Cole, J.C., Hartshorn, M.J., Murray, C.W., Nissink, J.W., Taylor, R.D., and Taylor, R. (2005) Modeling water molecules in protein–ligand docking using GOLD. *Journal of Medicinal Chemistry*, **48**, 6504–6515.

123 Huang, N. and Shoichet, B.K. (2008) Exploiting ordered waters in molecular docking. *Journal of Medicinal Chemistry*, **51**, 4862–4865.

124 Englebienne, P. and Moitessier, N. (2009) Docking ligands into flexible and solvated macromolecules. 4. Are popular scoring functions accurate for this class of proteins? *Journal of Chemical Information and Modeling*, **49**, 1568–1580.

125 Bissantz, C., Schalon, C., Guba, W., and Stahl, M. (2005) Focused library design in GPCR projects on the example of 5-HT (2c) agonists: comparison of structure-based virtual screening with ligand-based search methods. *Proteins*, **61**, 938–952.

126 Evers, A., Hessler, G., Matter, H., and Klabunde, T. (2005) Virtual screening of biogenic amine-binding G-protein coupled receptors: comparative evaluation of protein- and ligand-based virtual screening protocols. *Journal of Medicinal Chemistry*, **48**, 5448–5465.

127 Hawkins, P.C., Skillman, A.G., and Nicholls, A. (2007) Comparison of shape-matching and docking as virtual screening tools. *Journal of Medicinal Chemistry*, **50**, 74–82.

128 McGaughey, G.B., Sheridan, R.P., Bayly, C.I., Culberson, J.C., Kreatsoulas, C., Lindsley, S., Maiorov, V., Truchon, J.F., and Cornell, W.D. (2007) Comparison of topological, shape, and docking methods in virtual screening. *Journal of Chemical Information and Modeling*, **47**, 1504–1519.

129 de Graaf, C. and Rognan, D. (2008) Selective structure-based virtual screening for full and partial agonists of the beta2 adrenergic receptor. *Journal of Medicinal Chemistry*, **51**, 4978–4985.

130 Kasam, V., Zimmermann, M., Maass, A., Schwichtenberg, H., Wolf, A., Jacq, N., Breton, V., and Hofmann-Apitius, M. (2007) Design of new plasmepsin inhibitors: a virtual high throughput screening approach on the EGEE grid. *Journal of Chemical Information and Modeling*, **47**, 1818–1828.

131 Degliesposti, G., Kasam, V., Da Costa, A., Kang, H.K., Kim, N., Kim, D.W., Breton, V., Kim, D., and Rastelli, G. (2009) Design and discovery of plasmepsin II inhibitors using an automated workflow on large-scale grids. *ChemMedChem*, **4**, 1164–1173.

Part Two
Challenges

Virtual Screening. Edited by C. Sotriffer

ISBN: 978-3-527-32636-5

7
The Challenge of Affinity Prediction: Scoring Functions for Structure-Based Virtual Screening

Christoph Sotriffer and Hans Matter

7.1
Introduction

The purpose of virtual screening is to provide hits with novel chemical structure as a starting point for lead optimization after careful assessment of their optimization potential [1].

Structure-based virtual screening works on the premise of shape and interaction complementarity of the ligand with its putative target binding site, for which experimental 3D structures or validated homology models are available. Using docking algorithms combined in various ways with other filters (e.g., drug-likeness, physiochemical properties, binding site constraints, pharmacophore models, and molecular similarity), compounds are selected that have a high likelihood to interact with the target. To this end, the first step is to generate a proposed binding conformation (pose) using validated docking engines. These poses need to be sorted to identify the conformation that is closest to an experimental binding pose. Subsequently, the free energy of binding (ΔG°) for a particular conformation of a single compound interacting with the protein has to be estimated to rank the ligands and select those with the highest chance for biological activity. Approaches providing such estimates of affinity are, thus, of utmost importance in virtual screening. Normally, this pose ranking and affinity estimation is carried out with the help of scoring functions. Scoring functions are approximate mathematical models for predicting the strength of the noncovalent interaction between two binding partners. Such functions also guide the conformational and orientational search of the ligand in the binding cavity during the docking process.

This chapter focuses on different aspects of scoring functions for affinity prediction and pose ranking. First, we will outline the physicochemical background of current scoring approaches. As different scoring functions were recently reviewed [2–4] and their performance was extensively compared [5–8], we will provide only a brief overview of the different scoring function classes and focus on unique features and applications. Hence, we outline novel strategies and computational tools with an impact on improving the success rate in scoring protein–ligand interactions.

Virtual Screening. Edited by C. Sotriffer

ISBN: 978-3-527-32636-5

Finally, we will provide an account of integrating these functions into virtual screening workflows and a critical discussion of caveats.

7.2
Physicochemical Basis of Protein–Ligand Recognition

Thermodynamically, intermolecular interactions and protein–ligand complex formation are governed by the change in Gibbs free energy, ΔG. If ΔG is negative, the corresponding process or reaction can occur spontaneously. According to the Gibbs–Helmholtz equation, $\Delta G = \Delta H - T\Delta S$, the Gibbs free energy is composed of an enthalpic and a temperature-dependent entropic contribution, either of which can individually favor or disfavor protein–ligand binding. The free energy of binding at standard conditions, ΔG°, is correlated with the logarithm of the equilibrium binding constant, $\Delta G^\circ = RT \ln K_d$, where R is the gas constant and T is the temperature. As an experimental measure of affinity, K may be obtained either as a dissociation constant (K_d) or as an inhibition constant (K_i).

At the simplest level, the association between two binding partners is both entropically disfavored due to the loss of translational and rotational degrees of freedom and enthalpically favored due to the interactions formed upon association. However, there is much more involved in protein–ligand complex formation, mostly because the interaction partners are flexible systems and the association occurs in aqueous solution.

The enthalpic contributions favoring the binding process arise first of all from the direct interaction between the protein and the ligand. The various interaction types and forces are described here in more detail. In general, these interactions are driven by steric and electrostatic complementarity [9], as revealed by the analysis of experimental complex structures of tightly bound ligands. Imperfect fitting, causing "holes" at the protein–ligand interface [10], tends to reduce binding affinity. Analysis of available data from protein–ligand complexes indicates that unpaired buried polar groups strongly disfavor high-affinity binding as only few buried polar groups are not involved in hydrogen-bonding interactions in proteins [11]. Solvent should also be considered as polar groups are usually solvated prior to association and interact with individual water molecules via a network of hydrogen bonds. Thus, complex formation requires desolvation, and the water molecules are stripped off. If then a desolvated polar group is not paired with an appropriate functional group in the complex, the desolvation enthalpy cost is not counterbalanced, resulting in an unfavorable contribution to affinity. The precise energetic balance of these individual processes is difficult to estimate as it critically depends on the fact whether polar groups are solvent exposed or buried in a lipophilic binding site.

Water plays further important roles with respect to enthalpy and entropy. Interactions between hydrophobic partners are favorable in water as the association reduces the net hydrophobic surface in contact with the polar solvent, thus reducing structured and constrained water around the solutes and providing positive association entropy. Hence, this release of ordered water molecules is an entropy-driven process. Although the effect per atomic surface segment is relatively small, its contribution to protein–ligand interaction can be significant due to the large number of hydrophobic contacts in a complex. Another enthalpic contribution arises from the release of water molecules in lipophilic binding sites, which then form strong hydrogen bonds with bulk water. The lipophilic contribution to binding affinity is often proportional to the lipophilic surface area buried in the solvent.

Intramolecular effects based on conformational degrees of freedom can affect both enthalpy and entropy of binding. The bound ligand is normally observed in an energetically favorable conformation [12], which, however, does not necessarily correspond to the global minimum of the isolated molecule. Any energy difference between the preferred conformation both in the free and in the bound state leads to an unfavorable enthalpic contribution. The entropic contributions are related to the loss of conformational degrees of freedom as it can normally be assumed that much of the ligand's conformational flexibility is frozen upon binding. Often, increased binding affinities have been reported by constraining the inhibitor to a conformation that is recognized by the protein binding site, thus lowering the entropic barrier to complex formation; in some cases, significant contributions can be attributed to such a reduction in conformational flexibility [13]. The actual entropy loss per internal rotatable bond clearly depends on the tightness of the complex and the residual flexibility of the ligand in the bound state. Obviously, the same enthalpic and entropic considerations also apply to the protein, but it is much less straightforward to estimate the size or even the sign of these contributions for the macromolecular binding partner.

In order to achieve extremely high ligand affinities, optimization of both enthalpy and entropy contributions should be considered. One of the main obstacles in the exploration of structure–activity relationships (SAR) in congeneric series originates from the phenomenon of enthalpy/entropy compensation [14–16], that is, favorable changes in binding enthalpy are compensated by opposite changes in entropy and vice versa, resulting only in small changes in affinity. In experimental studies supported by X-ray structures, where a single hydrogen bond partner in the protein–ligand interface was replaced, it was shown that destabilization was due to loss in entropy. Thus, the formation of particular hydrogen bond interactions can be enthalpically unfavorable, but entropically favorable! Such an entropy gain has been reported to be due to replacement of water molecules by the ligand [17].

What are now the different types of forces that govern the direct interaction between a protein and a ligand? For ligands of pharmaceutical interest, protein–ligand binding usually occurs through noncovalent interactions. The physical basis of these interactions is generally well established through the theories of electromagnetic forces or, on a more fundamental level, of quantum mechanics. For macromolecules and liquid phases, however, direct application of these theories is significantly complicated by the size and complexity of the systems, in which a large number of fluctuating particles simultaneously interact and influence each other. Principles from classical mechanics and heuristic models are therefore commonly used as an approximation to describe protein–ligand interactions in aqueous solution.

The primary forces acting between a protein and a ligand are all of electrostatic nature. Interactions between explicit charges, dipoles, induced dipoles, and higher electric multipoles lead to phenomena that are usually referred to as salt bridges, hydrogen bonds, or van der Waals interactions. In simplified classifications, only the charge–charge interaction is called electrostatic. It leads to long-range attractive forces for partners with charge complementarity. Many drug-like molecules and binding sites of target proteins contain charged molecular substructures at physiological pH. This often leads to the observation of ionic interactions determining the binding mode in protein–ligand complexes. The strength of this interaction depends on the distance between the two charges and the dielectricity constant (Coulomb's law); a more accurate treatment of charge effects and electrostatic interactions is provided by the formalism of the Poisson–Boltzmann (PB) equation [18, 19].

Although charge–dipole and dipole–dipole interactions are weaker and less far reaching than charge–charge interactions, they are important in protein–ligand complexes. The formation of protein–ligand complexes also involves charge redistribution, either within one molecule (polarization) or within both partners (charge transfer). Inductive polarization occurs when a temporary dipole is induced in a nonpolar group by the field of a permanently charged dipole or ion [9]. Charge transfer interactions take place when electron donors and acceptors are sufficiently close in space to allow electron transfer. Although both effects occur frequently upon ligand recognition, they are often omitted from simple estimations of interaction energy or binding affinity.

Hydrogen bonds are essential biostructural motifs that are best described as electrostatic interaction between two electronegative centers and a hydrogen atom covalently bound to one partner. The hydrogen bond directionality arises from steric effects and an anisotropic, mutually polarized charge distribution. The strength of hydrogen bonds can be estimated by electrostatic and van der Waals forces without explicit additional terms for their calculation [20]. The consistency of experimental values for the contribution of an intramolecular hydrogen bond to protein stability suggests some additivity [21–23]. However, the contribution of hydrogen bonds to binding affinity strongly depends on solvation and desolvation effects (as mentioned above). Weak hydrogen bonding networks, with the CH−O hydrogen bond as the most prominent example, might also contribute to protein structure stabilization or protein–ligand recognition, but their actual contribution is still a matter of debate [24–28].

Important interactions also occur between nonpolar parts of molecules, preferably at short distances. These are due to dispersion or "London" forces, which are weakly attractive intermolecular forces. A tight surface fit between nonpolar ligand and binding site areas leads to significant intermolecular forces through the summation of many individual short-range contributions.

Weakly polar interactions in proteins and protein–ligand complexes are frequently phenomenologically analyzed and classified in terms of the interacting partners [29]. This especially includes interactions with π-systems, such as the NH–π, OH–π, or CH–π interaction [30, 31], aromatic–aromatic interactions (parallel π–π stacking versus edge-to-face interaction), and the cation–π interaction [32]. All of these can mostly be rationalized in terms of electrostatic interactions outlined above, that is, they involve interactions between monopoles, dipoles, and quadrupoles (permanent and induced).

Regarding the π–π interaction, 60% of protein aromatic side chains are involved in aromatic–aromatic pairs with particular geometrical requirements, 80% of which form networks with more than three interacting partners [33, 34]. These networks are important for tertiary structure stabilization and might also influence ligand recognition. A detailed analysis of pairs of aromatic amino acids in a representative set of 505 nonhomologous X-ray structures of proteins indicates that the corresponding aromatic rings have a preferred intermolecular structure; they are oriented in an off-centered parallel orientation [34] that is more stable than a T-shaped structure.

Cation–π interactions are another important motif dominated by electrostatic interactions [32, 35] within mainly hydrophobic subsites. A stabilizing interaction takes place between cations such as ammonium ions and electron-rich π-systems of neighboring aromatic rings. A recent study on factor Xa inhibitors revealed the importance of a quaternary ammonium ion for high binding affinity in the S4 subpocket formed by three aromatic rings, namely, Phe, Tyr, and Trp. The experimentally observed low affinity for the primary ammonium ion also suggests negligible cation–π interactions between Lys and Trp [36], in agreement with the statistical preferences from the analysis of the PDB [32].

As another phenomenological class, interactions with halogens deserve special attention. The introduction of halogens to enhance binding affinity and modulate pharmacokinetic properties is well established in lead optimization [37, 38]. In particular, organic fluorine is often used as bioisosteric hydrogen or oxygen replacement [39, 40] and has been investigated in detail, including its effects on nonbonded interactions in hydrophobic cavities and polar interactions. In general, fluorinated molecules interact with their targets revealing similar binding poses compared to nonfluorinated analogues, while the chemical properties of the C−F bond influences binding affinities. Furthermore, fluorine is able to alter the basicity of neighboring functionalities, thus modulating polar interactions, salt bridges, and cation–π interactions [37], as exemplified in carbonic anhydrase II inhibitors [41]. The importance of C−F···C=O interactions to binding affinity was demonstrated by systematically decorating thrombin inhibitors with fluorine [42]. A very detailed review of these and related weak orthogonal multipolar interactions is given by Diederich and coworkers. [43].

In addition, increasing experimental evidence indicates that organic chlorine and bromine atoms are favorably involved in discrete noncovalent dipolar protein–ligand interactions, termed "halogen bonding," and thus significantly contribute to binding affinity in molecular recognition [44–47]. Noncovalent interactions between Cl/Br and aromatic rings in proteins open a new way to manipulate molecular recognition. Recently, the nature of these interactions with hydrophobic aromatic rings in proteins was investigated to understand their contribution to binding affinity [48]. A systematic study on nonbonded contacts in the protein database both for Cl–π [48, 49] interactions and for bromine and chlorine in small-molecule crystal structures [48]

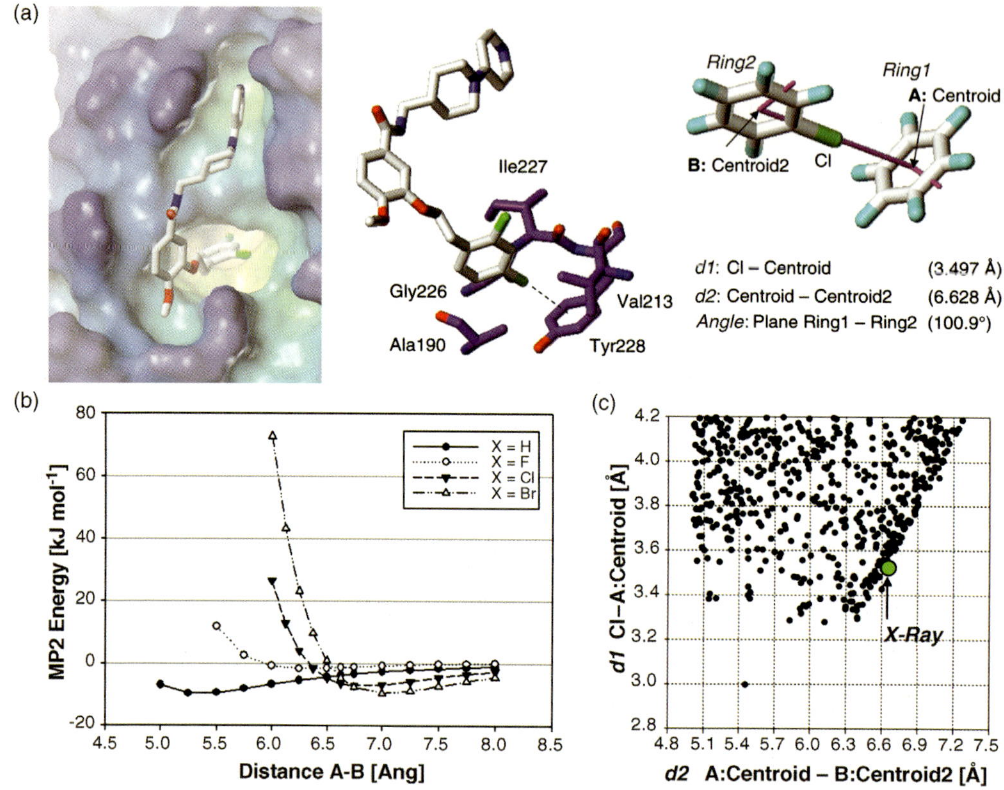

Figure 7.1 Investigation on halogen–π interactions by X-ray structural analysis, database searching, and *ab initio* calculations reveals a significant contribution to binding affinity [48]. (a) Chlorine–π interaction present in the X-ray structure of a 3-oxybenzamide-based inhibitor in complex with human factor Xa (K_i = 18 nM, resolution = 2.7 Å). The characteristic Cl ··· Tyr228 interaction geometry was then used for *ab initio* calculations and database searches in the Cambridge Crystallographic Database (CSD). (b) Plot of MP2 interaction energies (kJ/mol) versus nonbonded interaction distance A–B (Å) for *ab initio* calculations of four heterodimers with H (●), F (○), Cl (▼), and Br (△) as aromatic substituents approaching the second aromatic ring. (c) Scatter plots of distance Cl ··· centroid on the *y*-axis versus distance centroid2 ··· centroid on the *x*-axis (right) from 458 hits in the CSD. The interaction geometry from the fXa/3-oxybenzamide complex is highlighted.

revealed geometrical preferences of this contact (Figure 7.1). Directional preferences of the Cl ··· ring centroid interaction were found with a distribution of almost "edge-to-face"-shaped orientations with interplanar angle between 60 and 90°. Furthermore, it was shown that introduction of halogen atoms at distinct positions of two factor Xa inhibitor series consistently improves the free energy of binding by interaction to the plane of a tyrosine aromatic ring system [48]. This motif, first reported in 1998 [50], was then identified as very important contributor to high affinity in serine proteases [51–56].

In principle, all these interactions and contributions would have to be taken into account when estimating the affinity. Present approaches, however, hardly consider all possible interaction terms explicitly. Rather, they rely on implicit methods (such as the knowledge-based scoring functions) or on a set of generally dominant terms (such as the empirical scoring function). Especially the weakly polar interactions described above are often not explicitly accounted for. Nevertheless, the binding affinity is typically modeled as a sum of individual terms describing the different intermolecular interaction types, the conformational energy, and possibly some entropic components. This is usually based on the assumption of additivity, which constitutes a reasonable starting point for affinity estimation methods, but is not strictly valid for protein–ligand interactions [57].

7.3 Classes of Scoring Functions

Although experimental data on protein–ligand interactions are sometimes difficult to interpret, additive linear models generally provide a useful first approximation for the empirical development of scoring functions. A more rigorous treatment would require time-consuming simulations with the consideration of all involved molecules. These demanding computational approaches can yield reasonably accurate binding free energy differences, but they can be applied only to a limited number of compounds, preferably sharing the same scaffold. The processing of large databases in virtual screening or millions of configurations in docking needs faster and, thus, simpler schemes for estimating protein–ligand interactions. The resulting scoring functions allow to guide flexible docking algorithms and rank ordering series of docked molecules. Although substantial progress was reported in the field of docking and scoring, the accuracy of scoring functions is still not sufficient to guarantee reasonably reliable predictions.

There are three general classes of scoring functions, which will be briefly discussed in the following section, namely, force field-based approaches, knowledge-based methods, and regression-based empirical scoring functions. As empirical and knowledge-based scoring functions have extensively been reviewed in the literature (see, for example, Refs [2–4]), only their main features will be presented here. Computationally more demanding force field-based methods are now more often incorporated in virtual screening strategies for rescoring and will be put into perspective by comparison to faster approaches.

7.3.1 Force Field-Based Methods

Empirical force fields are based on classical mechanics and on the assumption that the conformational and interaction energy of a molecular system can be expressed as a sum of many individual contributions, such as bond-stretching, angle-bending, torsional, electrostatic, and van der Waals interaction terms. While molecular mechanics (MM) force field methods are much faster than quantum mechanical (QM) approaches, the quality of the energy evaluations critically depends on empirical parameters. These parameters are commonly derived from physical measurements or *ab initio* calculations; but they are not based on binding affinity data. The need for empirical parameterization generally restricts the applicability range of a certain force field to particular molecule classes. Accordingly, in the context of scoring functions, force fields parameterized explicitly for the description of biomolecules are of prime interest, such as AMBER [58] or CHARMM [59].

For scoring protein–ligand interactions, the total free energy of binding is approximated by the force field estimate of the gas phase enthalpy of binding, typically computed as a sum of all intermolecular van der Waals and electrostatic interactions between the binding partners; the intramolecular (strain) energy is also frequently included. The earliest docking approaches, such as DOCK [60] and GOLD [61], used related force fields.

To provide a better approximation of the binding free energy, the desolvation energies of ligand and protein are sometimes taken into account using implicit solvation methods. Solvation and some entropic factors can be implicitly accounted for by adding either a continuum solvent Poisson–Boltzmann (PB) [62] or a generalized Born (GB) [63] term for polar solvation, and a solvent-accessible surface area (SA) term for nonpolar solvation. The intermolecular force field terms and desolvation terms may then be used as descriptors for calibrating an empirical scoring function, for example, the RankScore function [64]. More commonly, force field and desolvation terms are directly combined without further calibration on experimental binding affinities. This methodology is referred to as MM–PBSA [65] or MM–GBSA [66]. It is computationally expensive (in particular the MM–PBSA approach) and, thus, only useful for rescoring of preselected poses.

Stahl and coworkers demonstrated that MM–PBSA can be efficiently used to distinguish between low- and high-affinity ligands if the affinity differs by at least two orders of magnitude in IC_{50} [67]. They could also show that the standard averaging over a molecular dynamics (MD) trajectory can be replaced by simple energy minimization without significantly reducing the discrimination power.

The MM–PBSA approach was used to examine in detail the binding affinities of a set of biotin analogues for avidin [68]. This study indicated only minor dependence on the employed force field, but mixing of force fields for the MD sampling and the MM–PBSA calculation is not recommended. The same group improved the approach to predict the entropic term in MM–PBSA [69] by introducing a geometrically fixed buffer region outside the truncated protein. This results in a significantly reduced standard deviation of the calculation by a factor of 2–4, which ensures that the entropy term no longer limits the precision of the MM/PBSA predictions. Other groups aimed to improve the computational efficiency of this approach by using an implicit GB solvation model during MD to enhance conformational sampling, by using an efficient Poisson–Boltzmann solver, and by using distributed computing [70]. Using this efficient protocol, reasonable correlations of relative free binding energies with experimental data were reported for 18 urokinase inhibitors. In a larger application of this workflow to 308 small-molecule ligands in complex with urokinase, PTP-1B, and Chk-1, significant correlations with experimental affinities were observed ($r = 0.72–0.83$) [71].

In another recent comparative study, the effectiveness of a high-throughput MM–PBSA rescoring function is evaluated on different test sets [72]. In contrast to the previous study, only single, minimized protein–ligand complexes using a rigid protein approximation were employed. The authors show that in terms of sampling during docking, a shape-based contact score is sufficient (e.g., DOCK contact). For regenerating X-ray complexes, the MM–PBSA rescoring did not improve results over MM rescoring, while surface area and solvation terms did not improve the discrimination of further poses of a single ligand. Within a retrospective virtual screening investigation, a minor improvement in terms of the number of actives in the ranked database was found. From both studies, it appears that rapid scoring schemes followed by MM–PBSA rescoring is a reasonable approach, but might require an improved treatment of protein–ligand interactions by full minimization of a flexible protein–ligand complex or a treatment using adequate MD sampling.

The similar MM–GBSA approach has been shown to improve early enrichment rates in the virtual screening of large compound databases [66]. Again, the authors applied only simple energy minimization using the OPLS-AA force field [73] with the generalized Born implicit solvent model.

The use of an MM–GBSA function was also successfully applied to rescore docked ligand poses in a study by Lyne *et al.*, resulting in a correct ranking of multiple series of congeneric kinase inhibitors for different targets [74]. In our own work, this correlation was reproduced for one example of this study, namely, the published p38 kinase inhibitors (MM–GBSA in Maestro 8.0, Schrödinger Inc.) using carefully selected poses on the basis of the PDB structure 2bak and a rigid protein treatment during minimization. Treating the protein as flexible around the ligands significantly reduces the predictivity. Interestingly, addition of related p38 kinase inhibitors to the same scaffold reported by the same group [75] led to inferior results for both the static and the flexible protein treatment, which indicates that this MM–GBSA correlation is predictive only within a narrow structural neighborhood (Figure 7.2).

A further evaluation of the MM–GBSA rescoring for pharmacologically relevant targets including CDK2, factor Xa, thrombin, and HIV-RT revealed a remarkable agreement between experimental affinities and predictions, even if based only on energy minimization for the investigated protein–ligand X-ray structures [76]. The authors point out that in theory the lack of MD sampling would not allow the protein binding site to sufficiently relax after docking diverse scaffolds, while in practice this problem could be minimized when evaluating congeneric series. On the other hand, the standard averaging over MD trajectories might introduce additional noise due to still imperfect sampling or some force field limitations.

A study comparing MM–PBSA and MM–GBSA on 45 PTP-1B inhibitors demonstrated reasonable agreement with experimental binding affinities ($r = 0.87$), with MM–PBSA being slightly inferior [77]. Interestingly, for this example the empirical X-Score scoring function [78] (see below) was found to produce equally good results on complex geometries from either docking or ensembles from MD simulations [77].

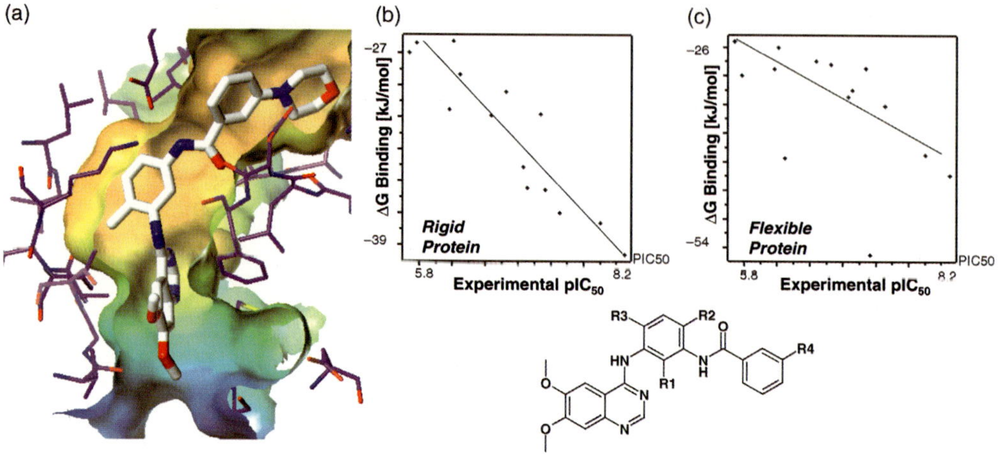

Figure 7.2 Prediction of relative binding affinities using MM–GBSA on a series of aminoquinazoline-based p38 kinase inhibitors [74]. (a) Binding mode of an aminoquinazoline interacting with p38 kinase in the DFG-out conformation (pdb code: 2bak). The ligand was docked into the binding site; the pose is similar to the X-ray structure of the related inhibitor in 2bak. The protein is shown with a MOLCAD solvent-accessible surface. (b) Internal MM–GBSA validation using 14 analogues from this series docked into the binding site using QXP2.0 [112] and rigid protein treatment during the employed MM–GBSA protocol. Experimental versus predicted binding affinity shows a good correlation for this series ($r^2 = 0.801$). (c) Same series with flexible protein treatment in a sphere of 8 Å around the reference ligand. This setup significantly lowers the correlation ($r^2 = 0.335$). Adding additional inhibitors to the same scaffold reported by the same group [75] resulted in a lower prediction for static ($r^2 = 0.326$) and flexible protein treatment ($r^2 = 0.222$), suggesting that the MM–GBSA correlation holds only in a narrow structural environment for this series.

Another interesting study by Graves *et al.* reported on the use of model binding sites in the buried cores of proteins generated by carefully designed point mutations [79]. These cavities can bind small ligands and thus allow to explore specific intermolecular interactions, again using MM–GBSA rescoring after docking. Interestingly, the employed rescoring was not only found to rescue many false negatives but also introduced more false positives.

In a comparative study by Pearlman [80], MM–PBSA was shown to perform relatively poorly for a congeneric series of 16 p38 MAP kinase inhibitors compared to computationally more demanding free energy calculations and did not reveal any advantage over empirical scoring functions. This led him to conclude that one should be selective in applying MM–PBSA and that for systems amenable to other free energy approaches, application of these approaches may be preferred. Furthermore, he demonstrated that additional approximations to speed up the calculations led to inferior results.

Further research in this area might transform MM–PBSA into a useful tool for standard evaluation of binding poses, while advances in computational power might extend applicability of this approach to a larger number of already preselected compounds or binding poses. However, the controversial results in the literature and the authors' own less encouraging experience call for a careful validation of any MM–PBSA workflow for the protein of interest before application to ranking novel molecules. Altering protonation states between inhibitors, attaching larger substituents to a core fragment, or significant deviations from lead structure binding modes might cause significantly reduced predictivity. The careful analysis of protein binding sites and model systems providing insight into the energetic contributions will hopefully lead to a final picture of the general caveats and the usefulness of this approach.

The linear interaction energy (LIE) method represents a compromise between the more rigorous and computationally demanding free energy perturbation (FEP) calculations and the simple scoring functions. In contrast to FEP, LIE uses only initial and final states of the binding event of a single ligand to calculate binding free energies [81]. Hence, this method is computationally much less demanding than FEP, as no intermediate states are required to estimate binding affinities but still slow due to the sampling of phase space for the two states considered. In a recent study, Stjernschantz *et al.* presented an automated LIE procedure for lead optimization, and for 3 of the 4 systems studied, this approach outperformed 10 different scoring functions [82]. Another study on 22 CK2 inhibitors [83] also highlighted LIE as an efficient approach for binding affinity estimation.

Jorgensen and coworkers generalized this method to include not only the interaction energies of the ligands in the solvated complex and the unbound state but also relevant descriptors capturing protein–ligand interactions (hydrogen bond counts, rotatable bonds, and various surface area contributions) in a multivariate regression analysis [84, 85]. Huang and Caflisch have developed a computationally more efficient workflow named LIECE, which replaces MD sampling with a simple energy minimization of the ligand and combines LIE with a PB description of electrostatics [86].

7.3.2
Empirical Scoring Functions

Empirical scoring functions are based on the evaluation of localized, chemically intuitive interactions between the ligand and the protein in a noncovalent complex. Following the assumption of additivity, they decompose the affinity into a series of individual contributions believed to be important for the overall free energy of binding (see above). Each contribution term is based on a descriptor multiplied by a weighting coefficient. In general, this weighting coefficient is determined by a mathematical fit to a training set of experimental affinities for experimental protein–ligand complexes using statistical algorithms. The descriptors depend on the structural features of the complex and aim to capture essential geometric characteristics of the interaction. Typically, terms accounting for hydrogen bonds, ionic interactions, surface complementarity, and certain entropic contributions are included. However, empirical scoring functions show significant differences both in the number and type of descriptors applied in the equation and with respect to the size and composition of the training set. Details about individual parameterizations have been summarized and commented in several reviews [2, 87–90].

A list of the most common and most recent empirical scoring functions described in the literature is provided in the Appendix (Appendix A: Software Overview, Section "Scoring functions"). It should be noted that some of the functions listed there exist in different software implementations (as, for example, ChemScore). Furthermore, a single name may represent multiple function variants developed by the same authors (as, for example, in the case of X-Score and SFCscore). The list also includes functions that contain force field terms, but since these are multiplied by a weighting coefficient calibrated on experimental affinities, the functions should be classified as empirical (occasionally, they are referred to as "semiempirical" scoring functions). Finally, some of the functions (e.g., ScreenScore) follow a consensus scoring approach (as discussed in detail in Section 7.4.3), which means that the ultimate score is obtained from the combined application of at least two functions.

Many variants exist with respect to different descriptors. Hydrogen bonds are often scored by counting the number of donor–acceptor pairs that fall into a given distance and angle range favorable for hydrogen bonding. The count is generally scaled by a function that accounts for deviations from ideal standard values. Most functions consider all types of hydrogen bonds equivalently, but some attempts have been made to distinguish between different donor–acceptor functional group pairs. Reducing the weight of hydrogen bonds localized at the solvent-exposed rim of a binding site can be a useful concept to avoid false positives in virtual screening. This can be achieved by multiplying the hydrogen bond contribution with a factor that depends on the accessibility of the involved protein counter group [91].

The empirical AIScore adds new hydrogen-bonding terms from *ab initio* quantum chemical calculations to an established scoring function [92]. Charged and resonance-assisted hydrogen bond energies for 19 different donor and 34 acceptor types were implemented and fitted in addition to hydrophobic interactions to experimental data. Furthermore, the treatment of multifurcated hydrogen bonds was improved.

Ionic interactions are handled in a way similar to hydrogen bonds. Long-distance charge–charge interactions are usually neglected, and it is thus more appropriate to refer to salt bridges or charge-assisted hydrogen bonds. Some functions assign a stronger weight to salt bridges than neutral hydrogen bonds, but this bears the danger that highly charged molecules receive overestimated scores. Interactions of negatively charged functional groups with metal ions in a protein binding pocket are generally treated in a distance-dependent manner. Details of the specific coordination geometry are neglected in most of the functions (exceptions are, for example, the scoring functions of eHITS [93] and SLIDE [94]).

Hydrophobic interactions are usually calibrated to the number of protein–ligand contacts or the size of the contact surface buried upon complex formation. By assigning a hydrophobicity character to the atoms or surface patches, more specific contact counts or surface measures can be obtained, such as hydrophobic–hydrophobic contacts as favorable and hydrophobic–hydrophilic contacts as unfavorable contributions to binding affinity.

Simple entropy terms attempt to account for the restriction of conformational degrees of freedom of the ligand upon complex formation. A crude but useful estimate of this contribution is the number of rotatable bonds of a ligand. More sophisticated estimates try to take into account the degree of buriedness and immobilization of the atoms connected by the corresponding single bond. This is based on the assumption that parts of the ligand that are not completely buried or immobilized will contribute less to the conformational entropy loss.

Many functions have particular terms that distinguish them from other members of the class. For example, the GlideXP scoring function [95] based on ChemScore [96] includes both a grid-based water desolvation energy term and terms that account for specific protein–ligand structural motifs that provide "exceptionally large contributions" to enhance binding affinity (e.g., hydrophobic enclosure, where a lipophilic portion of a ligand is enclosed on opposite sides by lipophilic protein atoms). This scoring function and the associated docking protocol have been developed to reproduce experimental affinities for a set of 198 complexes and to yield significant database enrichments against relevant targets.

Because of the reliance on a limited sample of available experimental data for training, empirical functions may exhibit nontransferability issues, and it can be difficult to know what each term accounts for and to assess where errors arise. The success of empirical scoring functions is, in fact, limited both by the amount and consistency of experimental protein–ligand complexes and by the consistency and quality of the biological data used for regression analysis. This problem points to a major source of uncertainty in most empirically derived functions. Moreover, experimental protein–ligand complex structures are mostly available for high-affinity ligands, but not for chemically related analogues with low (or no) binding affinity.

7.3.3
Knowledge-Based Scoring Functions

By means of statistical analyses of interatomic contacts, knowledge-based methods try to capture the knowledge about protein–ligand binding that is implicitly stored in large structural databases. The method is founded on the assumption that close intermolecular interactions between certain atom types or functional groups occurring more frequently than expected by random or seen in an average distribution are likely to be energetically favorable and should therefore enhance the binding affinity [97, 98]. In contrast, for less frequently observed contacts, repulsive or unfavorable interaction between two atom types is anticipated. The mathematical formulation is based on the inverse Boltzmann law that allows to calculate "potentials of mean force" from the statistical probability distribution in the analyzed ensemble of experimental structures. The distance-dependent atom pair potentials thus obtained can then be used to score a protein–ligand complex. Most notably, knowledge-based potentials are derived exclusively from structural data; their derivation does not depend on experimental affinity data. Nevertheless, with respect to affinity correlation the best functions show similar performance as other approaches. It should be noted, though, that knowledge-based scoring functions show best performance in pose prediction and identification of native binding modes [8, 99].

The statistical analysis of a large number of complexes in the PDB database led to the generation of knowledge-based scoring functions such as SMoG [100],

Bleep [101], PMF [102, 103], and DrugScore [104] (cf. Appendix A: Software Overview, Section "Scoring functions"). The functions differ with respect to the number of complexes used for derivation, the precise functional form, the definition of the reference state, the distance range taken into consideration, and the number of different atom types. Another variant in derivation is given by the inclusion of information about protein atom mobility based on isotropic B-factors [105]. A general limitation of all functions is the rare occurrence of certain atom types (e.g., halogen atoms) in the presently available protein–ligand complex structures, preventing the derivation of statistically significant atom pair potentials for these types. This point has been addressed by the development of a new variant of the DrugScore function, DrugScore^{CSD}. Instead of using the PDB, it is based on data generated from the crystal packing of small organic molecules available through the Cambridge Structural Database [99]. The highly resolved small-molecule structures provide relevant contact data across a better balanced distribution of atom types found in drug-like molecules and produce potentials of superior statistical significance and improved performance in different scoring scenarios. Based exclusively on protein–ligand complexes from the PDB, the PMF function has also been rederived using a 10-fold larger data set, and an improved performance was observed for many test sets [103].

The original DrugScore and PMF were compared with a novel atom–atom potential derived from a database of protein–ligand complexes – the Astex statistical potential (ASP) [106]. The ASP approach was also used to construct a targeted scoring function for CDK2 that produced significantly improved enrichment rates compared to the original ASP function. As might be expected, it was demonstrated that the more structures are used in the construction of the targeted function, the better the overall results are.

7.4 Interesting New Approaches to Scoring Functions

There are several approaches to address the issue of scoring and to improve the performance of scoring functions in terms of pose prediction and affinity correlation. A selection of recent developments is discussed in the next section.

7.4.1 Improved Treatment of Hydrophobicity and Dehydration

The scoring function HYDE by Rarey and coworkers [107] estimates binding affinities from only two terms that account for dehydration of polar and nonpolar groups in the protein–ligand interface and use a modified treatment of hydrogen bonding. These terms are based on log *P*-derived atomic increments to estimate dehydration and hydrogen-bonding free energies. Furthermore, the atomic accessibility is included in the calculation. The dehydration term highlights that some atoms contribute favorably while others are detrimental to the overall score. Hence, some hydrogen bond partners are penalized upon dehydration, unless they are able to compensate this loss by a new intermolecular hydrogen bond with excellent geometry and thus high energetic contribution. Thus, the dehydration of polar atoms in narrow binding pockets is less expensive than the dehydration of solvent-exposed atoms, which is consistent with experimental data [107]. In contrast, most scoring functions focus on favorable interactions, as penalties are difficult to include due to a lack of X-ray structures and biological data for weak binders.

The HYDE score is target independent and is reported to provide a classification of compounds in high- and low-affinity ligands. In general, HYDE represents a generally applicable and thermodynamically sensible cutoff score for identification of binders. HYDE may be superior to other scoring functions in this respect, and validation of HYDE by prospective screens with different targets would represent significant progress.

The destabilizing effect from dehydration of a hydrogen-bond partner buried in an apolar environment upon complex formation has been described [108], but it is often ignored. Other studies also highlight the beneficial effect of including dehydration of polar groups [109]. In particular, the HINT force field estimates the contribution of pair interactions from log *P*-values of corresponding surface elements, depending on their interatomic distances [110].

Using ChemScore [96], the effect of scaling hydrogen bond, metal–ligand, and hydrophobic interactions was systematically investigated on the basis of buriedness of intermolecular interactions in protein–ligand complexes [111]. Buriedness was expressed using receptor density scaling (RDS), as defined by the number of heavy atoms around an interaction. Optimization of scaled ChemScore terms using buriedness from experimental X-ray data and docked inactive ligands significantly improved the ability to discriminate actives from inactives. These modified ChemScore terms penalize interactions with flexible outer walls or loops of the binding site; they adjust hydrogen-bond strengths in solvent-exposed surface areas when there is competition with solvent for favorable H-bond interactions.

Kroemer and coworkers [109] reported the development of empirical scoring functions by combining force field-based descriptors from QXP [112] and descriptors based on solvent accessible surface area, thereby accounting for conformational entropy and desolvation of both ligand and receptor upon forming the complex. The protein solvent-accessible surface descriptor to capture entropic contributions has been derived by Murphy and Freire from some protein–protein complexes [113]. A particularly effective descriptor besides this one was the change in polar and nonpolar solvent-accessible surface area for the ligand and in negatively charged hydrophilic and hydrophobic solvent-accessible protein surface area. These descriptors led to significant improvements in affinity prediction for 24 test complexes, while the force field-based descriptors alone were superior in binding pose identification.

The main stabilizing contribution to protein–ligand interactions in this approach represents the removal of apolar groups from bulk water, mainly driven by changes in solvent entropy upon binding. An interesting work described a simple method for assessing the contribution of solvent entropy changes on binding affinity in intermolecular complexes [114]. This approach considers the changes in orientational degrees of freedom of a self-associating arbitrary solvent caused by complex formation of solutes. Systematic placement of solvent surrounding a ligand by arbitrary rules estimates the degree of order imposed by solvation. Computed changes in this degree of order upon complex formation were shown to correlate well with observed binding affinities of complexes in aqueous solutions.

Abel *et al.* reported the development of a novel and computationally efficient descriptor of solvent contribution to the ligand binding free energy [115]. This descriptor captures the effect of ligands displacing solvent molecules from a protein binding site. In a validation study using factor Xa inhibitor complexes, the free energy differences between congeneric pairs of ligands were correctly estimated, while binding site features were elucidated with respect to the hydration of the factor Xa site relevant to the SAR of inhibitors.

7.4.2
Development and Validation of SFCscore

One of the most recent additions to the list of available scoring functions is given by the SFCscore functions [116]. These empirical scoring functions have been developed through a concerted effort between academia and the pharmaceutical industry (the *Scoring Function Consortium*, SFC). The consortium enabled to harness some of the experimental structure and affinity data available in the participating pharmaceutical companies, thereby leading to training sets of unprecedented size and quality. More than 850 well-resolved complex structures with affinity data were obtained through the data collection procedure from corporate and public sources and used to set up different training sets for the calibration of new regression-based scoring functions. Over 60 different descriptors were evaluated for all complexes, including terms accounting for interactions with and among aromatic ring systems as well as many surface-dependent terms.

In total, eight different functions were obtained and extensively tested. Internal cross-validation suggested highly predictive functions. Due to the growth and availability of the PDBbind database [117, 118], extensive unbiased validation on external test sets could be carried out and comparison of the performance with 14 other scoring functions was possible [6]. Overall, the SFCscore functions revealed superior performance in the large comparative tests of affinity prediction. Good performance was also observed with respect to pose prediction from docking poses generated for 22 different target proteins [116].

Although most other scoring functions were outperformed in terms of affinity prediction, a really major leap could not be observed. Most of the remaining deficiencies may be attributed to problems inherent to the simple empirical approach, which tries to predict the affinity of a protein–ligand complex from one single configuration, without consideration of the solvent, the unbound state of the two molecules, and their flexibility. Furthermore, despite all efforts of compiling a high-quality data set, structure and affinity data bear unavoidable inherent experimental errors. For example, binding modes may depend on crystallization conditions, protonation states are not apparent from the structure, and affinity values can strongly depend on the measurement conditions, such as pH and salt concentration.

These factors can hardly be eliminated in a large generic data set of heterogeneous protein–ligand complexes. Based on these fundamental problems, it is likely that for such data sets average prediction errors significantly below 1.0 pK units may be very difficult if not impossible to achieve. Evaluation of the SFCscore functions has shown that the development of empirical functions appears to converge to this limit with respect to the prediction error.

7.4.3 Consensus Scoring

To augment the performance of individual functions, concepts of consensus scoring were developed, which aim to account for the complexity of molecular recognition by relying on multiple individual schemes derived from different physical phenomena. These concepts were shown to be useful to improve the overall performance in docking [5, 119, 120]. Pioneered by Charifson *et al.* [119], predictions from individual functions are combined to rank poses. This approach often leads to an increased performance in hit rates, primarily by decreasing the number of false positives [119]. However, such a decrease might eliminate some true positives, which are favorably scored in only one scoring function. Hence, any workflow for virtual screening needs to compare the performance of individual functions versus consensus schemes for individual targets.

Consensus scoring has been implemented by using multiple functions for rescoring a set of docking poses for each ligand. Further investigations aim to establish the performance of consensus techniques in various scenarios and to determine the best approach for fusion of individual scores [121, 122].

Some work on consensus scoring in ligand-based virtual screening has indicated that much of the improvement from combining scores originates from the fact that different methods have different systematic errors [123]. It has also been shown on a theoretical basis that the combination of individual functions improves the enrichment of true actives only if each individual function is distinctive and has already a high performance [124].

Therefore, additional improvement may be obtained by repeating the entire docking process using multiple methods rather than simply rescoring. The GFscore method uses a nonlinear neural network to combine five scoring functions [125]. Another approach, the bootstrap-based consensus method (BBCS), is based on ensemble learning from multiple scorings with the same functional form but different energy parameter sets [126]. The SeleX-CS consensus scoring algorithm has recently been introduced to address the problem of initial parameter settings in a consensus approach and the use of true inactives [127]. Another strategy combines X-ray information with docking poses by a genetic algorithm to optimize functions based on binding property data from multiple docking runs [128]. These methods often require additional training sets or computational expense, but some form of the original sum rank method still appears to be practical for real-life problems.

An interesting alternative was reported by Vigers and Rizzi [129] to eliminate systematic ligand-specific scoring errors. They propose to use a simple statistical correction called multiple active site correction (MASC) as "reference score" for a ligand against a diverse range of binding pockets. For any actual binding site, the score then can be compared with the MASC reference score. If a significantly higher score is obtained for the active site of interest, such a compound is more likely to represent a true active. This process, however, requires profiling a candidate database by docking all members into a diverse set of proteins. This might not always be feasible, even if this only has to be done once for a routinely used virtual screening library.

7.4.4 Tailored Scoring Functions

Empirical scoring functions are typically derived from a more or less balanced collection of protein–ligand complexes. Systematic studies [130] have confirmed previous observations that although substantial enrichment is sometimes obtained, this is not common for all targets. Instead, for some targets the enrichments are worse than random selection. The limited accuracy in ranking by affinity prompted some research groups to tailor these functions for the protein of interest with an appropriate training set. Hence, existing scoring functions are augmented with features specific for particular binding sites. An overview of these targeted functions has recently been given [131]. In general, targeted functions are based on established functions that are extended, recalibrated, or augmented by specific terms or filters.

Gohlke and Klebe developed the AFMoC procedure [132] for tailored scoring functions based on the DrugScore [104] knowledge-based pair potentials. The generic DrugScore fields derived from the entire PDB are adapted to a single protein binding site by incorporating information from known ligands (Figure 7.3). While the formalism is similar to CoMFA (comparative molecular field analysis) [133], the AFMoC fields originate from an analysis of the protein and not from the ligands alone. A regularly spaced grid is placed over the binding site and knowledge-based pair potentials between protein atoms and ligand atom probes are mapped on the grid intersections resulting in "potential fields." In a statistical analysis, these atom-type specific interaction fields are correlated with binding affinities, producing weighting factors for each field value. Significant improvements for affinity prediction were reported compared to global potentials.

The conceptually similar COMBINE approach by Wade and coworkers [134] is based on the analysis of force field energy terms per residue to describe interaction differences of a congeneric series. The predictive regression equations were reported to find application in structure-based design [135–137].

Another approach based on statistical analysis of residue-specific protein–ligand interaction terms is named TScore [138]. Here, individual protein–ligand interactions are evaluated for each residue within 8 Å around the ligand. Force field-based descriptors are replaced by Chemscore [96] and PLP [139] terms for hydrogen bonds, lipophilicity, and steric contact. Its application to a series of factor Xa inhibitors resulted in a predictive tailored scoring function with 52 selected descriptors after PLS analysis ($q^2 = 0.64$, $r^2 = 0.83$). This concept allows a visual interpretation of

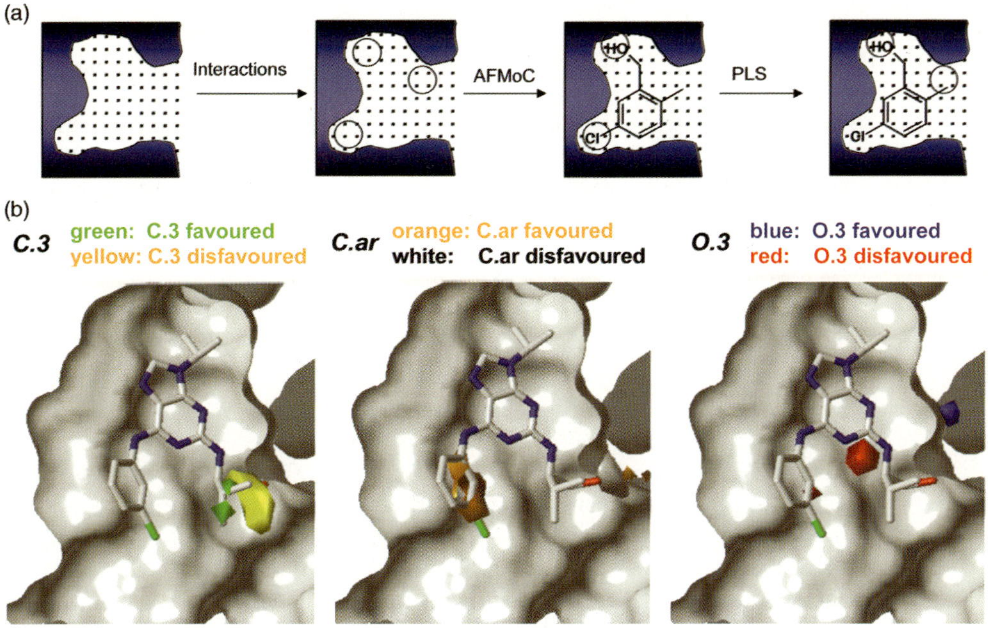

Figure 7.3 Development and application of customized scoring functions. (a) Individual steps during generation of tailored scoring functions using the AFMoC procedure [132], which integrates protein- and ligand-derived descriptors and results in statistical models on protein–ligand interactions for estimation of binding affinity. On a predefined grid, favorable protein interactions with particular ligand atom types are precomputed. These are adapted by incorporating information from a series of docked or crystallized ligands. A statistical analysis using PLS usually leads to models highlighting both favorable and unfavorable contributions. (b) Chemical interpretation of an AFMoC model for a series of 86 substituted purines as CDK-2 inhibitors [206]. The derived PLS model ($q^2 = 0.52$, $r^2 = 0.80$) indicates favorable and unfavorable regions for particular atom types, as shown for C.3, C.ar and O.3, and the CDK-2/purvalanol A complex (PDB code 1ckp). The CDK-2 binding site is represented as MOLCAD solvent-accessible surface.

statistical results based on coloring residues by their importance in the model. However, the applicability of similar approaches might be limited to analogues from related chemotypes. Hence, global scoring function predictions are often integrated into the targeted function, with the aim to be applicable beyond the narrow analogue series investigated, for example, in the case of AFMoC and TScore (Figure 7.4).

The AutoShim approach uses PLS analysis based on affinities for a training set to add single-point pharmacophores in a protein cavity for correction [140]. These pharmacophore points are weighted by PLS coefficients to augment interactions of particular importance, thus adjusting a general scoring function toward a particular target cavity.

Other attempts are based on tailor-made empirical functions by adding descriptors and determine weights for these novel plus the known terms using appropriate statistics and a training set of several ligands. Retraining of a function using focused

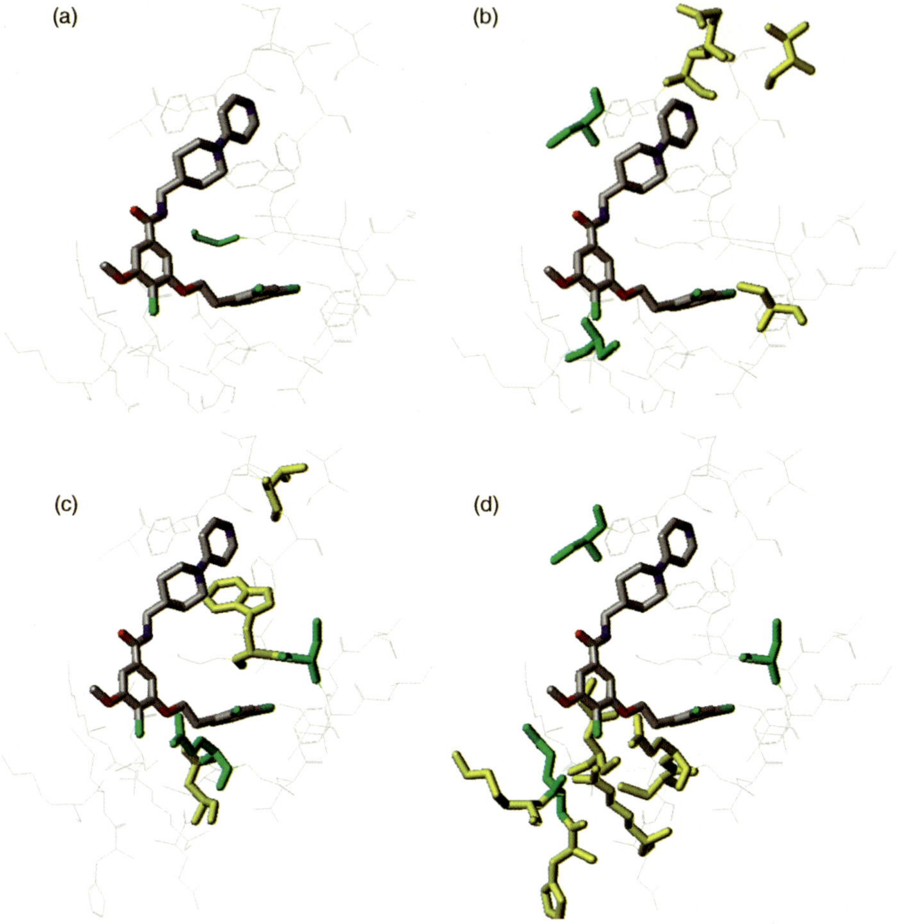

Figure 7.4 Chemical interpretation of the customized scoring function TScore developed for a series of 80 3-oxybenzamide-based factor Xa inhibitors [55]. Key amino acids in the factor Xa binding site linked to affinity are extracted from the resulting PLS model ($q^2 = 0.64$, $r^2 = 0.83$). Green indicates favorable affinity contributions of an amino acid-based interaction term, while negative contributions of a residue are shown in yellow. (a) Residue-based Chemscore hydrogen bond term; (b) residue-based Chemscore lipophilic term; (c) residue-based PLP hydrogen bond term; (d) residue-based PLP steric term.

data for a protein often improves the discrimination for this target and might also assist in understanding the structure–activity relationship. Such a retraining is based on adjusting weights for individual terms of a function, as described, for example, by Rognan *et al.* [141] and Murray *et al.* [142], both starting from ChemScore [96].

In a similar fashion, Catana and Stouten [143] developed multiple functions based on QXP protein–ligand interaction terms [112]. The concept was also applied for improving a force field-based scoring function for CDK-2 using short MD simulations based on quantum-refined force fields [144]. Here, the statistical analysis of global interaction energy terms, hydrogen-bonding changes, and the number of rotatable bonds produced adjusted coefficients for individual contributions to a target-specific function.

The supervised scoring model (SSM), as proposed by Teramoto and Fukunishi [145], applies supervised learning to optimize the FlexX scoring function for particular targets. An approximate linear correction term between the binding affinity and the root mean square deviation (RMSD) of a docked ligand pose is derived by docking selected compounds for a target and using the deviation from the experimental pose for statistical analysis with random forests. Using these modifications of a global empirical scoring function, the authors report a significantly enhanced enrichment, especially of the top ranks of the virtual screening database.

Targeted scoring functions for knowledge-based potentials have been described, for example, for ASP [106]. They combine interatomic contact data for a global set of protein–ligand complexes with data from a large collection of complexes of a single target. This limits the applicability of the concept to targets with a wealth of structural information.

Pham and Jain [146, 147] reported on the recalibration of the Surflex-Dock scoring function by including artificial "negative data" from computer-generated nonbinding poses and inactive compounds for a particular target, with the aim to understand unfavorable binding contributions. The scoring functions for individual targets were optimized by sampling parameter space and observing changes in prediction accuracy. Finally, the standard function was augmented by adding particular constraints and terms accounting for decoys.

The target-specific optimization method (TOP) by Seifert focuses entirely on discrimination between actives and decoys [148]. Enrichment factors were shown to be insufficient to evaluate the discrimination properties of a scoring function. In contrast, analysis of variance techniques (ANOVA) is superior to quantify the discriminatory power with respect to binders and inactives [149]. This optimization using ANOVA on distributions of docking scores for actives and inactives starts from the empirical function implemented in the docking program ProPose. However, as sometimes there is no reliable quantification of "nonbinding" and no structural information for weak ligands available, a correct calibration remains difficult in these cases.

7.4.5 Structural Interaction Fingerprints

The residue-based SIFt (structural interaction fingerprints) methodology, as introduced by Singh and coworkers [150], calculates an interaction fingerprint of a pose by encoding seven interactions between the ligand and each residue in the active site, in analogy to COMBINE [134] and TScore [138]. A recent review summarizes applications and improvements of this concept to docking and filtering [151]. Although SIFt is not a scoring function *per se*, it extracts molecular interaction information and converts it to binary fingerprints. These fingerprints may then be used either to aid analysis of virtual screening data by mining or filtering or for similarity searching between protein–ligand complexes. The authors demonstrated the use of similarity searching and clustering of this bit-string information to identify poses with similar interaction pattern. This allows to compute SIFt-based enrichment scores by identification of molecules with an interaction pattern similar to that of a particular lead series.

This concept was applied both for organizing and analyzing the structural information in the protein kinase family and for virtual screening [152]. Its extension to a profile-SIFt by measuring the conservation of interactions in reference protein–ligand complexes was effective for filtering and ranking by comparing this profile with SIFts from individual docking solutions [152]. Recently, the concept has also been applied to fragment docking [153] in order to measure the conservation of interaction of novel molecular probes. Further additions by Kelly and Mancera have successfully encoded information about strength and geometric grouping of hydrogen-bonding interactions in this fingerprint [154].

Recently, the structural interaction fingerprint concept has been extended, by introducing weighted SIFts, to capture the relative importance of different binding interactions [155]. These weights were determined by machine learning; they again provide insight into essential protein–ligand interactions and might be applied as tailored residue-based scoring function.

7.5 Comparative Assessment of Scoring Functions

Obviously, thorough comparative evaluations are of utmost importance not only for selection and application but also for improvement of scoring functions. Unfortunately, practically relevant and truly unbiased comparative assessments are by no means trivial to achieve, as documented by many studies in the recent literature (cf. [156] and references therein).

The difficulties encountered are manifold, in particular with respect to the performance in virtual screening. First of all, none of the test sets compiled so far has yet reached the status of a commonly accepted standard benchmarking set against which any new method would have to be evaluated. This is in part related to the problems in compiling such data sets, including the availability of a sufficient amount of suitable experimental structures and affinity data [166] and a consensus of what constitutes a reasonable diversity. In evaluating scoring functions, it is, in fact, important to use a diverse set of binding sites, each of which challenges the scoring function in different ways. With respect to virtual screening, the generation of sufficiently large [131], nontrivial, and realistic decoy sets is a major challenge. Nevertheless, very useful data sets have started to appear (e.g., [8, 157, 158]), and recommendations for the compilation of new test sets and the improvement of existing ones have been defined [156, 159, 160]. Other problems of comparative studies include the selection of appropriate, statistically valid metrics and the corresponding error estimates for the evaluation of both the results (such as RMSD values, correlation coefficients, enrichment factors, and AUC of ROC curves; cf. [161–164] for a detailed discussion and [165] for a suggested statistical framework to analyze virtual screening results) and the issues of data sharing with respect to the detailed settings used in preparing the structures and running the programs [156]. This last point is important not only for reproducibility and comparability in general but also for evaluation in virtual screening in order to allow separation of the scoring function quality from other factors in the workflow. In fact, while virtual screening is able to enrich hit molecules in ranked lists of relatively small size, there is often little correlation between experimental affinity and predicted score. Enrichment calculations (often based on *a priori* classification of molecules into "actives" and "inactives") reflect both the quality of the entire virtual screening workflow, including the mandatory target and ligand preparation, and the quality of docking plus the scoring assessment. Often the experimental validation of compounds assumed to be inactive is not available in public databases. Furthermore, there is no guarantee that the correct conformation was sampled during docking and this best pose has also the best scoring prediction [166].

Despite all these difficulties and limitations, valuable large-scale assessments of scoring function performance are already available. An instructive compilation of comparative studies has been presented by Moitessier *et al.* [167], and further evaluations have appeared since then (e.g., [8, 168–170]). In the following section, we focus primarily on two of the most comprehensive studies at the moment, which have been conducted by Warren *et al.* [157] and Cheng *et al.* [8].

In general, three aspects are of interest when evaluating the performance of scoring functions. (1) Pose prediction: this is the ability to detect native or near-native poses among a set of solutions generated by docking ("docking power"); (2) virtual screening: this refers to the ability to rank compounds and/or separate actives from inactives ("ranking power"); and (3) affinity prediction: this indicates the ability to predict the actual affinity of compounds ("scoring power"). In theory, with access to the true ΔG° value from scoring, all problems could be solved simultaneously with the same accuracy; in contrast, current scoring functions have clear strengths and weaknesses with respect to these three issues.

The group of Wang has been active in the field of comparative scoring function evaluation since 2003 when they published an assessment of scoring functions for pose prediction [171]. Due to their work on the PDBbind database [117], they were later able to provide large data sets with affinity values for assessing the scoring power. The first study of this kind appeared in 2004 [6], which also formed the basis for evaluation of more recently developed scoring functions such as SFCscore [116]. The availability of such data sets constituted a major advance in the field since the formerly very limited size and diversity of affinity test sets may have led to far too optimistic estimates of the actual scoring power. In the most recent update, the Wang group has presented a refined test set of 195 diverse, high-quality structures to assess docking power, ranking power, and scoring power at the same time and in a way that the evaluations are independent of the context of docking or virtual screening [8]. Briefly, the currently best functions reach the following values: (1) close to 80% success rate in detecting a near-native pose (RMSD < 2 Å) as top-ranked result; (2) correlation with experimental affinity of ~0.65 in terms of Pearson correlation coefficient for the entire data set, and between 0.34 and 0.82 for four target-specific data sets; and (3) 58% success rate in ranking power, as assessed by the ability to correctly rank the low-, medium-, and high-affinity ligand of a certain target for all 65 targets in the data set, based on the true experimental binding mode. Thus, while respectable success rates are obtained in pose prediction, the correlation with experimental affinity is disappointingly weak for all functions (despite the fact that the test set is spoiled with some training set complexes for various functions).

Warren *et al.* [157] presented an evaluation closely related to the virtual screening context. With an impressive effort, this study was performed under the most unbiased and practically relevant scenario possible. Altogether, 10 docking programs and 37 scoring functions were tested against 8 proteins of 7 target types. With respect to pose prediction, 19 docking protocols (i.e., 10 docking programs with 1–5 scoring variants) were tested on 136 structurally known complexes of the 7 targets. The success rates in identifying the pose closest to the crystal conformation considerably varied across the targets and protocols, with best values close to 75% and many results of less than 10%. Nevertheless, for five of the seven target types, at least one protocol was able to identify poses within 2 Å of the crystallographic conformation for ≥40% of the complexes. With respect to virtual screening for lead identification, for six of the seven targets at least one docking program/scoring function combination showed an enrichment factor ≥5 at 10% of the rank-ordered compound list. However, performance across diverse targets was inconsistent. Furthermore, troubling cases of lack of correlation between the ability to reproduce binding modes and the enrichment in virtual screening were observed. As commented by Leach *et al.* [166], enrichment may be due to screening out compounds that are wrong for the target rather than selecting those that are right; thus, it would appear that virtual screening has advanced to the point where it can distinguish between sensible and unlikely candidate ligands, but distinguishing among the sensible ones remains a major challenge. Finally, with respect to affinity prediction for lead optimization, "the data revealed that there is no statistically significant correlation between measured affinity and any of the scoring functions evaluated across all eight protein targets examined" [157]. Indeed, the by far best correlation coefficient observed for a single target and scoring function combination had an absolute value of 0.57. This highlighted the major shortcoming of current scoring functions, indicating that we are still far apart from a correct estimate of the Gibbs free energy of binding. As summarized by the authors, "The fault was not in the reproduction of the experimentally observed binding mode by the docking programs or in the ability to differentiate active ligands from decoys, but in the inability of the current scoring functions to distinguish, differentiate, and quantify the sometimes subtle differences that can change ligand affinity from highly potent to inactive" [157].

Clearly, there is still much need for improvement of scoring functions, and tailored strategies beyond the application of a single score list of a standard scoring function must be recommended for virtual screening applications.

7.6
Tailoring Scoring Strategies in Virtual Screening

7.6.1
Toward a Strategy for Applying Scoring Functions

Decision making in drug discovery critically depends on quality and timeliness of computational results. In order to impact research and provide qualified answers, they need to be reliable and fast. Consequently, a robust algorithm providing reliable results but not within a realistic timeframe will not impact a decision on which compounds to explore next. In contrast, methods with fast but low-quality results will find application only as early filters rather than for advanced decision making for prioritization of subsequent synthesis goals.

The application of scoring functions is fast, but does not always result in a significant correlation with binding affinities across a diverse set of scaffolds. This prompted many research groups to develop improved functions and smart post-processing schemes. Several strategies for successful integration of scoring functions into virtual screening workflows have been discussed in the literature. In view of those discussions, this section will provide practical hints for the planning phase of a virtual screening experiment.

To allow rapid screening of large compound databases, a cascaded scoring scheme is often applied. There are many ways to reduce the number of compounds for docking and scoring by prefiltering. It is often done using simple molecular or physicochemical properties [172] or including a prescreening based on ligand similarity [173, 174]. Such filters are sometimes followed by the application of pharmacophore models and/or docking constraints in the binding site. Other methods to focus on relevant compounds include only general considerations of "lead-likeness" [175] for molecules.

The careful preparation and analysis of a binding site might provide further information on critical success factors for virtual screening. This could include the comparison of different experimental conformations from X-ray structures of the same or related proteins. Furthermore, consensus positions of water molecules and key consensus pharmacophore interactions should be considered for building filters or constraints for docking or postprocessing. If such an analysis reveals untypical interactions like a halogen– or cation–π interaction, adequate or adapted scoring functions and postprocessing tools should be employed. Key interactions from known protein–ligand complexes could be included as pharmacophore filters, constraints, or subsite occupancy requirements [176]. For some prominent target families, certain key interactions are obvious, such as H-bonds for hinge binding in protein kinases, S1-site occupation for serine protease, metal interactions for matrix metalloproteinases (MMPs), or aspartyl binding for aspartyl proteases. However, while producing better enrichment rates by filtering out false positives, the filters might also reduce the number of true actives due to novel, unexpected modes of interactions, as in the case of nonmetal-complexing MMP ligands [177].

There is no fundamental reason why a single scoring function should be used to identify the most adequate ligand conformation *and* rank order ligands. Rather, it is possible to define a multistep strategy to decouple these tasks. For docking and pose evaluation, simple scoring functions are often used as a rapid filter for the entire database, focusing on relevant poses and molecules first. These poses are then subjected to different rescoring approaches, where computationally more demanding methods could find an application. While some scoring functions are integrated in docking engines, postprocessing of poses should always be considered provided docking exhaustively samples conformational space. After pose selection, the ranking step may use a computationally even more demanding scoring procedure, such as MM–PBSA, MM–GBSA, or FEP calculations for preselected poses only. A retrospective validation step might be useful at this stage, as there is no consensus about a single protocol that might work for many different binding sites.

7.6.2
Retrospective Validation Prior to Prospective Virtual Screening

One of the requirements prior to virtual screening is to identify the most adequate scoring function for a new binding site. Rigorous retrospective validation prior to large-scale application in a prospective virtual screening campaign is mandatory to select the tools with optimal performance for a certain target or a certain problem. Any validation, however, depends on the availability of reference molecules. Accordingly, information on ligands for the investigated target is required, from literature, patent information, or other sources, like a preliminary experimental screening.

A validation study needs to focus on both aspects of virtual screening, namely, the selection of correct poses for a particular binding site and the ranking of these poses by affinity. The availability of many different functions allows integrating them in automated scoring and postprocessing workflows to evaluate which one shows the highest degree of predictivity in terms of pose prediction and affinity ranking plus enrichment rates. The best functions for both tasks are possibly not the same, which opens the question whether a cascaded scoring process or a consensus of two (or more) functions might provide more favorable results. According to literature and own experience, there is no general workflow. Different tools and their integration could result from validation studies. Certainly, obtaining good enrichment is qualitatively more challenging than reproducing crystallographic poses, both in terms of algorithmic efficiency and in terms of scoring function accuracy.

Critical questions to be addressed upon validation pertain to the treatment of receptor flexibility, the inclusion of ligand and receptor strain energies, and the treatment of water and solvation effects. Technical issues of implementation must be solved in parallel, like the correct preparation of protein structures (including protonation states, treatment of missing residues, and binding site definitions) or the conversion of file formats, which could significantly differ between scoring functions. The initial planning phase also needs to consider which metric of success is appropriate for a given problem in a validation study (cf. Section 7.5 and references therein).

7.6.3 Lessons Learned: Improvements in Scoring Evaluations

After initial validation studies and application of a virtual screening workflow, a first round of experimental testing in a high-quality biological assay is useful to identify actives for a particular target protein. In general, high-quality rather than rapid assay settings are favored for virtual screening to reduce the risk of experimental false negatives. Such an early experimental feedback is desirable and might lead to an iterative virtual screening protocol. On the basis of initial results, key components of the virtual screening workflow can be reevaluated. Furthermore, this new information might allow to generate scoring functions tailored toward a better discrimination of actives and inactives. Some examples of customized functions were discussed above. Such a novel function can be used to rescore already existing poses and select new interesting analogues for experimental testing.

If there is an initial enrichment of known actives, statistical approaches might also be able to augment the separation. To improve recovery of experimental true actives after docking, Klon *et al.* reported a simple machine learning procedure employing 2D fingerprints and docking scores [178]. Using a few known actives at the top of the scored poses and the rest of the ligands as poorly docked, the docking score predetermines, in the absence of known activity, what are likely to be active or inactive poses. When docking alone enriches the initial collection, the application of a naïve Bayes classifier was able to improve this enrichment. The authors concluded that such an approach could be applied without knowing the activity of all compounds and results in superior enrichment of known actives compared to the use of scoring alone. Krumrine *et al.* [179] applied a similar argument in reranking docking hits as informed by initial docking hit distribution in their chemical neighborhood. Those poses from clusters with many other hits are presumed to be true positives more likely than docking hits from poorly scoring clusters, although such a strategy might work only in the absence of nonsystematic errors for a particular scaffold. Sullivan and Martin pointed out that predictive QSAR models on docking scores for compounds with *a priori* unknown experimental affinity might be generated for correction of scores for some random errors introduced in the scoring process [180].

These strategies for reanalyzing hitlists when information is available is seen as an effective way of maximizing the impact of a virtual screen, but it critically depends on the integration of computational and biochemical testing efforts with compound logistics.

7.6.4 Postfiltering Results of Virtual Screenings

Due to deficiencies in scoring, additional filters like topological properties of poses are often employed to support selection of virtual hits for testing. This could include the steric complementarity to the binding site, the complementarity of matching polar and lipophilic surface areas or any mismatches of them, and other improper ligand geometries, accounting for high ligand strain energy.

However, all advanced scoring and rescoring schemes are likely not to replace the last step in virtual screening, namely, the visual inspection of a few hundreds or more poses by an experienced computational or medicinal chemist. This step serves as final filter to select those compounds with the best interaction profile. High-end computer graphics combined with adequate visualization of key interactions and bookkeeping possibilities have greatly enhanced the interactive selection of interesting poses and molecules. This is a very time-consuming and tedious procedure, which ensures that selected molecules indeed bind in a physically meaningful way and show expected properties. The impact of scoring schemes is to preselect molecules for this final inspection and to provide some detailed insight into the nature and putative strength of any protein–ligand interaction. Advances in the generation of sophisticated scoring schemes will then allow to focus even more on promising molecules and geometries as a starting point for experimental testing and structure-based design.

7.7 Caveats for Development of Scoring Functions

7.7.1 General Points

In several comparative studies, it has been shown that while docking programs were successful in generating poses with acceptable geometries close to the experimental structure, virtual screening did not always lead to acceptable hit rates. As it has been demonstrated, the accurate estimation of binding free energies for diverse ligands is difficult. Predicting binding affinities might be possible only if a tailored scoring function is applied to congeneric ligands, while for diverse databases and targets not included in scoring function training, the achievable prediction accuracy is only moderate (at best ~1.0–1.5 pKi units). Some of the underlying issues will be discussed in this section.

One fundamental problem is related to the accuracy of calculated protein–ligand interaction terms plus desolvation penalties. Any estimation of the free energy of binding results from subtraction of large energetic terms computed for individual interactions, leading to a relatively small number for the binding affinity. Different levels of accuracy in estimating the interaction terms are observed and errors here cannot be assumed to compensate. Furthermore, as pointed out by Tirado-Rives and Jorgensen, the actual *window of activity* in virtual screening is rather small, as the free energy difference between a potent inhibitor (e.g., 50 nM) and the experimental detection limit (~100 μM) is only ~18.5 kJ/mol [181], while weak hits often show a binding affinity of only ~10 μM. Ligands typically do not bind in their lowest-energy conformation and there is a loss of conformational degrees of freedom upon binding. The authors have addressed the free energy change for this "conformer focusing" and could show that uncertainties from this source significantly contribute to the error in virtual screening for rank ordering diverse compounds.

7.7.2
Biological Data

For the development of regression-based functions and for testing knowledge- and force field-based methods, balanced biological data, preferably from one laboratory, are essential. In general, the experimental settings for determining binding affinities and crystal structures should be comparable in terms of pH, concentrations, and other parameters. Any experimental value included in a regression analysis should reliably reflect the true free energy of binding. The usual experimental data from biochemical experiments are expressed in terms of IC_{50} values and can be compared only under certain assumptions, like identical concentrations of the involved molecular partners [182]. Measuring K_i values for kinases, for example, requires many experimental data points for variation of ATP and inhibitor concentrations and is, thus, done only for selected compounds. Accordingly, although K_i values are clearly preferable to IC_{50} data, only the latter might be available for many targets. More systematic compilations and measurements reflecting actual binding affinities are thus required to generate balanced data sets for method development. Caution has to be taken to unveil the true mechanism of binding, as IC_{50} values can significantly differ from K_i values and could include systematic artifacts. Further restrictions concern the accuracy of experimentally determined binding affinities, in particular for compounds with very low solubility, high plasma protein binding, or only moderate stability under experimental conditions. For cell-based assays, membrane permeability might also influence experimental data. Additional accounts of problems with experimental data have appeared in the recent literature [183, 184].

There is no general solution to the issue of data availability, consistency, and comparability, especially for the desirable broad set of protein targets and ligands, requiring many different assays under a multitude of conditions, which probably do not always reflect only the true protein–ligand recognition event. In addition, the development of improved scoring functions also requires more fundamental physicochemical measurements for a broad set of structures, including ligand solvation energies and pK_a values for proteins.

7.7.3
Structural Data on Protein–Ligand Complexes and Decoy Data Sets

One of the limitations of many scoring functions is that they are derived from crystal structures of extremely potent ligands, while structural or affinity information about less active analogues is often not available as they typically do not progress in a lead optimization program. Structural data on weak and unfavorable protein–ligand interactions are sparse since experimental X-ray structures of low-affinity ligands are more difficult to obtain and less interesting to project teams. Those available often suffer from lower resolution or structural disorder.

Furthermore, it is important to reflect on limitations of protein crystal structures [185], which are partially due to errors in reported structures [186, 187] and significant experimental limitations. Among these are the effects of protein flexibility [188], the existence of multiple binding modes [189, 190], protonation effects [191–193], also influencing binding modes [194], and the occurrence of tautomers [193, 195]. With respect to ligand binding, it must also be kept in mind that some of the experimental structure data are affected by crystal contacts, which can now easily be detected with software tools like ReliBase [196]. Interestingly, a recent study showed that 36% of the ligands in the PDBbind 2007 database are influenced by these contacts, which might affect the performance of scoring functions as well [197].

It has recently been shown that ligand bias can contribute significantly to the number of false positives in scoring [198]. Some scoring functions favor more complex molecules due to additive descriptors in their underlying mathematical functions, which led to the proposal of different normalization and rescoring approaches [199]. In order to overcome these limitations for virtual screening validation, data sets combining ligands with comparable physicochemical properties were proposed. The recent database of useful decoys (DUD) consists of 40 targets including published ligands and decoy compounds [158]. The decoys have been chosen such that they differ in topology from the binder, but have similar distributions of physicochemical parameters in order to avoid artificial enrichments. Although the creation of balanced data sets with comparable property distributions is a significant step forward in scoring function development and validation, it is difficult to guarantee that all decoy molecules do indeed not bind to the target of interest. Hence, careful and consistent data sets are required to take full advantage of this concept. Similar considerations hold for binding pose decoys, as it is not always known whether a second conformation is indeed able to bind to a cavity; the conformational equilibrium might be hidden or could be influenced by crystallization.

7.7.4
Cooperativity and Other Model Deficiencies

Some of the more fundamental limitations of current scoring functions are based on significant model deficiencies and assumptions with respect to important factors in molecular recognition, such as ligand desolvation and intramolecular entropy effects. It also includes the fact that noncovalent protein–ligand interactions are normally treated as additive, an assumption not always applicable. In fact, noncovalent interactions are often either mutually reinforced (positively cooperative) or weakened (negative cooperativity). Ligands can improve their affinity when the motion within a receptor site is reduced (positively cooperative binding); such an organization occurs with a benefit in binding (favorable enthalpy) and a limitation in internal dynamics (entropy penalty). In contrast, negative cooperativity induces converse effects, namely, a less efficient packing (cost in enthalpy) and a benefit in entropy [200].

Interestingly, additivity of ligand SARs is also often assumed. Studies on combinatorial libraries for different target families have revealed that only half of them exhibit additive behavior [201]. Methods for computationally detecting cooperativity and incorporating them into scoring schemes are still missing.

Moreover, there is the issue of flexibility, which is addressed by methodologies such as molecular dynamics simulations in combination with experimental data. Changes in protein and ligand flexibility and the associated entropic effects on the binding free energy are difficult to estimate. By using isothermal titration calorimetry, it was shown, for example, that some inhibitors of carbonic anhydrase II are not rigidly fixed in the binding pocket, but a considerable degree of residual entropy remains in the bound ligand [202]. The use of NMR spectroscopy also allowed to detect that more than one conformation for a p38 kinase/inhibitor complex exists in solution, in contrast to the "rigid" complex observed in the crystal. Apparently, the ATP-pocket is highly flexible even after ligand binding [203]. A comparison between molecular dynamics simulations and experimental NMR backbone relaxation times for protein structures provided some evidence that intraprotein hydrogen bonds in specific loop and turn regions are stabilized by electronic polarization, which might be critical for the dynamical stability of these local structures in proteins [204]. These and other effects influencing the internal stability of proteins and its relationship to protein–ligand binding entropy remain to be investigated in comparative studies in order to stimulate further development of practicable scoring schemes.

The uncertainty regarding the role of water molecules in the active site and the balance between enthalpy and entropy add to this problem. Studies by Homans and his group have shown that for a hydrophobic model protein pocket, ligand binding is not driven by the entropy gain of solvent water, but rather by favorable dispersion interactions arising from suboptimal hydration of this pocket [205]. Here, optimization for ligand-shape complementarity might offer a useful design principle.

For most of these topics, it is too early to judge whether they will mature into reliable scoring techniques with significant impact on structure-based virtual screening. However, significant improvements in these fields are expected.

7.8 Conclusions

Identification of novel lead structures and their optimization into drug candidates is one of the key technologies in today's drug discovery efforts. Several computational and medicinal chemistry approaches have been successfully applied to this problem. As virtual screening is gaining importance in drug discovery complementary to HTS, the need for a reliable scoring function or reliable workflows integrating multiple of these functions and filter criteria becomes pressing.

In this chapter, we have shown that the reality of protein–ligand interactions is still far too complex to be correctly captured with *in silico* approaches for rapid prediction of the binding free energy. Simpler schemes work to a certain degree, and a variety of methods exist for estimating binding affinities. Clearly, the neglect of important contributions to the protein–ligand recognition event still leads to unsatisfactory predictions in too many cases. Nevertheless, the field has witnessed significant improvements that allow reasonable binding pose prediction and affinity estimation under certain prerequisites. Hence, it is of utmost importance to be aware of the concepts and limitations of the applied scoring functions in order to select those with a high probability of success for prospective applications to novel protein binding sites in virtual screening. Since several aspects play together in virtual screening applications, project-specific validation of the entire workflow is essential.

With the increasing availability of computational resources, many physically relevant interactions, in particular with respect to entropic contributions, may be integrated into future scoring workflows. In addition, quantum chemistry and molecular dynamics may lead to further enhancement of current approaches. Access to larger and more balanced experimental data sets might allow, in future, to study the influence of particular interaction terms in more detail. More efforts along these lines can be realistically expected to result in significant improvements toward a reliable estimation of binding free energies in protein–ligand complexes.

Acknowledgment

The authors would like to thank Christian Buning, Clemens Giegerich, Stefan Güssregen (Sanofi-Aventis), and Gerhard Klebe (University of Marburg) for stimulating discussions on several aspects of this chapter.

References

1 Baringhaus, K.H. and Matter, H. (2004) Efficient strategies for lead optimization by simultaneously addressing affinity, selectivity and pharmacokinetic parameters, in *Methods and Principles in Medicinal Chemistry: Cheminformatics in Drug Discovery* (ed. T.I. Oprea), Wiley-VCH verlag GmbH, Weinheim, pp. 333–379.

2 Böhm, H.J. and Stahl, M. (2002) The use of scoring functions in drug discovery applications, in *Reviews in Computational Chemistry*, vol. 18 (eds K.B. Lipkowitz and D.B. Boyd), John Wiley & Sons Inc., New York, pp. 41–87.

3 Gohlke, H. and Klebe, G. (2002) Approaches to the description and prediction of the binding affinity of small-molecule ligands to macromolecular receptors. *Angewandte Chemie – International Edition in English*, **41**, 2644–2676.

4 Rajamani, R. and Good, A.C. (2007) Ranking poses and structure-based lead discovery and optimization: current trends in scoring function development. *Current Opinion in Drug Discovery & Development*, **10**, 308–315.

5 Stahl, M. and Rarey, M. (2001) Detailed analysis of scoring functions for virtual screening. *Journal of Medicinal Chemistry*, **44**, 1035–1042.

6 Wang, R., Lu, Y., Fang, X., and Wang, S. (2004) An extensive test of 14 scoring functions using the PDBbind refined set of 800 protein–ligand complexes. *Journal of Chemical Information and Computer Sciences*, **44**, 2114–2125.

7 Ferrara, P., Gohlke, H., Price, D.J., Klebe, G., and Brooks, C.L. (2004)

Assessing scoring functions for protein–ligand interactions. *Journal of Medicinal Chemistry*, **47**, 3032–3047.

8 Cheng, T., Li, X., Li, Y., Liu, Z., and Wang, R. (2009) Comparative assessment of scoring functions on a diverse test set. *Journal of Chemical Information and Modeling*, **49**, 1079–1093.

9 Andrews, P.R. (1993) Drug–receptor interactions, in *3D-QSAR in Drug Design. Theory, Methods and Applications*, ESCOM, Leiden, NL, pp. 13–40.

10 Stahl, M. and Böhm, H.-J. (1998) Development of filter functions for protein–ligand docking. *Journal of Molecular Graphics & Modelling*, **16**, 121–132.

11 McDonald, I.K. and Thornton, J.M. (1994) Satisfying hydrogen bonding potential in proteins. *Journal of Molecular Biology*, **238**, 777–793.

12 Butler, K.T., Luque, F.J., and Barril, X. (2009) Toward accurate relative energy predictions of the bioactive conformation of drugs. *Journal of Computational Chemistry*, **30**, 601–610.

13 Khan, A.R., Parrish, J.C., Fraser, M.E., Smith, W.W., Bartlett, P.A., and James, M.N.G. (1998) Lowering the entropic barrier for binding conformationally flexible inhibitors to enzymes. *Biochemistry*, **37**, 16839–16845.

14 Dunitz, J.D. (1995) Win some, lose some: enthalpy–entropy compensation in weak molecular interactions. *Chemistry & Biology*, **2**, 709–712.

15 Luque, I. and Freire, E. (2002) Structural parametrization of the binding enthalpy of small ligands. *Proteins*, **49**, 181–190.

16 Freire, E. (2008) Do enthalpy and entropy distinguish first in class from best in class? *Drug Discovery Today*, **13**, 869–874.

17 Dunitz, J. (1994) The entropic cost of bound water in crystals and biomolecules. *Science*, **264**, 670

18 Warwicker, J. and Watson, H.C. (1982) Calculation of the electric potential in the active site cleft due to α-helix dipoles. *Journal of Molecular Biology*, **157**, 671–679.

19 Davis, M.E. and McCammon, J.A. (1990) Electrostatics in biomolecular structure and dynamics. *Chemical Reviews*, **90**, 509–521.

20 Dauber, P. and Hagler, A.T. (1980) Crystal packing, hydrogen bonding, and the effect of crystal forces on molecular conformation. *Accounts of Chemical Research*, **13**, 105–112.

21 Morgan, B.P., Scholtz, J.M., Ballinger, M.D., Zipkin, I.D., and Bartlett, P.A. (1991) Differential binding energy: a detailed evaluation of the influence of hydrogen bonding and hydrophobic groups on the inhibition of thermolysin by phosphorus-containing inhibitors. *Journal of the American Chemical Society*, **113**, 297–307.

22 Shirley, B.A., Stanssens, P., Hahn, U., and Pace, C.N. (1992) Contribution of hydrogen bonding to the conformational stability of ribonuclease T1. *Biochemistry*, **31**, 725–732.

23 Obst, U., Banner, D.W., Weber, L., and Diederich, F. (1997) Molecular recognition at the thrombin active site: structure-based design and synthesis of potent and selective thrombin inhibitors and the X-ray structures of two thrombin inhibitors. *Chemistry & Biology*, **4**, 287–295.

24 Derewenda, Z.S., Lee, L., and Derewenda, U. (1995) The occurrence of C=H···O hydrogen bonds in proteins. *Journal of Molecular Biology*, **252**, 248–262.

25 Scheiner, S., Kar, T., and Gual, Y. (2001) Strength of the CαH···O hydrogen bond of amino acid residues. *The Journal of Biological Chemistry*, **276**, 9832–9837.

26 Vargas, R., Garza, J., Dixon, D.A., and Hay, B.P. (2000) How strong is the C−H···O=C hydrogen bond? *Journal of the American Chemical Society*, **122**, 4750–4755.

27 Yohannan, S., Faham, S., Yang, D., Grosfeld, D., Chamberlain, A.K., and Bowie, J.U. (2004) A Cα−H···O hydrogen bond in a membrane protein is not stabilizing. *Journal of the American Chemical Society*, **126**, 2284–2285.

28 Pierce, A.C., Sandretto, K.L., and Bemis, G.W. (2002) Kinase inhibitors and the case for CH···O hydrogen bonds in protein–ligand binding. *Proteins*, **49**, 567–576.

29 Burley, S.K. and Petsko, G.A. (1998) Weakly polar interactions in proteins. *Advances in Protein Chemistry*, **39**, 125–189.
30 Tsuzuki, S., Honda, K., Uchimaru, T., Mikami, M., and Tanabe, K. (2000) Origin of the attraction and directionality of the NH/π interaction: comparison with OH/π and CH/π interactions. *Journal of the American Chemical Society*, **122**, 11450–11458.
31 Brandl, M., Weiss, M.S., Jabs, A., Suhnel, J., and Hilgenfeld, R. (2001) CH–π interactions in proteins. *Journal of Molecular Biology*, **307**, 357–377.
32 Gallivan, J.P. and Dougherty, D.A. (1999) Cation–π interactions in structural biology. *Proceedings of the National Academy of Sciences of the United States of America*, **96**, 9459–9464.
33 Burley, S.K. and Petsko, G.A. (1985) Aromatic–aromatic interaction: a mechanism of protein structure stabilization. *Science*, **229**, 23–28.
34 McGaughey, G.B., Gagné, M., and Rappé, A.K. (1998) π-Stacking interactions. Alive and well in proteins. *The Journal of Biological Chemistry*, **273**, 15458–15463.
35 Dougherty, D.A. and Stauffer, D.A. (1990) Acetylcholine binding by a synthetic receptor: implications for biological recognition. *Science*, **250**, 1558–1560.
36 Salonen, L.M., Bucher, C., Banner, D.W., Haap, W., Mary, J.-L., Benz, J., Kuster, O., Seiler, P., Schweizer, W.B., and Diederich, F. (2009) Cation–π interactions at the active site of factor Xa: dramatic enhancement upon stepwise N-alkylation of ammonium ions. *Angewandte Chemie – International Edition in English*, **48**, 811–814.
37 Böhm, H.-J., Banner, D., Bendels, S., Kansy, M., Kuhn, B., Müller, K., Obst-Sander, U., and Stahl, M. (2004) Fluorine in medicinal chemistry. *ChemBioChem*, **5**, 637–643.
38 Hagmann, W.K. (2008) The many roles for fluorine in medicinal chemistry. *Journal of Medicinal Chemistry*, **51**, 4359–4369.
39 Schweizer, E., Hoffmann-Röder, A., Scharer, K., Olsen, J.A., Fah, C., Seiler, P., Obst-Sander, U., Wagner, B., Kansy, M., and Diederich, F. (2006) A fluorine scan at the catalytic center of thrombin: C−F, C−OH, and C−OMe bioisosterism and fluorine effects on pK_a and log D values. *ChemMedChem*, **1**, 611–621.
40 Shah, P. and Westwell, A.D. (2007) The role of fluorine in medicinal chemistry. *Journal of Enzyme Inhibition and Medicinal Chemistry*, **22**, 527–540.
41 Maren, T.H. and Conroy, C.W. (1993) A new class of carbonic anhydrase inhibitor. *The Journal of Biological Chemistry*, **268**, 26233–23239.
42 Olsen, J.A., Banner, D.W., Seiler, P., Wagner, B., Tschopp, T., Obst-Sander, U., Kansy, M., Müller, K., and Diederich, F. (2004) Fluorine interactions at the thrombin active site: protein backbone fragments H−Cα−C=O comprise a favorable C−F environment and interactions of C−F with electrophiles. *ChemBioChem*, **5**, 666–675.
43 Paulini, R., Müller, K., and Diederich, F. (2005) Orthogonal multipolar interactions in structural chemistry and biology. *Angewandte Chemie – International Edition in English*, **44**, 1788–1805.
44 Metrangolo, P., Meyer, F., Pilati, T., Resnati, G., and Terraneo, G. (2008) Halogen bonding in supramolecular chemistry. *Angewandte Chemie – International Edition in English*, **47**, 6114–6127.
45 Auffinger, P., Hays, F.A., Westhof, E., and Ho, P.S. (2004) Halogen bonds in biological molecules. *Proceedings of the National Academy of Sciences of the United States of America*, **101**, 16789–16794.
46 Politzer, P., Lane, P., Concha, M.C., Ma, Y., and Murray, J.S. (2007) An overview of halogen bonding. *Journal of Molecular Modeling*, **13**, 305–311.
47 Lu, Y., Shi, T., Wang, Y., Yang, H., Yan, X., Luo, X., Jiang, H., and Zhu, W. (2009) Halogen bonding: a novel interaction for rational drug design? *Journal of Medicinal Chemistry*, **52**, 2854–2862.
48 Matter, H., Nazaré, M., Güssregen, S., Will, D.W., Schreuder, H., Bauer, A., Urmann, M., Ritter, K., Wagner, M.,

and Wehner, V. (2009) Evidence for C−Cl/C−Br π-interactions as an important contribution to protein–ligand binding affinity. *Angewandte Chemie – International Edition in English*, **48**, 2911–2916.

49 Imai, Y.N., Inoue, Y., Nakanishi, I., and Kitaura, K. (2008) Cl–π interactions in protein–ligand complexes. *Protein Science: A Publication of the Protein Society*, **7**, 1129–1137.

50 Tucker, T.J., Brady, S.F., Lumma, W.C., Lewis, S.D., Gardell, S.J., Naylor-Olsen, A.M., Yan, Y., Sisko, J.T., Stauffer, K.J., Lucas, B.J., Lynch, J.J., Cook, J.J., Stranieri, M.T., Holahan, M.A., Lyle, E.A., Baskin, E.P., Chen, I.W., Dancheck, K.B., Krueger, J.A., Cooper, C.M., and Vacca, J.P. (1998) Design and synthesis of a series of potent and orally bioavailable noncovalent thrombin inhibitors that utilize nonbasic groups in the P1 position. *Journal of Medicinal Chemistry*, **41**, 3210–3219.

51 Adler, M., Kochanny, M.J., Ye, B., Rumnenik, G., Light, D.R., Biancalana, S., and Whitlow, M. (2002) Crystal structures of two potent nonamidine inhibitors bound to factor Xa. *Biochemistry*, **41**, 15514–15523.

52 Maignan, S., Guilloteau, J.-P., Choi-Sledeski, Y.M., Becker, M.R., Ewing, W.R., Pauls, H.W., Spada, A.P., and Mikol, V. (2003) Molecular structures of human factor Xa complexed with ketopiperazine inhibitors: preference for a neutral group in the S1 pocket. *Journal of Medicinal Chemistry*, **46**, 685–690.

53 Roehrig, S., Straub, A., Pohlmann, J., Lampe, T., Pernerstorfer, J., Schlemmer, K.-H., Reinemer, P., and Perzborn, E. (2005) Discovery of the novel antithrombotic agent 5-chloro-*N*-({(5S)-2-oxo-3-[4-(3-oxomorpholin-4-yl)phenyl]-1,3-oxazolidin-5-yl}methyl)thiophene-2-carboxamide (BAY 59–7939): an oral, direct factor Xa inhibitor. *Journal of Medicinal Chemistry*, **48**, 5900–5908.

54 Shi, Y., Sitkoff, D., Zhang, J., Klei, H.E., Kish, K., Liu, E.C.-K., Hartl, K.S., Seiler, S.M., Chang, M., Huang, C., Youssef, S., Steinbacher, T.E., Schumacher, W.A., Grazier, Y., Pudzianowski, A., Apedo, A., Doscenza, L., Yanchunas, J., Stein, P.D., and Atwal, K.S. (2008) Design, structure–activity relationships, X-ray crystal structure, and energetic contributions of a critical P1 pharmacophore:3-chloroindole-7-yl-based factor Xa inhibitors. *Journal of Medicinal Chemistry*, **51**, 7541–7551.

55 Matter, H., Will, D.W., Nazaré, M., Schreuder, H., Laux, V., and Wehner, V. (2005) Structural requirements for factor Xa inhibition by 3-oxybenzamides with neutral P1 substituents: combining X-ray crystallography, 3D-QSAR and tailored scoring functions. *Journal of Medicinal Chemistry*, **48**, 3290–3312.

56 Nazaré, M., Will, D.W., Matter, H., Schreuder, H., Ritter, K., Urmann, M., Essrich, M., Bauer, A., Wagner, M., Czech, J., Lorenz, M., Laux, V., and Wehner, V. (2005) Probing the subpockets of factor Xa reveals two binding modes for inhibitors based on a 2-carboxyindole scaffold: a study combining structure–activity relationship and X-ray crystallography. *Journal of Medicinal Chemistry*, **48**, 4511–4525.

57 Dill, K.A. (1997) Additivity principles in biochemistry. *The Journal of Biological Chemistry*, **272**, 701–704.

58 Weiner, S.J., Kollman, P.A., Nguyen, D.T., and Case, D.A. (1986) An all atom force field for simulations of proteins and nucleic acids. *Journal of Computational Chemistry*, **7**, 230–252.

59 Brooks, B.R., Bruccoleri, R.E., Olafson, B.D., Swaminathan, D.J.S.S., and Karplus, M. (1983) A program for energy minimization and dynamics calculations. *Journal of Computational Chemistry*, **4**, 187–217.

60 Kuntz, I.D., Blaney, J.M., Oatley, S.J., Langridge, R., and Ferrin, T.E. (1982) A geometric approach to macromolecule–ligand interactions. *Journal of Molecular Biology*, **161**, 269–288.

61 Jones, G., Willett, P., Glen, R.C., Leach, A.R., and Taylor, R. (1997) Development and validation of a genetic algorithm for flexible docking. *Journal of Molecular Biology*, **267**, 727–748.

62 Baker, N.A. (2005) Biomolecular applications of Poisson–Boltzmann methods, in *Reviews in Computational Chemistry*, vol. 21 (eds K.B. Lipkowitz, R. Larter, and T.R. Cundari), John Wiley & Sons Inc., pp. 349–379.

63 Ghosh, A., Rapp, C.S., and Friesner, R.A. (1998) Generalized Born model based on a surface integral formulation. *The Journal of Physical Chemistry. B*, **102**, 10983–10990.

64 Englebienne, P. and Moitessier, N. (2009) Docking ligands into flexible and solvated macromolecules. 5. Force-field-based prediction of binding affinities of ligands to proteins. *Journal of Chemical Information and Modeling*, **49**, 2564–2571.

65 Kollman, P.A., Massova, I., Reyes, C., Kuhn, B., Huo, S., Chong, L., Lee, M., Lee, T., Duan, Y., Wang, W., Donini, O., Cieplak, P., Srinivasan, J., Case, D.A., and Cheatham, T.E. (2000) Calculating structures and free energies of complex molecules: combining molecular mechanics and continuum models. *Accounts of Chemical Research*, **33**, 889–897.

66 Huang, N., Kalyanaraman, C., Irwin, J.J., and Jacobson, M.P. (2006) Physics-based scoring of protein–ligand complexes: enrichment of known inhibitors in large-scale virtual screening. *Journal of Chemical Information and Modeling*, **46**, 243–253.

67 Kuhn, B., Gerber, P., Schulz-Gasch, T., and Stahl, M. (2005) Validation and use of the MM–PBSA approach for drug discovery. *Journal of Medicinal Chemistry*, **48**, 4040–4048.

68 Weis, A., Katebzadeh, K., Soderhjelm, P., Nilsson, I., and Ryde, U. (2006) Ligand affinities predicted with the MM/PBSA method: dependence on the simulation method and the force field. *Journal of Medicinal Chemistry*, **49**, 6596–6606.

69 Kongsted, J. and Ryde, U. (2009) An improved method to predict the entropy term with the MM/PBSA approach. *Journal of Computer-Aided Molecular Design*, **23**, 63–71.

70 Brown, S.P. and Muchmore, S.W. (2007) Rapid estimation of relative protein–ligand binding affinities using a high-throughput version of MM–PBSA. *Journal of Chemical Information and Modeling*, **47**, 1493–1503.

71 Brown, S.P. and Muchmore, S.W. (2009) Large-scale application of high-throughput molecular mechanics with Poisson–Boltzmann surface area for routine physics-based scoring of protein–ligand complexes. *Journal of Medicinal Chemistry*, **52**, 3159–3165.

72 Thompson, D.C., Humblet, C., and Joseph-McCarthy, D. (2008) Investigation of MM–PBSA rescoring of docking poses. *Journal of Chemical Information and Modeling*, **48**, 1081–1091.

73 Kaminski, G.A., Friesner, R.A., Tirado-Rives, J., and Jorgensen, W.L. (2001) Evaluation and reparametrization of the OPLS-AA force field for proteins via comparison with accurate quantum chemical calculations on peptides. *The Journal of Physical Chemistry B*, **105**, 6474–6487.

74 Lyne, P.D., Lamb, M.L., and Saeh, J.C. (2006) Accurate prediction of the relative potencies of members of a series of kinase inhibitors using molecular docking and MM–GBSA scoring. *Journal of Medicinal Chemistry*, **49**, 4805–4808.

75 Cumming, J.G., McKenzie, C.L., Bowden, S.G., Campbell, D., Masters, D.J., Breed, J., and Jewsbury, P.J. (2004) Novel potent and selective anilinoquinazoline and anilinopyrimidine inhibitors of p38 MAP kinase. *Bioorganic & Medicinal Chemistry Letters*, **14**, 5389–5394.

76 Guimarães, C.R.W. and Cardozo, M. (2008) MM–GB/SA rescoring of docking poses in structure-based lead optimization. *Journal of Chemical Information and Modeling*, **48**, 958–970.

77 Zhang, X., Li, X., and Wang, R. (2009) Interpretation of the binding affinities of PTP1B inhibitors with the MM–GB/SA method and the X-score scoring function. *Journal of Chemical Information and Modeling*, **49**, 1033–1048.

78 Wang, R., Lai, L., and Wang, S. (2002) Further development and validation of empirical scoring functions for structure-based binding affinity prediction. *Journal of Computer-Aided Molecular Design*, **16**, 11–26.

79 Graves, A.P., Shivakumar, D.M., Boyce, S.E., Jacobson, M.P., Case, D.A., and Shoichet, B.K. (2008) Rescoring docking hit lists for model cavity sites: predictions and experimental testing. *Journal of Molecular Biology*, **377**, 914–934.

80 Pearlman, D.A. (2005) Evaluating the molecular mechanics Poisson–Boltzmann surface area free energy method using a congeneric series of ligands to p38 MAP kinase. *Journal of Medicinal Chemistry*, **48**, 7796–7807.

81 Åqvist, J., Medina, C., and Samuelsson, J.E. (1994) A new method for predicting binding affinity in computer-aided drug design. *Protein Engineering*, **7**, 385–391.

82 Stjernschantz, E., Marelius, J., Medina, C., Jacobsson, M., Vermeulen, N.P., and Oostenbrink, C. (2006) Are automated molecular dynamics simulations and binding free energy calculations realistic tools in lead optimization? An evaluation of the linear interaction energy (LIE) method. *Journal of Chemical Information and Modeling*, **46**, 1972–1983.

83 Bortolato, A. and Moro, S. (2007) In *silico* binding free energy predictability by using the linear interaction energy (LIE) method: bromobenzimidazole CK2 inhibitors as a case study. *Journal of Chemical Information and Modeling*, **47**, 572–582.

84 Rizzo, R.C., Tirado-Rives, J., and Jorgensen, W.L. (2001) Estimation of the binding affinities for HEPT and nevirapine analogues with HIV-1 reverse transcriptase via Monte Carlo simulations. *Journal of Medicinal Chemistry*, **44**, 145–154.

85 Tominaga, Y. and Jorgensen, W.L. (2004) General model for estimation of the inhibition of protein kinases using Monte Carlo simulations. *Journal of Medicinal Chemistry*, **47**, 2534–2549.

86 Huang, D. and Caflisch, A. (2004) Efficient evaluation of binding free energy using continuum electrostatics solvation. *Journal of Medicinal Chemistry*, **47**, 5791–5797.

87 Böhm, H.J. and Stahl, M. (1999) Rapid empirical scoring functions in virtual screening applications. *Medicinal Chemistry Research*, **9**, 445–462.

88 Tame, J.R.H. (1999) Scoring functions: a view from the bench. *Journal of Computer-Aided Molecular Design*, **13**, 99–108.

89 Oprea, T.I. and Marshall, G.R. (1998) Receptor-based prediction of binding affinities, in *3D-QSAR in Drug Design*, vol. **2** (eds H. Kubinyi, G. Folkers, and Y.C. Martin), Kluwer Academic Publishers, Dordrecht, NL, pp. 35–61.

90 Brooijmans, N. and Kuntz, I.D. (2003) Molecular recognition and docking algorithms. *Annual Review of Biophysics and Biomolecular Structure*, **32**, 335–373.

91 Stahl, M. (2000) Modifications of the scoring function in FlexX for virtual screening applications. *Perspectives in Drug Discovery and Design*, **20**, 83–98.

92 Raub, S., Steffen, A., Kämper, A., and Marian, C.M. (2008) AIScore: chemically diverse empirical scoring function employing chemical binding energies of hydrogen-bonded complexes. *Journal of Chemical Information and Modeling*, **48**, 1492–1510.

93 Zsoldos, Z., Szabo, I., Szabo, Z., and Johnson, A.P. (2003) Software tools for structure based rational drug design. *Journal of Molecular Structure (THEOCHEM)*, **666–667**, 659–665.

94 Schnecke, V. and Kuhn, L.A. (2000) Virtual screening with solvation and ligand-induced complementarity. *Perspectives in Drug Discovery and Design*, **20**, 171–190.

95 Friesner, R.A., Murphy, R.B., Repasky, M.P., Frye, L.L., Greenwood, J.R., Halgren, T.A., Sanschagrin, P.C., and Mainz, D.T. (2006) Extra precision glide: docking and scoring incorporating a model of hydrophobic enclosure for protein–ligand complexes. *Journal of Medicinal Chemistry*, **49**, 6177–6196.

96 Eldridge, M.D., Murray, C.W., Auton, T.R., Paolini, G.V., and Mee, R.P. (1997) Empirical scoring functions: I. The development of a fast empirical scoring function to estimate the binding affinity of ligands in receptor complexes. *Journal of Computer-Aided Molecular Design*, **11**, 425–445.

97 Gohlke, H. and Klebe, G. (2001) Statistical potentials and scoring

functions applied to protein–ligand binding. *Current Opinion in Structural Biology*, **11**, 231–235.

98 Verdonk, M.L. and Mooij, W.T.M. (2008) Knowledge-based methods in structure-based design, in *Computational and Structural Approaches to Drug Discovery, The RSC Biomolecular Sciences Series* (eds R.M. Stroud and J. Finer-Moore), RSC Publishing, pp. 111–126.

99 Velec, H.F.G., Gohlke, H., and Klebe, G. (2005) DrugScoreCSD-knowledge-based scoring function derived from small molecule crystal data with superior recognition rate of near-native ligand poses and better affinity prediction. *Journal of Medicinal Chemistry*, **48**, 6296–6303.

100 Ishchenko, A.V. and Shakhnovich, E.I. (2002) SMall Molecule Growth 2001 (SMoG2001): an improved knowledge-based scoring function for protein–ligand interactions. *Journal of Medicinal Chemistry*, **45**, 2770–2780.

101 Mitchell, J.B.O., Laskowski, R.A., Alex, A., and Thornton, J.M. (1999) BLEEP: a potential of mean force describing protein–ligand interactions: I. Generating the potential. *Journal of Computational Chemistry*, **20**, 1165–1177.

102 Muegge, I. and Martin, Y. (1999) A general and fast scoring function for protein–ligand interactions: a simplified potential approach. *Journal of Medicinal Chemistry*, **42**, 791–804.

103 Muegge, I. (2006) PMF scoring revisited. *Journal of Medicinal Chemistry*, **49**, 5895–5902.

104 Gohlke, H., Hendlich, M., and Klebe, G. (2000) Knowledge-based scoring function to predict protein–ligand interactions. *Journal of Molecular Biology*, **295**, 337–356.

105 Yang, C.-Y., Wang, R., and Wang, S. (2006) M-Score: a knowledge-based potential scoring function accounting for protein atom mobility. *Journal of Medicinal Chemistry*, **49**, 5903–5911.

106 Mooij, W.T.M. and Verdonk, M.L. (2005) General and targeted statistical potentials for protein–ligand interactions. *Proteins*, **61**, 272–287.

107 Reulecke, I., Lange, G., Albrecht, J., Klein, R., and Rarey, M. (2008) Towards an integrated description of hydrogen bonding and dehydration: decreasing false positives in virtual screening with the HYDE scoring function. *ChemMedChem*, **3**, 885–897.

108 Savage, H.J., Elliott, C.J., Freeman, C.M., and Finney, J.L. (1993) Lost hydrogen bonds and buried surface area: rationalizing stability in globular proteins. *Journal of the Chemical Society: Faraday Transactions*, **89**, 2609–2617.

109 Giordanetto, F., Cotesta, S., Catana, C., Trosset, J.-Y., Vulpetti, A., Stouten, P.F.W., and Kroemer, R.T. (2004) Novel scoring functions comprising QXP, SASA, and protein side-chain entropy terms. *Journal of Chemical Information and Computer Sciences*, **44**, 882–893.

110 Kellogg, G.E., Burnett, J.C., and Abraham, D.J. (2001) Very empirical treatment of solvation and entropy: a force field derived from log $P_{o/w}$. *Journal of Computer-Aided Molecular Design*, **15**, 381–393.

111 O'Boyle, N.M., Brewerton, S.C., and Taylor, R. (2008) Using buriedness to improve discrimination between actives and inactives in docking. *Journal of Chemical Information and Modeling*, **48**, 1269–1278.

112 McMartin, C. and Bohacek, R.S. (1997) QXP: powerful, rapid computer algorithms for structure-based drug design. *Journal of Computer-Aided Molecular Design*, **11**, 333–344.

113 Murphy, K.P. and Freire, E. (1992) Thermodynamics of structural stability and cooperative folding behavior in proteins. *Advances in Protein Chemistry*, **43**, 313–361.

114 Doweyko, A.M. and Johnson, S.R. (2006) A novel method to simulate the hydrophobic effect and its application to the ranking of host/guest complexes. *Journal of Chemical Information and Modeling*, **46**, 2563–2573.

115 Abel, R., Young, T., Farid, R., Berne, B.J., and Friesner, R.A. (2008) Role of the active-site solvent in the thermodynamics of factor Xa ligand binding. *Journal of the American Chemical Society*, **130**, 2817–2831.

116 Sotriffer, C.A., Sanschagrin, P., Matter, H., and Klebe, G. (2008) SFCscore: scoring functions for affinity prediction of protein–ligand complexes. *Proteins*, **73**, 395–419.

117 Wang, R., Fang, X., Lu, Y., and Wang, S. (2004) The PDBbind database: collection of binding affinities for protein–ligand complexes with known three-dimensional structures. *Journal of Medicinal Chemistry*, **47**, 2977–2980.

118 Wang, R., Fang, X., Lu, Y., Yang, C.Y., and Wang, S. (2005) The PDBbind database: methodologies and updates. *Journal of Medicinal Chemistry*, **48**, 4111–4119.

119 Charifson, P.S., Corkery, J.J., Murcko, M.A., and Walters, W.P. (1999) Consensus scoring: a method for obtaining improved hit rates from docking databases of three-dimensional structures into proteins. *Journal of Medicinal Chemistry*, **42**, 5100–5109.

120 Clark, R.D., Strizhev, A., Leonard, J.M., Blake, J.F., and Matthew, J.B. (2002) Consensus scoring for ligand/protein interactions. *Journal of Molecular Graphics & Modelling*, **20**, 281–295.

121 Oda, A., Tsuchida, K., Takakura, T., Yamaotsu, N., and Hirono, S. (2006) Comparison of consensus scoring strategies for evaluating computational models of protein–ligand complexes. *Journal of Chemical Information and Modeling*, **46**, 380–391.

122 Yang, J.M., Chen, Y.F., Shen, T.W., Kristal, B.S., and Hsu, D.F. (2005) Consensus scoring criteria for improving enrichment in virtual screening. *Journal of Chemical Information and Modeling*, **45**, 1134–1146.

123 Baber, J.C., Shirley, W.A., Gao, Y., and Feher, M. (2006) The use of consensus scoring in ligand-based virtual screening. *Journal of Chemical Information and Modeling*, **46**, 277–288.

124 Yang, J.-M., Chen, Y.-F., Shen, T.-W., Kristal, B.S., and Hsu, D.F. (2005) Consensus scoring criteria for improving enrichment in virtual screening. *Journal of Chemical Information and Modeling*, **45**, 1134–1146.

125 Betzi, S., Suhre, K., Chetrit, B., Guerlesquin, F., and Morelli, X. (2006) GFscore: a general nonlinear consensus scoring function for high throughput docking. *Journal of Chemical Information and Modeling*, **46**, 1704–1712.

126 Fukunishi, H., Teramoto, R., Takada, T., and Shimada, J. (2008) Bootstrap-based consensus scoring method for protein–ligand docking. *Journal of Chemical Information and Modeling*, **48**, 988–996.

127 Bar-Haim., S., Aharon, A., Ben-Moshe, T., Marantz, Y., and Senderowitz, H. (2009) SeleX-CS: a new consensus scoring algorithm for hit discovery and lead optimization. *Journal of Chemical Information and Modeling*, **49**, 623–633.

128 Smith, R., Hubbard, R.E., Gschwend, D.A., Leach, A.R., and Good, A.C. (2003) Analysis and optimization of structure-based virtual screening protocols (3). New methods and old problems in scoring function design. *Journal of Molecular Graphics & Modelling*, **22**, 41–53.

129 Vigers, G.P.A. and Rizzi, J.P. (2004) Multiple active site corrections for docking and virtual screening. *Journal of Medicinal Chemistry*, **47**, 80–89.

130 Cummings, M.D., DesJarlais, R.L., Gibbs, A.C., Mohan, V., and Jaeger, E.P. (2005) Comparison of automated docking programs as virtual screening tools. *Journal of Medicinal Chemistry*, **48**, 962–976.

131 Seifert, M.H.J. (2009) Targeted scoring functions for virtual screening. *Drug Discovery Today*, **14**, 562–569.

132 Gohlke, H. and Klebe, G. (2002) DrugScore meets CoMFA: adaptation of fields for molecular comparison (AFMoC) or how to tailor knowledge-based pair-potentials to a particular protein. *Journal of Medicinal Chemistry*, **45**, 4153–4170.

133 Cramer, R.D., Patterson, D.E., and Bunce, J.E. (1988) Comparative molecular field analysis (CoMFA). 1. Effect of shape on binding of steroids to carrier proteins. *Journal of the American Chemical Society*, **110**, 5959–5967.

134 Ortiz, A.R., Pisabarro, M.T., Gago, F., and Wade, R.C. (1995) Prediction of drug binding affinities by comparative binding

energy analysis. *Journal of Medicinal Chemistry*, **38**, 2681–2691.

135 Ortiz, A.R., Pastor, M., Palomer, A., Cruciani, G., Gago, F., and Wade, R.C. (1997) Reliability of comparative molecular field analysis models: effects of data scaling and variable selection using a set of human synovial fluid phospholipase A2 inhibitors. *Journal of Medicinal Chemistry*, **40**, 1136–1148.

136 Perez, C., Pastor, M., Ortiz, A.R., and Gago, F. (1998) Comparative binding energy analysis of HIV-1 protease inhibitors: incorporation of solvent effects and validation as a powerful tool in receptor-based drug design. *Journal of Medicinal Chemistry*, **41**, 836–852.

137 Wang, T. and Wade, R.C. (2001) Comparative binding energy (COMBINE) analysis of influenza neuraminidase–inhibitor complexes. *Journal of Medicinal Chemistry*, **44**, 961–971.

138 Matter, H., Will, D.W., Nazaré, M., Schreuder, H., Laux, V., and Wehner, V. (2005) Structural requirements for factor Xa inhibition by 3-oxybenzamides with neutral P1 substituents: combining X-ray crystallography, 3D-QSAR, and tailored scoring functions. *Journal of Medicinal Chemistry*, **48**, 3290–3312.

139 Gehlhaar, D.K., Verkhivker, G.M., Rejto, P.A., Sherman, C.J., Fogel, D.B., Fogel, L.J., and Freer, S.T. (1995) Molecular recognition of the inhibitor AG-1343 by HIV-1 protease: conformationally flexible docking by evolutionary programming. *Chemistry & Biology*, **2**, 317–324.

140 Martin, E.J. and Sullivan, D.C. (2008) AutoShim: empirically corrected scoring functions for quantitative docking with a crystal structure and IC_{50} training data. *Journal of Chemical Information and Modeling*, **48**, 861–872.

141 Rognan, D., Lauemoller, S.L., Holm, A., Buus, S., and Tschinke, V. (1999) Predicting binding affinities of protein ligands from three-dimensional models: application to peptide binding to class I major histocompatibility proteins. *Journal of Medicinal Chemistry*, **42**, 4650–4658.

142 Murray, C.W., Auton, T.R., and Eldridge, M.D. (1998) Empirical scoring functions. II. The testing of an empirical scoring function for the prediction of ligand–receptor affinities and the use of Bayesian regression to improve the quality of the model. *Journal of Computer-Aided Molecular Design*, **12**, 503–519.

143 Catana, C. and Stouten, P.F.W. (2007) Novel, customizable scoring functions, parameterized using N-PLS, for structure-based drug discovery. *Journal of Chemical Information and Modeling*, **47**, 85–91.

144 Ferrara, P., Curioni, A., Vangrevelinghe, E., Meyer, T., Mordasini, T., Andreoni, W., Acklin, P., and Jacoby, E. (2006) New scoring functions for virtual screening from moleculat dynamics simulations with a Quantum-Refined Force-Field (QRFF-MD). Application to cyclin-dependent kinase 2. *Journal of Chemical Information and Modeling*, **46**, 254–263.

145 Teramoto, R. and Fukunishi, H. (2007) Supervised scoring models with docked ligand conformations for structure-based virtual screening. *Journal of Chemical Information and Modeling*, **47**, 1858–1867.

146 Pham, T.A. and Jain, A.N. (2006) Parameter estimation for scoring protein–ligand interactions using negative training data. *Journal of Medicinal Chemistry*, **49**, 5856–5868.

147 Pham, T.A. and Jain, A.N. (2008) Customizing scoring functions for docking. *Journal of Computer-Aided Molecular Design*, **22**, 269–286.

148 Seifert, M.H.J. (2009) Robust optimization of scoring functions for a target class. *Journal of Computer-Aided Molecular Design*, **23**, 633–644.

149 Seifert, M.H. (2006) Assessing the discriminatory power of scoring functions for virtual screening. *Journal of Chemical Information and Modeling*, **46**, 1456–1465.

150 Deng, Z., Chuaqui, C., and Singh, J. (2004) Structural Interaction Fingerprint (SIFt): a novel method for analyzing three-dimensional protein–ligand binding interactions. *Journal of Medicinal Chemistry*, **47**, 337–344.

151 Brewerton, S.W. (2008) The use of protein–ligand interaction fingerprints in docking. *Current Opinion in Drug Discovery & Development*, **11**, 356–364.

152 Chuaqui, C., Deng, Z., and Singh, J. (2005) Interaction profiles of protein kinase–inhibitor complexes and their application to virtual screening. *Journal of Medicinal Chemistry*, **48**, 121–133.

153 Marcou, G. and Rognan, D. (2007) Optimizing fragment and scaffold docking by use of molecular interaction fingerprints. *Journal of Chemical Information and Modeling*, **47**, 195–207.

154 Kelly, M.D. and Mancera, R.L. (2004) Expanded interaction fingerprint method for analyzing ligand binding modes in docking and structure-based design. *Journal of Chemical Information and Computer Sciences*, **44**, 1942–1951.

155 Nandigam, R.K., Kim, S., Singh, J., and Chuaqui, C. (2009) Position specific interaction dependent scoring technique for virtual screening based on weighted protein–ligand interaction fingerprint profiles. *Journal of Chemical Information and Modeling*, **49**, 1185–1192.

156 Jain, A.N. and Nicholls, A. (2008) Recommendations for evaluation of computational methods. *Journal of Computer-Aided Molecular Design*, **22**, 133–139.

157 Warren, G.L., Andrews, C.W., Capelli, A.M., Clarke, B., LaLonde, J., Lambert, M.H., Lindvall, M., Nevins, N., Semus, S.F., Senger, S., Tedesco, G., Wall, I.D., Woolven, J.M., Peishoff, C.E., and Head, M.S. (2006) A critical assessment of docking programs and scoring functions. *Journal of Medicinal Chemistry*, **49**, 5912–5931.

158 Huang, N., Shoichet, B.K., and Irwin, J.J. (2006) Benchmarking sets for molecular docking. *Journal of Medicinal Chemistry*, **49**, 6789–6801.

159 Hawkins, P.C.D., Warren, G.L., Skillman and, A.G., and Nicholls, A. (2008) How to do an evaluation: pitfalls and traps. *Journal of Computer-Aided Molecular Design*, **22**, 179–190.

160 Irwin, J.J. (2008) Community benchmarks for virtual screening. *Journal of Computer-Aided Molecular Design*, **22**, 193–199.

161 Cole, J.C., Murray, C.W., Nissink, J.W.M., Taylor, R.D., and Taylor, R. (2005) Comparing protein–ligand docking programs is difficult. *Proteins*, **60**, 325–332.

162 Jain, A.N. (2008) Bias, reporting, and sharing: computational evaluations of docking methods. *Journal of Computer-Aided Molecular Design*, **22**, 201–212.

163 Kirchmair, J., Markt, P., Distinto, S., Wolber, G., and Langer, T. (2008) Evaluation of the performance of 3D virtual screening protocols: RMSD comparisons, enrichment assessments, and decoy selection: what can we learn from earlier mistakes? *Journal of Computer-Aided Molecular Design*, **22**, 213–228.

164 Nicholls, A. (2008) What do we know and when do we know it? *Journal of Computer-Aided Molecular Design*, **22**, 239–255.

165 Zhao, W., Hevener, K.E., White, S.W., Lee, R.E., and Boyett, J.M. (2009) A statistical framework to evaluate virtual screening. *BMC Bioinformatics*, **10**, 225

166 Leach, A.R., Shoichet, B.K., and Peishoff, C.E. (2006) Prediction of protein–ligand interactions. Docking and scoring: Successes and gaps. *Journal of Medicinal Chemistry*, **49**, 5851–5855.

167 Moitessier, N., Englebienne, P., Lee, D., Lawandi, J., and Corbeil, C.R. (2008) Towards the development of universal, fast and highly accurate docking/scoring methods: a long way to go. *British Journal of Pharmacology*, **153**, S7–S26.

168 Kim, R. and Skolnick, J. (2008) Assessment of programs for ligand binding affinity prediction. *Journal of Computational Chemistry*, **29**, 1316–1331.

169 Enyedy, I.J. and Egan, W.J. (2008) Can we use docking and scoring for hit-to-lead optimization? *Journal of Computer-Aided Molecular Design*, **22**, 161–168.

170 Englebienne, P. and Moitessier, N. (2009) Docking ligands into flexible and solvated macromolecules. 4. Are popular scoring functions accurate for this class of proteins? *Journal of Chemical Information and Modeling*, **49**, 1568–1580.

171 Wang, R., Lu, Y., and Wang, S. (2003) Comparative evaluation of 11 scoring

functions for molecular docking. *Journal of Medicinal Chemistry*, **46**, 2287–2303.

172 Oprea, T.I. and Matter, H. (2004) Integrating virtual screening in lead discovery. *Current Opinion in Chemical Biology*, **8**, 349–358.

173 Vidal, D., Thormann, M., and Pons, M. (2006) A novel search engine for virtual screening of very large databases. *Journal of Chemical Information and Modeling*, **46**, 836–843.

174 Zavodszky, M.I., Rohatgi, A., Van Voorst, J.R., Yan, H., and Kuhn, L.A. (2009) Scoring ligand similarity in structure-based virtual screening. *Journal of Molecular Recognition*, **22**, 280–292.

175 Hann, M.M. and Oprea, T.I. (2004) Pursuing the leadlikeness concept in pharmaceutical research. *Current Opinion in Chemical Biology*, **8**, 255–263.

176 Jansen, J.M. and Martin, E.J. (2004) Target-biased scoring approaches and expert systems in structure-based virtual screening. *Current Opinion in Chemical Biology*, **8**, 359–364.

177 Matter, H. and Schudok, M. (2004) Recent advances in the design of matrix metalloprotease inhibitors. *Current Opinion in Drug Discovery & Development*, **7**, 513–535.

178 Klon, A.E., Glick, M., Thoma, M., Acklin, P., and Davies, J.W. (2004) Finding more needles in the haystack: a simple and efficient method for improving high-throughput docking results. *Journal of Medicinal Chemistry*, **47**, 2743–2749.

179 Krumrine, J.R., Maynard, A.T., and Lerman, C.L. (2005) Statistical tools for virtual screening. *Journal of Medicinal Chemistry*, **48**, 7477–7481.

180 Sullivan, D.C. and Martin, E.J. (2008) Exploiting structure–activity relationships in docking. *Journal of Chemical Information and Modeling*, **48**, 817–830.

181 Tirado-Rives, J. and Jorgensen, W.L. (2006) Contribution of conformer focusing to the uncertainty in predicting free energies for protein–ligand binding. *Journal of Medicinal Chemistry*, **49**, 5880–5884.

182 Cheng, Y.-C. and Prusoff, W.H. (1973) Relationship between the inhibition constant (K_i) and the concentration of inhibitor which causes 50 per cent inhibition (I_{50}) of an enzymatic reaction. *Biochemical Pharmacology*, **22**, 3099–3108.

183 Shoichet, B.K. (2006) Interpreting steep dose–response curves in early inhibitor discovery. *Journal of Medicinal Chemistry*, **49**, 7274–7277.

184 Ferreira, R.S., Bryant, C., Ang, K.K.H., McKerrow, J.H., Shoichet, B.K., and Renslo, A.R. (2009) Divergent modes of enzyme inhibition in a homologous structure–activity series. *Journal of Medicinal Chemistry*, **52**, 5005–5008.

185 Davis, A.M., Teague, S.J., and Kleywegt, G.J. (2003) Application and limitations of X-ray crystallographic data in structure-based ligand and drug design. *Angewandte Chemie – International Edition in English*, **42**, 2718–2736.

186 Hooft, R.W.W., Vriend, G., Sander, C., and Abola, E.E. (1996) Errors in protein structures. *Nature*, **381**, 272

187 Nissink, J.W.M., Murray, C., Hartshorn, M., Verdonk, M.L., Cole, J.C., and Taylor, R. (2002) A new test set for validating predictions of protein–ligand interaction. *Proteins*, **49**, 457–471.

188 Cozzini, P., Kellogg, G.E., Spyrakis, F., Abraham, D.J., Costantino, G., Emerson, A., Fanelli, F., Gohlke, H., Kuhn, L.A., Morris, G.M., Orozco, M., Pertinhez, T.A., Rizzi, M., and Sotriffer, C.A. (2008) Target flexibility: an emerging consideration in drug discovery and design. *Journal of Medicinal Chemistry*, **51**, 6237–6255.

189 Mattos, C. and Ringe, D. (1993) Multiple binding modes, in *3D QSAR in Drug Design. Theory, Methods and Applications* (ed. H. Kubinyi), Springer, pp. 226–254.

190 Maignan, S., Guilloteau, J.-P., Choi-Sledeski, Y.M., Becker, M.R., Ewing, W.R., Pauls, H.W., Spada, A.P., and Mikol, V. (2003) Molecular structures of human factor Xa complexed with ketopiperazine inhibitors: preference for a neutral group in the S1 pocket. *Journal of Medicinal Chemistry*, **46**, 685–690.

191 Steuber, H., Czodrowski, P., Sotriffer, C.A., and Klebe, G. (2007) Tracing changes in protonation: a prerequisite to factorize thermodynamic data of inhibitor binding to aldose reductase. *Journal of Molecular Biology*, **373**, 1305–1320.

192 Milletti, F., Storchi, L., and Cruciani, G. (2009) Predicting protein pK_a by environment similarity. *Proteins*, **76**, 484–495.

193 Ten Brink, T. and Exner, T.E. (2009) Influence of protonation, tautomeric, and stereoisomeric states on protein–ligand docking results. *Journal of Chemical Information and Modeling*, **49**, 1535–1546.

194 Stubbs, M.T., Reyda, S., Dullweber, F., Moller, M., Klebe, G., Dorsch, D., Mederski, W.W.K.R., and Wurziger, H. (2002) pH-Dependent binding modes observed in trypsin crystals: lessons for structure-based drug design. *ChemBioChem*, **46**, 685–690.

195 Milletti, F., Storchi, L., Sforna, G., Cross, S., and Cruciani, G. (2009) Tautomer enumeration and stability prediction for virtual screening on large chemical databases. *Journal of Chemical Information and Modeling*, **49**, 68–75.

196 Hendlich, M., Bergner, A., Günther, J., and Klebe, G. (2003) Relibase: design and development of a database for comprehensive analysis of protein–ligand interactions. *Journal of Molecular Biology*, **326**, 607–620.

197 Søndergaard, C.R., Garrett, A.E., Carstensen, T., Pollastri, G., and Nielsen, J.E. (2009) Structural artifacts in protein–ligand X-ray structures: implications for the development of docking scoring functions. *Journal of Medicinal Chemistry*, **52**, 5673–5684.

198 Jacobsson, M. and Karlen, A. (2006) Ligand bias of scoring functions in structure-based virtual screening. *Journal of Chemical Information and Modeling*, **46**, 1334–1343.

199 Carta, G., Knox, A.J.S., and Lloyd, D.G. (2007) Unbiasing scoring functions: a new normalization and rescoring strategy. *Journal of Chemical Information and Modeling*, **47**, 1564–1571.

200 Williams, D.H., Stephens, E., O'Brien, D.P., and Zhou, M. (2004) Understanding noncovalent interactions: ligand binding energy and catalytic efficiency from ligand-induced reductions in motion within receptors and enzymes. *Angewandte Chemie – International Edition in English*, **43**, 6596–6616.

201 Patel, Y., Gillet, V.J., Howe, T., Pastor, J., Oyarzabal, J., and Willett, P. (2008) Assessment of additive/nonadditive effects in structure–activity relationships: implications for iterative drug design. *Journal of Medicinal Chemistry*, **51**, 7552–7562.

202 Stockmann, H., Bronowska, A., Syme, N.R., Thompson, G.S., Kalverda, A.P., Warriner, S.L., and Homans, S.W. (2008) Residual ligand entropy in the binding of p-substituted benzenesulfonamide ligands to bovine carbonic anhydrase II. *Journal of the American Chemical Society*, **130**, 12420–12426.

203 Honndorf, V.S., Coudevylle, N., Laufer, S., Becker, S., and Griesinger, C. (2008) Dynamics in the p38α MAP kinase-SB203580 complex observed by liquid-state NMR spectroscopy. *Angewandte Chemie – International Edition in English*, **47**, 3548–3551.

204 Tong, Y., Chang, G., Mei, Y., and Zhang, J.Z.H. (2009) Simulation of NMR data reveals that proteins' local structures are stabilized by electronic polarization. *Journal of the American Chemical Society*, **131**, 8636–8641.

205 Homans, S.W. (2007) Water, water everywhere – except where it matters? *Drug Discovery Today*, **12**, 534–539.

206 Naumann, T. and Matter, H. (2002) Structural classification of protein kinases using 3D molecular interaction field analysis of their ligand binding sites: target family landscapes. *Journal of Medicinal Chemistry*, **45**, 2366–2378.

8
Protein Flexibility in Structure-Based Virtual Screening: From Models to Algorithms

Angela M. Henzler and Matthias Rarey

8.1
How Flexible Are Proteins? – A Historical Perspective

Researchers' view of binding a ligand to a receptor has changed fundamentally over the last century – mainly from Fischer's lock and key principle in 1894 where the protein is considered as rigid scaffold [1] to the *induced fit effect* in 1958 that regards the protein to be a flexible object [2]. Since then, the idea of proteins' dynamic behavior upon ligand binding has gained acceptance. However, the detailed mechanisms behind the events themselves remain unresolved. Over the last decade, the kind of protein flexibility upon binding had been under discussion, and today, the debate is still going on [3–8]. As a result, some models have been hypothesized able to describe mechanisms and types of moves that proteins have to undergo. The discussion motivates flexibility models of structure-based drug design. They depict the basis of protein–ligand docking techniques treating both molecules flexibly and thus affect structure-based virtual screening (VS) as well.

8.1.1
Ligand Binding Is Coupled with Protein Conformational Change

Koshland's concept of the *induced fit* was able to overcome limitations of the former rigid and shape-based theory. Even if there is no shape complementarity, why shouldn't a ligand with good interactions fit into a pocket offering enough space? Koshland argued that substrates bind prior to subsequent side chain reorientations. Thus, the protein gains its precise fit and improves protein–ligand interactions. He emphasized that protein–ligand fitting mostly occurs as a result of structural changes induced by the ligand. The aspect explains why molecules revealing no shape complementarity to the apoprotein structure can nevertheless interact [2]. Although the induced fit theory is frequently used to explain protein's dynamic behavior, the concept lacks to describe each aspect of the binding event. Do only ligands offering enough binding strength to form an initially stable complex induce a protein adaptation? The limitations motivated researchers to doubt the long-established theory of induced protein–ligand fitting in turn [9].

Virtual Screening. Edited by C. Sotriffer

ISBN: 978-3-527-32636-5

An alternative view of protein dynamics upon binding suggests the mechanism of *conformational selection* [10]. Essentially, it assumes the conformational change to occur before ligand binding. The ligand selectively binds to one out of a population of preexisting conformations. Therefore, ligands not able to form strong interactions may also find an adequately shape-matching counterpart. That proteins do not exist in a single, unique conformation was supposed by Frauenfelder among others [11]. After extensive studies of heme proteins, he yielded valuable insights into protein dynamics. All possible conformations of a protein can be represented via points in a $3N$-dimensional space (where N is the number of atoms). A hypersurface in this space assigns each structure a specific energy value – the energy landscape of protein conformations. Valleys therein represent favorable low-energy conformations, while hills are associated with protein's reluctantly adopted conformations. As the energy landscape is complex and rugged, with many hills and valleys of varying height and gradients, Frauenfelder had the notion that a biomolecule can assume multiple of nearly isoenergetic conformations. These conformations significantly differ from each other, but all are close to a common average structure. A conformational change depicts a protein motion from one to another energetic favorable state that corresponds to a jump from one valley to the other. This energy landscape perspective of protein motion was soon transferred to explain protein folding [12] and the process of ligand binding as well [13–15]. The concept of an energy landscape laid the foundation to describe flexible proteins as ensembles of different conformational states. The model is consistent with different kinds of considered structural variations, irrespectively. Together with the mechanism of conformational selection, it explains phenomena such as broad-range ligand binding or binding various ligand orientations [16].

Even if conformational selection is more appropriate to explain special binding events, the well-established induced fit concept is not outdated and keeps its legitimation. Each of both pathways may be pursued: in case of conformational selection, the ligand binds selectively to one of the macromolecule's low populated conformations; while in case of an induced fit, the ligand binds to the predominating conformation of the macromolecule. Which path is chosen mainly depends on ligand and protein concentration [17].

8.1.2
Types of Flexibility

Besides investigating the basic binding mechanisms, the first key step toward modeling protein flexibility in structure-based design applications is to elucidate the various types of flexibility in proteins and their individual importance for ligand binding.

Many protein binding sites seem to have a dual character. Luque and Freire recognized regions in binding sites of enzymes with higher and lower structural stability. The latter mainly occur in loops [3]. The border region seems to be more flexible than the binding site core, caused by more flexible solvent-accessible residues. However, the border may stabilize upon ligand binding and enclose parts of the ligand [4]. Catalytic residues mostly appear in regions with high structural stability and their reorientation can result in an improved contribution to binding affinity. Gutteridge and Thornton recognized that catalytic residues of enzymes perform slight side chain motions, while the protein backbone shows only marginal adaptation. Major side chain moves mainly occur on protein surface [5]. Najmanovich *et al.* also considered the side chain flexibility of binding sites. They detected only three or less flexible side chains in 85% of considered proteins. Large and polar amino acid residues were more flexible than others and a correlation of backbone and side chain reorientation could not be observed [6]. These observations suggest that only a restricted number of side chains are significantly affected by conformational changes upon ligand binding.

Comparisons of flexible and rigid proteins helped Gunasekaran and Nussinov to discover that rigid proteins have highly polar sites opposed to binding sites with large backbone moves that show rather hydrophobic residue pair interactions [7]. Brylinski and Skolnick considered the question what kind of conformational changes are triggered by ligand binding in general, for which they compared apo- and holoproteins extracted from the Protein Data Bank (PDB) [18]. Even if they recognized flexibility of domains, backbone, loops, as well as that of side chains, they mainly concentrate on the analysis of global structural changes. These preferably occur in multidomain proteins by large-scale hinge-bending movements. Backbone variations of globular structures can be nearly neglected [8]. The question for which degree of flexibility one should account for is complicated by the proclamation that the PDB is biased toward rigid proteins. Experimental structure determination preferably captures conformations shifted toward environmental conditioned low-energy states [19]. Therefore, existing flexibility analysis and pose prediction methods that are often validated by PDB structures should be considered carefully.

It still remains unclear which type of motions, in general, have to be considered to model ligand binding. All in all, the discussion about the observations of flexible proteins suggests the existence of three types of proteins – nearly rigid proteins that show slight side chain motions upon ligand binding, while other structural components are rather rigid; flexible proteins that reveal side chain as well as relatively large loop, backbone, and domain rearrangements; and finally, intrinsically unstable proteins that conclude folding only in presence of their ligand [20].

8.2 Flexible Protein Handling in Protein–Ligand Docking

For consideration of protein flexibility in structure-based VS, one has to intrude into underlying docking engines of the process. Here, we want to provide the readership with an overview of the state-of-the-art flexible–protein–flexible–ligand docking that we term as *fully flexible docking*. Several authors have already reviewed and discussed the procedures [21–23]. In literature, algorithmic details and the type of flexibility are often criteria for classification of docking methods; however, they have not been focused here to a great extent. It can be observed that the mentioned mechanistic flexibility models have major impact on the development of docking algorithms. Docking techniques that either follow the conformational selection or that perform induced fit have emerged.

Fully flexible docking is rather a workflow of several separated processes than it is an all-in-one process: docking techniques following the conformational selection theory mainly introduce protein flexibility in a preprocessing step via ensemble generation. It often goes hand in hand with analysis of protein flexibility. Ensemble-based docking engines perform a proper protein conformer selection and ligand placement granting optimal complementary fit. Alternatively, the docking stage follows an induced fit concept that is mainly driven by strong electrostatic interactions. In this case, the engine roughly fits the ligand into a single site. Deviations from optimal geometry and steric overlap are accepted, but induced fit docking demands a refinement stage that forces the protein to rearrange for ligand accommodation.

For clarity, we follow the depicted scheme in Figure 8.1 to describe essential flexible protein handling techniques of docking applications. The computational approaches are characterized according to the stage when they account for protein conformational change. The section thus starts with methods that perform conformational selection and introduces approaches for protein flexibility analysis and ensemble generation. Ensemble-based docking methodologies are examined further. The section continues with consideration of docking methods that do not expect ensembles and solely rely on input of a single protein structure. Some of these induced fit docking techniques need approaches for pose refinement that are also summarized. At the end of this chapter, we will conclude to briefly consider these techniques for their application in structure-based VS in retrospect.

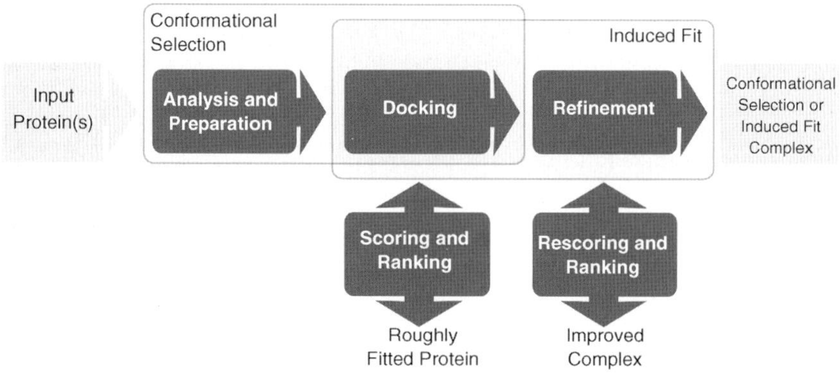

Figure 8.1 Protein flexibility can be incorporated in several docking stages: before, while, or after ligand placement. Preliminary to docking, flexibility analysis identifies flexible parts. The information obtained is used for adequate receptor conformational sampling. The docking stage explores the conformational space of the ligand and/or the protein. A scoring function guides the docking to a roughly fitted ligand that may clash with the protein. Complex refinement takes place posterior to docking.

8.2.1
Docking Following Conformational Selection

Some docking approaches conform to the paradigm to describe the protein as an ensemble of differently populated conformational states in equilibrium. Such ensemble-based docking techniques represent the targeted protein via multiple input structures, each of them showing another conformational state. The ensemble should adequately reflect the target's spectrum of flexibility. Protein flexibility analysis can help to identify rigid and variable protein parts and to decide which of them should be directed to 3D structural sampling (Figure 8.2). Ensemble generation methods sample the conformational space and extract the most relevant representatives to participate in the ensemble description before ensemble-based docking methodologies select the state most complementary to the ligand.

8.2.1.1 **Protein Flexibility Analysis and Protein Ensemble Generation**

Ensembles may originate from different sources. Experimental structure determination via NMR or X-ray crystallography [24] provides various conformations ready to serve as input for ensemble-based docking techniques [48]. Not always these sources offer structures of the target of interest due to the involved high effort or experimental obstacles. A practical alternative is to build up an ensemble from snapshots of molecular dynamics (MD) simulations. Certainly, in this case some questions arise – most importantly, how to adjust the simulation parameters and how to extract representative snapshots from the trajectory? Answers cannot be given in general as researchers tune the parameters following their own philosophy. Furthermore, it is almost not possible to compare different settings as only the docking result can serve as a measure of quality. The docking success, in turn, is greatly influenced by the performance of many components like the docking engine and the scoring function. MD simulations are frequently used to prepare ensembles and the snapshots may also serve to generate receptor-based pharmacophore models [26, 27]. *Relaxed complex schemes* are docking protocols that employ MD simulations to extract snapshots as an initial preparation step [28, 29]. Modeling extended motions via MD simulation, for example, global backbone rearrangements of apoproteins, is usually impracticable as it requires intensive simulations to gather the snapshots. Nevertheless, it is possible to circumvent this hurdle by accelerated simulations. A recently introduced method, for example, places resins into the site to enforce pocket stretching during the simulation [30].

Besides the MD-based approaches, Monte Carlo (MC)-based conformational sampling can be employed to establish an ensemble describing protein's equilibrium state. Generally, detailed simulations in which the structure is embedded in discrete water molecules are impracticable. Implicit solvent simulations are used to approximate protein dynamics in aqueous solution. Reduced coarse-grained multistep simulation may accelerate the simulation but quickly reach limits with respect to simulation time reduction and accuracy [31, 32]. Spatial coarse-graining techniques may gain further runtime improvement, as the target has not necessarily to be treated in high atomic resolution to model its dynamics. Particularly, if larger molecules and extended motions are considered, the resolution of the calculation can be reduced. Under the assumption that strong electrostatic interactions almost hinder intradomain motions, it is possible to consider only rigid domains and their rearrangements [33]. Techniques that identify rigid and flexible parts in proteins and detect molecular hinges are thus useful tools to constrain the protein to relevant conformational sampling [34–36]. In contrast, if the target is supposed to be rather rigid and the dynamics is restricted to only a few binding site residues, a selection of a minimal amount of side chains and sampling rotamers may be better suited to focus on detailed motions in ligand binding [37–40].

Minimized structures gained from MD simulations are also often basis of *normal mode analysis* (NMA) [41–43]. NMA assumes that all atoms harmonically oscillate around their equilibrium points. The oscillations defined by frequency and amplitude (normal mode) are extracted and reflect directions of internal protein motions. Given all its normal modes, the entire protein motion can be expressed as a superposition of modes. The modes with lowest frequency correspond to rather delocalized motions in proteins in which a large number of atoms oscillate in coordinated motion with considerable amplitude. Modes with higher frequency represent more localized motions. Linear combinations of the most relevant normal modes can be employed to depict essential protein motions. Stepwise displacement of atoms of the original structure along the modes can be applied to build up an ensemble of relevant protein conformations [44, 45].

Another approach generates ensembles with prior knowledge of already known binders. Under the assumption that a target binds ligands, showing similar shape complementarity, even the docking technique itself can be used to gain different protein conformations. Placing the given ligands into the site, ignoring some steric hindrance and optimizing the protein structure afterward, facilitates the search of novel ligands that are similar to the already known ones. A small-scale VS can also help to identify relevant receptor conformations with good enrichment that finally may participate in an ensemble-based large-scale VS experiment [46, 47]. If a set of protein structures originated from experimental or computational methods is already given, a geometrical point of view may also help to reduce the set and to select the most relevant conformations. In this situation, only those structures should contribute to the ensemble that share a similar core region [25].

8.2.1.2 **Ensemble-Based Docking Techniques**

Ensemble-based docking techniques consider a broad spectrum of flexibility. Multiple structures with different side chain conformers, loops, or backbone arrangements may contribute to the ensemble. The docking procedure selects the appropriate counterpart and fits the given ligand. In principle, it is possible to perform sequential docking against each protein representative serving as a separate target for which an appropriate ligand pose has to be identified. The final result may then be either the highest ranked pose or the results of all docking runs that are merged to create an averaged complex structure. Sequential docking is common practice even if it is a quite inefficient way to introduce protein flexibility. Furthermore, novel protein conformations that result from combining structural elements

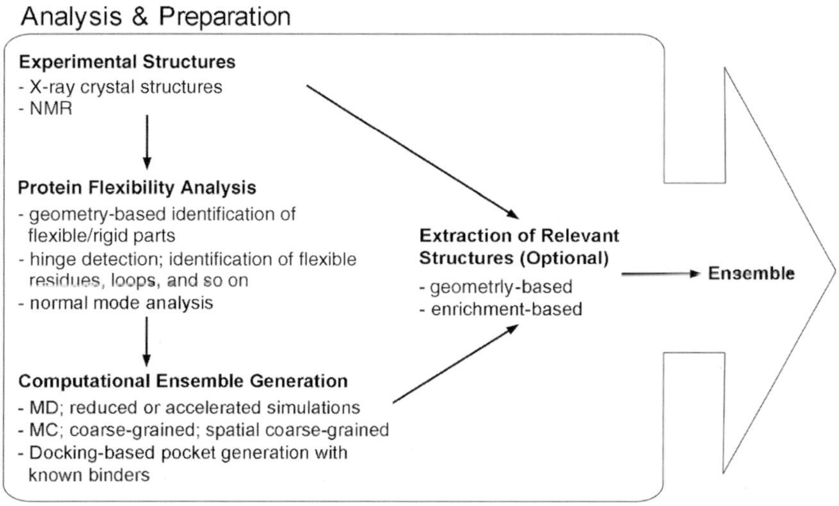

Figure 8.2 Summary of methods for protein flexibility analysis and ensemble preparation.

of the individual protein conformations are omitted by this procedure. Thus, over the last few years, novel ensemble-based approaches emerged and conventional rigid protein docking programs were extended to handle protein ensembles with the intent to evaluate the ensemble in a single docking run. Essentially, the methods fall into three categories. Some docking approaches rely on affordable search strategies to accelerate the evaluation of the ensemble space and select the most probable protein conformation. Others join the ensemble structures to a united protein structure to avoid multiple evaluation of similar protein regions and to consider only dissimilar regions individually. The last category of approaches utilizes ensemble-representative 3D grids to enable fast energy evaluation.

Ensemble-Based Optimal Structure Selection It is possible to avoid iterative docking against each protein ensemble member if one accepts not necessarily to select the ensemble structure most complementary to the ligand. Then heuristic search strategies can select at least well-fitting ensemble structures. Several docking approaches exist that accomplish heuristic ensemble structure selection, for example, one method based on a SIMPLEX local optimization procedure. The algorithm introduces an extra parameter m that references one protein conformation of the ensemble. The parameter is optimized to selecting the best suited structure then [49]. An integer index that identifies a single conformation in an ensemble stack is incorporated as variable in another MC-based docking approach. This allows to randomly switch from one structure to the other during global optimization of the ligand placement [50]. Besides that, genetic algorithms may also select an optimal fitting protein structure. A protein–ligand complex is then encoded in a chromosome. Individual flexible side chains and the rest of the protein are represented via digits in separate genes. Genetic operators randomly change side chain conformations and select the remaining protein part from the initial population of multiple input structures [51]. Finally, another procedure can be applied if previous docking results are present, and, thus, preferred protein conformations of ligands are known beforehand. This knowledge can be used to train a binary decision tree using QSAR classification. The decision tree can be used to select the appropriate ensemble conformation for novel molecules [52].

Targeting a United Protein Structure The second category of docking approaches utilizes a united protein description. A disadvantage of the above-mentioned optimization procedures is that they have to evaluate protein–ligand interactions in a redundant fashion. A characteristic feature of ensembles is that each pair of protein conformations shows regions with high structural similarity. In these regions, it is dispensable to evaluate interactions multiple times. A merged protein structure with a constant core region thus avoids redundant scoring and multiple protein conformations can be indirectly evaluated in a single docking run.

An application that follows this strategy is FlexE [53] that extends the docking tool FlexX [54] for protein ensemble handling. It utilizes FlexX's incremental construction algorithm to place the ligand fragment by fragment into the active site. Opposed to FlexX, FlexE places the ligand into a united protein description. Variable side chain and backbone parts are kept in clusters of alternative conformations. After each construction step, all possible interactions between the partially placed ligands and all conformations of the united protein structure are determined and an optimal collection of conformations of all protein parts is selected. Based on this selection, each partial solution is scored. The final solution, that is, the high-scoring ligand pose placed into the optimal protein structure, is reconstructed from the partial placements. A graph-based algorithm recombines the clustered conformations to form a novel valid protein structure regardless of the structure the protein parts originally stem from.

Another docking approach describes the ensemble in a similar fashion by a composite representation: one conformation for the rigid part, multiple for each of the flexible parts [55]. Orientations of the ligand molecule are sampled and matched to hot spots in the binding site. Complementarity of a certain ligand configuration is calculated based on its interaction with the independent receptor parts. For each ligand configuration, a depth-first search is first performed to check if at least one receptor conformation can accommodate the ligand without steric hindrance. If so, the ligand is scored for each component of the composite representation. The optimal receptor conformation is assembled using the best-fit conformation of each flexible receptor region.

The ensemble handling via a united protein structure assumes that mobile protein regions, such as side chains and loops, move independently and can be combined to form novel protein conformations. Thus, the approaches not only select the best fitting protein structure of the ensemble but may also construct a novel recombined best suited protein conformation.

Docking with United Ensemble Grids The precalculation of a three-dimensional grid that stores the potential interaction energy for ligand atoms at each grid point enables a fast energy evaluation of ligand poses during docking. Potential grids can also be employed in ensemble docking approaches to accelerate the pose evaluation in the same way. Therefore, energetic contributions of individual protein conformations have to be joined into a single generalized energetic description for the complete flexible protein. There exist several strategies to generate ensemble-based potential grids [55–58]. One strategy merges multiple energy grids generated from individual input structures into a single energy-average grid. An alternative way is to superimpose initially the ensemble structures and geometrically average the different conformations to gain a single average structure. This can then be used for the geometry-based calculation of a single average grid. Optionally, the individual contribution of an ensemble structure may be weighted. The composite grid avoids the evaluation of each ensemble structure, and thus, it requires only a single docking run. Due to the averaging process, the resulting energies are, however, only approximate.

In situ cross-docking joins multiple grids to one single grid to overcome sequential docking calculations [59]. The ensemble grids are aligned next to each other and high energy values are assigned to the border regions between each neighboring pair of grids. The procedure allows to handle the ensemble simultaneously in one docking run where the ligand explores the aligned grids. The technique therefore avoids the averaging of grids resulting in a more objective ligand evaluation.

A recently introduced interesting method utilizes an elastic potential grid [60]. Contrary to the already mentioned grid-based methods, the grid intended for docking is an irregular three-dimensional potential grid. Initially, a regular grid is generated from one of the input structures. The remaining input structures are used to deform the grid by displacement of grid intersection points according to protein movements represented by the remaining input structures. The precalculated potential field values are kept constant during deformation. During a docking run, protein–ligand interactions are determined by interpolation of neighboring grid points of the deformed grid.

8.2.2
Induced Fit Docking: Single-Structure-Based Docking Techniques

Contrary to ensemble-based docking, induced fit docking needs only a single input protein structure. The change in protein conformation is implemented after the ligand is placed into the binding pocket. The ligand itself, of course, may also experience a conformational change. In induced fit docking applications, often ligand and protein conformational spaces are explored consecutively. The uncoupled flexibility treatment of ligand and protein avoids a combined conformational search and thus combinatorial explosion of the underlying search space. Nevertheless, many approaches follow a quasi-simultaneous ligand and protein conformational search for the induced fit complex. They have to restrict the complex search space to become affordable. In the following, we first consider docking techniques that change ligand and protein conformations consecutively before looking at those that change the conformations simultaneously during the docking run.

8.2.2.1 Consecutive Ligand and Protein Conformational Change

In general, two different kinds of protein pocket adaptations may occur: In one case, the pocket is too narrow, but interactions between ligand and target structure are strong enough to overcome initial steric hindrance, which is eliminated afterward by protein pocket adaptation. In the other case, the pocket is too wide. The ligand binds, but to promote a stronger binding the interaction geometries have to be optimized. The pocket refines its structure and encloses the ligand. Induced fit docking techniques should imitate this behavior, that is, initially ignore possible steric hindrance and refine the complex structure afterward.

Soft Docking Implementations To ignore steric hindrance and to allow the ligand to intrude into the site even if it does not offer room enough, soft docking techniques may be used. The term *soft docking* generally covers techniques that implicitly model protein flexibility by permitting the ligand to partially penetrate receptor's binding site surface.

In 1991, Jiang and Kim developed the first approach that utilizes such a soft receptor [61]. The algorithm places target and ligand in an equally spaced 3D grid and describes the shapes of both molecules by cubes of grid size dimensions. A cube may be defined as surface or volume cube depending on whether it intersects the molecular surface. A translation is defined by a vector that results in at least one coinciding pair of surface cubes, one from each molecule. The algorithm enumerates all of these translations. For pose evaluation, protein–ligand surface cube matches are rewarded, whereas surface–volume cube overlaps are punished. The cube size decides the softness of the target. Larger cube size allows the ligand to overlap more with the target structure, whereas smaller cubes rather restrict ligand intrusion.

A similar geometric approach assigns intrinsic values to grid points to describe the surface, interior, and exterior volumes of the molecules. Shape matches are determined by calculating correlation functions. The correlation values indicate surface match, penetration, or no contact at all [62]. This method is especially successful in protein–protein docking applications and belongs to the standard approaches in this field.

Receptor surface penetration of the ligand is also modeled via manipulation of scoring functions. To soften the target structure, repulsive ligand–receptor interactions are attenuated. Common practice is to adjust the Lennard-Jones potential that models van der Waals interactions. The softening is often realized by replacing the original Lennard-Jones 12–6 potential with a 9–6 potential [63, 64]. The modification leads to flattening the steepness of the repulsion term. Thus, closer atom contacts become less restrictive and steric hindrance by side chains that prevent ligands from intrusion into the binding site is avoided. Other approaches soften the energy function in a similar fashion, but switch between hard and soft potentials for varying interatomic distances [65].

Soft receptors are an easy and efficient way to model a certain degree of protein flexibility. Their major disadvantage is certainly a substantial lack of accuracy. Usually, soft docking is the initial step of an induced fit workflow before a complex refinement occurs.

Complex Refinement For complete induced fit modeling, an optimization of the roughly fitted complex is required subsequently. Many induced fit docking approaches already integrate a final refinement stage. For docking approaches that do not integrate, herein some refinement methods are proposed that can easily succeed the actual docking process.

To improve the efficiency of adjusting side chain rotamers, Schaffer and Verkhivker implemented a postdocking side chain optimization procedure using the dead-end elimination (DEE) algorithm, followed by local minimizations and energy evaluations of all generated DEE solutions [66].

A molecular mechanics optimization allows partial to full atom flexibility of the protein through an energy minimization of the protein–ligand complexes and can be used for postprocessing of docked poses. In favor of that, various minimization methods ranging from a steepest descent to a genetic algorithm can be used [67]. A refinement of docked protein–ligand structures may be gained by amplitude optimization of elastic network normal modes as well [68]. Elastic networks suppose that the energy of the system can be described by a network of simple harmonic pair potentials [69]. Normal mode calculation under this assumption does not result in physically meaningful frequencies, but at least the low-frequency modes are in good agreement with modes derived from classical force fields that are normally used for mode determination. Afterward, the energy refinement can be performed along the normal mode amplitudes as degrees of freedom [70].

Approaches That Consecutively Place Ligands and Optimize the Resulting Complex Induced fit docking approaches usually integrate a complex refinement stage.

The docking program SLIDE optimizes side chains after the ligand is roughly placed into the site. The placement is guided by a set of interaction template points [71]. Ligand–side chain collisions are cleaned up assuming the *minimal rotation hypothesis*. Accordingly, the large side chain rearrangements that occupy many atoms have rather the potential to cause new steric clashes than slight residue adjustments [72]. SLIDE was further expanded to identify flexible and rigid parts of the protein and to introduce backbone deformations into the docking calculation [73].

A local induced fit motion is sampled by ADAM docking in combination with an energy minimization. ADAM utilizes a vdW-offset 3D grid. To enlarge the pocket uniformly, the potential curve is shifted that allows the atoms to get closer. The structure optimization covers side chains and ligand movements. The energy minimization is performed with the L-BFGS method [74].

Sherman *et al.* [75] developed an induced fit docking protocol as follows. Defined rules initially help to select presumably flexible residues in the binding site and replaces them by the amino acid alanine. A soft docking with this manipulated receptor places the ligand into the site. Finally, the docking protocol resubstitutes the alanines by the original side chains and predicts their low-energy conformations in presence of the soft docked ligand. To evaluate ligand poses, the protocol redocks the ligand with a hard potential and rescores the complex accounting for the refinement energy.

8.2.2.2 Simultaneous Ligand and Protein Conformational Change

Some methods try to avoid the postprocessing of generated docking solutions and shift the handling of receptor flexibility toward the actual docking stage. It leads to docking approaches where ligand and receptor experience a quasi-simultaneous conformational exploration. For this coupled ligand–receptor conformational search to be precise, in fact full MD simulations of the complete complex system should be performed and extended motions considered. Due to the prolonged simulation time that is required for such a full simulation, the technique remains impracticable or can only be performed up to an extremely restricted extent with approximations [77]. As in docking approaches that consider only ligand flexibility, heuristic searches and a reduction of the number of degrees of freedom help to enhance fully flexible docking techniques. Some of the techniques are introduced in the following.

Monte Carlo Simulated Docking Some induced fit docking approaches search for the docked complex in a probabilistic MC-based manner. Several of them introduce variables associated with protein degrees of freedom into the MC cycle. The variables are evaluated by energetic terms and optimized for protein–ligand fit. Early methods were restricted to consider only side chain flexibility [78], but soon extended to treat flexible loops as well [79]. Other approaches direct the docking with a geometric-based method initially [80], or rather follow a coarse-grained multistep conformational exploration that may combine the MC search with other optimization techniques, such as genetic algorithms, or gradient-based methods. Recently, backbone flexibility could also be incorporated into the docking stage [81]. Stochastic tunneling also performs an MC-based random walk, but every time a new local minimum is identified it flattens the regions of the potential energy surface that lie significantly above the local minimum [82]. Therefore, it "tunnels" through energy barriers and avoids that the process get stuck unnecessarily in other local minima of similar but higher energy. FlexScreen [83] implements the stochastic tunneling for protein–ligand docking and was recently extended to randomly rotate dihedrals of selected side chains in the MC cycle that was successfully applied in VS [84].

Docking Methods That Explore Side Chain Rotamers Many proteins show only slight movements of usually 6–12 binding site residues, their backbones remain almost rigid. Conformational changes of so-called *gatekeeper residues* can reveal hidden subpockets upon ligand binding. A plausible restriction to sample protein flexibility is to use a limited number of critical degrees of freedom and consider only movements of binding site residues. Several of such semiflexible approaches were proposed that explore side chain and ligand conformations simultaneously, while the docking engine optimally fits the ligand into the site [85, 86]. A genetic algorithm may also dock a flexible ligand to a semiflexible protein with selected side chain flexibility. The side chains–ligand complex may be encoded in the individuals of the genetic algorithm [87, 88]. Often the side chain conformational space is restricted to rotamer libraries of low-energy side chain conformations [89, 90]. Leach and Lemon combined the dead-end elimination and the A^* algorithm to explore the conformational space of a ligand and a rotamer library simultaneously [38].

Docking with Collective Degrees of Freedom Instead of explicit modeling macromolecular flexibility with native degrees of freedom, one can alternatively depict protein motions by use of collective degrees of freedom. Structure variations along collective degrees of freedom represent compact protein motions that result from a simultaneous change of a subset of receptor's native degrees of freedom. A collective protein representation enables the modeling of extended protein motions, including loop and domain rearrangements without dramatic increase of computational cost.

Modes of protein motion determined by harmonic dynamics or principal component analysis (PCA) serve to describe essential collective motions and they can be introduced directly into the docking procedure. Most conformational variations are captured approximately by a few essential modes. Included as additional variables in protein–ligand docking, they can be optimized and thus the collective protein motions and ligand conformations are simultaneously explored [91–93].

Another concept to account for essential motions of the target structure in protein–ligand docking is that of molecular hinges. The hinge bending approach models large conformational changes via points specifically placed into the protein structure that allow relative movements of domains or substructural units [94].

An interesting data structure, called flexibility tree, can be employed in the search for the docked complex structure and it allows to combine several flexibility techniques [95]. The data structure hierarchically encodes the flexibility of a protein in variables that allow several protein parts to experience different kinds of moves. Flexibility of domains may be described via normal mode or hinge motions, and side chains are allowed to explore rotameric states. Flexibility trees for protein and ligand are implemented in FlipDock that provides a genetic algorithm to optimize the variables to gain an induced fit complex [96].

8.2.3
Integrated Docking Approaches

Conformational selection as well as induced fit may depict rather two overdrawn extrema of the binding event. The reality may be better reflected by a model that lies somewhere in between. A combination of an ensemble-based technique with a soft docking and a complex refinement procedure enables implementation of an intermediate approach to agree with conformational selection and induced fit at the same time. In fact there exist methods that realize both concepts. The relaxed complex methods already mentioned in Section 8.2.1.1 that combine molecular dynamics methods with ensemble docking techniques also belong to that category of integrated approaches. They utilize MD simulations not only for ensemble generation but also for postprocessing of the docked complexes to implement an induced fit [28, 29, 97, 98]. Besides them, there exist other integrated approaches [99–101]. Exemplarily, we describe two methods in the following.

Fleksy [102] is a docking protocol that incorporates the FlexE docking [53] engine already described in Section 8.2.1.2. Given an experimental input structure, the protocol generates multiple receptor conformations to introduce receptor flexibility. For rule-based identified or alternatively user-defined residues, it extracts some most

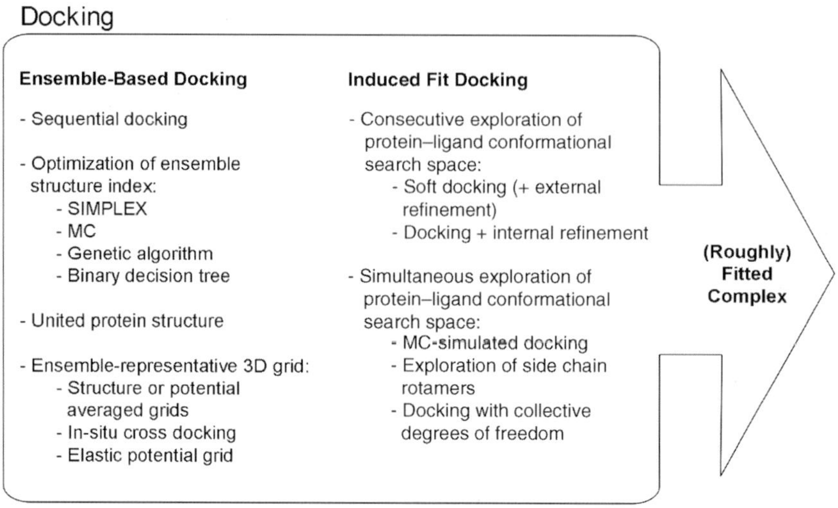

Figure 8.3 Summary of methods for fully flexible docking.

probable rotamers from a rotamer library. The resulting ensemble of receptor conformations is directed to FlexE that performs a soft docking against the united protein structure. The complexes of the best performing poses are rebuilt and forwarded to a complex-minimization stage [103]. Finally, the minimized complexes are rescored according to a consensus score. The highest ranked solution is finally supposed to be the optimal complementary complex.

SCARE [76] systematically replaces pairs of neighboring residues by alanines intending to remove the area of the site that hinders the ligand to intrude. It thus generates an ensemble consisting of multiple gapped pocket versions. The ligand is docked to each pocket version and the best scoring pocket is directed to a refinement stage in which the backbone with the original side chains is optimized and rescored.

8.3 Flexible Protein Handling in Docking-Based Virtual Screening

The aim of protein–ligand docking is to predict the pose that a ligand will adopt upon binding. Moreover, docking would like to estimate the binding free energy. In contrast to that, the docking engine that accomplishes a virtual screening has to fulfill a slight different task. The prediction of the optimal complex geometry is less in focus. In fact, docking each compound from a library, it has to decide which of them will probably bind and which will not. This requires a scoring function that ranks the compounds, optimally, according to their binding free energy. Furthermore, the docking engine has to evaluate a library sometimes containing hundreds of thousands of compounds and therefore it should screen rapidly to ensure a high-throughput of the process.

Fully flexible docking methods are a step toward more reliable compound assessment. For their application in structure-based virtual screening, some effects have to be considered that result from the introduction of protein flexibility. The following sections retrospectively consider the above-mentioned fully flexible docking approaches in respect to their efficiency and ability to discriminate binders from nonbinders.

8.3.1
Efficiency of Fully Flexible Docking Approaches in Retrospective

To make library evaluation affordable, a fast docking engine is an absolute premise. In general, modeling target flexibility is counter-productive for the acceleration of the docking calculation. For computational methods, the time limiting step is the modeling of protein conformational change. However, with respect to VS, the increase of computational costs mainly depends on in which docking stage the flexibility is introduced – prior, during, or posterior to the actual docking run. An introduction of target flexibility as a preprocessing step is rather affordable than postprocessing. In the former case, the expensive conformational change has to be modeled only once and the prepared target structure can be reused in later VS experiments. In the latter case, the whole range of complexed library compounds should be optimized individually for an objective ligand evaluation. This implicates that docking approaches following conformational selection should be more efficient for the employment in VS. If the ensemble is already generated, the runtime scales at most linearly with ensemble size that may be further reduced by using grids, united protein structures, or sophisticated search algorithms.

The practicability of an induced fit docking technique in VS mainly depends on the degree of flexibility of the considered target structure. The docking stage in consecutive induced fit approaches, that is, the soft docking stage, is quite efficient. The costly step is that of complex optimization afterward. Nevertheless, approaches optimizing only a restricted set of side chain conformations may be affordable too, either in consecutive or simultaneous fully flexible docking. They are successful for protein targets with small deviations in the three-dimensional structure and they are practicable in VS experiments up to moderate library size. However, for targets with more elaborate movements, restricted induced fit docking will fail to identify the correct ligand pose. In such cases, approaches are needed that sample a broader conformational space, but they are hardly applicable in VS as their induced fit modeling is quite expensive. Thus, VS of targets with inherently extended motions can be carried out only for extremely small-scale libraries and under approximations that in fact results in a loss of accuracy.

Integration of ensemble and induced fit docking may extract and combine the best of both worlds. If input structures are provided, ensemble-based docking may be more appropriate to handle extended elaborate motions, while simple slight motions are well treated by induced fit docking [63]. Furthermore, various filtering techniques for the generation of target-constrained compound libraries or pharmacophore-guided screening may help to enhance the throughput of VS approaches. In addition, multistep VS that initially performs a crude but fast, before it ends with a precise compound evaluation of only the best ranked compounds, of previous steps accelerates the screening further.

8.3.2
Discrimination of Binders and Nonbinders

A docking engine for VS purposes has not to be only fast but also accurate. The introduction of protein flexibility into docking procedures increases the chance to find a receptor in the correct conformational state as ensembles and allowed ligand–receptor overlaps offer more room in the binding pocket to accommodate a particular pose. Nevertheless, flexible receptor docking also reduces the selectivity of the docking process as a wider variety of compounds that not necessarily have to be ligands are able to fit into the more relaxed protein representation. This has a dramatic effect on the VS process. Compared to rigid receptor screening, a flexible receptor screening will generate valid poses for more library compounds [104].

Docking approaches evaluate the generated ligand poses by a scoring function that ideally reflects the binding affinity of the small molecule and guides the docking process to identify the probably best binding ligand pose. However, for a VS, the scoring function has not only to identify the best pose of the individual compounds but also to decide if well-fitting compounds are indeed hits. For efficiency reasons, pose evaluation and thus scoring have to be fast to become affordable in VS. Therefore, applicable scoring functions mostly account for simple binding-productive intermolecular interactions and neglect other hard to calculate terms. Assuming a rigid receptor, simple energetic functions might be adequate to score ligands, but the scoring function in flexible receptor docking has to assess the goodness of protein conformations as well. Unfavorable energetic contributions caused by uncomfortable protein conformations may overcome binding-productive contributions. As a result, when not accounting for them in flexible receptor VS, the predicted receptor conformation is implicitly overestimated and the compound falsely declared being a binder. Similarly, if weak intermolecular interactions are detected but the internal energy of the protein facilitates ligand binding, the compound is falsely predicted being a nonbinder. The controversy between the preservation of accuracy and ensuring rapidness of scoring functions lead to work-arounds to handle the problem. For example, it is sensible to rescore the best complexes more extensively after ligand placement using accurate scoring functions. It helps to maximize the selection of the most active ligands and to minimize false positive predictions.

8.4
Summary

Approaches for fully flexible docking either follow a conformational selection or an induced fit concept (Figure 8.3). Ensemble docking implements the principle of conformational selection and relies on the protein structural change occurring before the ligand binds to the protein. The ensemble of input protein conformations represents the range of moves that the targeted protein may adapt and that considers efficiently global protein moves. In contrast, induced fit docking modifies the protein conformation upon docking and therefore expects a single input protein conformation. The docking engine has to accept an initially unfavorable protein conformation, therefore, induced fit docking starts with a rough ligand placement. A subsequent protein refinement stage forces a structure adaptation toward a complex with better shape complementarity. However, the refinement stage should be restricted to involve rather local protein structure adjustment in order to retain it affordable. A combination of the complementary ensemble and induced fit docking methodologies offer the possibility to presumably model a more realistic binding event and to account for global and local protein flexibility at the same time.

Thus, first promising methods for fully flexible protein–ligand docking are already available. For their application in virtual screening, however, prediction accuracy and efficiency of the methods still leave room for improvement. A key role for further success must be attached to scoring functions able to take protein conformational changes into account in order to reliably discriminate binders from nonbinders of flexible proteins. Here, we focused on the theoretical background of techniques for fully flexible docking and discussed critical aspects that arise in the virtual screening of flexible targets. We refer to Chapter 9 that provides and discusses interesting examples for the application of fully flexible docking in virtual screening.

References

1 Fischer, E. (1894) Einfluss der Configuration auf die Wirkung der Enzyme. *Berichte der Deutschen Chemischen Gesellschaft*, **27** (3), 2985–2993.

2 Koshland, D. (1958) Application of a theory of enzyme specificity to protein synthesis. *Proceedings of the National Academy of Sciences of the United States of America*, **44** (2), 98–104.

3 Luque, I. and Freire, E. (2000) Structural stability of binding sites: consequences for binding affinity and allosteric effects. *Proteins*, **41** (Suppl. 4), 63–71.

4 Zhang, H., Zhang, T., Chen, K., Shen, S., Ruan, J., and Kurgan, L. (2009) On the relation between residue flexibility and local solvent accessibility in proteins. *Proteins*, **76** (3), 617–636.

5 Gutteridge, A. and Thornton, J. (2004) Conformational change in substrate binding, catalysis and product release: an open and shut case? *FEBS Letters*, **567** (1), 67–73.

6 Najmanovich, R., Kuttner, J., Sobolev, V., and Edelman, M. (2000) Side-chain flexibility in proteins upon ligand binding. *Proteins*, **39** (3), 261–268.

7 Gunasekaran, K. and Nussinov, R. (2007) How different are structurally flexible and rigid binding sites? Sequence and structural features discriminating proteins that do and do not undergo conformational change upon ligand binding. *Journal of Molecular Biology*, **365** (1), 257–273.

8 Brylinski, M. and Skolnick, J. (2008) What is the relationship between the global structures of apo and holo proteins? *Proteins*, **70** (2), 363–377.

9 Bosshard, H.R. (2001) Molecular recognition by induced fit: how fit is the concept? *News in Physiological Sciences*, **16** (4), 171–173.

10 Berger, C., Weber-Bornhauser, S., Eggenberger, J., Hanes, J., Plückthun, A., and Bosshard, H.R. (1999) Antigen recognition by conformational selection. *FEBS Letters*, **450** (1–2), 149–153.

11 Frauenfelder, H., Sligar, S.G., and Wolynes, P.G. (1991) The energy landscapes and motions of proteins. *Science*, **254** (5038), 1598–1603.
12 Onuchic, J.N. (1997) Contacting the protein folding funnel with NMR. *Proceedings of the National Academy of Sciences of the United States of America*, **94** (14), 7129–7131.
13 Kumar, S., Ma, B., Tsai, C.J., Wolfson, H., and Nussinov, R. (1999) Folding funnels and conformational transitions via hinge-bending motions. *Cell Biochemistry and Biophysics*, **31** (2), 141–164.
14 Ma, B., Kumar, S., Tsai, C.J., and Nussinov, R. (1999) Folding funnels and binding mechanisms. *Protein Engineering*, **12** (9), 713–720.
15 Verkhivker, G.M., Bouzida, D., Gehlhaar, D.K., Rejto, P.A., Freer, S.T., and Rose, P.W. (2002) Complexity and simplicity of ligand–macromolecule interactions: the energy landscape perspective. *Current Opinion in Structural Biology*, **12** (2), 197–203.
16 Tsai, C.J., Ma, B., and Nussinov, R. (1999) Folding and binding cascades: shifts in energy landscapes. *Proceedings of the National Academy of Sciences of the United States of America*, **96** (18), 9970–9972.
17 Hammes, G.G., Chang, Y.-C., and Oas, T.G. (2009) Conformational selection or induced fit: a flux description of reaction mechanism. *Proceedings of the National Academy of Sciences of the United States of America*, **106** (33), 13737–13741.
18 Bernstein, F.C., Koetzle, T.F., Williams, G.J., Meyer, E.F., Brice, M.D., Rodgers, J.R., Kennard, O., Shimanouchi, T., and Tasumi, M. (1977) The Protein Data Bank. A computer-based archival file for macromolecular structures. *European Journal of Biochemistry*, **80** (2), 319–324.
19 Kirchmair, J., Markt, P., Distinto, S., Schuster, D., Spitzer, G.M., Liedl, K.R., Langer, T., and Wolber, G. (2008) The Protein Data Bank (PDB), its related services and software tools as key components for *in silico* guided drug discovery. *Journal of Medicinal Chemistry*, **51** (22), 7021–7040.
20 Cozzini, P., Kellogg, G.E., Spyrakis, F., Abraham, D.J., Costantino, G., Emerson, A., Fanelli, F., Gohlke, H., Kuhn, L.A., Morris, G.M., Orozco, M., Pertinhez, T.A., Rizzi, M., and Sotriffer, C.A. (2008) Target flexibility: an emerging consideration in drug discovery and design. *Journal of Medicinal Chemistry*, **51** (20), 6237–6255.
21 Teodoro, M. and Kavraki, L. (2003) Conformational flexibility models for the receptor in structure based drug design. *Current Pharmaceutical Design*, **9** (20), 1635–1648.
22 Barril, X. and Fradera, X. (2006) Incorporating protein flexibility into docking and structure-based drug design. *Expert Opinion on Drug Discovery*, **1** (4), 335–349.
23 Totrov, M. and Abagyan, R. (2008) Flexible ligand docking to multiple receptor conformations: a practical alternative. *Current Opinion in Structural Biology*, **18** (2), 178–184.
24 Furnham, N., Blundell, T., DePristo, M., and Terwilliger, T. (2006) Is one solution good enough? *Nature Structural & Molecular Biology*, **13** (3), 184–185.
25 Bolstad, E.S.D. and Anderson, A.C. (2009) In pursuit of virtual lead optimization: pruning ensembles of receptor structures for increased efficiency and accuracy during docking. *Proteins*, **75** (1), 62–74.
26 Carlson, H.A., Masukawa, K.M., Rubins, K., Bushman, F.D., Jorgensen, W.L., Lins, R.D., Briggs, J.M., and McCammon, J.A. (2000) Developing a dynamic pharmacophore model for HIV-1 integrase. *Journal of Medicinal Chemistry*, **43** (11), 2100–2114.
27 Meagher, K.L., Lerner, M.G., and Carlson, H.A. (2006) Refining the multiple protein structure pharmacophore method: consistency across three independent HIV-1 protease models. *Journal of Medicinal Chemistry*, **49** (12), 3478–3484.
28 Lin, J.-H., Perryman, A.L., Schames, J.R., and McCammon, J.A. (2002) Computational drug design

accommodating receptor flexibility: the relaxed complex scheme. *Journal of the American Chemical Society*, **124** (20), 5632–5633.

29 Amaro, R., Baron, R., and McCammon, J. (2008) An improved relaxed complex scheme for receptor flexibility in computer-aided drug design. *Journal of Computer-Aided Molecular Design*, **22** (9), 693–705.

30 Withers, I.M., Mazanetz, M.P., Wang, H., Fischer, P.M., and Laughton, C.A. (2008) Active site pressurization: a new tool for structure-guided drug design and other studies of protein flexibility. *Journal of Chemical Information and Modeling*, **48** (7), 1448–1454.

31 Nilmeier, J. and Jacobson, M. (2008) Multiscale Monte Carlo sampling of protein sidechains: application to binding pocket flexibility. *Journal of Chemical Theory and Computation*, **4** (5), 835–846.

32 Shehu, A., Kavraki, L.E., and Clementi, C. (2009) Multiscale characterization of protein conformational ensembles. *Proteins*, **76** (4), 837–851.

33 Gohlke, H. and Thorpe, M.F. (2006) A natural coarse graining for simulating large biomolecular motion. *Biophysical Journal*, **91** (6), 2115–2120.

34 Jacobs, D.J., Rader, A.J., Kuhn, L.A., and Thorpe, M.F. (2001) Protein flexibility predictions using graph theory. *Proteins*, **44** (2), 150–165.

35 Thorpe, M.F., Lei, M., Rader, A.J., Jacobs, D.J., and Kuhn, L.A. (2001) Protein flexibility and dynamics using constraint theory. *Journal of Molecular Graphics & Modelling*, **19** (1), 60–69.

36 Lei, M., Zavodszky, M.I., Kuhn, L.A., and Thorpe, M.F. (2004) Sampling protein conformations and pathways. *Journal of Computational Chemistry*, **25** (9), 1133–1148.

37 Dunbrack, R.L. and Karplus, M. (1994) Conformational analysis of the backbone-dependent rotamer preferences of protein sidechains. *Nature Structural Biology*, **1** (5), 334–340.

38 Leach, A.R. and Lemon, A.P. (1998) Exploring the conformational space of protein side chains using dead-end elimination and the A* algorithm. *Proteins*, **33** (2), 227–239.

39 Anderson, A.C., O'Neil, R.H., Surti, T.S., and Stroud, R.M. (2001) Approaches to solving the rigid receptor problem by identifying a minimal set of flexible residues during ligand docking. *Chemistry & Biology*, **8** (5), 445–457.

40 Hartmann, C., Antes, I., and Lengauer, T. (2007) IRECS: a new algorithm for the selection of most probable ensembles of side-chain conformations in protein models. *Protein Science*, **16** (7), 1294–1307.

41 Wilson, E.B., Decius, J., and Cross, P. (1955) (eds) *Molecular Vibrations: The Theory of Infrared and Raman Vibrational Spectra*, McGraw-Hill Book Co., New York.

42 Brooks, B. and Karplus, M. (1983) Harmonic dynamics of proteins: normal modes and fluctuations in bovine pancreatic trypsin inhibitor. *Proceedings of the National Academy of Sciences of the United States of America*, **80** (21), 6571–6575.

43 Tirion, M.M. (1996) Large amplitude elastic motions in proteins from a single-parameter, atomic analysis. *Physical Review Letters*, **77** (9), 1905–1908.

44 Cavasotto, C.N., Kovacs, J.A., and Abagyan, R.A. (2005) Representing receptor flexibility in ligand docking through relevant normal modes. *Journal of the American Chemical Society*, **127** (26), 9632–9640.

45 Rueda, M., Bottegoni, G., and Abagyan, R. (2009) Consistent improvement of cross-docking results using binding site ensembles generated with elastic network normal modes. *Journal of Chemical Information and Modeling*, **49** (3), 716–725.

46 Cavasotto, C.N. and Abagyan, R.A. (2004) Protein flexibility in ligand docking and virtual screening to protein kinases. *Journal of Molecular Biology*, **337** (1), 209–225.

47 Rao, S., Sanschagrin, P.C., Greenwood, J.R., Repasky, M.P., Sherman, W., and Farid, R. (2008) Improving database enrichment through ensemble docking. *Journal of Computer-Aided Molecular Design*, **22** (9), 621–627.

48 Bolstad, E.S.D. and Anderson, A.C. (2008) In pursuit of virtual lead optimization: the role of the receptor structure and ensembles in accurate docking. *Proteins*, **73** (3), 566–580.

49 Huang, S.-Y. and Zou, X. (2007) Ensemble docking of multiple protein structures: considering protein structural variations in molecular docking. *Proteins*, **66** (2), 399–421.

50 Bottegoni, G., Kufareva, I., Totrov, M., and Abagyan, R. (2009) Four-dimensional docking: a fast and accurate account of discrete receptor flexibility in ligand docking. *Journal of Medicinal Chemistry*, **52** (2), 397–406.

51 Corbeil, C.R., Englebienne, P., and Moitessier, N. (2007) Docking ligands into flexible and solvated macromolecules. 1. Development and validation of FITTED 1.0. *Journal of Chemical Information and Modeling*, **47** (2), 435–449.

52 Hritz, J., de Ruiter, A., and Oostenbrink, C. (2008) Impact of plasticity and flexibility on docking results for cytochrome P450 2D6: a combined approach of molecular dynamics and ligand docking. *Journal of Medicinal Chemistry*, **51** (23), 7469–7477.

53 Claussen, H., Buning, C., Rarey, M., and Lengauer, T. (2001) FlexE: efficient molecular docking considering protein structure variations. *Journal of Molecular Biology*, **308** (2), 377–395.

54 Rarey, M., Kramer, B., Lengauer, T., and Klebe, G. (1996) A fast flexible docking method using an incremental construction algorithm. *Journal of Molecular Biology*, **261** (3), 470–489.

55 Wei, B., Weaver, L., Ferrari, A., Matthews, B., and Shoichet, B. (2004) Testing a flexible-receptor docking algorithm in a model binding site. *Journal of Molecular Biology*, **337** (5), 1161–1182.

56 Knegtel, R.M., Kuntz, I.D., and Oshiro, C.M. (1997) Molecular docking to ensembles of protein structures. *Journal of Molecular Biology*, **266** (2), 424–440.

57 Osterberg, F., Morris, G., Sanner, M., Olson, A., and Goodsell, D. (2002) Automated docking to multiple target structures: incorporation of protein mobility and structural water heterogeneity in AutoDock. *Proteins*, **46** (1), 34–40.

58 Schapira, M., Abagyan, R., and Totrov, M. (2003) Nuclear hormone receptor targeted virtual screening. *Journal of Medicinal Chemistry*, **46** (14), 3045–3059.

59 Sotriffer, C.A. and Dramburg, I. (2005) "In situ cross-docking" to simultaneously address multiple targets. *Journal of Medicinal Chemistry*, **48** (9), 3122–3125.

60 Kazemi, S., Krüger, D.M., Sirockin, F., and Gohlke, H. (2009) Elastic potential grids: accurate and efficient representation of intermolecular interactions for fully flexible docking. *ChemMedChem*, **4** (8), 1264–1268.

61 Jiang, F. and Kim, S. (1991) "Soft docking": matching of molecular surface cubes. *Journal of Molecular Biology*, **219** (1), 79–102.

62 Katchalski-Katzir, E., Shariv, I., Eisenstein, M., Friesem, A.A., Aflalo, C., and Vakser, I.A. (1992) Molecular surface recognition: determination of geometric fit between proteins and their ligands by correlation techniques. *Proceedings of the National Academy of Sciences of the United States of America*, **89** (6), 2195–2199.

63 Ferrari, A.M., Wei, B.Q., Costantino, L., and Shoichet, B.K. (2004) Soft docking and multiple receptor conformations in virtual screening. *Journal of Medicinal Chemistry*, **47** (21), 5076–5084.

64 Erickson, J.A., Jalaie, M., Robertson, D.H., Lewis, R.A., and Vieth, M. (2004) Lessons in molecular recognition: the effects of ligand and protein flexibility on molecular docking accuracy. *Journal of Medicinal Chemistry*, **47** (1), 45–55.

65 Vieth, M., Hirst, J.D., Kolinski, A., and Brooks, C.L., III (1998) Assessing energy functions for flexible docking. *Journal of Computational Chemistry*, **19** (14), 1612–1622.

66 Schaffer, L. and Verkhivker, G.M. (1998) Predicting structural effects in HIV-1 protease mutant complexes with flexible ligand docking and protein side-chain optimization. *Proteins*, **33** (2), 295–310.

67 Pencheva, T., Lagorce, D., Pajeva, I., Villoutreix, B.O., and Miteva, M.A. (2008) AMMOS: automated molecular mechanics optimization tool for *in silico* screening. *BMC Bioinformatics*, **9**, 438.

68 Lindahl, E. and Delarue, M. (2005) Refinement of docked protein–ligand and protein–DNA structures using low frequency normal mode amplitude optimization. *Nucleic Acids Research*, **33** (14), 4496–4506.

69 Hinsen, K. (1998) Analysis of domain motions by approximate normal mode calculations. *Proteins*, **33** (3), 417–429.

70 Lindahl, E., Azuara, C., Koehl, P., and Delarue, M. (2006) NOMAD-Ref: visualization, deformation and refinement of macromolecular structures based on all-atom normal mode analysis. *Nucleic Acids Research*, **34** (Web Server issue), W52–W56.

71 Schnecke, V. and Kuhn, L.A. (1999) Database screening for HIV protease ligands: the influence of binding-site conformation and representation on ligand selectivity. *Proceedings of the International Conference on Intelligent Systems for Molecular Biology*, 242–251.

72 Zavodszky, M. and Kuhn, L. (2005) Side-chain flexibility in protein–ligand binding: the minimal rotation hypothesis. *Protein Science*, **14** (4), 1104–1114.

73 Zavodszky, M.I., Lei, M., Thorpe, M.F., Day, A.R., and Kuhn, L.A. (2004) Modeling correlated main-chain motions in proteins for flexible molecular recognition. *Proteins*, **57** (2), 243–261.

74 Mizutani, M.Y., Takamatsu, Y., Ichinose, T., Nakamura, K., and Itai, A. (2006) Effective handling of induced-fit motion in flexible docking. *Proteins*, **63** (4), 878–891.

75 Sherman, W., Day, T., Jacobson, M.P., Friesner, R.A., and Farid, R. (2006) Novel procedure for modeling ligand/receptor induced fit effects. *Journal of Medicinal Chemistry*, **49** (2), 534–553.

76 Bottegoni, G., Kufareva, I., Totrov, M., and Abagyan, R. (2008) A new method for ligand docking to flexible receptors by dual alanine scanning and refinement (SCARE). *Journal of Computer-Aided Molecular Design*, **22** (5), 311–325.

77 Mangoni, M., Roccatano, D., and Nola, A.D. (1999) Docking of flexible ligands to flexible receptors in solution by molecular dynamics simulation. *Proteins*, **35** (2), 153–162.

78 Abagyan, R., Totrov, M., and Kuznetsov, D. (1994) ICM: a new method for protein modeling and design – applications to docking and structure prediction from the distorted native conformation. *Journal of Computational Chemistry*, **15** (5), 488–506.

79 Bastard, K., Thureau, A., Lavery, R., and Prévost, C. (2003) Docking macromolecules with flexible segments. *Journal of Computational Chemistry*, **24** (15), 1910–1920.

80 Taylor, R.D., Jewsbury, P.J., and Essex, J.W. (2003) FDS: flexible ligand and receptor docking with a continuum solvent model and soft-core energy function. *Journal of Computational Chemistry*, **24** (13), 1637–1656.

81 Davis, I.W. and Baker, D. (2009) RosettaLigand docking with full ligand and receptor flexibility. *Journal of Molecular Biology*, **385** (2), 381–392.

82 Wenzel, W. and Hamacher, K. (1999) Stochastic tunneling approach for global minimization of complex potential energy landscapes. *Physical Review Letters*, **82** (15), 3003–3007.

83 Merlitz, H. and Wenzel, W. (2002) Comparison of stochastic optimization methods for receptor–ligand docking. *Journal of Physical Chemistry Letters*, **362** (3–4), 271–277.

84 Kokh, D.B. and Wenzel, W. (2008) Flexible side chain models improve enrichment rates in *in silico* screening. *Journal of Medicinal Chemistry*, **51** (19), 5919–5931.

85 Leach, A.R. (1994) Ligand docking to proteins with discrete side-chain flexibility. *Journal of Molecular Biology*, **235** (1), 345–356.

86 Desmet, J., Wilson, I.A., Joniau, M., Maeyer, M.D., and Lasters, I. (1997) Computation of the binding of fully flexible peptides to proteins with flexible

side chains. *The FASEB Journal*, **11** (2), 164–172.

87 Jones, G., Willett, P., Glen, R.C., Leach, A.R., and Taylor, R. (1997) Development and validation of a genetic algorithm for flexible docking. *Journal of Molecular Biology*, **267** (3), 727–748.

88 Morris, G.M., Huey, R., Lindstrom, W., Sanner, M.F., Belew, R.K., Goodsell, D.S., and Olson, A.J. (2009) AutoDock4 and AutoDockTools4: automated docking with selective receptor flexibility. *Journal of Computational Chemistry*, **30** (16), 2785–2791.

89 Dunbrack, R.L. and Karplus, M. (1993) Backbone-dependent rotamer library for proteins. Application to side-chain prediction. *Journal of Molecular Biology*, **230** (2), 543–574.

90 Lovell, S.C., Word, J.M., Richardson, J.S., and Richardson, D.C. (2000) The penultimate rotamer library. *Proteins*, **40** (3), 389–408.

91 Tatsumi, R., Fukunishi, Y., and Nakamura, H. (2004) A hybrid method of molecular dynamics and harmonic dynamics for docking of flexible ligand to flexible receptor. *Journal of Computational Chemistry*, **25** (16), 1995–2005.

92 Zacharias, M. (2004) Rapid protein–ligand docking using soft modes from molecular dynamics simulations to account for protein deformability: binding of FK506 to FKBP. *Proteins*, **54** (4), 759–767.

93 May, A. and Zacharias, M. (2008) Protein–ligand docking accounting for receptor side chain and global flexibility in normal modes: evaluation on kinase inhibitor cross docking. *Journal of Medicinal Chemistry*, **51** (12), 3499–3506.

94 Sandak, B., Wolfson, H.J., and Nussinov, R. (1998) Flexible docking allowing induced fit in proteins: insights from an open to closed conformational isomers. *Proteins*, **32** (2), 159–174.

95 Zhao, Y., Stoffler, D., and Sanner, M. (2006) Hierarchical and multi-resolution representation of protein flexibility. *Bioinformatics (Oxford, England)*, **22** (22), 2768–2774.

96 Zhao, Y. and Sanner, M. (2007) FLIPDock: docking flexible ligands into flexible receptors. *Proteins*, **68** (3), 726–737.

97 Alonso, H., Bliznyuk, A.A., and Gready, J.E. (2006) Combining docking and molecular dynamic simulations in drug design. *Medicinal Research Reviews*, **26** (5), 531–568.

98 Wong, C. (2008) Flexible ligand-flexible protein docking in protein kinase systems. *Biochimica et Biophysica Acta*, **1784** (1), 244–251.

99 Spassov, V.Z., Yan, L., and Flook, P.K. (2007) The dominant role of side-chain backbone interactions in structural realization of amino acid code. ChiRotor: a side-chain prediction algorithm based on side-chain backbone interactions. *Protein Science*, **16** (3), 494–506.

100 Koska, J., Spassov, V.Z., Maynard, A.J., Yan, L., Austin, N., Flook, P.K., and Venkatachalam, C.M. (2008) Fully automated molecular mechanics based induced fit protein–ligand docking method. *Journal of Chemical Information and Modeling*, **48** (10), 1965–1973.

101 Jain, A.N. (2009) Effects of protein conformation in docking: improved pose prediction through protein pocket adaptation. *Journal of Computer-Aided Molecular Design*, **23** (6), 355–374.

102 Nabuurs, S., Wagener, M., and De Vlieg, J. (2007) A flexible approach to induced fit docking. *Journal of Medicinal Chemistry*, **50** (26), 6507–6518.

103 Krieger, E., Koraimann, G., and Vriend, G. (2002) Increasing the precision of comparative models with YASARA NOVA: a self-parameterizing force field. *Proteins*, **47** (3), 393–402.

104 Barril, X. and Morley, S.D. (2005) Unveiling the full potential of flexible receptor docking using multiple crystallographic structures. *Journal of Medicinal Chemistry*, **48** (13), 4432–4443.

9
Handling Protein Flexibility in Docking and High-Throughput Docking: From Algorithms to Applications

Claudio N. Cavasotto

9.1
Introduction: Docking and High-Throughput Docking in Drug Discovery

For the last two decades, experimental high-throughput screening (HTS) of in-house or commercially available compound collections was the method of choice of the pharmaceutical industry for hit/lead identification [1, 2]. However, its failure to deliver according to the expectations, coupled with the cost of HTS experiments, led to the development and use of computational methods in this task [3]. Thus, a variety of *in silico* methods rooted in physical principles and/or experimental knowledge became available for different purposes, including but not limited to the prioritization of sublibraries of compounds for experimental evaluation [4, 5]. The use of a three-dimensional (3D) structural representation of the target paved the way for structure-based approaches, such as docking-based virtual screening [4–6], structure-based lead optimization [7], design of target-specific virtual chemical libraries [8, 9], characterization of ligand–receptor interactions at an atomic level [10], and probing structure–function relationships [11] among others. It has been reported that a large amount of money could be saved in drug discovery projects if target structural information is used in the early stages of hit/lead development [12]. This, coupled with the growth of experimentally determined structures and the advances in homology modeling [11], has triggered the wide use of structure-based methods in drug discovery [13].

If the experimental structure of a ligand–receptor complex is not available, this may be *in silico* modeled through ligand docking. The sequential process of docking a virtual chemical library and assigning a "score" to each compound – which measures the likelihood of binding – is usually referred to as high-throughput docking (HTD) or structure-based virtual screening (SBVS). The main goal of HTD is to prioritize the compound library such that only those compounds with a high chance of binding to the protein proceed for experimental testing. HTD also provides a 3D representation of the candidates complexed with the target.

The first attempt to predict nonnative ligand–receptor complexes goes back to 1976, when Beddell *et al.* [14] developed handmade representations of the protein

Virtual Screening. Edited by C. Sotriffer

ISBN: 978-3-527-32636-5

structure in an attempt to design compounds that fit into hemoglobin. Since the early 1980s, when the first computer docking methods were developed [15, 16], there has been an active development and improvement of docking and HTD methods (for review, cf. Refs [5, 6, 17]).

As a necessary condition, a HTD program should incorporate a good conformational sampling of the ligand in the field of the receptor, a reliable scoring function (able to discriminate potential binders from nonbinders), and should be computationally affordable. However, an inadequate representation of the system may certainly limit the performance of docking and HTD methods. The most common problems are uncertainty in the protonation states of ligand and residues due to induced pK_a changes, inclusion/exclusion of ions and water molecules in the binding site [18], flipping of asparagines and glutamines, errors in assignment of histidine tautomer states, and not accounting for protein flexibility, since most docking methods were developed based on Fischer's [19] theory of lock and key, that is, using a rigid representation of the receptor.

In this chapter, we will present case studies where docking and HTD methods accounting for protein flexibility were used in the context of drug discovery/design or lead optimization projects. This will be preceded by a theoretical analysis of the problem, followed by concrete examples of docking failures stemming from neglecting protein flexibility.

9.2 The Challenge of Accounting for Protein Flexibility in Docking

9.2.1 Theoretical Understanding of the Problem

The first step toward accounting for target flexibility in docking is the correct understanding of the physical foundation of ligand–protein association. The first theory to explain ligand binding was the "lock and key" mechanism, proposed by Emil Fischer in 1894 [19], by which the ligand fits into the receptor like the key into a lock, thus demanding shape complementarity. However, this explanation falls short to explain the fact of structurally different bound and unbound proteins. In 1958, Koshland proposed the "induced fit" theory [20, 21], whereby the ligand and protein structures adapt to each other in the process of binding. This theory assumes that the protein is partially flexible, whose final conformation is "induced" by the substrate binding to it. These two theories would describe two types of binding processes: if the unbound and bound states are structurally similar, then the binding process can be understood in terms of the "lock and key" theory. But when there is significant structural change in the receptor upon binding, then the "induced fit" theory would explain protein flexibility in the context of ligand binding.

Recently, the notion of preexisting protein conformations was used to rationalize binding events based on the concept of folding funnels [22, 23]. According to this theory, the native state of the protein may not be represented by a single conformation, but by a structural ensemble of low-energy conformations in thermodynamical equilibrium. Thus, the energy landscape of a flexible protein is characterized by a multiminima rugged bottom, with low-energy barriers separating the equilibrium conformers. The lower the barriers, the more accessible the different conformations are. In this context, ligands would select the most favorable protein conformation to bind, thus shifting the equilibrium toward that receptor conformer that optimizes ligand binding (conformer selection). In the case of well-defined native states, little change would be expected upon ligand binding (lock and key event). Studies on antigen–antibody binding [24, 25], and protein–protein binding [26] have shown that bound conformations are present in the unbound conformational ensemble.

In this way, binding site flexibility could be better rationalized not from the fact that the protein receptor can adapt to diverse ligands but from its prior existence as an ensemble in thermodynamical equilibrium, with several quasi-isoenergetic different conformations that ligands select upon binding. As Van Regenmortel pointed out, the ligand determines the structural conformation of the binding site, not much by inducing it, but by selecting the conformer that optimizes the interaction (conformer selection) [27]. Based on experimental evidence [28], we could say that the most accurate description of the ligand binding process would be a two-step process: the conformer selection stage of partially fitting structures, followed by an "induced fit" stage, where minor adjustments take place within binding site. Thus, structural changes upon ligand binding take place within the preexisting conformational ensemble. In the context of this theory, Ikeguchi *et al.* described the ligand binding process in terms of linear response theory (LRT), whereby receptor structural changes upon ligand binding can be represented as the perturbation that the ligand induces on the receptor unbound conformational states [29].

9.2.2
Docking Failures Due to Protein Flexibility

There is mounting evidence that many receptors exhibit flexibility upon ligand binding (see Ref. [30] for a thorough review). Inspection of the PDB reveals cases of large- and small-scale movements upon ligand binding. In HIV protease [31], it is observed as large displacement of the "flaps" upon ligand binding; in p38 MAP kinase, a large-scale loop rearrangement takes place upon binding of picomolar inhibitor BIRB 796 [32]; a similar behavior was observed in c-Abl kinase (Figure 9.1); and DHFR exhibits a loop displacement of more than 7 Å upon ligand binding [33, 34]. However, in other cases, the flexibility exhibited upon ligand binding is modest, sometimes just the displacement of a single "gatekeeper" residue [35, 36]. It was reported that in $\sim$85% of cases, three or less binding site residues show conformational changes upon ligand binding [37]. However, since even small structural changes can lead to an energy change of 14 kJ/mol [38], it is reasonable to expect that, in many cases, variations in the binding site structure will have an influence on docking outcomes.

The impact of receptor flexibility on docking is usually assessed by cross-docking experiments, whereby a series of ligands is docked to all their corresponding

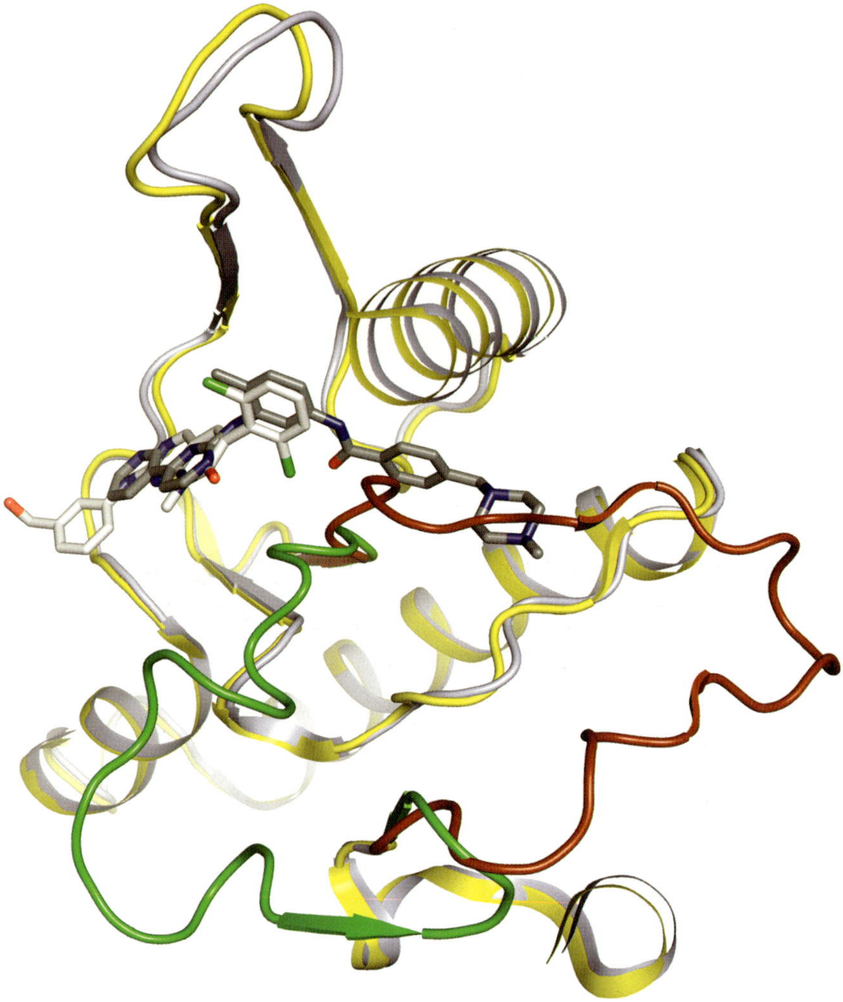

Figure 9.1 Large loop rearrangement in c-Abl protein kinase. ATP-competitive ligand PD1663 26 (light gray carbon atoms) binds to the receptor with the activation loop (brown) in the "in" position (PDB 1OPJ, yellow ribbon). However, larger compound imatinib (dark gray carbon atoms) is able to bind only after the activation loop (green) rearranges to the "out" position (PDB 1OPK, light blue ribbon). Color code for noncarbon atoms: oxygen, red; nitrogen, blue; chlorine, green. Figure prepared with pyMol (www.pymol.org).

cocrystallized structures, and their RMSD determined. Murray *et al.* [38] reported cross-docking experiments on three enzymes: thrombin, thermolysin, and neuraminidase. Self-docking (docking the ligand to the cocrystallized structure) achieved a success rate of 76%, while this was reduced to 49% in the case of cross-docking. Working on 10 rigid structures of HIV-1 protease, Bouzida *et al.* [31] also showed the limitations of ignoring protein flexibility in docking.

Cavasotto and Abagyan [39] reported cross-docking and HTD experiments on a set of 33 protein kinases. The success rate of self-docking (100%) dropped to ~70% when cross-docking was performed, following the same trend observed by Murray *et al.* [38]. However, the fraction of ligands that were both correctly cross-docked *and* ranked within the top 10% in a small-scale HTD experiment was ~49%, which has to be compared with the ~70% obtained just by doing cross-docking. This clearly shows that at least in protein kinases, SBVS is more sensitive to target flexibility than ligand docking. From a structural point of view, flexibility of the gly-rich loop and/or changes at the side chain level were responsible for the failures in cross-docking in the studied kinases (Figure 9.2).

Using four different docking methods (DOCK [40], FlexX [41], GOLD [42] and CDOCKER [43]), Erickson *et al.* [44] studied the impact of several structural factors on ligand docking, including protein flexibility. The authors found a fall in the success rate when docking to "average" or apo (unbound) structures, being this correlated

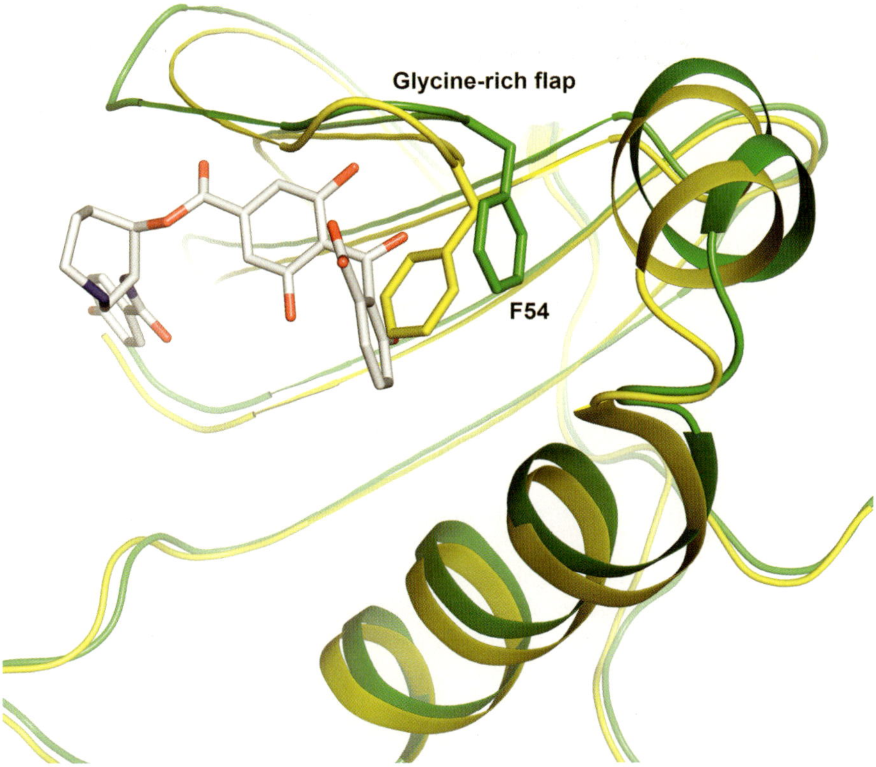

Figure 9.2 Failures in docking due to protein flexibility. Balanol (gray carbon atoms) cannot dock to the adenosine-bound structure of PKA (PDB 1BKX, yellow ribbon) due to clashes with the gly-rich loop, especially with F54. A midrange rearrangement of the gly-rich loop (PDB 1BX6, green ribbon) allows balanol to dock into the target structure. Color code: oxygen, red; nitrogen, blue. Figure prepared with pyMol (www.pymol.org).

with the degree of protein flexibility upon ligand binding. Cross-docking studies of nonnucleoside inhibitors of HIV reverse transcriptases (HIV-NNRTI) to 18 crystal structures also showed a decreased performance when compared to self-docking results [45].

9.3
Accounting for Protein Flexibility in Docking-Based Drug Discovery and Design

The examples provided in the previous section (and others reported elsewhere [46–48]) clearly show the need to account for protein flexibility in docking methods, especially in HTD, by incorporating side chain and backbone flexibility in the binding site. Although there has recently been active developments in this field (cf. Refs [46–50] for a review), a relatively small number of concrete applications of flexible ligand–flexible receptor docking methods in the context of large-scale screening of virtual chemical libraries have been reported. It should be noted that although some methods are too computationally demanding to account for target flexibility in the large-scale HTD, they can still be used for docking a smaller number of molecules, which could be very important at the lead optimization stage.

In this section, we report the application of docking methods incorporating protein flexibility in concrete drug discovery and design projects (cf. Table 9.1). These applications will be grouped according to the type of approach followed to account for target flexibility in docking:

1) Receptor ensemble-based methods, in which several target structures are used as input for docking. In this case, target flexibility (represented by the ensemble of structures) is accounted for prior to the docking procedure, and protein and ligand flexibility are dealt with in a sequential way: protein first, ligand second. This category includes docking to multiple receptor structures or receptor ensemble docking (RED) and docking using ensemble-based optimal structure selection, ensemble-based united protein representation, or ensemble-based potential grids.
2) Single-structure-based methods, in which protein flexibility could be accounted for implicitly (representing the target structure by soft potential maps) or explicitly. In the latter case, the ligand and receptor conformational space could be explored simultaneously (stochastic-based energy optimization docking methods, docking using side chain rotamers, docking using collective degrees of freedom, or molecular dynamics (MD) methods) or sequentially (methods in which protein relaxation follows ligand docking, such as molecular mechanics/Poisson–Boltzmann surface area (MM/PBSA) rescoring). Hybrid methods such as the induced fit docking (IFD) [51] fall also into this category.
3) Multilevel methods, where protein flexibility is accounted for at least in two independent stages of the docking protocol. This is the case of the relaxed complex scheme (RCS) [52, 53], in which an ensemble of unbound target structures is generated by MD and then used to dock a small chemical library

Table 9.1 Applications of docking-based methods incorporating target flexibility at different stages of the drug discovery/design process.

Target	Computational tool	Type of approach	Primary objective	Binding affinity of discovered or optimized ligands	Reference
Aldose reductase	DOCK [40]	Receptor ensemble-based docking	Discovery of new ligands	Low/mid μM	[55]
T4 lysozyme L99A/M102Q	DOCK [40]	Receptor ensemble-based docking	Discovery of new ligands	Low mM	[59]
BACE-1	AutoDock	Receptor ensemble-based docking	Discovery of new ligands	N/A	[60]
PPARγ	GLIDE [61]	Receptor ensemble-based docking	Discovery of new ligands	Low μM	[62]
Asparaginyl-tRNA synthetase	SLIDE [63, 64]	Single-structure-based docking	Discovery of new ligands	μM	[65]
Toxoplasma gondii adenosine kinase	Induced fit docking [51]	Single-structure-based docking	Assessing ligand binding mode	Low μM	[67]
MDM2	Induced fit docking [51]	Single-structure-based docking	Assessing ligand binding mode	nM–μM	[70]
ALK5	GOLD [42]	Single-structure-based docking	SAR data rationalization	N/A	[71]
VEGF	AutoDock/AMBER [72]	Single-structure-based docking	Lead optimization	Low nM	[73]
BoNTAe	MD (AMBER [72])	Single-structure-based docking	Lead optimization	High nM	[74]
Plasmepsin II	BEAR [76]	Single-structure-based docking	Lead optimization	Low nM–low μM	[75]
Aldose reductase 2	DOCK [40]/MD (AMBER [72])	Single-structure-based docking	Drug discovery/lead optimization	Low μM	[77]
RNA-editing ligase	RCS [52, 53]	Multilevel	Drug discovery	Low μM	[78]
Melanin-concentrating hormone receptor-1	Ligand-steered binding site modeling [11, 82]	Homology modeling	Homology modeling/ discovery of new ligands	Low μM	[82]
Cannabinoid receptor-2	Ligand-steered binding site modeling [11, 82]	Homology modeling	SAR data rationalization	N/A	[80, 81]
Neurokinin-1 receptor	Ligand-supported homology modeling [83]	Homology modeling	Homology modeling/ discovery of new ligands	Sub-μM	[84]

using a fast rigid receptor docking tool. Selected complex conformations are then subjected to a refinement/rescoring using a MM/PBSA approach, thus accounting for protein flexibility again at the refinement stage.

4) Docking-based methods used in homology modeling. In this case, flexible docking is used to refine models of binding sites, thus mimicking protein flexibility upon ligand binding.

9.3.1 Receptor Ensemble-Based Docking Methods

One promising strategy to account for target flexibility in SBVS is the use of multiple receptor conformations (MRCs) to perform sequential docking, and then combine the results in a meaningful way. This receptor ensemble docking approach was successfully tested in several systems [39, 54–56]. The target structures can be chosen from experimental sources [57, 58] or *in silico* generated by MD [52, 53] or MC methods [39, 54].

At the initial stage of the project, and if several experimental structures are available, a small-scale HTD using a structural ensemble of the target, followed by cross-docking and enrichment factor analysis, could guide the decision as to whether or not it is critical to actually account for target flexibility in a large-scale HTD. It was shown that using two or three representative structures as a target ensemble, better RMSD and enrichment factors can be obtained for protein kinases [39]. HTD results were combined using the *merging and shrinking* procedure that, for each compound, keeps the best rank among those corresponding to different structures in the ensemble. This procedure was tested on 21 groups of 2 or 3 protein kinase complexes by measuring changes in the enrichment factor, obtaining an improvement of approximately twofold when the top 1%, 5%, and 10% of the ranked database was evaluated. Since a soft representation of the receptor was used in the above-mentioned study, it can be concluded that at least in the case of protein kinases, RED performs better than single-structure soft-grid rigid docking. This was the same conclusion reached by Ferrari *et al.* [55] while investigating the performance of soft grid docking versus RED in HTD on two cavity sites of T4 lysozyme and aldose reductase. The former undergoes small but important structural changes upon ligand binding, while the latter undergoes large structural changes. The Available Chemicals Directory (ACD) seeded with known ligands was screened against those targets, and it was found that, when one structure is used, although rigid docking using a soft representation of the target outperforms docking using a hard representation, this is reversed when MRCs are used. In an attempt to assess the predictability of this approach, six top-ranking molecules of aldose reductase from the RED, which ranked poorly in the soft docking calculation, were prioritized for experimental testing. Four out of six exhibited enzymatic inhibition in the low micromolar range.

Working on a modified version of DOCK, a novel algorithm combining multiple flexible regions from experimental structures into a set of discrete receptor conformations was developed to incorporate flexibility into structure-based drug discovery [59]. This method scales linearly and not exponentially with the number of degrees of freedom. This protocol was first evaluated on a hydrophobic binding site of the L99A mutant of T4 lysozyme, using the ACD library seeded with known binders. Initial calculations showed that large decoy molecules ranked better than small known binders, which clearly affected the quality of the enrichment factor. To achieve proper differentiation between known binders and "decoy" compounds, a receptor conformational energy weighting term was incorporated. The same type of calculations performed on thymidylate synthase also showed the better performance of the protocol incorporating receptor flexibility versus single structure docking. To test the predictability of this approach, the ACD library was screened against a polar binding site of a T4 mutant (L99A/M102Q). Eighteen new molecules that were predicted to bind and change the conformation of the binding site were tested experimentally, identifying 14 binders among them. These identified binders were also cocrystallized and it was observed a very good correlation between the actual ligand binding poses and the predicted ones.

Inhibition of β-secretase (BACE-1) is an attractive strategy for anti-Alzheimer therapy. However, a rational approach to this has been hindered by the flexibility of this protein. In a recent contribution [60], a RED approach was undertaken to discover new BACE-1 inhibitors. This was accomplished by performing HTD of the NCI database using AutoDock (http://autodock.scripps.edu) in two ways: first, through HTD on an ensemble of static X-ray BACE-1 structures, thus accounting for target flexibility through MRCs; second, by combining the above-mentioned structures to generate a single structure that encoded the protein motion and performing HTD on this averaged structure. The latter approach was accomplished by combining energy maps using an energy weighting scheme. The authors reported that *in vitro* testing of top-ranking compounds led to the discovery of new leads.

A RED approach was used to screen a library of natural products against PPARγ, a target involved in many diseases, including type II diabetes mellitus. HTD was performed with GLIDE [61] onto two PPARγ crystal structures (cf. Figure 9.3), and it revealed 29 potential agonists [62]. Six flavonoids were identified in a PPARγ transcriptional activity assay, and one of these six displayed low micromolar activity, $EC_{50} = 2.9\ \mu M$. To further structurally characterize the ligands' mechanism of action, induced fit docking [51] was performed, showing evidence that five active flavonoids induce conformational change in the receptor upon binding.

9.3.2
Single-Structure-Based Docking Methods

Seven classes of micromolar inhibitors of the enzyme Brugia malayi asparaginyl-tRNA synthetase (AsnRS), a target for antiparasitic drug design, were discovered using SLIDE software [63, 64], which docks flexible ligands to a binding site, followed by side chain relaxation. Seven classes of compounds were found to exhibit micromolar inhibitory activity toward the enzyme [65], while relative affinities predicted by SLIDE acceptably correlate with the ranking in experimental testing. Some analogues to one of the classes of ligands, the long side chain variolins, cannot

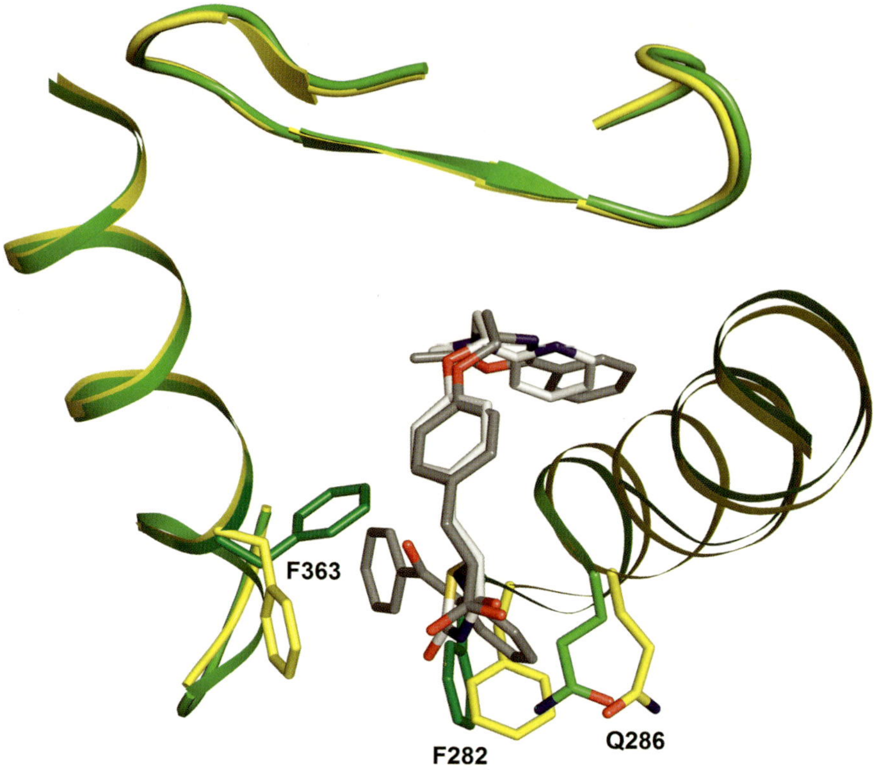

Figure 9.3 Side chain flexibility in nuclear receptor PPARγ. Comparing crystal structures 1FM6 and 1FM9, it is observed that three residues exhibit marked flexibility in the PPARγ binding site: F282, Q286, and F363. The cocrystallized ligands are also displayed, clearly showing how cross-docking of those ligands would fail. These two structures were used to discover novel PPARγ agonists using a receptor ensemble docking approach with GLIDE [62]. Protein ribbon and carbon atoms color code: 1FM6: green; 1FM9: yellow. Ligands carbon atoms color code: 1FM6: light gray; 1FM9, dark gray. Color code for noncarbon atoms: oxygen, red; nitrogen, blue. Figure prepared with pyMol (www.pymol.org).

be docked into the adenosyl pocket of AsnRS closed conformation due to steric clashes, though the short side chain variolins could dock. The authors hypothesized that the reason for this was the mobility of the motif 2 loop, which allows long side chain variolins to bind in the adenosine site. Modeling loop flexibility using rigidity-optimized conformational kinetics [66] (ROCK) indeed confirmed this hypotheses. Thus, combining ROCK and SLIDE could provide an interesting approach to incorporate flexibility at the backbone and side chain level in docking-based drug design.

A series of N^6-benzyladenosine analogues were synthesized and evaluated for binding affinity on *Toxoplasma gondii* adenosine kinase, a relevant target for anti-toxoplasma agents [67]. Among the tested analogues, N^6-(2,4-dimethoxybenzyl) adenosine displayed favorable antitoxoplasma activity (low micromolar) without host toxicity. Schrodinger's induced fit [51, 68] was used to assess the binding mode of N^6-benzyladenosine analogues. Molecular modeling revealed that the enhanced binding of N^6-(2,4-dimethoxybenzyl)adenosine correlates with the favorable van der Waals interaction of hydrophobic residues Y169, F201, L46, and L142 with the benzyl moiety of the ligand. The binding energy trend of N^6-(2,4-dimethoxybenzyl)adenosine and other two N^6-benzyladenosine analogues was also correctly estimated by induced fit docking and energy minimization.

Five nonpeptide, small-molecule inhibitors of the human MDM2 – p53 protein–protein interaction were discovered using the dynamic pharmacophore method [69]. Although not a docking-based method, the dynamic pharmacophore uses input from MRCs to create a pharmacophore model that accounts for protein flexibility; that model is then used to virtual screen large chemical libraries. Docking of the five discovered inhibitors with IFD suggested that the inhibitors mimicked the binding residues F19, W23, and L26 of p53 [70]. The docking poses also predicted enhanced ligand–receptor hydrogen bond interaction within the binding cleft.

Studying the inhibition of the transforming growth factor beta type 1 receptor (ALK5) and its selectivity against ALK4/ALK7 with nitrogenous heterocycle compounds – 1,2,4-trisubstituted imidazoles and 1,3,5-trisubstituted pyrazoles, two molecules showed a relative potent inhibition toward ALK5 and weak cytotoxicity, with an acceptable selectivity versus ALK4/ALK7 (10 times better than the known ALK5 inhibitor SB431 542) [71]. In order to assess the structural determinants of ligand binding, the binding mode of one of the best inhibitors was determined using flexible docking with GOLD 3.1 and setting the side chains of K232 and D351 flexible. Several tight ligand–ALK5 interactions were predicted, obtaining a correct rationalization of SAR data.

The vascular endothelial growth factor (VEGF) is implicated in uncontrolled angiogenesis, thus becoming a relevant drug target. Papakyriakou *et al.* performed docking (using AutoDock) and MD (using AMBER [72]) studies on potent members of the anthranilamide class of VEGFR-2 inhibitors [73]. Molecular recognition patterns observed from the computational modeling that accounted for receptor flexibility in implicit aqueous environment guided the design and synthesis of new analogues from existing scaffolds by altering their steric and electronic characteristics. Experimental evaluation of these analogues showed several novel VEGFR-2 low nanomolar inhibitors with less cytotoxic effects and more potent than the parent compounds.

Botulism, a neuroparalytic life-threatening disease, is caused by the botulinum neurotoxin serotype A (BoNTA). Although antibodies are effective in preventing the extracellular toxin to continue the intoxication process, they have no effect on prior intoxicated neurons. Targeting the BoNTA endopeptidase (BoNTAe) could be a valid alternative, since its inhibition may potentially neutralize the intracellular BoNTA. Pang *et al.* performed molecular dynamics (using AMBER) of a low micromolar inhibitor complexed with BoNTAe to guide lead optimization. They found a serotype-selective, small-molecule, high-nanomolar competitive inhibitor of BoNTAe, nearly an order of magnitude more potent than its parent compound [74]. This was also aided by a synthesis-based computer-aided molecular design protocol, which incorporates synthetic feasibility into the design, in addition to binding energy and selectivity.

Plasmepsin II, a *Plasmodium falciparum* aspartic protease, is an important drug target in the fight against malaria. In fact, effective plasmepsin inhibitors could serve as an alternative strategy alone or in synergy with other existing antimalarial drugs. Degliesposti *et al.* [75] performed a postprocessing refinement of a HTD of commercially available libraries using BEAR [76], a refinement/rescoring protocol that incorporates protein flexibility through MD simulations, which also allows to compute binding free energy estimation using MM–PBSA and MM–GBSA. Among the top-ranking compounds, four chemotypes were highly populated: *N*-alkoxyamidines, guanidines, amides, and ureas and thioureas. Thirty representative molecules of each cluster were selected for further bioevaluation, taking into account their binding free energy and key ligand–plasmepsin interactions. Inhibition experiments based on FRET substrate degradation showed that 26 out of the 30 tested compounds inhibited plasmepsin II between the low nanomolar and low micromolar range.

Targeting aldose reductase (ALR2), a relevant target for the treatment of diabetes, Rastelli *et al.* [77] performed rigid receptor HTD using DOCK of the NCI library (127 000 compounds), followed by experimental testing for ALR2 binding and selectivity toward ALR1. Five of the tested compounds showed activity in the micromolar range toward ALR2. The structures of the complexes between the five inhibitors and ALR2 were determined and refined using modeling and MD simulations (AMBER) and were used to guide lead optimization. Starting with a micromolar hit ($IC_{50} = 42\,\mu M$) and after rounds of synthesis, a compound showing 10-fold improve in binding affinity and 10-fold better selectivity toward ALR1 was found. The binding mode was also in agreement with SAR data rationalization.

9.3.3
Multilevel Methods

Recently, druglike inhibitors of the RNA-editing ligase 1 (REL1) enzyme, a drug target relevant to tropical and subtropical diseases, were developed by using a structure-based drug design procedure incorporating target flexibility [78]. Starting from a HTD using the NCI Diversity Set on the REL1 X-ray structure using AutoDock4 program, the 30 best ranking compounds predicted to interact with REL1's ATP-binding site were further refined with the RCS method [52, 53], which redocks compounds to a structural ensemble of the target generated through MD considering explicit solvation. After filtering the candidates according to druglike filters, two out of eight compounds displayed micromolar affinity toward REL1. A further similarity search against the full NCI library and the RCS refinement of the best candidates gave two out of six REL1 inhibitors with $IC_{50} \sim 1\,\mu M$. Three of the most promising compounds also displayed a considerable degree of selectivity toward RNA ligases. A similar approach had also been used to predict potential ligands targeting the avian influenza virus subtype H5N1, a potential pandemic threat resistant to antiviral drugs [79].

9.3.4
Homology Modeling

As an obvious consequence of protein flexibility, different ligands are sometimes observed to bind to different binding site conformations. This, in fact, is the reason why many cross-docking experiments fail. In such cases, modeling of the binding site with a nonnative ligand can be achieved with many of the single-structure-based docking methods. As it has been shown, this could be a valuable tool for lead optimization purposes or to generate structurally different target structures to be used in a HTD context [39].

Extending this idea, the ligand-steered homology modeling method uses existing ligands to shape and optimize the binding site through a docking-based stochastic global energy minimization procedure [11]. In this case, the target to be modeled and the structural template are different proteins. The goal is to generate a 3D representation of the complex to rationalize SAR data [80, 81], to guide lead optimization, or to use the target model structure with HTD purposes. This approach was tested on the melanin-concentrating hormone receptor-1 (MCH-R1), a target for antiobesity drugs [82]. A HTD performed on ligand-steered developed models and followed by experimental testing resulted in six low micromolar compounds. A related approach had been presented by Klebe and coworkers in the context of homology modeling, where information about ligand binding was incorporated in the modeling process by user-defined ligand–protein restraints derived from manual placement or rigid docking [83]; models thus generated were used to virtually screen a chemical library against the neurokinin-1 receptor, discovering submicromolar binders [84].

9.4
Conclusions

Accounting for protein flexibility in docking and high-throughput docking in an efficient and affordable way still remains a major hurdle in computer-aided drug discovery. In recent years, several new strategies incorporating the flexibility of the target in docking-based methods have been developed and evaluated, but a relative small number of actual applications of these new tools in the context of drug discovery and design have been published. In this chapter, we presented the theoretical foundation of the problem of docking with target flexibility and a number of cases where docking clearly failed for ignoring this effect. This was followed by examples of drug discovery/design or lead optimization projects where docking and HTD methods accounting for target flexibility were successfully used. The review of this limited number of cases available shows that, so far, the use of the receptor ensemble-based approach perhaps remains the most promising approach to discover novel ligands. For *in silico* guided lead optimization, promising results were obtained by using refinement by molecular dynamics. The lack of extensive validation of many of the docking-based methods incorporating target flexibility, coupled with the reduced number of successful applications of those methods to concrete drug discovery and/or lead optimization cases, shows that more effort is still needed to come up with an approach that is computationally affordable and yet accurate enough to be used in a predictive way.

References

1 Entzeroth, M. (2003) Emerging trends in high-throughput screening. *Current Opinion in Pharmacology*, **3**, 522–529.

2 Mahapatra, A. (2008) Screening for success. *ACS Chemical Biology*, **3**, 449–450.

3 Phatak, S.S., Stephan, C.C., and Cavasotto, C.N. (2009) High-throughput and *in silico* screenings in drug discovery. *Expert Opinion on Drug Discovery*, **4**, 947–959.

4 Kontoyianni, M., Madhav, P., Suchanek, E., and Seibel, W. (2008) Theoretical and practical considerations in virtual screening: a beaten field? *Current Medicinal Chemistry*, **15**, 107–116.

5 Cavasotto, C.N. and Orry, A.J. (2007) Ligand docking and structure-based virtual screening in drug discovery. *Current Topics in Medicinal Chemistry*, **7**, 1006–1014.

6 Kitchen, D.B., Decornez, H., Furr, J.R., and Bajorath, J. (2004) Docking and scoring in virtual screening for drug discovery: methods and applications. *Nature Reviews. Drug Discovery*, **3**, 935–949.

7 Lundstrom, K. (2007) Structural genomics and drug discovery. *Journal of Cellular and Molecular Medicine*, **11**, 224–238.

8 Orry, A.J., Abagyan, R.A., and Cavasotto, C.N. (2006) Structure-based development of target-specific compound libraries. *Drug Discovery Today*, **11**, 261–266.

9 Schnur, D.M. (2008) Recent trends in library design: "rational design" revisited. *Current Opinion in Drug Discovery & Development*, **11**, 375–380.

10 Blundell, T.L., Sibanda, B.L., Montalvao, R.W., Brewerton, S., Chelliah, V., Worth, C.L., Harmer, N.J., Davies, O., and Burke, D. (2006) Structural biology and bioinformatics in drug design: opportunities and challenges for target identification and lead discovery. *Philosophical Transactions of the Royal Society of London. Series B, Biological Sciences*, **361**, 413–423.

11 Cavasotto, C.N. and Phatak, S.S. (2009) Homology modeling in drug discovery: current trends and applications. *Drug Discovery Today*, **14**, 676–683.

12 Stevens, R.C. (2004) Long live structural biology. *Nature Structural & Molecular Biology*, **11**, 293–295.

13 Jorgensen, W.L. (2004) The many roles of computation in drug discovery. *Science*, **303**, 1813–1818.

14 Beddell, C.R., Goodford, P.J., Norrington, F.E., Wilkinson, S., and Wootton, R. (1976) Compounds designed to fit a site of known structure in human hemoglobin. *British Journal of Pharmacology*, **57**, 201–209.

15 Kuntz, I.D., Blaney, J.M., Oatley, S.J., Langridge, R., and Ferrin, T.E. (1982) A geometric approach to macromolecule–ligand interactions. *Journal of Molecular Biology*, **161**, 269–288.

16 Goodford, P.J. (1985) A computational procedure for determining energetically favorable binding sites on biologically important macromolecules. *Journal of Medicinal Chemistry*, **28**, 849–857.

17 Sperandio, O., Miteva, M.A., Delfaud, F., and Villoutreix, B.O. (2006) Receptor-based computational screening of compound databases: the main docking-scoring engines. *Current Protein & Peptide Science*, **7**, 369–393.

18 Corbeil, C.R., Englebienne, P., and Moitessier, N. (2007) Docking ligands into flexible and solvated macromolecules. 1. Development and validation of FITTED

1.0. *Journal of Chemical Information and Modeling*, **47**, 435–449.

19 Fischer, E. (1894) Einfluss der configuration auf die wirkung derenzyme. *Berichte der Deutschen Chemischen Gesellschaft*, **27**, 2985–2993.

20 Koshland, D.E., Jr. (1995) The key-lock theory and the induced fit theory. *Angewandte Chemie, International Edition*, **33**, 2375–2378.

21 Koshland, D.E., Jr. (1958) Application of a theory of enzyme specificity to protein synthesis. *Proceedings of the National Academy of Sciences of the United States of America*, **44**, 98–123.

22 Ma, B., Kumar, S., Tsai, C.J., and Nussinov, R. (1999) Folding funnels and binding mechanisms. *Protein Engineering*, **12**, 713–720.

23 Tsai, C.J., Kumar, S., Ma, B., and Nussinov, R. (1999) Folding funnels, binding funnels, and protein function. *Protein Science*, **8**, 1181–1190.

24 Berger, C., Weber-Bornhauser, S., Eggenberger, J., Hanes, J., Pluckthun, A., and Bosshard, H.R. (1999) Antigen recognition by conformational selection. *FEBS Letters*, **450**, 149–153.

25 James, L.C., Roversi, P., and Tawfik, D.S. (2003) Antibody multispecificity mediated by conformational diversity. *Science*, **299**, 1362–1367.

26 Tobi, D. and Bahar, I. (2005) Structural changes involved in protein binding correlate with intrinsic motions of proteins in the unbound state. *Proceedings of the National Academy of Sciences of the United States of America*, **102**, 18908–18913.

27 Van Regenmortel, M.H. (1999) Molecular recognition in the post-reductionist era. *Journal of Molecular Recognition*, **12**, 1–2.

28 Bosshard, H.R. (2001) Molecular recognition by induced fit: how fit is the concept? *News in Physiological Sciences*, **16**, 171–173.

29 Ikeguchi, M., Ueno, J., Sato, M., and Kidera, A. (2005) Protein structural change upon ligand binding: linear response theory. *Physical Review Letters*, **94**, 078102.

30 Teague, S.J. (2003) Implications of protein flexibility for drug discovery. *Nature Reviews. Drug Discovery*, **2**, 527–541.

31 Bouzida, D., Rejto, P.A., Arthurs, S., Colson, A.B., Freer, S.T., Gehlhaar, D.K., Larson, V., Luty, B.A., Rose, P.W., and Verkhivker, G.M. (1999) Computer simulations of ligand–protein binding with ensembles of protein conformations: a Monte Carlo study of HIV-1 protease binding energy landscapes. *International Journal of Quantum Chemistry*, **72**, 73–84.

32 Pargellis, C., Tong, L., Churchill, L., Cirillo, P.F., Gilmore, T., Graham, A.G., Grob, P.M., Hickey, E.R., Moss, N., Pav, S., and Regan, J. (2002) Inhibition of p38 MAP kinase by utilizing a novel allosteric binding site. *Nature Structural Biology*, **9**, 268–272.

33 Cody, V., Galitsky, N., Rak, D., Luft, J.R., Pangborn, W., and Queener, S.F. (1999) Ligand-induced conformational changes in the crystal structures of *Pneumocystis carinii* dihydrofolate reductase complexes with folate and NADP(+). *Biochemistry*, **38**, 4303–4312.

34 Schweitzer, B.I., Dicker, A.P., and Bertino, J.R. (1990) Dihydrofolate-reductase as a therapeutic target. *The FASEB Journal*, **4**, 2441–2452.

35 Smith, G.M., Alexander, R.S., Christianson, D.W., McKeever, B.M., Ponticello, G.S., Springer, J.P., Randall, W.C., Baldwin, J.J., and Habecker, C.N. (1994) Positions of His-64 and a bound water in human carbonic-anhydrase-II upon binding three structurally related inhibitors. *Protein Science*, **3**, 118–125.

36 Kryger, G., Silman, I., and Sussman, J.L. (1999) Structure of acetylcholinesterase complexed with E2020 (Aricept (R)): implications for the design of new anti-Alzheimer drugs. *Structure*, **7**, 297–307.

37 Najmanovich, R., Kuttner, J., Sobolev, V., and Edelman, M. (2000) Side-chain flexibility in proteins upon ligand binding. *Proteins*, **39**, 261–268.

38 Murray, C.W., Baxter, C.A., and Frenkel, A.D. (1999) The sensitivity of the results of molecular docking to induced fit effects: application to thrombin, thermolysin and neuraminidase. *Journal of Computer-Aided Molecular Design*, **13**, 547–562.

39 Cavasotto, C.N. and Abagyan, R.A. (2004) Protein flexibility in ligand docking and virtual screening to protein kinases. *Journal of Molecular Biology*, **337**, 209–225.

40 Meng, E.C., Shoichet, B.K., and Kuntz, I.D. (1992) Automated docking with grid-based energy evaluation. *Journal of Computational Chemistry*, **13**, 505–524.

41 Rarey, M., Kramer, B., Lengauer, T., and Klebe, G. (1996) A fast flexible docking method using an incremental construction algorithm. *Journal of Molecular Biology*, **261**, 470–489.

42 Jones, G., Willett, P., and Glen, R.C. (1995) Molecular recognition of receptor sites using a genetic algorithm with a description of desolvation. *Journal of Molecular Biology*, **245**, 43–53.

43 Wu, G.S., Robertson, D.H., Brooks, C.L., and Vieth, M. (2003) Detailed analysis of grid-based molecular docking: a case study of CDOCKER – a CHARMm-based MD docking algorithm. *Journal of Computational Chemistry*, **24**, 1549–1562.

44 Erickson, J.A., Jalaie, M., Robertson, D.H., Lewis, R.A., and Vieth, M. (2004) Lessons in molecular recognition: the effects of ligand and protein flexibility on molecular docking accuracy. *Journal of Medicinal Chemistry*, **47**, 45–55.

45 Daeyaert, F., de Jonge, M., Heeres, J., Koymans, L., Lewi, P., Vinkers, M.H., and Janssen, P.A. (2004) A pharmacophore docking algorithm and its application to the cross-docking of 18 HIV-NNRTI's in their binding pockets. *Proteins*, **54**, 526–533.

46 Cozzini, P., Kellogg, G.E., Spyrakis, F., Abraham, D.J., Costantino, G., Emerson, A., Fanelli, F., Gohlke, H., Kuhn, L.A., Morris, G.M., Orozco, M., Pertinhez, T.A., Rizzi, M., and Sotriffer, C.A. (2008) Target flexibility: an emerging consideration in drug discovery and design. *Journal of Medicinal Chemistry*, **51**, 6237–6255.

47 Barril, X. and Fradera, X. (2006) Incorporating protein flexibility into docking and structure-based drug design. *Expert Opinion on Drug Discovery*, **1**, 335–349.

48 Cavasotto, C.N. and Singh, N. (2008) Docking and high throughput docking: successes and the challenge of protein flexibility. *Current Computer-Aided Drug Design*, **4**, 221–234.

49 B-Rao, C., Subramanian, J., and Sharma, S.D. (2009) Managing protein flexibility in docking and its applications. *Drug Discovery Today*, **14**, 394–400.

50 Corbeil, C.R. and Moitessier, N. (2009) Docking ligands into flexible and solvated macromolecules. 3. Impact of input ligand conformation, protein flexibility, and water molecules on the accuracy of docking programs. *Journal of Chemical Information and Modeling*, **49**, 997–1009.

51 Sherman, W., Day, T., Jacobson, M.P., Friesner, R.A., and Farid, R. (2006) Novel procedure for modeling ligand/receptor induced fit effects. *Journal of Medicinal Chemistry*, **49**, 534–553.

52 Lin, J.H., Perryman, A.L., Schames, J.R., and McCammon, J.A. (2002) Computational drug design accommodating receptor flexibility: the relaxed complex scheme. *Journal of the American Chemical Society*, **124**, 5632–5633.

53 Lin, J.H., Perryman, A.L., Schames, J.R., and McCammon, J.A. (2003) The relaxed complex method: accommodating receptor flexibility for drug design with an improved scoring scheme. *Biopolymers*, **68**, 47–62.

54 Cavasotto, C.N., Kovacs, J.A., and Abagyan, R.A. (2005) Representing receptor flexibility in ligand docking through relevant normal modes. *Journal of the American Chemical Society*, **127**, 9632–9640.

55 Ferrari, A.M., Wei, B.Q., Costantino, L., and Shoichet, B.K. (2004) Soft docking and multiple receptor conformations in virtual screening. *Journal of Medicinal Chemistry*, **47**, 5076–5084.

56 Duca, J.S., Madison, V.S., and Voigt, J.H. (2008) Cross-docking of inhibitors into CDK2 structures. 1. *Journal of Chemical Information and Modeling*, **48**, 659–668.

57 Barril, X. and Morley, S.D. (2005) Unveiling the full potential of flexible receptor docking using multiple crystallographic structures. *Journal of Medicinal Chemistry*, **48**, 4432–4443.

58 Knegtel, R.M., Kuntz, I.D., and Oshiro, C.M. (1997) Molecular docking to ensembles of protein structures. *Journal of Molecular Biology*, **266**, 424–440.

59 Wei, B.Q., Weaver, L.H., Ferrari, A.M., Matthews, B.W., and Shoichet, B.K. (2004) Testing a flexible-receptor docking algorithm in a model binding site. *Journal of Molecular Biology*, **337**, 1161–1182.

60 Cosconati, S., Huey, R., Marinelli, L., Novellino, E., Goodsell, D.S., and Olson, A.J. (2008) Identification of novel β-secretase inhibitors through the inclusion of protein flexibility in virtual screening calculations. *The FASEB Journal*, **22**, 791.8.

61 Friesner, R.A., Murphy, R.B., Repasky, M.P., Frye, L.L., Greenwood, J.R., Halgren, T.A., Sanschagrin, P.C., and Mainz, D.T. (2006) Extra precision glide: docking and scoring incorporating a model of hydrophobic enclosure for protein–ligand complexes. *Journal of Medicinal Chemistry*, **49**, 6177–6196.

62 Salam, N.K., Huang, T.H., Kota, B.P., Kim, M.S., Li, Y., and Hibbs, D.E. (2008) Novel PPAR-gamma agonists identified from a natural product library: a virtual screening, induced-fit docking and biological assay study. *Chemical Biology & Drug Design*, **71**, 57–70.

63 Schnecke, V. and Kuhn, L.A. (2000) Virtual screening with solvation and ligand-induced complementarity. *Perspectives in Drug Discovery and Design*, **20**, 171–190.

64 Schnecke, V., Swanson, C.A., Getzoff, E.D., Tainer, J.A., and Kuhn, L.A. (1998) Screening a peptidyl database for potential ligands to proteins with side-chain flexibility. *Proteins*, **33**, 74–87.

65 Sukuru, S.C., Crepin, T., Milev, Y., Marsh, L.C., Hill, J.B., Anderson, R.J., Morris, J.C., Rohatgi, A., O'Mahony, G., Grotli, M., Danel, F., Page, M.G., Hartlein, M., Cusack, S., Kron, M.A., and Kuhn, L.A. (2006) Discovering new classes of Brugia malayi asparaginyl-tRNA synthetase inhibitors and relating specificity to conformational change. *Journal of Computer-Aided Molecular Design*, **20**, 159–178.

66 Zavodszky, M.I., Lei, M., Thorpe, M.F., Day, A.R., and Kuhn, L.A. (2004) Modeling correlated main-chain motions in proteins for flexible molecular recognition. *Proteins*, **57**, 243–261.

67 Kim, Y.A., Sharon, A., Chu, C.K., Rais, R.H., Al Safarjalani, O.N., Naguib, F.N., and el Kouni, M.H. (2007) Synthesis, biological evaluation and molecular modeling studies of *N*6-benzyladenosine analogues as potential anti-toxoplasma agents. *Biochemical Pharmacology*, **73**, 1558–1572.

68 Sherman, W., Beard, H.S., and Farid, R. (2006) Use of an induced fit receptor structure in virtual screening. *Chemical Biology & Drug Design*, **67**, 83–84.

69 Carlson, H.A., Masukawa, K.M., and McCammon, J.A. (1999) Method for including the dynamic fluctuations of a protein in computer-aided drug design. *Journal of Physical Chemistry A*, **103**, 10213–10219.

70 Bowman, A.L., Nikolovska-Coleska, Z., Zhong, H., Wang, S., and Carlson, H.A. (2007) Small molecule inhibitors of the MDM2-p53 interaction discovered by ensemble-based receptor models. *Journal of the American Chemical Society*, **129**, 12809–12814.

71 Li, X., Wang, L., Long, L., Xiao, J., Hu, Y., and Li, S. (2009) Synthesis and biological evaluation of 1,2,4-trisubstituted imidazoles and 1,3,5-trisubstituted pyrazoles as inhibitors of transforming growth factor beta type 1 receptor (ALK5). *Bioorganic & Medicinal Chemistry Letters*, **19**, 4868–4872.

72 Case, D.A., Cheatham, T.E., 3rd, Darden, T., Gohlke, H., Luo, R., Merz, K.M., Jr., Onufriev, A., Simmerling, C., Wang, B., and Woods, R.J. (2005) The Amber biomolecular simulation programs. *Journal of Computational Chemistry*, **26**, 1668–1688.

73 Papakyriakou, A., Katsarou, M.E., Belimezi, M., Karpusas, M., and Vourloumis, D. (2009) Discovery of potent vascular endothelial growth factor

receptor-2 inhibitors. *ChemMedChem*, **5**, 118–129.

74 Pang, Y.P., Vummenthala, A., Mishra, R.K., Park, J.G., Wang, S., Davis, J., Millard, C.B., and Schmidt, J.J. (2009) Potent new small-molecule inhibitor of botulinum neurotoxin serotype A endopeptidase developed by synthesis-based computer-aided molecular design. *PLoS One*, **4**, e7730.

75 Degliesposti, G., Kasam, V., Da Costa, A., Kang, H.K., Kim, N., Kim, D.W., Breton, V., Kim, D., and Rastelli, G. (2009) Design and discovery of plasmepsin II inhibitors using an automated workflow on large-scale grids. *ChemMedChem*, **4**, 1164–1173.

76 Rastelli, G., Degliesposti, G., Del Rio, A., and Sgobba, M. (2009) Binding estimation after refinement, a new automated procedure for the refinement and rescoring of docked ligands in virtual screening. *Chemical Biology & Drug Design*, **73**, 283–286.

77 Rastelli, G., Ferrari, A.M., Costantino, L., and Gamberini, M.C. (2002) Discovery of new inhibitors of aldose reductase from molecular docking and database screening. *Bioorganic & Medicinal Chemistry Letters*, **10**, 1437–1450.

78 Amaro, R.E., Schnaufer, A., Interthal, H., Hol, W., Stuart, K.D., and McCammon, J.A. (2008) Discovery of drug-like inhibitors of an essential RNA-editing ligase in *Trypanosoma brucei*. *Proceedings of the National Academy of Sciences of the United States of America*, **105**, 17278–17283.

79 Cheng, L.S., Amaro, R.E., Xu, D., Li, W.W., Arzberger, P.W., and McCammon, J.A. (2008) Ensemble-based virtual screening reveals potential novel antiviral compounds for avian influenza neuraminidase. *Journal of Medicinal Chemistry*, **51**, 3878–3894.

80 Diaz, P., Phatak, S.S., Xu, J., Astruc-Diaz, F., Cavasotto, C.N., and Naguib, M. (2009) 6-Methoxy-*N*-alkyl isatin acylhydrazone derivatives as a novel series of potent selective cannabinoid receptor 2 inverse agonists: design, synthesis, and binding mode prediction. *Journal of Medicinal Chemistry*, **52**, 433–444.

81 Diaz, P., Phatak, S.S., Xu, J., Fronczek, F.R., Astruc-Diaz, F., Thompson, C.M., Cavasotto, C.N., and Naguib, M. (2009) 2,3-dihydro-1-benzofuran derivatives as a series of potent selective cannabinoid receptor 2 agonists: design, synthesis, and binding mode prediction through ligand-steered modeling. *ChemMedChem*, **4**, 1615–1629.

82 Cavasotto, C.N., Orry, A.J., Murgolo, N.J., Czarniecki, M.F., Kocsi, S.A., Hawes, B.E., O'Neill, K.A., Hine, H., Burton, M.S., Voigt, J.H., Abagyan, R.A., Bayne, M.L., and Monsma, F.J., Jr. (2008) Discovery of novel chemotypes to a G-protein-coupled receptor through ligand-steered homology modeling and structure-based virtual screening. *Journal of Medicinal Chemistry*, **51**, 581–588.

83 Evers, A., Gohlke, H., and Klebe, G. (2003) Ligand-supported homology modelling of protein binding-sites using knowledge-based potentials. *Journal of Molecular Biology*, **334**, 327–345.

84 Evers, A. and Klebe, G. (2004) Successful virtual screening for a submicromolar antagonist of the neurokinin-1 receptor based on a ligand-supported homology model. *Journal of Medicinal Chemistry*, **47**, 5381–5392.

10
Consideration of Water and Solvation Effects in Virtual Screening

Johannes Kirchmair, Gudrun M. Spitzer, and Klaus R. Liedl

10.1
Introduction

Water is the essence of life. While it is recognized as the essential medium for any being, its omnipresent and deep impact on life at the microscopic, atomic level is often underestimated or disregarded due to the complexity of its nature. In the field of virtual screening, expanding collections of easily accessible chemical compounds on the one hand and the increasing amount of structurally determined drug targets on the other hand ask for efficient virtual screening methods that simplify or even disregard some of the effects of water molecules on ligand binding. Obviously, the success of a virtual screening method is inherently connected to the simplifications and assumptions being made. Several aspects of the protein–ligand binding process are highly complex and make it fairly difficult to choose what kind of effects to consider in detail and which ones to approximate or to neglect. Moreover, even cutting-edge methods do not necessarily imply superior predictive power [1].

Thermodynamic effects on ligand binding affinity can roughly be divided into two classes: enthalpic contributions, which can be derived from electrostatic and van der Waals potentials by examining the distances between interacting groups, and entropic contributions, which arise from the dynamics of theses groups.

The binding of a ligand to a macromolecule is limited by a loss in rotational and translational entropy. Moreover, water molecules play a pivotal role during the binding process, acting as mediators of interactions between both binding partners, thereby significantly contributing to the overall thermodynamics of the system. Both ligand and protein need to strip off or at least to rearrange their solvation shell and water molecules during the approach of the ligand to the receptor. Ligands capable of displacing certain water molecules from the protein surface to the less-ordered solvent phase frequently show superior affinity to their target due to favorable entropic effects [2].

The binding free energy of a water molecule is determined by its close neighborhood. While tightly bound water molecules are primarily located in tight hydrophilic pockets where they form several H-bonds with the protein and ligand, weakly

Virtual Screening. Edited by C. Sotriffer

ISBN: 978-3-527-32636-5

bound water molecules are usually located in rather hydrophobic areas of the protein where H-bonding is limited by the surroundings. Barillari *et al.* analyzed the properties of protein-bound water molecules and found that the binding free energy of conserved water molecules is more favorable than that of water molecules displaced upon binding of small organic molecules [3].

Complexity arises from the combination and compensation of enthalpic and entropic effects, which depend on the geometry, charging, polarity and dynamics of the binding site. While it is feasible to compute enthalpic energies from the respective potentials, it is highly challenging to quantify dynamics and disorder and, hence, entropy. The assessment of the latter requires an explicit representation of the solvent molecules involved in the formation of a complex. Only an accurate calculation of entropic and enthalpic effects induced by water upon ligand binding allows to draw conclusions with respect to ligand design [3].

Water molecules can act as potential H-bond acceptors and donors and form up to a maximum of four H-bonds simultaneously. Their stability and localization becomes more pronounced with increasing number of H-bonding interactions [4, 5]. The large number of binding partners usually indicates a higher degree of conservation. Water molecules can act as a flexible connector for bridging noncovalent interactions between ligand and receptor [4]. They may alter the degree of hydrophobicity and the electrostatics of the binding site by interlinked and complex effects. Sleigh *et al.* [6] and Tame *et al.* [7] have demonstrated the important role of water in shielding electric charges, enabling both charged and hydrophobic ligands to bind to the peptide binding protein OppA. Moreover, water molecules influence structure and dynamics of the binding site region [8]. Water has also been shown to guide ligand specificity and affinity, as in the case of different kinds of substrates binding to L-arabinose-binding protein (ABP) [9] or serine proteases [10]. It can act as a discriminator of substrate and product (e.g., to enhance product release and, thus, to increase enzymatic turnover) [11] and serve as reagent and proton transporter in biochemical reactions [12–14]. The latter one points out the possible therapeutic potential of inhibitors designed to block such essential water molecules in the active site of an enzyme.

An interesting aspect of the protein–ligand binding process is how water exits cavities upon ligand binding. Studies on the dynamic behavior of an acetylcholine esterase system using a molecular dynamics (MD) approach has shown that for this target the substrate needs to approach the catalytic center of the protein through a deep, narrow gorge, which is in part filled with water in case there is no small molecule present [15]. These computational studies demonstrated sponge-like properties of this protein that allow water molecules to leave and enter the cavity at various locations.

Depending on the proximate neighborhood of water molecules, two very distinct aspects can be distinguished: individual water molecules mostly bound to the protein or ligand(s) and bulk water, providing the "matrix" for complex formation. In general, computational approaches tend to focus on only one of these two aspects, either assessing the affinity of a particular water molecule to the protein (in order to estimate the possibility of mediating interactions or displacement) or investigating solvation and desolvation effects of the ligand and the protein to estimate hydrophobic effects.

However, no clear distinction exists in the range between individually bound water molecules and bulk water. On the one extreme there are water molecules tightly bound by multiple H-bonds in deep, narrow, polar caverns of the protein. They may act, for example, as stabilizers of the protein conformation (the so-called structural water molecules) [16, 17], and therefore are often highly conserved. They may also form extensive H-bonding networks, linking several neighboring water molecules and protein or ligand moieties and, consequently, ensure protein function [18, 19]. With increasing size of water-filled cavities (active sites of specific enzymes < huge cavities of promiscuous metabolic enzymes such as CYP3A4 < pores of ion channels and membrane pumps), the water molecules become more disordered and, thus, easier to displace by approaching ligands [20, 21].

Surface water molecules are of particular importance to protein tertiary structure, that is, for the solvation of polar residues and the stabilization of neighboring equally charged groups [8]. The hydrophobic effect is widely accepted to arise from solvent reorganization [1], provides the driving force for protein folding [22, 23], and in many cases substantially contributes to protein–ligand binding [1, 24, 25]. It emerges from apolar surfaces that interrupt the network of favorable H-bonds that dominate bulk water. Water molecules in the vicinity of the apolar surface are likely to compensate lacking H-bonds by strengthening interactions with their neighbors, leading to more ordered water structures around the apolar surface. Whenever hydrophobic particles aggregate, burial of hydrophobic surfaces will release water molecules from ordered structures leading to a favorable change in entropy [24, 25]. Computational methods often roughly estimate the hydrophobic effect by the buried apolar surface area [25]. Significant influence of the protein surface on the surrounding water molecules is in general observable only for the first or second solvation shells [26] finally leading to the other extreme of water molecules, that is, bulk water.

Due to these various roles of water molecules it is hard to overestimate their importance in ligand binding [25, 27–29]. In order to appropriately investigate the process of protein–ligand binding, it is necessary to investigate three different states – the free ligand, the free protein, and the protein–ligand complex. The solvated ligand needs to strip off a portion of its water coat upon binding to the receptor and prevails in doing so only if the binding to its target is more favorable than remaining in the solvent [19, 30]. H-bonding interactions to the polar part of the ligand are geometrically considerably constrained, in particular with respect to their length. It is easy for water molecules of the solvation shells to meet the geometric requirements of the ligand's H-bonding moieties, whereas the fairly rigid protein environment may fail in doing so. Therefore, any deviation from the optimal spatial arrangement of H-bonds between the receptor and the ligand, even in the scale of a fraction of an Ångstrom, may be connected with a significant loss of affinity. As a rule of thumb, it is therefore advised to avoid any H-bonding acceptors and donors on the ligand side if they cannot be appropriately saturated by the environment of the binding site. The resulting apolar parts of the ligand then may contribute to the hydrophobic effect.

On the receptor side, water molecules may be dislodged upon ligand binding, which is likely to have a large impact on binding affinity. Considering the global consequences of this process, the same effects as for the ligand are decisive. Water molecules favor remaining close to polar groups whereas displacing them from an apolar surface area may enhance entropy-driven ligand binding [31]. However, this does not necessarily imply superior overall affinity for the ligand [32].

Water molecules at the interface of protein and ligand, mediating interactions, seem to be much more a common situation than an exception [33–35] and can be of comparable strength to direct interactions [29]. Lu *et al.* [4] have analyzed a large set of crystal structures of the PDBbind database [36] and found that three-quarters of the ligand-bound water molecules are interfacial water molecules (i.e., they are located between the ligand and the protein). The vast majority of investigated protein–ligand complexes shows at least a single water molecule to be involved in binding – an observation that is shared in studies by Klebe [33]. One of the most prominent examples where a systematic analysis and optimization of water-related effects on ligand binding resulted in highly potent drugs is given by HIV-1 protease (Figure 10.1).

At this point, the striking role of water for rational drug design should have become evident. In the following, we will discuss experimental and computational approaches for analyzing properties of water molecules, their scope, and limitations.

10.2 Experimental Approaches for Analyzing Water Molecules

X-ray crystallography is the most common experimental approach to derive 3D structures from biomolecules, with the Protein Data Bank [38] covering more than 60 000 structures. In order to derive 3D structural models, the electron density (ED) maps need to be interpreted in a multistep optimization workflow. An important quality benchmark is the resolution of the data, which is expressed in Ångstrom (Å). Generally speaking, protein structures resolved with low resolution (>2.5 Å) are likely to imply structural uncertainties that make them unsuitable for molecular modeling and computational approaches [39]. B-factors (also referred to as temperature factors) are displacement parameters that model the effects of static and dynamic disorder in the crystal and indicate the relative reliability of different parts of the model. The R-value is used to measure the ability of the structural model to explain the experimental data. As it is susceptible to overfitting, it should be combined with R_{free}, which is calculated from reflections that are not considered during model refinement [39]. While both R and R_{free} are only global quality measures [40], the real-space R-factor (RSR) [41] represents a local benchmark for the fit of data at residue level (e.g., one water molecule at a time). ED maps offer a thorough look on the data obtained from X-ray crystallographic experiments and their examination should be considered a crucial step before molecular modeling [4, 42–44].

Inherent limitations of the method and the refinement process bring about some ambiguities in water molecule identification. Due to their low electron density, hydrogen atoms are difficult to localize. Diffraction data of a resolution of about 0.8 Å or better is required to allow determination of their location. Unfortunately, such high resolution can be obtained only in rather a few cases. Consequently, direct

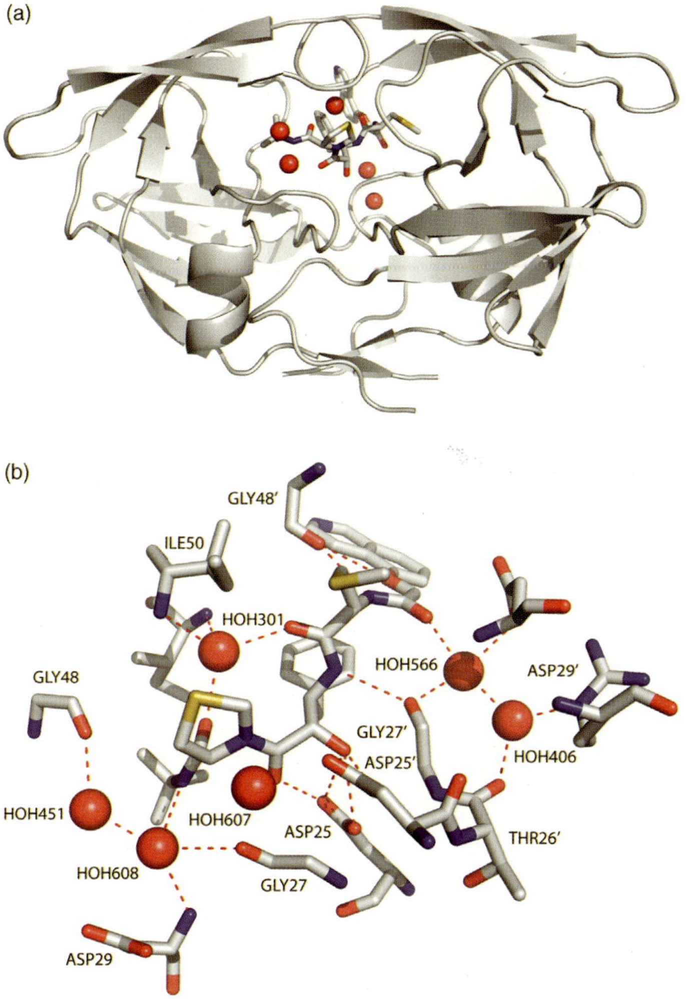

Figure 10.1 In order to reveal the enzymatic mechanism of HIV-1 protease, Adachi *et al.* [37] investigated the target structure in complex with a picomolar inhibitor (KNI-272) by high-resolution X-ray and neutron crystallography. (a) The active site of HIV-1 protease is located between two identical subunits. It includes the Asp-Thr-Gly sequence, which is common to aspartic proteases. (b) Several water molecules (including HOH301, HOH566, and HOH608) mediate interactions between inhibitor and HIV-1 protease (PDB 3fx5), forming interactions with key moieties such as Gly27 and the catalytically active Asp25′. These water molecules are located next to KNI-272 and, hence, are candidates for displacement by ligand binding. (c) The electron density maps confirm the presence of HOH301 when KNI-272 is bound. HOH301 mediates crucial interactions with Ile50 and Ile50′. Some nonpeptidic cyclic urea compounds displace this water molecule upon binding in order to enhance affinity to the target [31]. (d) Overlay of a cyclic urea inhibitor (blue color, PDB 1hvr) and the protein environment of 3fx5 (gray color). The figure highlights exact substitution of HOH301 by the urea moiety.

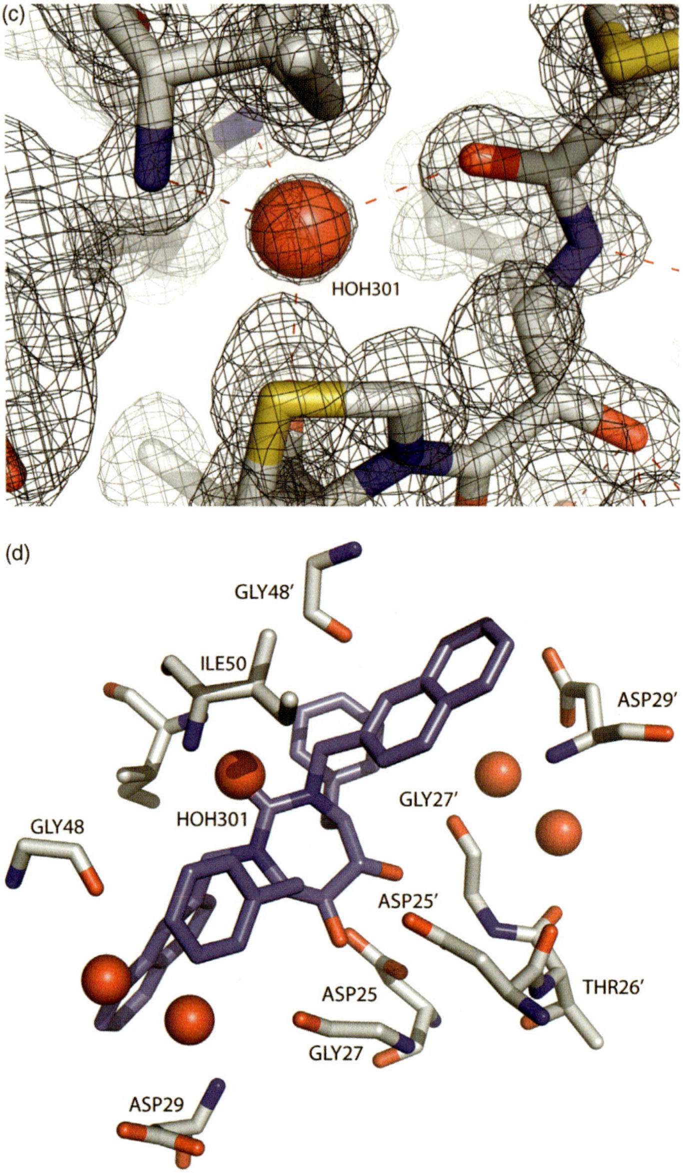

Figure 10.1 (*Continued*)

observation of both hydrogen bonds and tautomeric states is challenging. At resolutions common for determination of macromolecules (i.e., around 2 Å), further uncertainties about H-bonds arise from the isoelectronic character of oxygen and nitrogen atoms in glutamine and asparagine side chains [39]. H-bonding patterns may be helpful during the fairly subjective process of placing water molecules in ED maps. A water molecule having no interaction partners is usually considered to be an artifact. Still, many examples for noninteracting water molecules can be found in the PDB. Due to the nature of the most common benchmarks used to grade the quality of such models, crystallographers are tempted to legitimate unexplained electron density by the placement of water molecules in order to improve statistics [45, 46]. Differences in the interpretation of water positions can be identified even if the same high-resolution electron density is used for refinement by two different crystallographers, which highlights the possible uncertainties one is facing when working with X-ray-derived structural models [39]. Another drawback of X-ray structures is that they provide only an averaged mapping with limited information on the dynamics of the system under investigation.

B-factors are indicators for the mobility of water molecules present in crystal structures. Although B-factors *per se* are not comparable between different structures, they can be normalized and put in direct relation to the factors of the proximate molecular environment, providing valuable insight into the magnitude of interaction. In general, B-factors decrease with the number of H-bonding interactions formed. Brenk *et al.* [47], for example, have used the B-factor as an indicator for the degree of conservation of specific water molecules within the binding pocket and implemented these observations in a structure-based pharmacophore model (see below). Another aspect that can be directly assessed from investigating X-ray structures is the propensity of hydration at protein–ligand interfaces and the protein surface [48]. On the ligand side, positively charged nitrogens and negatively charged oxygens show the highest propensity for hydration at protein–ligand interfaces, followed by neutral heteroatoms. On the protein side, the charged side chains of Glu, Arg, Asp, and Lys show the most pronounced propensity [4]. A large analysis of water molecules around polar protein atoms shows that the probability distributions have characteristic shapes for different atoms rather than appearing randomly. High importance of water molecules for protein folding and stability is inferred from these results [48]. Another study showed that well-resolved internal water molecules are likely to be located proximate to residues that are not involved in α-helical or ß-sheet secondary structures and, thus, not forming direct intramolecular H-bonds [17]. A cluster analysis identified consensus water sites among serine proteases and assessed the impact on ligand specificity [10]. Mustata *et al.* [16] used clustering analysis to identify water molecules common in seven crystal structures of alanine racemase. With multiple X-ray structures, it could also be shown that water molecules can occupy the same positions in crystal structures of the same protein (complex) observed under different experimental conditions [49, 50] and with different ligands bound to its target [51–54]. The latter observation is particularly valuable to modelers, as it offers strong indications for highly conserved water molecules that can be exploited by rational design.

While X-ray crystallography identifies electron densities, the spallation neutron beam is diffracted by atomic nuclei. Thereby, neutron crystallography allows localization of hydrogen atom positions that usually cannot be observed in biological structures investigated by X-ray diffraction. The visibility of hydrogen atoms in neutron crystallography allows direct observation of H-bonding interactions, protonation states, catalytic mechanisms, and hydration states [55]. Consequently, a complete network of hydrogen-bonding D_2O molecules can be observed at the protein–solvent or protein–ligand interface. Chatake *et al.* [56] classified hydration water molecules by their shapes. They found triangular, short ellipsoids, long ellipsoids, and spherical peaks. The various shapes correspond to the number of atoms anchored by the formation of H-bonds. The amount of neutron diffraction data is still limited, although it would be very helpful for gaining new insight into the influence of water on protein structure and ligand binding. Limitations of the method arise from the large crystal size required for good results and from long data acquisition times needed to compensate for the low flux of available neutron beams [55]. An improvement can be expected together with technical development of the method.

NMR represents a powerful technology, which is complementary to X-ray crystallography, that supplies not only structural information on biomolecules but also dynamic information [57, 58]. However, the application of NMR for assessing water molecule properties is limited for several reasons. NMR requires large quantities of soluble, multiple labeled protein. The measurements are time consuming and limited in respect to protein size [44]. In contrast to X-ray models, NMR models usually consist of a collection of 10–25 conformations. These structural variations cannot always be ascribed clearly to true dynamics and can also result from underdetermination of the structure by the data [44]. Since the handling of multiple conformations in molecular modeling and virtual screening in particular is computationally expensive, in general one or a few representative conformations are selected from the experimentally determined conformational ensemble. Observation of ordered water molecules is hampered by exchange with bulk solvent in a timescale that is short compared to the NMR experiment. Usually, NMR methods will rather provide information on the average properties of solvent water molecules than giving detailed information on single water molecules [1].

Isothermal titration calorimetry (ITC) records the heat that is released (or absorbed) during stepwise addition of a ligand to a protein (or vice versa). Complexity of data interpretation arises from the number of potential sources of heat. Heat of dilution can be quantified by adding ligand after the saturation point. Heat resulting from changes in the protonation state can be identified by using buffers with different protonation enthalpy. Also, aggregation or structural changes may result in unexpected heat signals. Therefore, careful consideration of processes other than the one observed is crucial for data interpretation. The enthalpy change (ΔH) can be calculated from integration over heat signals. The binding constant K_b (and therefore the binding free energy ΔG°) is determined by nonlinear fitting of the curve described by the heat signals decreasing during the experiment. Once ΔG and ΔH are determined, the entropy change (ΔS) associated with the interaction can be calculated [59, 60]. Prediction of these values has proven to be difficult due to numerous contributions arising from protein, ligand, and solvent molecules. The key problem for rational drug design is to identify reliable correlations between structure, energetics, and dynamics. The possibility of detecting the full thermodynamic profile of an interaction within a few experiments leads to the establishment of ITC as standard for validating theoretical predictions of thermodynamic parameters [60].

However, entropy and enthalpy itself do not suffice for an in-depth understanding of a system, as the range of possible contributions of these parameters is large. But whenever predictions derived from structural data, perhaps enriched by molecular dynamics simulations, do not correspond to these values, this strongly indicates insufficiencies within the underlying hypotheses and lack of understanding of the system. Examples for experimental results that disagree with general expectations include hydrophobic interactions, which were found to be enthalpy driven, and entropy-driven H-bonds between ligand and protein [44]. Olsson *et al.* [59] launched the SCORPIO database, an online structure/calorimetry repository for protein interactions. By analyzing 254 protein–ligand complexes, they could confirm a correlation between binding affinity and increase in apolar surface area change, a relation that is well accepted in the field of drug design. Intriguingly, only a weak correlation was identified between affinity and changes in entropy, which is usually expected to occur because of the release of ordered solvent from apolar surface areas.

10.3 Computational Approaches for Analyzing Water Molecules

A considerable part of water molecules present in X-ray crystallographic models do play a decisive role in the binding free energies of a protein–ligand complex, but not all of them [2, 61]. Computational approaches can aid in differentiation and explanation of their contributions to the overall binding affinity. Today, a plethora of different techniques for assessing the impact of water molecules on ligand binding are available. Molecular dynamics simulations using explicit solvent models are certainly the most thorough approach, but there are also a number of fast computational models and algorithms available that allow an efficient assessment of water binding sites, as discussed below.

10.3.1 Molecular Dynamics Simulations

The observation of a system over a specific time period at atomic level causes a considerable data flood. It requires the calculation and recording of the full MD trajectory including all solvent molecules. Yet even more time consuming are analyses of the emerging data and, hence, efficient statistical methods are of utmost importance for elucidating information. Several different water models have been developed for the explicit consideration of solvation effects in MD simulations [62].

An inherent problem in rational drug design that is often addressed by MD simulation techniques is which water molecule could possibly be exploited for mediating interactions between a ligand and its target and which water molecules could be favorably displaced upon ligand binding. Analogous to X-ray data, B-factors can be determined for MD trajectories, indicating the degree of fluctuation of individual atoms. B-factors are usually lower for strongly bound water molecules compared to the bulk phase [63]. Another parameter reflecting the tightness of binding is the residence time of water molecules [64]. Brunne *et al.* [65] defined the residence time as the duration of stay of a water molecule within a given shell around a particular protein atom. The major drawback of this method is its need for a reference point on the protein side. In order to be able to measure residence times, we need to be able to precisely define the location of water molecules in the context of protein, which is a nontrivial task, considering conformational shifts of the protein and the immanent fluctuations of water molecules. Lounnas and Pettitt [63] used a grid-based approach to analyze the location and behavior of water molecules.

The radial distribution function is a traditional way of quantifying the local conservation of water molecules during MD simulations. While this measure is suitable for measuring water molecules around spherical elements, things turn out to be tricky for asymmetric, complex structures. Another possibility to statistically determine the location of a water molecule and therefore the hydration site is to average its position in relation to the coordinate frame [63]. However, applicability of this approach is limited in case of a flexible protein, as the high level of noise causes information loss.

Henchman and McCammon [66] countered these limitations by two statistical methods for extracting information on water molecules from flexible biomolecular environments. First, they define the time-averaged position (TAP). It comprises two parameters, the location and the lifetime. In order to avoid dependence on the protein frame, they define the position of water molecules only depending on the local protein environment of each individual water molecule (the averaged residue coordinate, ARC). TAP is then calculated using the ARC. The authors have shown that their combined ARC/TAP approach produces considerably improved water densities, filters noise and is independent of the alignment of the protein frames. There are two shortcomings: the arbitrary decision of which residues to define being part of the local protein environment and the limited applicability to only close distances from the target molecule.

Huang *et al.* [67] presented a clustering approach for identifying hydration sites by residence time after all frames of a trajectory are aligned by the protein backbone. The authors were able to detect a considerable overlap between the tightly bound water molecules identified on the basis of their MD simulation and crystallized water molecules. In contrast, Falconi *et al.* [68] reported only a low overlap between hydration sites determined by MD simulation and X-ray crystallography. Reasons for the lack of agreement could be the different timescales observed by their 1 ns MD simulation and the X-ray experiment. Also, it is not possible to see from X-ray data whether a specific water molecule has a long residence time or if it binds in the hydration site only for a short time but with frequent exchange. In their MD simulations, the water density peaks observed result from high exchange rates, which corroborates observations that there is no direct relation between occupancy (i.e., a measure for the probability of a water molecule being present at a specific locus) and residence time [69]. Besides other influences, one likely reason for lacking consensus between experimentally and computationally derived hydration sites could also be the influence of packing effects in crystal structures [63, 65, 69–71].

Further benchmarks for the mobility of water molecules include occupancy rates for specific hydration sites and intersite jump time [70] (i.e., jumps of water molecules between hydration sites). MD simulations have also been successfully employed for analyzing the relaxation behavior of hydration shells of protein atoms [64], for detecting favorable pathways for the exchange of bound water molecules with bulk water, and for analyzing their importance in the structural integrity of the protein [72, 73]. These, in part, rapid exchanges of bulk water molecules and water molecules of the interior of the protein indicate the considerable degree of flexibility of macromolecules.

Computational approaches for calculating interaction energy and hydration energy are highly challenging, and inevitably bear errors and insufficiencies. The entropic contributions resulting from changes in the water phase upon ligand binding are particularly problematic to quantify. Free energy perturbation (FEP) and thermodynamic integration (TI) are among the most popular and most reliable approaches for calculating the free energies of binding on the basis of molecular dynamics simulations, being able to predict free energies of binding within 1 kcal/mol in favorable cases [74]. These approaches circumvent a simulation of the physical association or dissociation of a ligand with its target by considering a thermodynamic cycle. Different ligands are mutated step-by-step into each other both in solution and bound to the target protein. While in general it is possible to consider solvation and desolvation effects, the exact quantification remains challenging. Drawbacks of FEP and TI are their high computational cost and the limitation to rather small ligand mutations, which is why they are mostly applied in the lead optimization phase instead of the early discovery phase.

Approximate free energy methods such as the linear interaction energy (LIE) or the molecular mechanics–Poisson Boltzmann surface area (MM-PBSA) approaches allow to estimate the free energy of binding with lower demands on computational power. The abstraction accepted by the LIE approach [75–77] is the reduction of complexity to parameterized equations. Thereby, hydrophobic interactions are represented by the surface area term and ligand–solvent interactions by the electrostatic term. A substantial drawback of this method is its need for a calibration set. Thus, LIE is limited to the prediction of relative free energies of binding of structurally related compounds. In contrast to LIE, the MM-PBSA approach [78–80] is not depending on the availability of a parameterization set. It calculates the free energy of binding based on three individual simulations: one with the ligand, one with the protein, and one with the protein–ligand complex. The free energy of binding is calculated by subtraction of the energies of the individual molecules from the protein–ligand complex. While in the MM-PBSA approach in general simulations are performed using explicit water representations, the calculation of the hydration effects is based on a continuum electrostatic model. For more details on free energy approaches, the reader may consult a review by Mancera [74].

Watermap [81–83] is one of the most recent approaches that allows to compute both enthalpy and entropy of hydration sites in protein systems. It is based on the application of the inhomogeneous solvation theory [84] in combination with a clustering technique to derive maps of hydration sites, which allows to analyze the hydration thermodynamics by applying explicit solvent MD simulations in the low nanosecond timescale.

10.3.2
Empirical and Implicit Considerations of Solvation Effects

As molecular dynamics simulations imply considerable demands on computation time and expertise, a collection of empirical and implicit methods for investigating water-induced effects on ligand binding have been developed. SuperStar, for example, uses information derived from experimental data to identify interaction sites in proteins [85, 86]. It generates propensity maps representing the distribution of one functional group around another found in small-molecule crystal structures. Success rates reported for the prediction of water positions around proteins are promising, in particular for those water positions that are well defined in the X-ray structure [86].

Schymkowitz *et al.* [87] applied the empirical Fold-X force field to derive the position of water molecules at proteins. The knowledge-based approach was parameterized using high-resolution crystal structures of proteins including solvent molecules. A PDB-derived knowledge base comprising four descriptors (i.e., atomic density and hydrophobicity, H-bonds, and crystallographic B-factors) is used by Consolv to predict water-mediated ligand interactions in proteins [88]. The decision-making process implemented in Consolv includes a k-nearest-neighbor (knn) classifier combined with a genetic algorithm. knn is used for classification of water molecules; the genetic algorithm allows to weight and optimize the contribution of the different parameters. Amadasi *et al.* [43] combine the HINT free energy scoring model [89] and the Rank algorithm [90] in order to identify water molecules that are likely to be displaced upon ligand binding. HINT takes into account the physicochemical and steric properties of the protein environment and provides an estimate of the global interaction energy with the surrounding water molecules. Rank classifies water molecules according to the number of H-bonds formed with non-water molecules purely in the geometric context. The information gained from both approaches was integrated using a pseudo-Bayesian statistical analysis. The authors found high success rates when analyzing pairs of high-resolution apo and holo X-ray structures using their model. Intriguingly, predictivity is considerably weaker for structures with resolution worse than 2.0 Å, which indicates the sensitivity of computational approaches to the accurate placement of water molecules in X-ray structural models.

A multivariate statistical regression analysis on water molecules in ligand-free binding pockets revealed four parameters to correlate with the probability that a specific water molecule is conserved during ligand binding: the B-factor, the solvent-contact surface area, the total H-bond energy, and the number of protein–water contacts [91]. These functions are implemented in WaterScore to discriminate between bound and displaceable water molecules during the structure-based drug design process. Conserved water molecules were found to be more immobile and deeply buried in crevices or grooves in the binding site than replaceable water molecules. Unfortunately, the approach considers only those water molecules that are present in the apo structure and are missing in the holo structure if they are not sterically displaced by the ligand, although it would be particularly useful to have a tool that is able to identify the water molecules that are favorable for displacement [3].

Taking into account the solvent-accessible surface area and the free energies of transfer for each individual atom, Eisenberg and McLachlan [22] reported a method for calculating the degree of conservation of water molecules in protein structures. Also, neural networks have been applied for investigating protein hydration sites [92].

Another way of assessing possible water positions is to calculate interaction energies for probe molecules at sample positions throughout and around the macromolecule, as it is done for GRID molecular interaction fields [93]. After careful parameterization of the water probe and with a sufficiently close grid spacing, the method is able to reproduce, check, and predict water positions found in X-ray structures [94, 95]. By default, water molecules are not regarded part of the protein. Wrong energy maps for other probes will result if an interaction-mediating water molecule is indeed removed from the protein prior to further field calculations. Placement of several water molecules has to be done in an iterative way starting with water assignment to the best positions and repeating the calculation. Thereby, cooperative effects of water on a network may be neglected. CS-Map is another computational mapping approach (computational solvent mapping of proteins) [96]. It has been developed to address shortcomings of earlier mapping methods such as the problem of obtaining too many energy minima on the protein surface. The implemented three-step procedure includes a rigid body search for favorable interaction sites, minimization and rescoring, and clustering and ranking. The authors report the successful identification of protein hydration sites considering van der Waals, electrostatic, and solvation effects.

10.4 Water-Sensitive Virtual Screening: Approaches and Applications

Despite the vital role of water molecules in protein–ligand binding, efforts considering the impact of the solvent are surprisingly rudimental. The common approach in virtual screening is still to ignore water molecules completely or to focus on a very few water molecules that are known to be crucial for ligand action. So far, only a few approaches attempt to explicitly consider the properties of specific water molecules and their influence on ligand binding, which we discuss in the following sections.

10.4.1 Protein–Ligand Docking

Docking a ligand into a protein pocket is a combinatorial problem. Algorithms are designed to cover the space of interactions as exhaustively as possible to avoid missing of relevant poses. Obviously, considering explicit water molecules in the binding interface dramatically increases the search space, as water molecules are partially replaced by the ligand [33, 97]. The binding site has a quite different shape and different interaction patterns, depending on the individual water molecules remaining in the pocket. One could even consider each possible selection of retained water molecules as a completely different docking problem [18, 34]. Water molecules in the binding pocket typically have more degrees of freedom for possible interactions than one would expect, for example, resulting from side-chain torsions of amino acids within the binding site. Thus, water molecules in the binding site can be seen as further complication in terms of protein flexibility (discussed in Chapters 8 and 9 of this book).

Hydration complicates the scoring of poses generated by docking algorithms [74, 98, 99]. At least, it is clear that completely neglecting solvation and desolvation effects would considerably distort ligand ranking [25]. Recently, continuum solvation models such as MM-PBSA and MM-GBSA [78–80] have become rather popular to rescore docking poses [30]. However, the errors in hydration free energy predicted by continuum solvation models for druglike molecules seem to be larger than expected [100].

As summarized in a recent review [101], there is no consensus in the scientific community on whether an explicit treatment of water molecules indeed enhances docking results with respect to a lower RMSD values when comparing the docking pose with the experimental structure. Although the RMSD may be appropriate for evaluating poses and is therefore widely used as benchmark parameter, it mainly covers enthalpic aspects of the interaction, neglecting entropic contributions. However, for applicability of a docking tool during virtual screening a complete ranking, that is a scoring by binding affinity, is necessary.

Force fields can rather reliably describe interaction energies between different molecules; however, taking into account entropic effects is a major challenge [29]. The highest entropic contributions of water molecules to binding affinity have to be expected from the displacement of water molecules that are weakly bound but highly ordered within the binding site [81]. Such water molecules typically fill hydrophobic pockets. Expulsion of such water molecules leads to strong entropic gains on binding. Whether a specific hydrophobic pocket leads to an ordered arrangement of water molecules strongly depends on the shape of the pocket. The prediction of such ordering processes is a major challenge complicating correct scoring.

An appropriate way to validate a scoring function should be the enrichment of a virtual screening campaign. Unfortunately, publications covering the treatment of water molecules and presenting enrichment values are less frequent than those applying redocking and using RMSD for validation.

Basically, there are three ways the docking programs tackle explicit water molecules. The first type of approaches tries to predict which water molecules are retained in a protein before docking the ligand. This corresponds to considering water molecules part of the protein [28, 102–107]. The second type of algorithms consider explicit water molecules simultaneously with the ligand degrees of freedom [108–113]. In this way, one might see water molecules treated as part of the ligand.

Finally, there are programs that add water molecules after potential ligand poses are found solely to improve the scoring [114–116]. Only in the first two approaches are the structural predictions influenced directly by the water molecules. Obviously, all three possibilities to include explicit water molecules in docking can modify the score of a ligand in comparison to a mere implicit treatment of solvation and desolvation. In doing so the challenge is to correctly quantify water contributions.

Adopting the first approach considering water molecules as part of the protein, an inclusion of explicit active site water molecules can improve the RMSD accuracy of docking poses as found in an extensive study on cytochrome P450 and thymidine kinase protein–ligand complexes [103]. In this investigation, both an ensemble of active site water molecules from X-ray structures and an ensemble predicted by a GRID-based protocol improved the RMSD accuracy using the programs AutoDock, FlexX, and GOLD. The established strategies were subsequently applied to the catalytic site prediction and virtual screening of cytochrome P450 2D6 substrates [102].

In silico ligand generation studies on neuraminidase, PARP, and CDK2 found strong influences of tightly bound water molecules on the prediction of the binding mode and the chemical diversity of designed ligands [28, 104, 105]. These investigations were extended to a large set of ligand–protein complexes containing water molecules in the binding site, and the inclusion of crystallographic water molecules significantly improved the accuracy of docking predictions [107]. Though, an evaluation of FRED, QXP/FLO, and GLIDE for the charged binding pocket in cytochrome C peroxidase found that the inclusion of a decisive water molecule in the binding pocket did not enhance the enrichment during virtual screening [117].

A rather simple way to dock a protein with variable explicit water molecules is to combine multiple interaction grids into a weighted average grid thus using a single grid representation of the target [106].

The second approach consists of algorithms that consider explicit water molecules simultaneously with the ligand degrees of freedom. The particle concept within FlexX [110] addresses the problem of placing discrete water molecules by precomputing and storing favorable positions of water molecules. During the incremental construction process of the ligand, the stored water positions are chosen if additional H-bonds to the ligand can be formed. However, the overall improvement in the docking results observed was small.

An implementation of displaceable explicit water molecules in GOLD [113] takes into account that displaced water molecules lead to a gain in rigid body translational and rotational entropy. The gain in entropy is accounted for by a target- and water-position-independent reward optimized for a training set of target–ligand complexes. When all X-ray water molecules within 6 Å of the ligand are explicitly considered, GOLD correctly predicts the binding modes of almost all complexes of a diverse set of high-resolution protein–ligand complexes [118]. However, the authors of the study mentioned warn that this success is not a good performance indicator as many of the water molecules are likely to be ligand specific.

An interesting approach was chosen in the program SLIDE [111] starting with observed water positions and allowing a translational displacement in case of collision with the ligand. Only when the collision cannot be resolved, the water molecule is removed from the binding site. There are algorithms that consider explicit water molecules during protein–protein docking [112] by removing water molecules from solvated biomolecules in a biased Monte Carlo procedure.

Bridging displaceable water molecules can also be considered simultaneously with the ligand degrees of freedom using genetic algorithms by encoding the possible occurrence and orientation into the chromosomes as implemented in FITTED [108]. The application to virtual screening of potential HCV polymerase inhibitors has been demonstrated successfully and benchmarked against other popular docking programs [108]. The authors found an improved structural accuracy of docking results by their approach to include displaceable water molecules in contrast to techniques implemented in the popular docking programs GOLD and FlexX, where the inclusion of displaceable water molecules did not improve results. However, none of the popular scoring functions seems to significantly benefit from consideration of explicit water molecules [109], implying that virtual screening does not benefit from taking into account explicit water molecules. To address this problem, new screening functions were developed resulting in significantly better performance if the development of the scoring function also relies on data from inactive compounds [119].

Finally, the third approach of adding water molecules after potential ligand poses are found is intended to improve scoring only. A simple algorithm implemented within DOCK considering individual water molecules independent and equally displaceable during scoring of poses [116] rarely degrades docking performance, but rather increases enrichment of half of the 24 targets from the DUD database [120].

In the development of GLIDE 2.5, it has been found to be advantageous to dock explicit water molecules into the binding site for each energetically competitive ligand pose [114]. This "water-scoring" technology allows to reject a higher fraction of false positives. GLIDE 4.0 XP further improves this approach by a sophisticated model for hydrophobic enclosures and correlated H-bonding motifs even allowing the correct prediction of the exceptionally large binding affinity of streptavidin to biotin [115]. Although the terms of the scoring are calculated with fast empirical functions, their basis is derived from physical chemistry principles.

10.4.2
Pharmacophore Modeling

Ligand-based pharmacophore models can be derived in an automated way by arranging the key interactions of active ligands in 3D space. Possibilities to consider and predict both the water-mediated interactions and the displacement of bound water from the binding site are very limited for this approach. Lloyd *et al.* [121] presented a hybrid technique, integrating ligand and structure-based treatment in order to address water molecules involved in protein–ligand binding. A ligand-based pharmacophore model of the binding site is derived from known active compounds;

tightly bound water molecules included in the X-ray structure of the binding site are identified using WaterScore. The ligand-based site model is matched to the actual protein structure including the binding site features by superposition. In this way, the ligand-based pharmacophore can be interpreted using the information gained from the assessment of the protein-bound water molecules, allowing to draw conclusions on water-mediated protein–ligand interactions and the sterical displacement of water molecules by ligands.

Structure-based pharmacophore modeling allows to explicitly consider water-mediated interactions and displacement of water molecules directly from experimental data on protein–ligand complexes. In this approach, water molecules are treated as part of the protein environment. Possible interactions of the solvent with the ligand and the protein environment are thereby considered with hydrogen bond donor and acceptor functionalities. The importance of such water-mediated H-bonds can be reflected by a weighting factor of the respective pharmacophore feature: the more certain the position of a water molecule is known, the higher should be the contribution of the respective pharmacophore feature(s) to the overall ligand–pharmacophore match. LigandScout [122–124] is a software suite that allows for automated pharmacophore elucidation from protein–ligand structures. It considers bound water molecules as elements of the protein environment and automatically detects water-mediated protein–ligand interactions. H-bonds formed between the ligand and the water molecules are incorporated to the pharmacophore model.

The work of the Klebe group on tRNA-guanine transglycosylase (TGT) is an illustrative example of iterative rational drug design and highlights the impact of water molecules on ligand binding and protein conformations. The inhibition of TGT is considered a promising therapeutic approach, lowering the virulence of bacteria causing Shigellosis. After the X-ray structure of the target became available in 1996 [125], compounds acting at the substrate binding site have been discovered by a *de novo* design approach [126]. These early inhibitors show a binding mode very similar to the one of the natural substrate. Brenk *et al.* [47] identified imidazole-fused pyridazinedione analogues that show a distinct binding mode introducing conformational changes within the TGT binding site and water-mediated H-bonds (Figure 10.2). A structure-based pharmacophore model was developed considering the H-bonding with a particular water molecule (W1) and virtual screening was successfully performed using a multistep workflow, including several hierarchical filters, pharmacophore-based screening using UNITY [127], and docking using FLEXX [128]. Pharmacophore-based virtual screening studies on this adapted protein conformation revealed novel chemical scaffolds active on TGT such as pteridine analogues [129] and quinazolinones [130]. For these structural classes water molecules (water displacement) represent a major aspect of ligand binding [131]. Further crystallographic investigations have shown that water molecules within the substrate binding pocket of TGT play a key role in substrate binding, catalysis, and conformational adaptation of the protein to the ligand [132, 133].

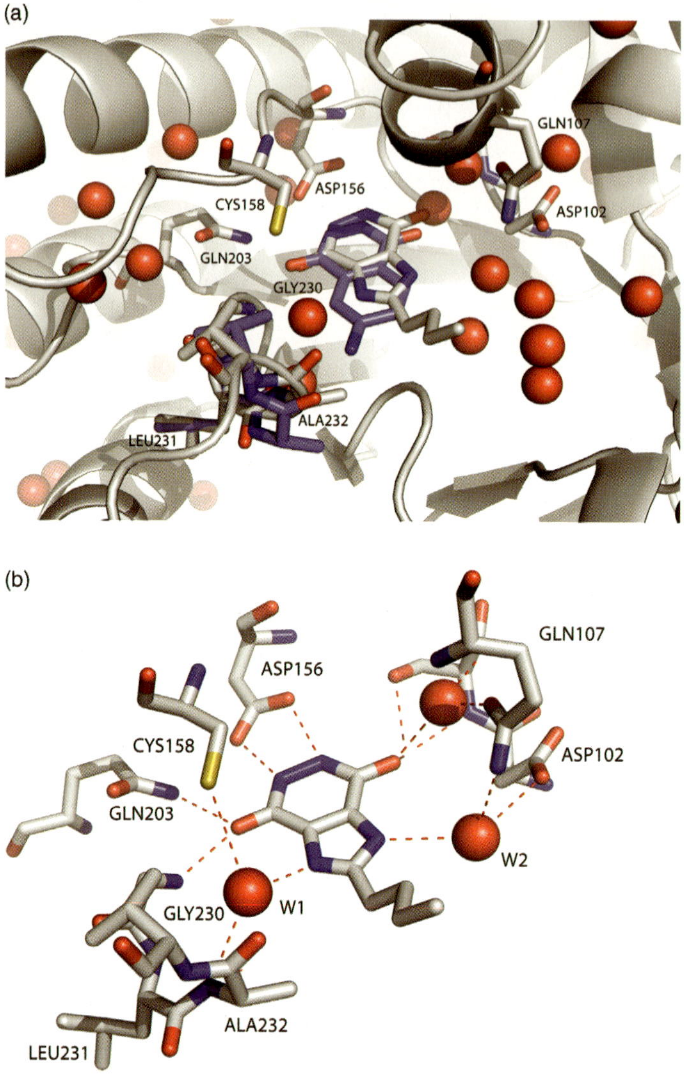

Figure 10.2 Rational design of tRNA-guanin transglycosylase (TGT) inhibitors. (a) Early developed phthalhydrazide-based inhibitors (Leu231 and Ala232 in blue color, PDB 1enu) show a binding mode that is very closely related to the one of the substrate. The imidazole-fused pyridazinedione analogues identified by Brenk *et al.* cause a flipping of the peptide bond at Leu231 to Ala232 (protein–ligand complex in gray color, PDB 1n2v). This new class of inhibitors establishes several water-mediated interactions: (b) W1 plays a key role in protein–ligand binding of pyridazinedione-based inhibitors, allowing the ligand to interact with Ala232 and Cys158. The low B-factor of this water molecule (which is comparable to the B-factors for its neighboring atoms) indicates full occupancy and rather strong binding. The pyridazinediones give rise to further side-chain shifts allowing the formation of H-bonds with Gln107 via another water molecule (W2).

10.5
Conclusions and Recommendations

Today, most of the time the impact of solvent on ligand binding is not adequately considered in molecular modeling and virtual screening. This is mostly due to the complexity of the effects involved and consequently limited by the high computational requirements for explicit consideration of water molecules. Therefore, even state-of-the-art structure-based and ligand-based virtual screening techniques rarely consider this aspect explicitly, but rather use implicit solvent models or try to estimate the solvent contribution from easily accessible parameters. For example, it is quite common to calculate the hydrophobic effect from the buried apolar surface area. Complexity arises from the mixture and compensation of enthalpic and entropic effects. To quantify them, one needs to know the exact physicochemical properties of water molecules at atomic level. Calculation of both the enthalpic penalty and the entropic benefit are challenging, as they depend on the binding pocket geometry, charge, polarity, and dynamics, on the ligand, and on other water molecules that could take part in a network.

Taking the necessary care, water positions can be reasonably derived both from X-ray data and from different mapping approaches. This information has been successfully employed to enhance structural predictions on ligand binding geometries in redocking studies. However, as soon as this structural information should be used for virtual screening, a decision is needed on which water molecules should be retained and which water molecules should be allowed to be replaced by a potential ligand. Virtual screening could not yet substantially benefit from considering explicit water molecules as for this purpose it would be necessary to predict the thermodynamic binding characteristics of individual water molecules that not only depend on enthalpic effects that usually dominate the localization of water molecules but also depend on entropic effects that substantially contribute to the free energy of binding. In principle, this information can be obtained by computer simulations; however, appropriate approaches are just emerging and need further validation by experimental techniques. The major challenge for reliable comparison of measured data and theoretical predictions is the decoupling of individual contributions to free energy of binding from experiments.

Still, there are several recommendations that could help consider water molecules and solvation effects in virtual screening. When using information on water molecules derived from X-ray data, it is very important to verify their position in the electron density directly, as the placement of water molecules may be arbitrary if not in the focus of the crystallographer. In addition, it is advisable to check whether the water molecule under consideration is confirmed by interaction partners in the structure. Computer simulations might help judge the mobility, ordering, and synergetic effects of specific water molecules.

Algorithms that explicitly consider water molecules' degrees of freedom during docking cannot reliably improve the virtual screening results; thus, responsibility for the treatment of explicit water molecules remains largely in the hand of the modeler, who needs to decide which water molecules to retain in the binding pocket. The impact of this decision cannot be underestimated, as water is essential to drug action and drug design.

References

1 Homans, S.W. (2007) Water, water everywhere: except where it matters? *Drug Discovery Today*, **12**, 534–539.

2 Hamelberg, D. and McCammon, J.A. (2004) Standard free energy of releasing a localized water molecule from the binding pockets of proteins: double-decoupling method. *Journal of the American Chemical Society*, **126**, 7683–7689.

3 Barillari, C., Taylor, J., Viner, R., and Essex, J.W. (2007) Classification of water molecules in protein binding sites. *Journal of the American Chemical Society*, **129**, 2577–2587.

4 Lu, Y.P., Wang, R.X., Yang, C.Y., and Wang, S.M. (2007) Analysis of ligand-bound water molecules in high-resolution crystal structures of protein–ligand complexes. *Journal of Chemical Information and Modeling*, **47**, 668–675.

5 Panigrahi, S.K. and Desiraju, G.R. (2007) Strong and weak hydrogen bonds in the protein–ligand interface. *Proteins: Structure, Function, and Bioinformatics*, **67**, 128–141.

6 Sleigh, S.H., Seavers, P.R., Wilkinson, A.J., Ladbury, J.E., and Tame, J.R.H. (1999) Crystallographic and calorimetric analysis of peptide binding to OppA protein. *Journal of Molecular Biology*, **291**, 393–415.

7 Tame, J.R.H., Murshudov, G.N., Dodson, E.J., Neil, T.K., Dodson, G.G., Higgins, C.F., and Wilkinson, A.J. (1994) The structural basis of sequence-independent peptide binding by OppA protein. *Science*, **264**, 1578–1581.

8 Brooks, C.L. and Karplus, M. (1989) Solvent effects on protein motion and protein effects on solvent motion: dynamics of the active-site region of lysozyme. *Journal of Molecular Biology*, **208**, 159–181.

9 Quiocho, F.A., Wilson, D.K., and Vyas, N.K. (1989) Substrate-specificity and affinity of a protein modulated by bound water-molecules. *Nature*, **340**, 404–407.

10 Sanschagrin, P.C. and Kuhn, L.A. (1998) Cluster analysis of consensus water sites in thrombin and trypsin shows conservation between serine proteases and contributions to ligand specificity. *Protein Science: A Publication of the Protein Society*, **7**, 2054–2064.

11 Fauman, E.B., Rutenber, E.E., Maley, G.F., Maley, F., and Stroud, R.M. (1994) Water-mediated substrate/product discrimination: the product complex of thymidylate synthase at 1.83 Å. *Biochemistry*, **33**, 1502–1511.

12 Garczarek, F. and Gerwert, K. (2006) Functional waters in intraprotein proton transfer monitored by FTIR difference spectroscopy. *Nature*, **439**, 109–112.

13 Luecke, H., Schobert, B., Richter, H.T., Cartailler, J.P., and Lanyi, J.K. (1999) Structure of bacteriorhodopsin at 1.55 Å resolution. *Journal of Molecular Biology*, **291**, 899–911.

14 Zhang, Z.D., Komives, E.A., Sugio, S., Blacklow, S.C., Narayana, N., Xuong, N.H., Stock, A.M., Petsko, G.A., and Ringe, D. (1999) The role of water in the catalytic efficiency of triosephosphate isomerase. *Biochemistry*, **38**, 4389–4397.

15 Gilson, M.K., Straatsma, T.P., McCammon, J.A., Ripoll, D.R., Faerman, C.H., Axelsen, P.H., Silman, I., and Sussman, J.L. (1994) Open back door in a molecular-dynamics simulation of acetylcholinesterase. *Science*, **263**, 1276–1278.

16 Mustata, G. and Briggs, J.M. (2004) Cluster analysis of water molecules in alanine racemase and their putative structural role. *Protein Engineering, Design and Selection*, **17**, 223–234.

17 Park, S. and Saven, J.G. (2005) Statistical and molecular dynamics studies of buried waters in globular proteins. *Proteins: Structure, Function, and Bioinformatics*, **60**, 450–463.

18 Hubbard, S.J. and Argos, P. (1994) Cavities and packing at protein interfaces. *Protein Science: A Publication of the Protein Society*, **3**, 2194–2206.

19 Smolin, N., Oleinikova, A., Brovchenko, I., Geiger, A., and Winter, R. (2005) Properties of spanning water networks at protein surfaces. *The Journal of Physical Chemistry B*, **109**, 10995–11005.

20 Helms, V. (2007) Protein dynamics tightly connected to the dynamics of surrounding and internal water molecules. *Journal of Chemical Physics and Physical Chemistry*, **8**, 23–33.

21 Poornima, C.S. and Dean, P.M. (1995) Hydration in drug design 1. Multiple hydrogen-bonding features of water molecules in mediating protein–ligand interactions. *Journal of Computer-Aided Molecular Design*, **9**, 500–512.

22 Eisenberg, D. and McLachlan, A.D. (1986) Solvation energy in protein folding and binding. *Nature*, **319**, 199–203.

23 Kuntz, I.D. and Kauzmann, W. (1974) Hydration of proteins and polypeptides. *Advances in Protein Chemistry*, **28**, 239–345.

24 Homans, S.W. (2007) Dynamics and thermodynamics of ligand–protein interactions, in *Bioactive Conformation I*, vol. **272, Topics in Current Chemistry** (ed. T. Peters), Springer, Berlin, pp. 51–82.

25 Shoichet, B.K., Leach, A.R., and Kuntz, I.D. (1999) Ligand solvation in molecular docking. *Proteins: Structure, Function, and Genetics*, **34**, 4–16.

26 Raschke, T.M. (2006) Water structure and interactions with protein surfaces. *Current Opinion in Structural Biology*, **16**, 152–159.

27 Cozzini, P., Fornabaio, M., Marabotti, A., Abraham, D.J., Kellogg, G.E., and Mozzarelli, A. (2004) Free energy of ligand binding to protein: evaluation of the contribution of water molecules by computational methods. *Current Medicinal Chemistry*, **11**, 3093–3118.

28 Garcia-Sosa, A.T., Firth-Clark, S., and Mancera, R.L. (2005) Including tightly-bound water molecules in *de novo* drug design. Exemplification through the *in silico* generation of poly (ADP-ribose) polymerase ligands. *Journal of Chemical Information and Modeling*, **45**, 624–633.

29 Li, Z. and Lazaridis, T. (2007) Water at biomolecular binding interfaces. *Physical Chemistry Chemical Physics*, **9**, 573–581.

30 Huang, N. and Jacobson, M.P. (2007) Physics-based methods for studying protein–ligand interactions. *Current Opinion in Drug Discovery & Development*, **10**, 325–331.

31 Lam, P.Y.S., Jadhav, P.K., Eyermann, C.J., Hodge, C.N., Ru, Y., Bacheler, L.T., Meek, J.L., Otto, M.J., Rayner, M.M., Wong, Y.N., Chang, C.H., Weber, P.C., Jackson, D.A., Sharpe, T.R., and Ericksonviitanen, S. (1994) Rational design of potent, bioavailable, nonpeptide cyclic ureas as HIV protease inhibitors. *Science*, **263** 380–384.

32 Mikol, V., Papageorgiou, C., and Borer, X. (1995) The role of water-molecules in the structure-based design of (5-hydroxynorvaline)-2-cyclosporine - synthesis, biological-activity, and crystallographic analysis with cyclophilin-A. *Journal of Medicinal Chemistry*, **38**, 3361–3367.

33 Klebe, G. (2006) Virtual ligand screening: strategies, perspectives and limitations. *Drug Discovery Today*, **11**, 580–594.

34 Gunther, J., Bergner, A., Hendlich, M., and Klebe, G. (2003) Utilising structural knowledge in drug design strategies: applications using Relibase. *Journal of Molecular Biology*, **326**, 621–636.

35 Hendlich, M., Bergner, A., Gunther, J., and Klebe, G. (2003) Relibase: design and development of a database for comprehensive analysis of protein–ligand interactions. *Journal of Molecular Biology*, **326**, 607–620.

36 Wang, R.X., Fang, X.L., Lu, Y.P., Yang, C.Y., and Wang, S.M. (2005) The PDBbind database: methodologies and updates. *Journal of Medicinal Chemistry*, **48**, 4111–4119.

37 Adachi, M., Ohhara, T., Kurihara, K., Tamada, T., Honjo, E., Okazaki, N.,

Arai, S., Shoyama, Y., Kimura, K., Matsumura, H., Sugiyama, S., Adachi, H., Takano, K., Mori, Y., Hidaka, K., Kimura, T., Hayashi, Y., Kiso, Y., and Kuroki, R. (2009) Structure of HIV-1 protease in complex with potent inhibitor KNI-272 determined by high-resolution X-ray and neutron crystallography. *Proceedings of the National Academy of Sciences of the United States of America*, **106**, 4641–4646.

38 Berman, H.M., Westbrook, J., Feng, Z., Gilliland, G., Bhat, T.N., Weissig, H., Shindyalov, I.N., and Bourne, P.E. (2000) The Protein Data Bank. *Nucleic Acids Research*, **28**, 235–242.

39 Davis, A.M., Teague, S.J., and Kleywegt, G.J. (2003) Application and limitations of X-ray crystallographic data in structure-based ligand and drug design. *Angewandte Chemie – International Edition in English*, **42**, 2718–2736.

40 Brunger, A.T. (1992) Free *R*-value: a novel statistical quantity for assessing the accuracy of crystal-structures. *Nature*, **355**, 472–475.

41 Jones, T.A., Zou, J.Y., Cowan, S.W., and Kjeldgaard, M. (1991) Improved methods for building protein models in electron-density maps and the location of errors in these models. *Acta Crystallographica. Section A, Foundations of Crystallography*, **47**, 110–119.

42 Kirchmair, J., Markt, P., Distinto, S., Schuster, D., Spitzer, G.M., Liedl, K.R., Langer, T., and Wolber, G. (2008) The Protein Data Bank (PDB), its related services and software tools as key components for *in silico* guided drug discovery. *Journal of Medicinal Chemistry*, **51**, 7021–7040.

43 Amadasi, A., Surface, J.A., Spyrakis, F., Cozzini, P., Mozzarelli, A., and Kellogg, G.E. (2008) Robust classification of 'relevant' water molecules in putative protein binding sites. *Journal of Medicinal Chemistry*, **51**, 1063–1067.

44 Davis, A.M., St-Gallay, S.A., and Kleywegt, G.J. (2008) Limitations and lessons in the use of X-ray structural information in drug design. *Drug Discovery Today*, **13**, 831–841.

45 Karplus, P.A. and Faerman, C. (1994) Ordered water in macromolecular structure. *Current Opinion in Structural Biology*, **4**, 770–776.

46 Meyer, E. (1992) Internal water-molecules and H-bonding in biological macromolecules: a review of structural features with functional implications. *Protein Science*, **1**, 1543–1562.

47 Brenk, R., Naerum, L., Gradler, U., Gerber, H.D., Garcia, G.A., Reuter, K., Stubbs, M.T., and Klebe, G. (2003) Virtual screening for submicromolar leads of tRNA-guanine transglycosylase based on a new unexpected binding mode detected by crystal structure analysis. *Journal of Medicinal Chemistry*, **46**, 1133–1143.

48 Matsuoka, D. and Nakasako, M. (2009) Probability distributions of hydration water molecules around polar protein atoms obtained by a database analysis. *The Journal of Physical Chemistry B*, **113**, 11274–11292.

49 Nakasako, M. (1999) Large-scale networks of hydration water molecules around bovine beta-trypsin revealed by cryogenic X-ray crystal structure analysis. *Journal of Molecular Biology*, **289**, 547–564.

50 Zhang, X.J. and Matthews, B.W. (1994) Conservation of solvent-binding sites in 10 crystal forms of T4-lysozyme. *Protein Science: A Publication of the Protein Society*, **3**, 1031–1039.

51 Faerman, C.H. and Karplus, P.A. (1995) Consensus preferred hydration sites in 6 FKBP12 drug complexes. *Proteins: Structure, Function, and Genetics*, **23**, 1–11.

52 Schwabe, J.W.R. (1997) The role of water in protein DNA interactions. *Current Opinion in Structural Biology*, **7**, 126–134.

53 Carrell, H.L., Glusker, J.P., Burger, V., Manfre, F., Tritsch, D., and Biellmann, J.F. (1989) X-ray-analysis of D-xylose isomerase at 1.9 Å: native enzyme in complex with substrate and with a mechanism-designed inactivator. *Proceedings of the National Academy of Sciences of the United States of America*, **86**, 4440–4444.

54 Lalonde, J.M., Bernlohr, D.A., and Banaszak, L.J. (1994) X-ray crystallographic structures of adipocyte

lipid-binding protein complexed with palmitate and hexadecanesulfonic acid: properties of cavity binding-sites. *Biochemistry*, **33**, 4885–4895.

55 Myles, D.A.A. (2006) Neutron protein crystallography: current status and a brighter future. *Current Opinion in Structural Biology*, **16**, 630–637.

56 Chatake, T., Ostermann, A., Kurihara, K., Parak, F.G., and Niimura, N. (2003) Hydration in proteins observed by high-resolution neutron crystallography. *Proteins: Structure, Function, and Genetics*, **50**, 516–523.

57 Otting, G., Liepinsh, E., and Wuthrich, K. (1991) Protein hydration in aqueous-solution. *Science*, **254**, 974–980.

58 Wiesner, S., Kurian, E., Prendergast, F.G., and Halle, B. (1999) Water molecules in the binding cavity of intestinal fatty acid binding protein: Dynamic characterization by water O-17 and H-2 magnetic relaxation dispersion. *Journal of Molecular Biology*, **286**, 233–246.

59 Olsson, T.S.G., Williams, M.A., Pitt, W.R., and Ladbury, J.E. (2008) The thermodynamics of protein–ligand interaction and solvation: insights for ligand design. *Journal of Molecular Biology*, **384**, 1002–1017.

60 Bjelic, S. and Jelesarov, I. (2008) A survey of the year 2007 literature on applications of isothermal titration calorimetry. *Journal of Molecular Recognition*, **21**, 289–311.

61 Lu, Y.P., Yang, C.Y., and Wang, S.M. (2006) Binding free energy contributions of interfacial waters in HIV-1 protease inhibitor complexes. *Journal of the American Chemical Society*, **128**, 11830–11839.

62 Dill, K.A., Truskett, T.M., Vlachy, V., and Hribar-Lee, B. (2005) Modeling water, the hydrophobic effect, and ion solvation. *Annual Review of Biophysics and Biomolecular Structure*, **34**, 173–199.

63 Lounnas, V. and Pettitt, B.M. (1994) A connected cluster of hydration around myoglobin: correlation between molecular-dynamics simulations and experiment. *Proteins: Structure, Function, and Genetics*, **18**, 133–147.

64 Bizzarri, A.R. and Cannistraro, S. (2002) Molecular dynamics of water at the protein–solvent interface. *The Journal of Physical Chemistry B*, **106**, 6617–6633.

65 Brunne, R.M., Liepinsh, E., Otting, G., Wuthrich, K., and Vangunsteren, W.F. (1993) Hydration of proteins: a comparison of experimental residence times of water-molecules solvating the bovine pancreatic trypsin-inhibitor with theoretical-model calculations. *Journal of Molecular Biology*, **231**, 1040–1048.

66 Henchman, R.H. and McCammon, J.A. (2002) Extracting hydration sites around proteins from explicit water simulations. *Journal of Computational Chemistry*, **23**, 861–869.

67 Huang, H.C., Jupiter, D., Qiu, M., Briggs, J.M., and VanBuren, V. (2008) Cluster analysis of hydration waters around the active sites of bacterial alanine racemase using a 2-ns MD simulation. *Biopolymers*, **89**, 210–219.

68 Falconi, M., Brunelli, M., Pesce, A., Ferrario, M., Bolognesi, M., and Desideri, A. (2003) Static and dynamic water molecules in Cu,Zn superoxide dismutase. *Proteins: Structure, Function, and Genetics*, **51**, 607–615.

69 Makarov, V.A., Andrews, B.K., Smith, P.E., and Pettitt, B.M. (2000) Residence times of water molecules in the hydration sites of myoglobin. *Biophysical Journal*, **79**, 2966–2974.

70 Henchman, R.H. and McCammon, J.A. (2002) Structural and dynamic properties of water around acetylcholinesterase. *Protein Science: A Publication of the Protein Society*, **11**, 2080–2090.

71 Makarov, V.A., Feig, M., Andrews, B.K., and Pettitt, B.M. (1998) Diffusion of solvent around biomolecular solutes: a molecular dynamics simulation study. *Biophysical Journal*, **75**, 150–158.

72 Bakowies, D. and van Gunsteren, W.F. (2002) Water in protein cavities: a procedure to identify internal water and exchange pathways and application to fatty acid-binding protein. *Proteins: Structure, Function, and Genetics*, **47**, 534–545.

73 Garcia, A.E. and Hummer, G. (2000) Water penetration and escape in proteins.

Proteins: Structure, Function, and Genetics, **38**, 261–272.

74 Mancera, R.L. (2007) Molecular modeling of hydration in drug design. *Current Opinion in Drug Discovery & Development*, **10**, 275–280.

75 Aqvist, J., Medina, C., and Samuelsson, J.E. (1994) New method for predicting binding-affinity in computer-aided drug design. *Protein Engineering*, **7**, 385–391.

76 Carlson, H.A. and Jorgensen, W.L. (1995) An extended linear-response method for determining free-energies of hydration. *The Journal of Physical Chemistry*, **99**, 10667–10673.

77 Hansson, T., Marelius, J., and Aqvist, J. (1998) Ligand binding affinity prediction by linear interaction energy methods. *Journal of Computer-Aided Molecular Design*, **12**, 27–35.

78 Kollman, P.A., Massova, I., Reyes, C., Kuhn, B., Huo, S.H., Chong, L., Lee, M., Lee, T., Duan, Y., Wang, W., Donini, O., Cieplak, P., Srinivasan, J., Case, D.A., and Cheatham, T.E. (2000) Calculating structures and free energies of complex molecules: combining molecular mechanics and continuum models. *Accounts of Chemical Research*, **33**, 889–897.

79 Massova, I. and Kollman, P.A. (1999) Computational alanine scanning to probe protein–protein interactions: a novel approach to evaluate binding free energies. *Journal of the American Chemical Society*, **121**, 8133–8143.

80 Srinivasan, J., Cheatham, T.E., Cieplak, P., Kollman, P.A., and Case, D.A. (1998) Continuum solvent studies of the stability of DNA, RNA, and phosphoramidate–DNA helices. *Journal of the American Chemical Society*, **120**, 9401–9409.

81 Young, T., Abel, R., Kim, B., Berne, B.J., and Friesner, R.A. (2007) Motifs for molecular recognition exploiting hydrophobic enclosure in protein–ligand binding. *Proceedings of the National Academy of Sciences of the United States of America*, **104**, 808–813.

82 Beuming, T., Farid, R., and Sherman, W. (2009) High-energy water sites determine peptide binding affinity and specificity of PDZ domains. *Protein Science: A Publication of the Protein Society*, **18**, 1609–1619.

83 Abel, R., Young, T., Farid, R., Berne, B.J., and Friesner, R.A. (2008) Role of the active-site solvent in the thermodynamics of factor Xa ligand binding. *Journal of the American Chemical Society*, **130**, 2817–2831.

84 Lazaridis, T. (1998) Inhomogeneous fluid approach to solvation thermodynamics. 1. Theory. *The Journal of Physical Chemistry B*, **102**, 3531–3541.

85 Verdonk, M.L., Cole, J.C., and Taylor, R. (1999) SuperStar: a knowledge-based approach for identifying interaction sites in proteins. *Journal of Molecular Biology*, **289**, 1093–1108.

86 Verdonk, M.L., Cole, J.C., Watson, P., Gillet, V., and Willett, P. (2001) SuperStar: improved knowledge-based interaction fields for protein binding sites. *Journal of Molecular Biology*, **307**, 841–859.

87 Schymkowitz, J.W.H., Rousseau, F., Martins, I.C., Ferkinghoff-Borg, J., Stricher, F., and Serrano, L. (2005) Prediction of water and metal binding sites and their affinities by using the Fold-X force field. *Proceedings of the National Academy of Sciences of the United States of America*, **102**, 10147–10152.

88 Raymer, M.L., Sanschagrin, P.C., Punch, W.F., Venkataraman, S., Goodman, E.D., and Kuhn, L.A. (1997) Predicting conserved water-mediated and polar ligand interactions in proteins using a K-nearest-neighbors genetic algorithm. *Journal of Molecular Biology*, **265**, 445–464.

89 Kellogg, G.E. and Abraham, D.J. (2000) Hydrophobicity: is Log$P_{(o/w)}$ more than the sum of its parts? *European Journal of Medicinal Chemistry*, **35**, 651–661.

90 Kellogg, G.E. and Chen, D.L. (2004) The importance of being exhaustive. Optimization of bridging structural water molecules and water networks in models of biological systems. *Chemistry & Biodiversity*, **1**, 98–105.

91 Garcia-Sosa, A.T., Mancera, R.L., and Dean, P.M. (2003) WaterScore: a novel

method for distinguishing between bound and displaceable water molecules in the crystal structure of the binding site of protein–ligand complexes. *Journal of Molecular Modeling*, **9**, 172–182.

92 Ehrlich, L., Reczko, M., Bohr, H., and Wade, R.C. (1998) Prediction of protein hydration sites from sequence by modular neural networks. *Protein Engineering*, **11**, 11–19.

93 Goodford, P.J. (1985) A computational-procedure for determining energetically favorable binding-sites on biologically important macromolecules. *Journal of Medicinal Chemistry*, **28**, 849–857.

94 Wade, R.C., Clark, K.J., and Goodford, P.J. (1993) Further development of hydrogen-bond functions for use in determining energetically favorable binding-sites on molecules of known structure: 1. Ligand probe groups with the ability to form 2 hydrogen-bonds. *Journal of Medicinal Chemistry*, **36**, 140–147.

95 Fornabaio, M., Spyrakis, F., Mozzarelli, A., Cozzini, P., Abraham, D.J., and Kellogg, G.E. (2004) Simple, intuitive calculations of free energy of binding for protein–ligand complexes. 3. The free energy contribution of structural water molecules in HIV-1 protease complexes. *Journal of Medicinal Chemistry*, **47**, 4507–4516.

96 Kortvelyesi, T., Dennis, S., Silberstein, M., Brown, L., and Vajda, S. (2003) Algorithms for computational solvent mapping of proteins. *Proteins: Structure, Function, and Genetics*, **51**, 340–351.

97 Kroemer, R.T. (2007) Structure-based drug design: docking and scoring. *Current Protein & Peptide Science*, **8**, 312–328.

98 Leach, A.R., Shoichet, B.K., and Peishoff, C.E. (2006) Prediction of protein–ligand interactions. Docking and scoring: successes and gaps. *Journal of Medicinal Chemistry*, **49**, 5851–5855.

99 Moitessier, N., Englebienne, P., Lee, D., Lawandi, J., and Corbeil, C.R. (2008) Towards the development of universal, fast and highly accurate docking/scoring methods: a long way to go. *British Journal of Pharmacology*, **1531**, S7–S26.

100 Kongsted, J., Soderhjelm, P., and Ryde, U. (2009) How accurate are continuum solvation models for drug-like molecules? *Journal of Computer-Aided Molecular Design*, **23**, 395–409.

101 Villacanas, O., Madurga, S., Giralt, E., and Belda, I. (2009) Explicit treatment of water molecules in protein–ligand docking. *Current Computer-Aided Drug Design*, **5**, 145–154.

102 de Graaf, C., Oostenbrink, C., Keizers, P.H.J., van der Wijst, T., Jongejan, A., and Vemleulen, N.P.E. (2006) Catalytic site prediction and virtual screening of cytochrome P450 2D6 substrates by consideration of water and rescoring in automated docking. *Journal of Medicinal Chemistry*, **49**, 2417–2430.

103 de Graaf, C., Pospisil, P., Pos, W., Folkers, G., and Vermeulen, N.P.E. (2005) Binding mode prediction of cytochrome P450 and thymidine kinase protein–ligand complexes by consideration of water and rescoring in automated docking. *Journal of Medicinal Chemistry*, **48**, 2308–2318.

104 Garcia-Sosa, A.T. and Mancera, R.L. (2006) The effect of a tightly bound water molecule on scaffold diversity in the computer-aided *de novo* ligand design of CDK2 inhibitors. *Journal of Molecular Modeling*, **12**, 422–431.

105 Mancera, R.L. (2002) De *novo* ligand design with explicit water molecules: an application to bacterial neuraminidase. *Journal of Computer-Aided Molecular Design*, **16**, 479–499.

106 Osterberg, F., Morris, G.M., Sanner, M.F., Olson, A.J., and Goodsell, D.S. (2002) Automated docking to multiple target structures: incorporation of protein mobility and structural water heterogeneity in AutoDock. *Proteins: Structure, Function, and Bioinformatics*, **46**, 34–40.

107 Roberts, B.C. and Mancera, R.L. (2008) Ligand–protein docking with water molecules. *Journal of Chemical Information and Modeling*, **48**, 397–408.

108 Corbeil, C.R., Englebienne, P., and Moitessier, N. (2007) Docking ligands into flexible and solvated macromolecules. 1. Development and validation of FITTED 1.0. *Journal of Chemical Information and Modeling*, **47**, 435–449.

109 Englebienne, P. and Moitessier, N. (2009) Docking ligands into flexible and solvated macromolecules. 4. Are popular scoring functions accurate for this class of proteins? *Journal of Chemical Information and Modeling*, **49**, 1568–1580.

110 Rarey, M., Kramer, B., and Lengauer, T. (1999) The particle concept: placing discrete water molecules during protein–ligand docking predictions. *Proteins: Structure, Function, and Genetics*, **34**, 17–28.

111 Schnecke, V. and Kuhn, L.A. (2000) Virtual screening with solvation and ligand-induced complementarity. *Perspectives in Drug Discovery*, **20**, 171–190.

112 van Dijk, A.D.J. and Bonvin, A. (2006) Solvated docking: introducing water into the modelling of biomolecular complexes. *Bioinformatics (Oxford, England)*, **22**, 2340–2347.

113 Verdonk, M.L., Chessari, G., Cole, J.C., Hartshorn, M.J., Murray, C.W., Nissink, J.W.M., Taylor, R.D., and Taylor, R. (2005) Modeling water molecules in protein–ligand docking using GOLD. *Journal of Medicinal Chemistry*, **48**, 6504–6515.

114 Friesner, R.A., Banks, J.L., Murphy, R.B., Halgren, T.A., Klicic, J.J., Mainz, D.T., Repasky, M.P., Knoll, E.H., Shelley, M., Perry, J.K., Shaw, D.E., Francis, P., and Shenkin, P.S. (2004) GLIDE: A new approach for rapid, accurate docking and scoring. 1. Method and assessment of docking accuracy. *Journal of Medicinal Chemistry*, **47**, 1739–1749.

115 Friesner, R.A., Murphy, R.B., Repasky, M.P., Frye, L.L., Greenwood, J.R., Halgren, T.A., Sanschagrin, P.C., and Mainz, D.T. (2006) Extra precision GLIDE: docking and scoring incorporating a model of hydrophobic enclosure for protein–ligand complexes. *Journal of Medicinal Chemistry*, **49**, 6177–6196.

116 Huang, N. and Shoichet, B.K. (2008) Exploiting ordered waters in molecular docking. *Journal of Medicinal Chemistry*, **51**, 4862–4865.

117 Deng, W. and Verlinde, C. (2008) Evaluation of different virtual screening programs for docking in a charged binding pocket. *Journal of Chemical Information and Modeling*, **48**, 2010–2020.

118 Hartshorn, M.J., Verdonk, M.L., Chessari, G., Brewerton, S.C., Mooij, W.T.M., Mortenson, P.N., and Murray, C.W. (2007) Diverse, high-quality test set for the validation of protein–ligand docking performance. *Journal of Medicinal Chemistry*, **50**, 726–741.

119 Englebienne, P. and Moitessier, N. (2009) Docking ligands into flexible and solvated macromolecules. 5. Force-field-based prediction of binding affinities of ligands to proteins. *Journal of Chemical Information and Modeling*, **49**, 2564–2571.

120 Huang, N., Shoichet, B.K., and Irwin, J.J. (2006) Benchmarking sets for molecular docking. *Journal of Medicinal Chemistry*, **49**, 6789–6801.

121 Lloyd, D.G., Garcia-Sosa, A.T., Alberts, I.L., Todorov, N.P., and Mancera, R.L. (2004) The effect of tightly bound water molecules on the structural interpretation of ligand-derived pharmacophore models. *Journal of Computer-Aided Molecular Design*, **18**, 89–100.

122 Wolber, G., Dornhofer, A.A., and Langer, T. (2006) Efficient overlay of small organic molecules using 3D pharmacophores. *Journal of Computer-Aided Molecular Design*, **20**, 773–788.

123 Wolber, G. and Langer, T. (2005) LigandScout: 3D pharmacophores derived from protein-bound ligands and their use as virtual screening filters. *Journal of Chemical Information and Modeling*, **45**, 160–169.

124 Wolber, G., Seidel, T., Bendix, F., and Langer, T. (2008) Molecule-pharmacophore superpositioning and pattern matching in computational drug design. *Drug Discovery Today*, **13**, 23–29.

125 Romier, C., Reuter, K., Suck, D., and Ficner, R. (1996) Crystal structure of tRNA-guanine transglycosylase: RNA modification by base exchange. *The EMBO Journal*, **15**, 2850–2857.

126 Gradler, U., Gerber, H.D., Goodenough-Lashua, D.M., Garcia, G.A., Ficner, R., Reuter, K., Stubbs, M.T., and Klebe, G. (2001) A new target for shigellosis: rational design and crystallographic studies of inhibitors of tRNA-guanine transglycosylase. *Journal of Molecular Biology*, **306**, 455–467.

127 Hurst, T. (1994) Flexible 3D searching: the directed tweak technique. *Journal of Chemical Information and Computer Science*, **34**, 190–196.

128 Rarey, M., Kramer, B., Lengauer, T., and Klebe, G. (1996) A fast flexible docking method using an incremental construction algorithm. *Journal of Molecular Biology*, **261**, 470–489.

129 Brenk, R., Gerber, H.D., Kittendorf, J.D., Garcia, G.A., Reuter, K., and Klebe, G. (2003) From hit to lead: *de novo* design based on virtual screening hits of inhibitors of tRNA-guanine transglycosylase, a putative target of shigellosis therapy. *Helvetica Chimica Acta*, **86**, 1435–1452.

130 Meyer, E.A., Brenk, R., Castellano, R.K., Furler, M., Klebe, G., and Diederich, F. (2002) De *novo* design, synthesis, and *in vitro* evaluation of inhibitors for prokaryotic tRNA-guanine transglycosylase: a dramatic sulfur effect on binding affinity. *ChemBioChem*, **3**, 250–253.

131 Brenk, R., Meyer, E.A., Reuter, K., Stubbs, M.T., Garcia, G.A., Diederich, F., and Klebe, G. (2004) Crystallographic study of inhibitors of tRNA-guanine transglycosylase suggests a new structure-based pharmacophore for virtual screening. *Journal of Molecular Biology*, **338**, 55–75.

132 Stengl, B., Meyer, E.A., Heine, A., Brenk, R., Diederich, F., and Klebe, G. (2007) Crystal structures of tRNA-guanine transglycosylase (TGT) in complex with novel and potent inhibitors unravel pronounced induced-fit adaptations and suggest dimer formation upon substrate binding. *Journal of Molecular Biology*, **370**, 492–511.

133 Stengl, B., Reuter, K., and Klebe, G. (2005) Mechanism and substrate specificity of tRNA-guanine transglycosylases (TGTs): tRNA-modifying enzymes from the three different kingdoms of life share a common catalytic mechanism. *ChemBioChem*, **6**, 1926–1939.

Part Three
Applications and Practical Guidelines

Virtual Screening. Edited by C. Sotriffer

ISBN: 978-3-527-32636-5

11
Applied Virtual Screening: Strategies, Recommendations, and Caveats

Dagmar Stumpfe and Jürgen Bajorath

11.1
Introduction

This chapter is focused on practical aspects of ligand-based virtual screening (LBVS), that is, computational screening of *in silico* formatted compound databases utilizing information from known active compounds as a starting point [1]. We will however not discuss the target structure-based screening techniques [2]. We will assume that the reader is familiar with the basic concepts underlying computational screening approaches such as appropriate molecular representations, chemical reference spaces, or distance relationships in chemical space that serve as a measure of similarity. Our main objectives will be to discuss principal aspects affecting the outcome of LBVS calculations, outline the applicability domain of LBVS methods, highlight opportunities and intrinsic limitations of these approaches, and comment on a few controversial issues. Much of these insights are based on experience values derived from practical LBVS applications, extensive comparisons of different computational methods in retrospective screening trials, and the review of many virtual screening studies. We will also comment on the interplay between computational and experimental compound screening and make some suggestions how to best analyze virtual screening results and select candidate compounds. Finally, two LBVS case studies originating from our laboratory will be discussed.

11.2
What Is Virtual Screening?

Regardless of the algorithms and search tools that are applied, the basic goal of LBVS is to utilize known active compounds as templates (or reference molecules), computationally screen large compound databases, select small sets of candidate compounds for experimental testing, and identify among them novel active compounds that structurally depart from the templates. Although many different methods have been developed or adapted for LBVS applications, this process is far from being routine and, to this date, generally not well understood with respect to its

Virtual Screening. Edited by C. Sotriffer

ISBN: 978-3-527-32636-5

advantages and disadvantages. Questionable studies have appeared, and continue to appear, in the literature and yet there are undisputed success stories, making it difficult to judge about the scientific value and reliability of virtual approaches. In fact, for the uninitiated observer, virtual screening might often still appear to be more of an art form (not to say "black magic") than rigorous science. Given this rather complex scientific environment, we are trying to better understand why LBVS methods succeed or fail and how to best select and apply them.

11.3 Spectrum of Virtual Screening Approaches

In the LBVS field, one can broadly distinguish between two basic categories of methods: similarity searching on one hand and compound classification on the other [3]. The popular similarity search tools as shown in Figure 11.1 include molecular fingerprints derived from molecular graphs (2D) or conformations (3D) [4, 5], pharmacophore models [6], simplified molecular graph representations [7],

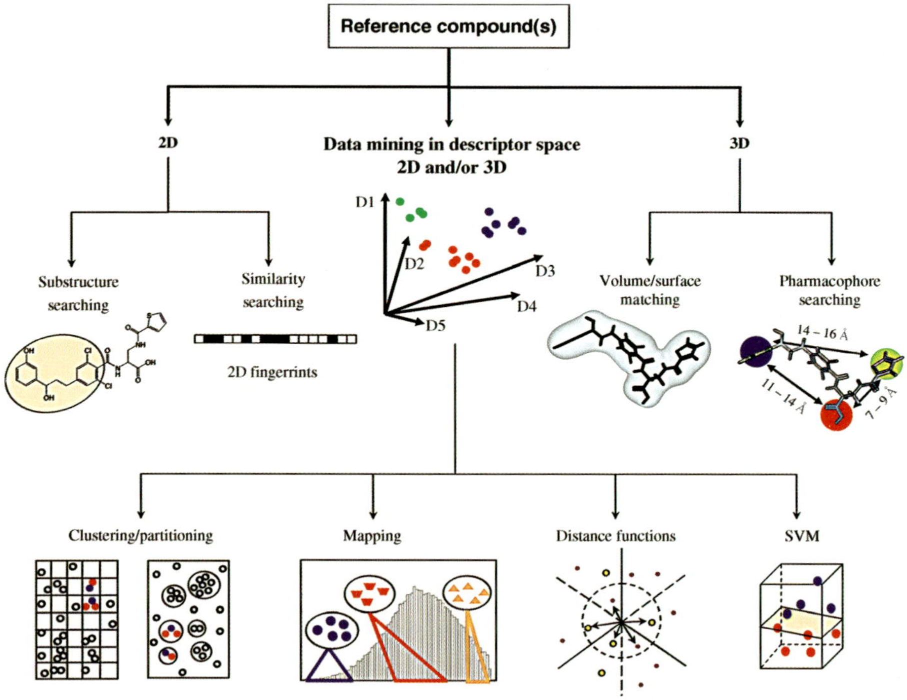

Figure 11.1 Ligand-based virtual screening methods. Exemplary computational methods for database screening are shown subdivided into techniques that are based on 2D or 3D compound representations, respectively, or that operate in chemical reference spaces formed by 2D or 3D descriptors.

or molecular shape queries [8, 9]. Although all these similarity search methods differ in their design, they have in common that they can be applied if only a single active reference compound is available. This is in contrast to compound classification methods that require multiple reference compounds as input. Compound classification approaches also include methods of very different character and complexity such as cluster analysis [10], cell-based [11, 12] or statistical partitioning [13, 14], and various machine learning approaches, for example, neural networks [15], self-organizing maps [16], or support vector machines (SVMs) [17, 18]. Although similarity search tools can be applied on the basis of individual reference molecules, their performance generally increases when multiple reference compounds are available, which then makes it possible to apply data fusion techniques to merge individual results [19]. Generally, the chemical information content of search calculations is increasing with the availability of multiple active reference compounds.

In addition to the two major categories of LBVS approaches, similarity searching and compound classification, database filtering techniques should also be added to the virtual screening spectrum. Rule-based filters that screen databases for compounds with desired (e.g., drug- or leadlike) or undesired (toxicity and instability) molecular properties are widely used, not to identify individual active compounds but rather to reduce the size of screening databases as much as possible for further studies using more sophisticated methods.

11.4
Molecular Similarity as a Foundation and Caveat of Virtual Screening

Despite substantial methodological differences, all LBVS approaches principally rely on the assessment of "similarity" between reference and database compounds. An intuitive assumption is that the more similar the molecules are, the more likely they share similar biological properties. However, similarity is essentially a subjective concept and whenever we change molecular representations and similarity measures [20], our perception of similarity also likely changes. Although there is no generally applicable way to evaluate and quantify molecular similarity, all LBVS approaches ultimately rely on the detection of "valid" similarity relationships between reference and database compounds. For this purpose, one would initially calculate a form of chemical similarity or structure/property resemblance. However, to further complicate matters, what we are really interested in is not chemical similarity *per se*, however evaluated, but rather potential similarity in the biological behavior of test compounds. Unfortunately, there are no generally applicable criteria or rules that tell us if molecular and biological similarity is related to each other. In fact, this relationship is often overlooked or even misunderstood. For example, in their seminal publication introducing the concept of "neighborhood behavior," Patterson *et al.* [21] established for one particular fingerprint (i.e., a specific molecular representation) that a Tanimoto coefficient (Tc) (quantifying fingerprint overlap) [4] of 0.85 corresponded to a high probability that two compounds shared similar biological activity. To date, this Tc threshold value is applied in many publications as a criterion for activity similarity, regardless of the fingerprints and similarity measures that are applied, although it has been shown that this threshold value is not a reliable indicator when other fingerprints are utilized [22]. It is indeed often overlooked that similarity threshold values are generally not transferable from one similarity search tool to another, but that they need to be reestablished through careful benchmarking for any combination of a similarity search tool and similarity metric. This equally applies to molecular descriptors such as 2D fingerprints and more sophisticated search tools such as pharmacophore or molecular shape representations. The key is that any chosen similarity threshold value must be activity relevant, which cannot be determined from first principles.

Similarity searching produces a compound database ranking in the order of decreasing calculated similarity to reference molecules that is usually based on pairwise comparisons. In contrast, compound classification methods such as clustering, partitioning, or machine learning techniques typically classify test compounds as "active" or "inactive," without a ranking scheme (although there are exceptions such as SVM-based compound ranking [23]). In these cases, distance relationships in chemical reference spaces are analyzed and proximity of database molecules to known active compounds serves as a measure of similarity and an indicator of bioactivity. Differences in the way similarity relationships are determined and expressed have important consequences for virtual screening and compound selection strategies, as further discussed below.

It should also be noted that one often applies different views of molecular similarity in LBVS. For example, a pharmacophore query that embodies the spatial arrangement of atoms or groups in molecules known or thought to be responsible for biological activity emphasizes "submolecular" or "local" similarity and requires prior knowledge. In contrast, the comparison of whole-molecule representations such as fingerprints, graphs, or arrays of property descriptors whose values define compound positions in chemical space account for "global" similarity. Here no assumption is made about those parts of molecules that might render them active and, accordingly, no knowledge about structure–activity relationships (SARs) is required. It is this global view of similarity that most LBVS methods rely on.

11.5
Goals of Virtual Screening

Any type of virtual screening ultimately aims at finding previously unknown molecules having a desired (specific) biological activity. However, one is rarely interested in finding compounds that are analogues of known active molecules. A simple substructure search in a database would be sufficient for this purpose. The major challenge of LBVS is to search for active compounds that structurally depart from reference molecules. This makes compound selection challenging. For example, going back to our similarity search example, simply selecting the top-ranked database compounds will not help to facilitate scaffold transitions. Rather, one needs to select compounds further down the ranking that structurally depart from the reference compounds. For this purpose, the notion of "global" similarity threshold values, or value ranges, that are biologically significant and delineate an "activity radius" (see below) around known active compounds is critical. However, for many widely used methods and search tools, measures of such activity radii have not been reported, often because the underlying problem might not be obvious to many practitioners in the field. Whether or not sufficient structural differences between reference and newly identified active compounds exist is often a matter of debate. The presence of different hierarchically derived molecular scaffolds [24] is often considered a criterion for success, but distinct molecular scaffolds might often be rather similar and only distinguished by, for example, a single heteroatom position. Therefore, scaffolds are further transformed into carbon skeletons that no longer contain bond order or heteroatom information, but reveal topological differences. Accordingly, active molecules producing distinct carbon skeletons are usually considered successful scaffold transitions made in the context of LBVS.

There might be different motivations to search for active compounds belonging to different structural classes. However, a major driver for the popularity of virtual screening techniques in pharmaceutical research is the desire to find active chemotypes that are sufficiently different from those reported by competitors so that independent intellectual property positions can be established. Furthermore, known active compounds that are difficult to access synthetically, have toxic effects, or yield "flat" SARs (i.e., are resistant to potency optimization through analogue generation) might need to be replaced with other chemotypes having a comparable biological activity profile, which is another prime application area for LBVS.

11.6 Applicability Domain

Essentially, all LBVS methods attempt to extrapolate from known active compounds and identify structurally increasingly diverse molecules having similar activity. This means that the targeted structure–activity relationships must be "continuous," that is, gradual changes in structure must be accompanied by moderate changes in biological activity, and the activity radius around an active compound must be populated with different chemotypes retaining similar activity. In contrast, any abrupt or "discontinuous" SAR behavior, that is, small structural modifications that cause a dramatic change or loss of biological activity, fall outside the application domain of LBVS methods. For example, closely related analogues where a small chemical change leads to a loss of activity must be recognized by any LBVS method as being "similar," although one compound is active, but the other is not. Thus, the presence of SAR discontinuity eliminates the continuous relationship between chemical and biological activity similarity on which LBVS methods are conceptually based. In contrast, SAR discontinuity is important for compound optimization where small chemical changes are introduced in order to catapult the potency of an active chemotype into the nanomolar range. Large-scale profiling of compound activity

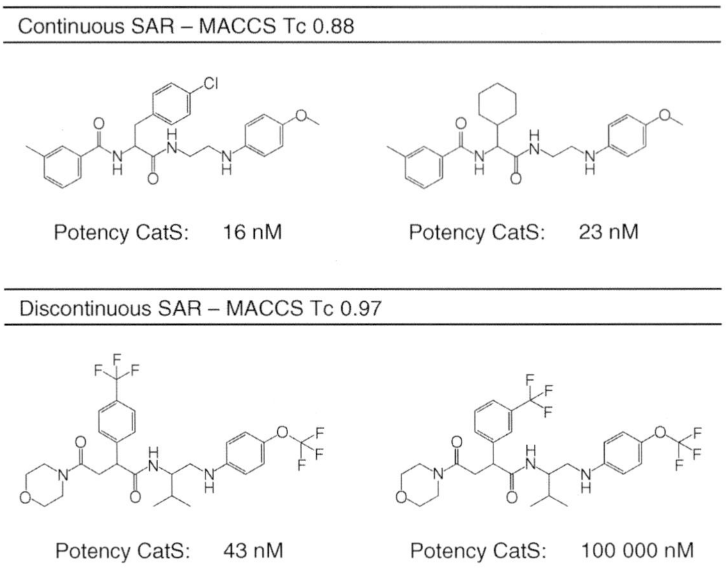

Figure 11.2 Heterogeneous SAR combining continuous and discontinuous SAR. Four cathepsin S inhibitors display different SAR behavior. Inhibitors related by a continuous SAR have comparable potency values despite structural variations (top). In the context of a discontinuous SAR, structurally similar inhibitors substantially differ in their potency for cathepsin S. Tc values calculated with MACCS structural keys are reported as a measure of molecular similarity.

classes has revealed that continuous and discontinuous SAR phenotypes are not mutually exclusive, and that the majority of SARs encoded in sets of active compounds are “heterogeneous” in nature [25], that is, they combine continuous and discontinuous elements as shown in Figure 11.2.

These SAR features can be rationalized using the intuitive concept of an “activity landscape,” that is, a 2D projection of chemical space with compound potency added as a third dimension [26]. The activity landscape underlying heterogeneous SARs is composed of smooth regions (where changes in chemical structure only lead to small or moderate changes in activity) that are intersected by steep “activity cliffs” (where small chemical changes cause dramatic potency alterations). Figure 11.3 shows such an activity landscape for a set of cathepsin K inhibitors.

LBVS methods can only be applied to screen smooth regions of such an activity landscape to identify alternative active chemotypes. If they map to the vicinity of an activity cliff, the opportunity exists to optimize these compounds. Importantly, however, the presence of SAR discontinuity severely limits the general applicability of LBVS methods. This can also be rationalized at the level of target proteins. If there is little or no variability in compound binding modes and no plasticity within a ligand binding site, a violation of critical receptor–ligand interactions caused, for example, by modification of a single functional group might not be permitted, giving rise to abrupt SAR behavior and strong discontinuity. In such instances, finding alternative active scaffolds is becoming a very difficult, if not impossible, task.

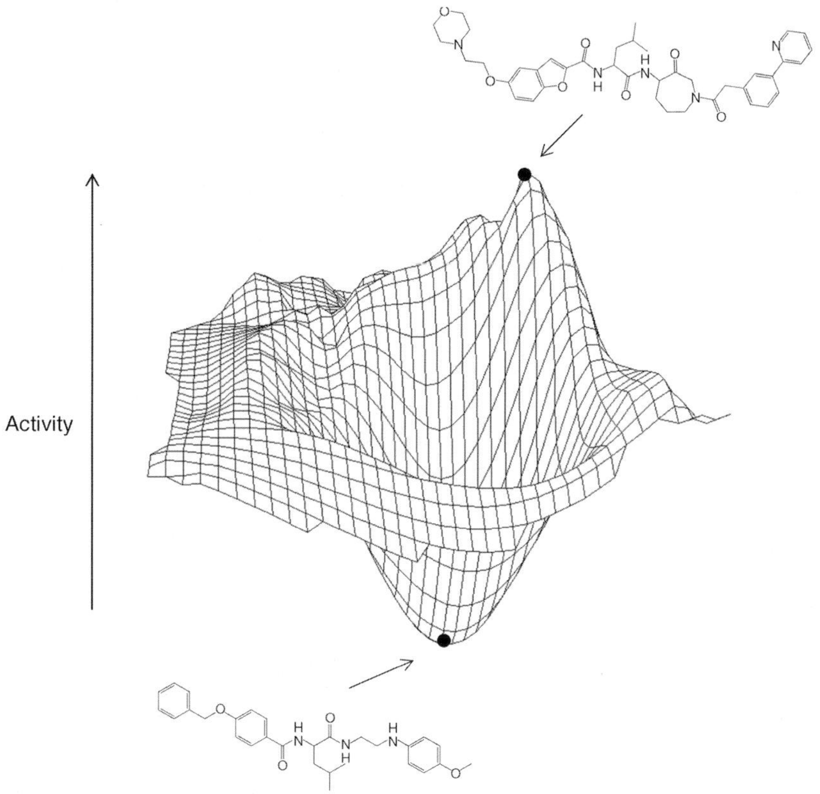

Figure 11.3 Activity landscape of a set of selective cathepsin K inhibitors (reference set from Section 11.14.2). Molecular structures of the most and least potent inhibitors are shown and their coordinates are indicated as black points in the landscape. Potency of the inhibitor is given by its pK_i or pIC$_{50}$ value. The chemical reference space was projected onto the *x*,*y*-plane through multidimensional scaling on the basis of MACCS Tc similarity. For clarity, only the *z*-axis (potency) is shown.

11.7 Reference and Database Compounds

At the beginning of any LBVS campaign, information about known active compounds must be surveyed and reference molecules selected. Typically, references are taken from the scientific or patent literature and hence represent highly optimized and potent leads or drug candidates. Accordingly, they are larger and more complex than average screening database compounds. This presents potential complications, depending on the LBVS methods that are applied. For example, for similarity searching using standard molecular fingerprints, the choice of highly complex reference molecules has been shown to generally present the most difficult search scenario, producing lowest hit rates, due to the bias introduced by molecular size and complexity [27, 28]. High fingerprint bit density produced by large and complex reference molecules leads to the preferential selection of database compounds of above-average size and often significantly increases false-positive rates. Accordingly, reference molecules are generally preferred that are comparable in size and complexity to average database compounds, for example, screening hits. However, screening hits are often not chosen because of their comparably low potency, which reflects another general misunderstanding of the LBVS approach, as further discussed below. For both similarity search and compound classification techniques, as many reference compounds as possible are typically chosen (if there are no specific reasons to exclusively focus on a particular chemotype) in order to maximize the SAR information content of LBVS calculations. It is important to select structurally diverse active compounds because analogue series only represent an individual scaffold and do not contribute relevant information (in fact, their inclusion might bias compound classification calculations toward the scaffold they represent). Similarity search methods are preferably applied in combination with data fusion techniques to make use of information provided by multiple reference molecules [5, 19]. In addition to known active compounds, machine learning methods applied in LBVS such as neural networks or support vector machines also require inactive compounds for learning. Confirmed inactive compounds are often more difficult to obtain than active reference molecules (if high-throughput screening (HTS) data sets are not available). Consequently, randomly selected database compounds are mostly used as negative training examples [23]. In general, this approximation is reasonable, but it presents another potential source of systematic prediction errors.

As long as 2D or relatively simple 3D molecular representations are utilized, most current LBVS methods can be readily applied to process very large source databases without substantial computational limitations. For example, version 8 of the popular public domain ZINC database [29] contains ~8.5 million *in silico* formatted compounds collected from vendor sources. Processing a database of this size is feasible for many current LBVS methods. However, results of virtual screening projects reported in the literature have also shown that databases of this size might not be essential for the identification of novel hits, provided the target is a "good" small-molecule target and tolerates the binding of diverse compounds (corresponding to the presence of "continuous" small-molecule SARs; see above).

Rule-based filtering techniques have become an integral part of LBVS campaigns to preselect compounds for screening that have druglike or, better, leadlike character [30] and remove compounds that are metabolically unstable, reactive, or contain toxic groups [31]. Compound filtering is computationally highly efficient and can be applied at different stages during the virtual screening process.

11.8
Biological Activity versus Compound Potency

Although some efforts have been made to include compound potency as a search parameter [32], LBVS methods generally treat biological activity in a qualitative manner, that is, reference compounds are not distinguished by potency differences.

Thus, weakly and highly potent reference compounds are regarded as "active" and separated from inactive compounds. This has some implications for the choice of reference compounds. Starting from highly optimized and potent compounds, if available, is intuitive, but will likely be negatively influenced by molecular complexity effects, as mentioned above. Weakly active compounds such as screening hits are less complex and might provide alternative starting points. Optimized leads might not necessarily provide an intrinsic advantage over more weakly potent compounds to find an alternative scaffold. Because compound potency is not taken into account during LBVS calculations, it is not possible to direct the search toward structurally distinct yet potent compounds. In fact, an observation generally made in LBVS is that most newly identified active compounds are only weakly potent, typically within the micromolar range, and rarely more potent than reference molecules. The activity landscape concept offers intuitive explanations for these observations. Optimized and highly potent compounds map to activity cliff regions or plateaus and departing from those structures very likely leads us into surrounding regions that are relatively flat and populated with weakly to moderately potent compounds including screening hits. Hence, the optimization aspect comes into play here. Active molecules identified by extrapolating from known reference structures are not chemically optimized, just like HTS hits, and generally serve as a starting point for further chemical exploration. From this point of view, obtaining a highly active new structure is a rather unlikely outcome for an LBVS campaign (although it occasionally might also happen).

11.9 Methodological Complexity and Compound Class Dependence

Many successful LBVS exercises are reported in the literature and probably many more are not published, especially those carried out in pharmaceutical settings. There is no doubt that LBVS, similar to structure-based virtual screening, produces hits against many different targets, although all LBVS methods are only approximate and error prone. What makes them often successful? Answering this question is not a trivial task. From systematic qualitative and quantitative SAR analysis, we have learned that many target proteins are promiscuous in their ligand binding properties and tolerant to continuous/heterogeneous SARs [33], thus providing a promising basis for LBVS. However, in reviewing practical LBVS applications, some general trends can be observed concerning the performance of LBVS methods that might be rather unexpected. Clearly, the computational complexity of different LBVS methods and the sophistication of chosen molecular representations do not scale with LBVS success rates. In some instances, different methodologies consistently identify novel active compounds and rather simple methods such as 2D fingerprints often produce as many, if not more, hits than approaches of much higher methodological complexity; in other cases, essentially all methods fail, regardless of their degree of sophistication. Moreover, there is a strong compound class dependence of the performance of LBVS methods. Different methods perform very differently on various compound classes [34], an observation that can also be made in benchmark calculations (that are otherwise only a poor indicator of expected LBVS performance in practical applications). It is essentially impossible to predict for a given target or compound class which LBVS methodology might be most promising. Here the type of chosen molecular representation often plays a rather critical role. Molecular features important for the biological activity of different compound classes might or might not be well captured by a given representation, for example, an array of molecular property descriptors, a certain fingerprint design, or a graph-based query. Furthermore, the question of whether 2D or 3D representations and LBVS methods are superior is debated for long time in the scientific literature. Clearly, molecules are active in three dimensions and hence 3D methods should have principal advantages. However, these expectations have not been confirmed in many comparative benchmarking studies where 2D-based approaches often perform better than 3D methods [35]. These findings are at least in part due to the fact that LBVS methodologies relying on putative binding conformations are much more vulnerable to prediction errors than many 2D approaches that are simpler and have "lower resolution," but are less error prone. For example, despite their simplicity, structural key-type fingerprints, which have a long history in chemical information science and database mining, have been surprisingly successful in many search situations [5, 36], probably because substructure patterns implicitly account for much SAR-relevant chemical information. Questions such as why a given LBVS method succeeds or fails or why it can treat some compound classes but not others are currently not well understood. We frequently see reports in the literature claiming that a particular virtual screening approach is "validated" because one or more active compounds have been identified when applying it. Often these are complex applications combining different methods in multiple steps and it usually remains unclear which of the reported calculations were essential for hit identification, again illustrating that reasons for success or failure of individual LBVS approaches are currently only poorly understood.

11.10 Search Strategies and Compound Selection

What are the criteria for planning and carrying out practical LBVS campaigns and for selecting candidate compounds? First of all, because method performance is generally highly variable and difficult to predict, different types of methodologies, utilizing different molecular representations, should be carried out in parallel; for example, different fingerprints for similarity searching together with machine learning methods. Figure 11.4 demonstrates alternative VS scenarios.

Similarity search tools produce database rankings, clustering or partitioning techniques identify database compounds that are grouped together with one or more reference molecules, and machine learning methods typically (but not always) yield class label predictions (i.e., "active" versus "inactive"). Applying different methods in parallel makes it attractive to consider a form of "consensus scoring" [37] to identify preferred candidate compounds. However, the heterogeneity of the

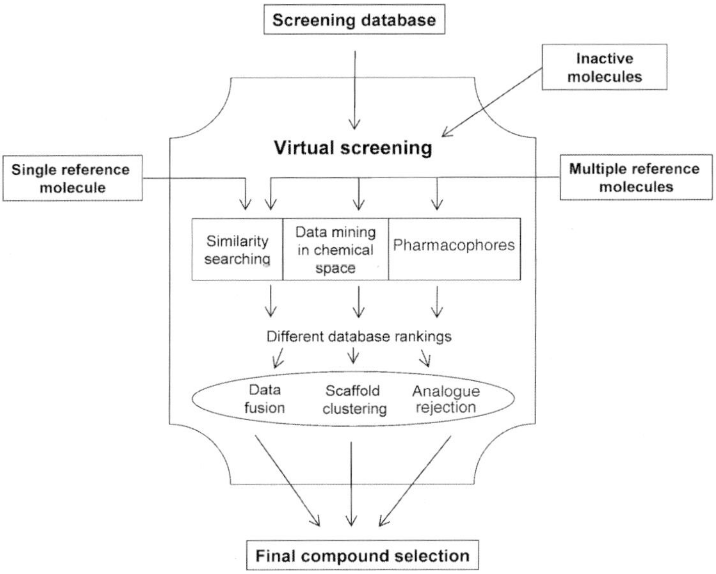

Figure 11.4 Virtual screening process. Depending on the available ligand information, different methods and strategies can be applied during a typical virtual screen, often in parallel.

readouts produced by different approaches requires searching for consensus patterns in different ways. Regardless of how consensus patterns are analyzed, one would be interested in candidate compounds that are recurrent in ranked lists and classified sets. However, given the strong compound class-dependent performance of LBVS methods, exclusively relying on consensus selections would be rather dangerous. For example, if one of the chosen methods succeeds but others fail, attractive compounds would likely be "averaged out." Consequently, for any of the applied methodologies, a number of preferred candidates, however determined, should also be selected individually. Thus, a database selection set combining consensus hits with candidates prioritized for each individual method is likely to provide the best basis for success.

What about selection set size? Both from an intellectual and a practical point of view, it is certainly an attractive exercise to computationally process millions of database compounds, select only a small candidate set, for example, a hundred or so, and hopefully identify one or more novel hits. However, the smaller the size of the selection set, the more likely the LBVS effort will fail, for more than one reason. First, one should consider that only a small number of hits for a given target will be available in a large database and that the vast majority of database compounds will be inactive, a situation akin to the well-known "needles in haystacks" scenario. Considering that all LBVS methodologies have disadvantages and only approximate prediction accuracy, a logical consequence is that most selected compounds will be false positives. Hence, it would often be an almost hopeless strategy to select only a handful of database compounds. For some LBVS methods such as mapping algorithms, it has been observed that active compounds are typically enriched in small compound selection sets, if the calculations succeed [38]. Provided that such insights are available, one might deliberately limit selection set size. However, these are exceptions rather than the rule, and in general such assumptions cannot be made. Accurately identifying individual active compounds is inconsistent with global accuracy limitations of LBVS. If successful, an LBVS campaign will yield a certain enrichment of active compounds over random selection and, from this point of view, selecting as many candidate compounds as possible for experimental evaluation would be meaningful. Of course, virtual screeners are often specifically asked to select a minimum number of candidates for testing in time-consuming and/or expensive assay systems (which is one of the attractions of the *in silico* approach for many experimentalists). However, one should be aware of the fact that the choice of very small compound selection sets is not consistent with the general accuracy limitations of current LBVS methods.

If an LBVS campaign suggests many candidate compounds that cannot be further prioritized, for example, because only class label predictions (i.e., active versus inactive) have been carried out, investigators often attempt to group these compounds according to their scaffolds or maximum common substructures and reduce the number of candidates by selecting a representative compound for each identified structural class. At first glance, this might look like a rational and plausible approach. However, it has a high risk of false-negative predictions. Why so? Even if a transition from reference compounds to a previously unobserved "active scaffold" has successfully been made, the possibility always exists that an individual compound representing this scaffold might be an inactive analogue, due to the presence of SAR discontinuity. Hence, if multiple candidate scaffolds are considered, it is always advisable to select at least a few analogues representing each scaffold. The probability that two, three, or more analogues representing an intrinsically active scaffold are all completely inactive is generally low, and thus by considering multiple analogues the probability of false-negative assignments might often be substantially reduced.

11.11
Virtual and High-Throughput Screening

From a scientific point of view, the interface between computational screening and HTS is of significant interest. The so-called sequential or iterative screening schemes have been designed to integrate computational and HTS efforts [39, 40]. The basic idea behind the sequential screening paradigm is to preselect a subset of a screening library by LBVS (or structure-based screening) that has a high probability to contain active compounds, subject these subsets to HTS, utilize newly identified hits as additional reference compounds for LBVS, carry out another round of virtual screening, test another subset, and so on. This strategy plays a major role in the strength of LBVS and is schematically demonstrated in Figure 11.5. Although LBVS is not sufficiently accurate to consistently identify active compounds in small selection sets, current LBVS methods are usually capable of enriching active compounds in subsets of, for example, 1–5% of a given database. For a screening

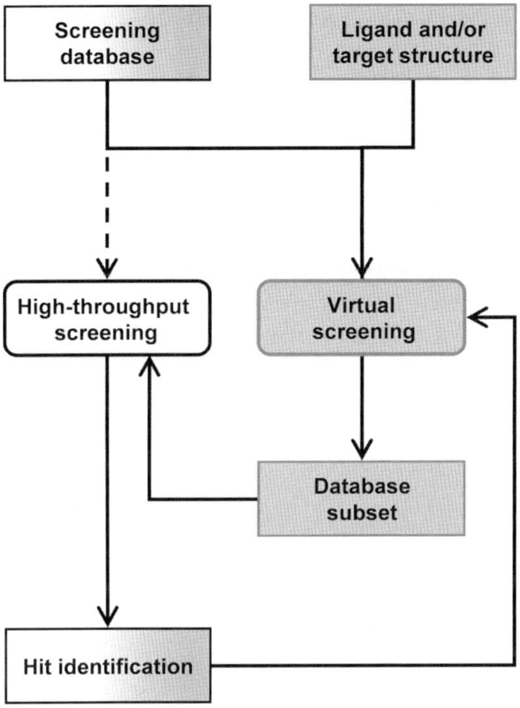

Figure 11.5 Sequential or iterative screening schemes to integrate computational and HTS efforts. Combining virtual screening and HTS in one or more iterations is expected to yield high hit rates while considerably reducing the experimental effort.

library containing a million compounds, an LBVS-selected subset of 10 000–50 000 compounds should be expected to contain a significant percentage of the available hits (otherwise, the applied methodology would essentially be of no use). In addition to the enrichment of active compounds, the deselection of compounds that are inconsistent with a given biological activity plays a major role in the reduction of the experimental efforts. Confirmed hits then further expand the knowledge base for LBVS and increase the probability of identifying additional hits in subsequent rounds.

In pilot studies, two to three iterations were often sufficient to achieve high hit rates; on average, experimental testing of ~10% of a screening library identified ~50% of the available hits [41]. Thus, if exhaustive hit identification is not essential, sequential screening schemes should in principle be highly attractive to reduce the experimental magnitude (and costs) of HTS projects. However, there have thus far only been limited activities in this area in pharmaceutical research (and only few publications). There are probably several reasons for this, including both technical and "philosophical" issues. Sequential screening has a few requirements that are often not straightforward to implement within a conventional HTS infrastructure, including, for example, the ability to cherry-pick compounds from screening plates.

It is technically often much easier to screen an entire plate than extract samples from it. Furthermore, high-throughput and virtual screeners typically represent different research philosophies and are rewarded for different types of accomplishments; the HTS scientist for screening increasing numbers of compounds more efficiently and, in contrast, the computational screener for reducing the number of candidate compounds as much as possible. In addition to technical constraints, this pseudo-competitive situation might explain why sequential screening schemes are currently not as far advanced in practice as one might hope for.

However, there are other areas where HTS and LBVS also complement each other. Computational screening is often applied to reevaluate screening libraries for compounds that are similar to attractive HTS hits in order to select candidates from the library (or other compound collections) for retesting. Furthermore, LBVS approaches are well suited to focus secondary libraries on selected active compounds. In this case, sets of similar molecules are identified in vendor or other compound sources in order to assemble moderately sized focused libraries for hit expansion.

11.12
Practical Applications: An Overview

Examples of practical LBVS applications carried out in our laboratory are given in Table 11.1. Since most of these projects were carried out in collaboration with pharmaceutical companies, the diverse biological targets studied here are not reported. Besides, for the purpose of our discussion, the nature of the targets is also not important. Rather, the results mirror some general trends we observed when practically applying 2D LBVS methods or combinations of 2D and 3D methods. In the majority of cases (12 of 14 projects), hits containing previously unobserved

Table 11.1 Practical LBVS applications.

Target protein	VS hit rate (%)	Active/assayed cpds
1	0.7	1/135
2	0.0	0/143
3	4.0	1/25
4	7.6	6/79
5	11.7	17/145
6	4.4	5/113
7	0.2	1/687
8	2.0	1/50
9	2.1	1/48
10	0.0	0/22
11	7.1	1/14
12	6.6	5/76
13	4.4	8/183
14	18.8	3/16

scaffolds were identified that were mostly active in the low micromolar range. Only a limited number of compounds (with 1 exception, fewer than 200), selected from virtually formatted vendor catalogues containing a total of 2–3 million compounds, were tested to identify novel active compounds. In a number of cases, only 50 or fewer compounds were evaluated and, as discussed above, such small selection sets are not necessarily a meaningful choice, given the intrinsic limitations of LBVS methods.

In these cases, more candidates were initially selected, but relatively only few of these compounds could ultimately be acquired for experimental evaluation. The results also show that although novel actives were identified in most cases, the number of hits was generally small; in six cases, only a single hit was identified. Thus, hit rates observed in these practical applications ranged from 0 to 18.8% (with an average of 5%) and were thus much lower than one would typically observe in retrospective benchmark trials using virtual screening methods. Clearly, experimental constraints and, in particular, compound availability play a role here, but the results also point at the often artificial nature of benchmark settings that do not realistically account for the potential of practical applications. Benchmark calculations are typically carried out using sets of optimized and highly potent compounds taken from databases or literature sources that are divided into reference and test sets. These test sets are then added to screening databases. Due to their larger size and modified molecular properties, leads or drug candidates are much easier to distinguish from average database compounds using similarity-based methods than screening hits, which renders the success rates of benchmarking calculations artificially high in many, if not all, instances.

In the following, two LBVS case studies will be discussed in greater detail: the identification of (1) an attractive antagonist of the lymphocyte function-associated antigen-1 (LFA-1) [42] and (2) target-selective inhibitors for cathepsin K (CatK) [43].

11.13 LFA-1 Antagonist

LFA-1 belongs to the integrin family of cell surface proteins, has two subunits α_L or CD11a and β_2 or CD18, and is expressed in normal and leukemia T cells [44]. It binds to the intercellular adhesion molecules (ICAM) -1, -2, and -3 of different cell types and these interactions have different functional consequences. The LFA-1/ICAM-1 complex plays, for example, an important role in mediating cellular adhesion. The α-subunit of LFA-1 contains a domain of 200 amino acids, the so-called I-domain [45], which is directly involved in ICAM-1 binding [46]. Several allosteric antagonists were discovered that interrupt this interaction and therefore indirectly inhibit cell adhesion. Allosteric antagonists bind to a site distant from the ligand binding site and prevent regular binding events through conformational effects. Most of the known allosteric antagonists for LFA-1 bind to a hydrophobic cleft in the I-domain and block a conformational transition of LFA-1 required for ICAM-1 binding [47, 48]. However, a single allosteric antagonist was identified to act through a different mechanism by binding at the interface between the α- and β-subunits. This antagonist, compound **1**,

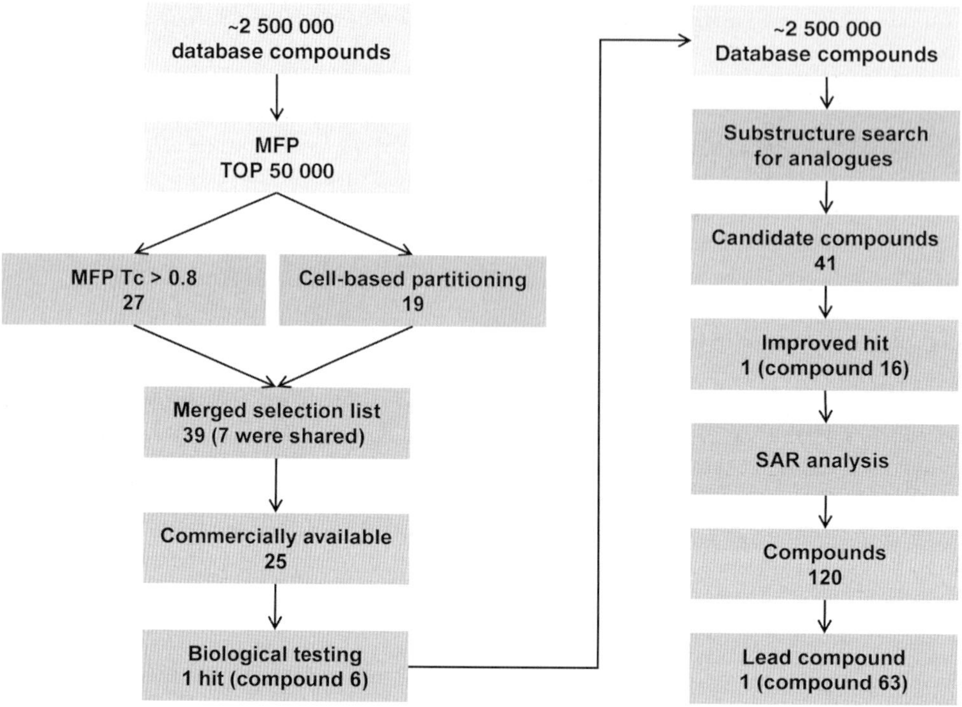

Figure 11.6 Searching for LFA-1 antagonists. The diagram summarizes the results of the LBVS and hit expansion process.

was highly potent with an IC_{50} value of 1.4 nM [49] and its unique mode of action was considered particularly attractive for a drug discovery effort. Therefore, this antagonist was used as the single reference compound in a LBVS campaign to search new LFA-1 antagonists. The molecular structure of compound **1** is shown in Figure 11.7.

11.13.1
Similarity Searching

A 2D "MiniFingerPrint" [50] was used for single-template similarity searching that consisted of fewer than 100 bit positions and combined value-range encoded property descriptors with binary structural fragment descriptors. A screening database of ~2 500 000 compounds collected from catalogues of several commercial vendors was searched and ranked by Tanimoto coefficient values relative to compound **1**. As illustrated in Figure 11.6, candidate molecules were chosen from the top-ranked 50 000 database compounds in two ways. First, all database molecules with a Tc above 0.8 were selected, resulting in only 27 compounds. Second, the top-ranked 50 000 compounds were subjected to cell-based partitioning calculations [51] using 5 different combinations of 1D/2D descriptors. All compounds that mapped at least in 2 of 5 calculations to the same cell as compound **1** were selected, leading to

19 molecules. Seven compounds were identified by both conventional similarity searching and partitioning. Thus, the final selection set consisted of only 39 compounds, 25 of which were commercially available and biologically tested.

In this case, additional test compounds with Tc values <0.80 relative to compound **1** could be easily selected from the similarity-based ranking. Similarity-based LBVS methods do not take mode of action information into account and hence the only information available for the search was the 2D structure of compound **1** and its property descriptor values.

11.13.2
Results and Further Calculations

The antagonistic effect of all 25 candidate compounds on LFA-1/ICAM-1 binding was tested in a competition enzyme-linked immunosorbent assay (ELISA). One weakly active compound was identified that blocked the interaction with an IC_{50} value of 70 μM (compound **6**). This compound was identified by similarity searching.

The scaffold of compound **6** was shared by several candidate compounds, but only compound **6** displayed measurable activity, thus illustrating the caveat associated with analogue selection (see above). For the hit expansion, a scaffold-based search for additional analogues was carried out in the screening, resulting in 41 compounds. Again, a single compound was found to be active with an IC_{50} value of 34.4 μM (compound **16**). SAR analysis was carried out by synthesizing 120 additional analogues displaying in part higher potency than compound **6**. The most potent analogue, compound **63**, had an IC_{50} value of 4.3 μM in the ELISA and 5.3 μM in a cell-based adhesion assay. The LBVS and hit expansion analysis is summarized in Figure 11.6, and Figure 11.7 illustrates the structural pathway leading to the most potent analogue.

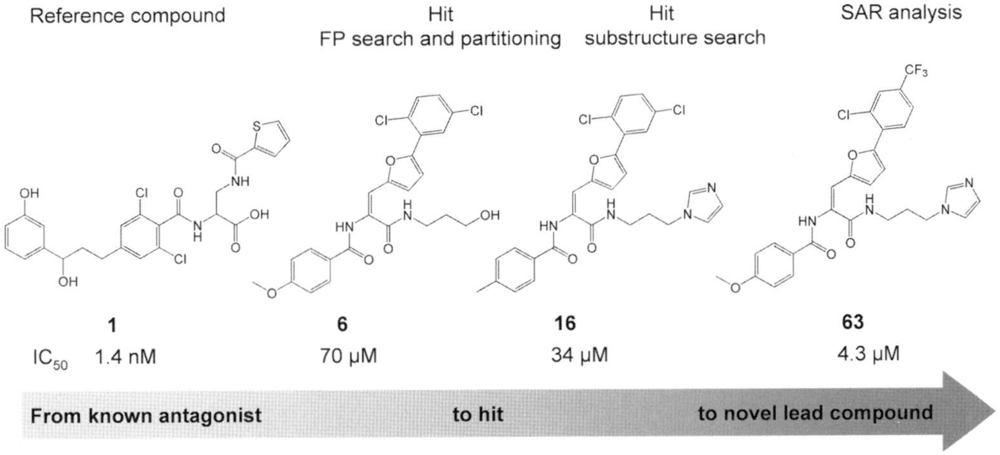

Figure 11.7 LFA-1 antagonist refinement. Active compounds obtained during the hit expansion and hit-to-lead stages are shown.

The observation that many analogues of the newly identified LFA-1 antagonist chemotype were inactive suggested the presence of substantial SAR continuity. Thus, the successful initial selection of compound **6** was fortuitous and the chemotype could have easily been missed. With its low micromolar potency, compound **63** was still ~1000-fold less potent than the reference compound. However, because immune cell surface receptor–ligand interactions are in general transient and only relatively weak, low micromolar potency is in these cases often sufficient for a lead to enter preclinical or even clinical evaluation. However, it should be noted that the detailed mechanism of action of the new antagonist chemotype represented by compound **63** was not determined in the context of our study. Thus, although we extrapolated from an LFA-1 antagonist with a unique mechanism of action, confirmed by an X-ray structure, it was by no means certain that compounds **6** and **63** acted through a similar mechanism because, as stated above, LBVS calculations did not take mode of action information into account.

11.14
Selectivity Searching

Structure–activity relationships can be transformed into structure–selectivity relationships (SSRs) when the biological activity of compounds against multiple targets is considered. The study of SSRs and the identification of small molecules that show differential selectivity patterns for individual targets within a protein family are of critical importance for chemical biology [52], chemogenomics [53], and drug discovery. Compound selectivity often results from differences in potency of a ligand or inhibitor against two or more targets. Whenever the potency significantly differs, a ligand is considered to be selective for one target over another. With the systematical evaluation of compounds having differential potency against multiple targets, SSRs can be formulated that add another level of complexity to SAR analysis. Recently, computational analyses of molecular selectivity and benchmark similarity searching for selective inhibitors, the so-called selectivity searching, were carried out with especially designed compound selectivity test systems [43, 54–57]. Inhibitor sets with potency information for two closely related protein targets were subdivided into sets containing selective molecules for one target and nonselective inhibitors for both targets based on the degree of their potency differences. For compound selectivity, a threshold of 50-fold lower potency for one target compared to another was applied and expressed as a selectivity ratio (SR) (the quotient of both potency values). Inhibitors were considered nonselective if SR values were between 0.1 and 10 (corresponding to 10-fold differences in potency) [56]. Compounds with 10- to 50-fold potency differences were not classified to avoid boundary effects.

Analysis of the assembled molecular test systems revealed rather complex SSR phenotypes. No obvious correlation between structural similarity and compound selectivity was detected in many instances [54, 56]. Structurally similar as well as structurally diverse compounds were found to be selective for the same target and ligands with distinct selectivity were related to each other by different degrees of

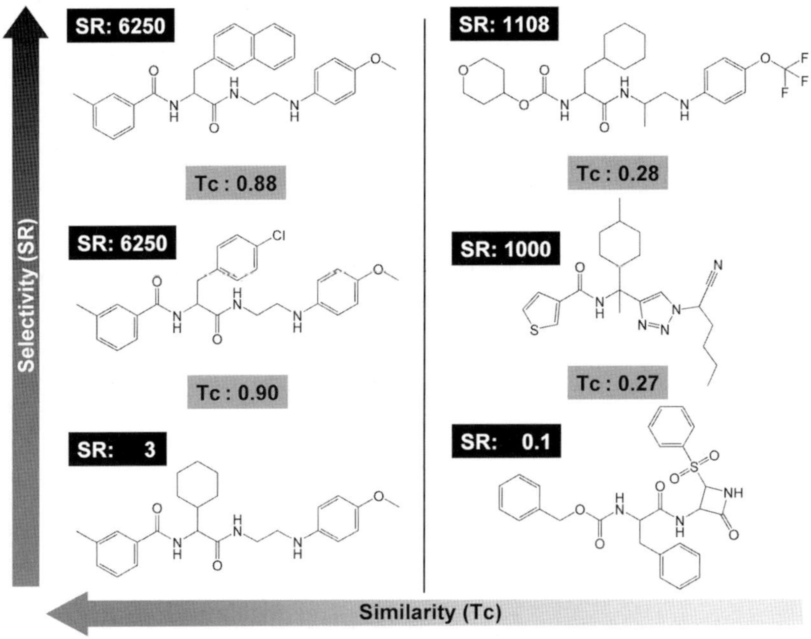

Figure 11.8 Different structure–selectivity relationships. Structurally similar as well as diverse molecules display different selectivity patterns in a set of cathepsin enzyme inhibitors. SR means selectivity ratio and is calculated as the quotient of the potency values of a ligand for cathepsin S over cathepsin K. As a measure of structural similarity, Tc reports pairwise MACCS Tanimoto coefficient values. Structures are taken from the "cat S/K 7–8 set" of Stumpfe *et al.* [56].

structural similarity. Such relationships are illustrated in Figure 11.8 that shows the variety of SSRs covered by one exemplary series of selective compounds. Despite the complexity of SSRs, in benchmark calculations, 2D fingerprints and support vector machines were successfully applied to identify target-selective compounds and significantly enrich selective compounds over nonselective and inactive molecules [55–58]. Thus, an interesting question has been whether or not this type of "selectivity searching" might also succeed in practical LBVS applications.

11.14.1 Selectivity Searching for Cathepsin K-Selective Inhibitors

For selectivity searching, three enzymes, cathepsins K, L, and S, were targeted and cathepsin K inhibitors selective for K over L and S were used as reference molecules in order to identify new cathepsin K-selective inhibitors [43].

The cathepsin enzymes are cysteine proteases belonging to the papain superfamily [59] and are closely related to each other with sequence identities of 56–60% (cathepsins K and L 60%, S and K 57%, and S and L 56% [60]). In addition to overall high sequence similarity, the active sites have a high degree of conservation.

Cathepsin inhibitors are typically substrate analogues containing a strong electrophilic group (a hallmark of these inhibitors), which covalently modify the active site cysteine. Recently, reversible covalent inhibitors have also been introduced with a less-reactive functional group, typically a nitrile, which renders these inhibitors reversible. However, these compounds still form a covalent yet reversible bond with the catalytic cysteine residue.

11.14.2
Selectivity Searching with 2D Fingerprints

For practical selectivity searching, 69 inhibitors with at least 50-fold selectivity for cathepsin K over S and L were selected as reference molecules. The search protocol involved two different in-house-developed LBVS approaches, as shown in Figure 11.9: a compound mapping algorithm termed DynaMAD [38] and a specialized type of molecular fingerprint consisting of compound class characteristic substructures, ACCS-FP [61].

Briefly, DynaMAD is designed to map database compounds to activity-specific consensus positions in chemical space representations of stepwise increasing dimensionality [38] and ACCS-FP is utilized in conventional fingerprint search calculations using multiple reference compounds [61].

Both search strategies reduced ~3.7 M ZINC database compounds [29] to two candidate lists containing 51 and 49 compounds, respectively. After visual inspection

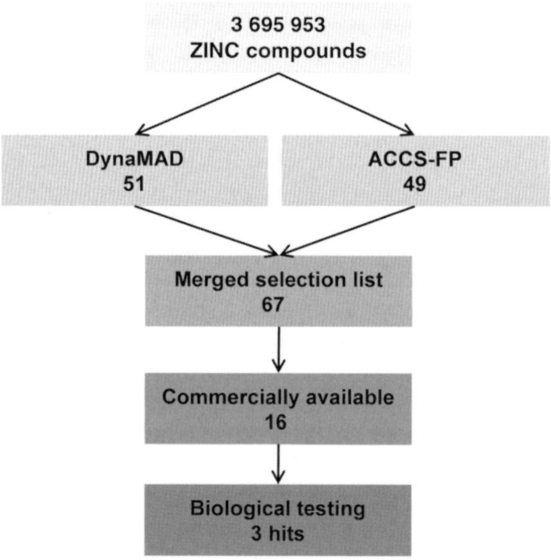

Figure 11.9 Practical selectivity searching. The diagram summarizes the results of selectivity searching for cathepsin K inhibitors, compound selection, and acquisition. As the compound database, a subset of the ZINC database was used [29].

(deletion of structurally too similar compounds) a combined selection set of 67 compounds remained. No candidate compound was identified by both strategies. Unfortunately, only 16 of 67 compounds were commercially available and could be purchased for biological testing.

11.14.3
Identification of Selective Inhibitors

After testing the compounds for enzyme inhibition in spectrophotometric assays for cathepsin S and L and in a fluorometric assay for cathepsin K, three new cathepsin K inhibitors could be identified, as shown in Figure 11.10.

The potency (IC_{50} values) of the hits was in the micromolar range, as typically observed for virtual screening hits [1, 39, 62], for the reasons discussed above. Compounds **1** and **2** were indeed found to have a cathepsin K-selective tendency because their potency difference is ~4–15-fold higher for cathepsin K compared to cathepsin S or L (**1** SR S/K 4.1 L/K 6.0, **2** SR S/K 4.4 L/K 14.7). Compound **3** had comparable IC_{50} values for cathepsin K, L, and S and was therefore not selective. The relatively low selectivity of compounds **1** and **2** was consistent with their relatively

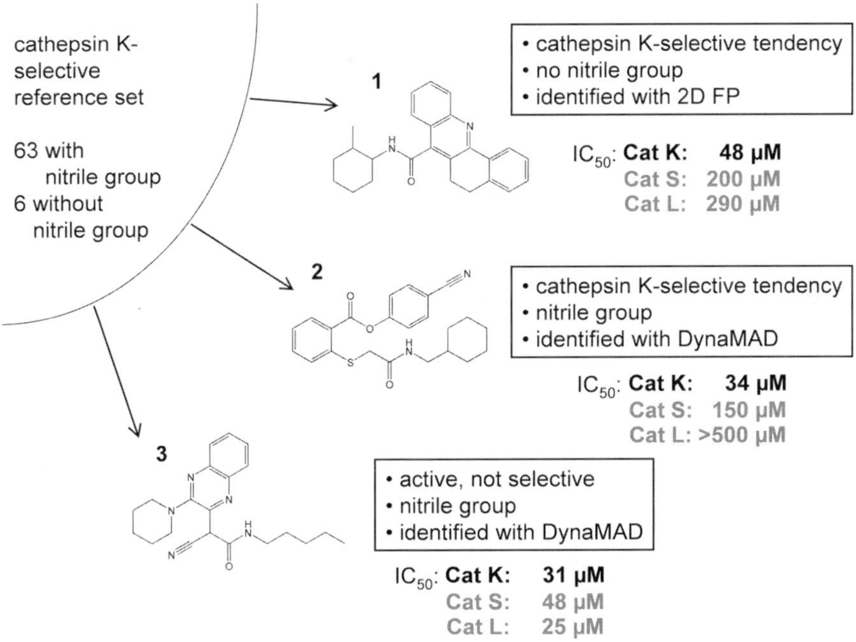

Figure 11.10 Cathepsin K inhibitors with target-selective tendency. The structures of 3 of 16 candidate compounds that inhibited cathepsin K, S, and L in different ways are shown. Compounds **1** and **2** display a cathepsin K-selective tendency, whereas compound **3** is comparably active against all three cathepsins. Measured IC_{50} values from experimental assay are given for each enzyme.

low potency. Further optimization of these hits would be expected to increase their potency values and selectivity ratios.

Compound **1** had very low structural similarity to known cathepsin inhibitors. Its maximum MACCS Tc value to reference set compounds was only 0.53. The corresponding values for compounds **2** and **3** were 0.79 and 0.80, respectively, which also indicate only limited structural similarity, below the level at which similarity in biological activity is typically expected [22]. Importantly, compound **1** contains no nitrile group and is the first cathepsin inhibitor identified lacking an electrophilic group that covalently (yet reversibly) modifies the enzyme. Hence, it is expected to act by a different noncovalent mechanism, which makes it attractive for further exploration.

Thus, in this case, global similarity-based LBVS methods successfully identified a new inhibitory chemotype that would not have been found had the known pharmacophore constraints taken into account.

11.15
Concluding Remarks

Ligand-based virtual screening methods are widely used for hit identification. The methodological spectrum of these methods is wide, ranging from rather simplistic fingerprint-based approaches to highly complex machine learning techniques. However, all these methods are approximate and much depends on the type of molecular representations that are utilized. Methodological complexity does not scale with virtual screening success; simpler is often better. Furthermore, all methods display a yet unpredictable compound class dependency that is again much influenced by chosen molecular representations. Hence, practical virtual screening protocols should best employ multiple methods of different design. Care must be taken to design compound selection strategies that take into account the potential strengths and weaknesses of different approaches and do not entirely rely on consensus approaches. Despite principal disadvantages that are integral to computational screening methods and caveats associated with specific applications and compound selection strategies, LBVS calculations have succeeded in many instances and often produced surprising results taking the many approximations into account that must usually be made. However, it remains often unclear why applied LBVS approaches succeed or fail or which methodological aspect or calculation conditions have truly been decisive for the identification of novel and structurally diverse hits. Thus, there is significant potential for future research beyond algorithm development and benchmarking to further explore these more principal questions.

Acknowledgments

We wish to thank Hanna Geppert for critical review of this chapter and Lisa Peltason for help with figures.

References

1 Bajorath, J. (2002) Virtual screening: methods, expectations, and reality. *Current Opinion in Drug Discovery & Development*, **2** (3), 24–28.

2 Klebe, G. (2006) Virtual ligand screening: strategies, perspectives and limitations. *Drug Discovery Today*, **11** (13–14), 580–594.

3 Stahura, F.L. and Bajorath, J. (2004) Virtual screening methods that complement HTS. *Combinatorial Chemistry & High Throughput Screening*, **7** (4), 259–269.

4 Willett, P. (2005) Searching techniques for databases of two- and three-dimensional structures. *Journal of Medicinal Chemistry*, **48** (13), 4183–4199.

5 Willett, P. (2006) Similarity-based virtual screening using 2D fingerprints. *Drug Discovery Today*, **11** (23–24), 1046–1053.

6 Mason, J.S., Good, A.C., and Martin, E.J. (2001) 3-D pharmacophores in drug discovery. *Current Pharmaceutical Design*, **7** (7), 567–597.

7 Gillet, V.J., Willet, P., and Bradshaw, J. (2003) Similarity searching using reduced graphs. *Journal of Chemical Information and Computer Sciences*, **43** (10), 338–345.

8 Cramer, R.D., Poss, M.A., Hernsmeier, M.A., Caulfield, T.J., Kowala, M.C., and Valentine, M.T. (1999) Prospective identification of biologically active structures by topomer shape similarity searching. *Journal of Medicinal Chemistry*, **42** (19), 3919–3933.

9 Hawkins, P.C., Skillman, A.G., and Nicholls, A. (2007) Comparison of shape-matching and docking as virtual screening tools. *Journal of Medicinal Chemistry*, **50** (1), 74–82.

10 Willett, P. (1987) *Similarity and Clustering in Chemical Information Systems*, Research Studies Press, Letchworth.

11 Pearlman, R.S. and Smith, K.M. (1998) Novel software tools for chemical diversity. *Perspectives in Drug Discovery and Design*, **9–11** (0), 339–353.

12 Godden, J.W. and Bajorath, J. (2004) Cell-based partitioning. *Methods in Molecular Biology*, **275**, 279–290.

13 Rusinko, A., Farmen, M., Lambert, C., Brown, P., and Young, S. (1999) Analysis of a large structure/biological activity data set using recursive partitioning. *Journal of Chemical Information and Computer Sciences*, **39** (6), 1017–1026.

14 Godden, J.W., Xue, L., and Bajorath, J. (2002) Classification of biologically active compounds by median partitioning. *Journal of Chemical Information and Computer Sciences*, **42** (5), 1263–1269.

15 Sadowski, J. (2000) Optimization of chemical libraries by neural networks. *Current Opinion in Chemical Biology*, **4** (3), 280–282.

16 Agrafiotis, D.K. and Xu, H. (2002) A self-organizing principle for learning nonlinear manifolds. *Proceedings of the National Academy of Sciences of the United States of America*, **99** (25), 15869–15872.

17 Warmuth, M.K., Liao, J., Rätsch, G., Mathieson, M., Putta, S., and Lemmen, C. (2003) Active learning with support vector machines in the drug discovery process. *Journal of Chemical Information and Computer Sciences*, **43** (2), 667–673.

18 Jorrissen, R.N. and Gilson, M.K. (2005) Virtual screening of molecular databases using a support vector machine. *Journal of Chemical Information and Modeling*, **45** (3), 549–561.

19 Hert, J., Willett, P., Wilton, D.J., Acklin, P., Azzaoui, K., Jacoby, E., and Schuffenhauer, A. (2004) Comparison of fingerprint-based methods for virtual screening using multiple bioactive reference structures. *Journal of Chemical Information and Computer Sciences*, **44** (3), 1177–1185.

20 Johnson, M.A. and Maggiora, G.M. (1990) *Concepts and Applications of Molecular Similarity* (eds M.A. Johnson and G.M. Maggiora), John Wiley & Sons, Inc., New York.

21 Patterson F D.E., Cramer, R.D., Fergusin, A.M., Clark, R.D., and Weinberger, L.E. (1996) Neighborhood behavior: a useful concept for validation of "molecular diversity" descriptors. *Journal of Medicinal Chemistry*, **39** (16), 3049–3059.

22 Martin, Y., Kofron, J., and Traphagen, L. (2002) Do structurally similar molecules

have similar biological activity? *Journal of Medicinal Chemistry*, **45** (19), 4350–4358.

23 Geppert, H., Horváth, T., Gärtner, T., Wrobel, S., and Bajorath, J. (2008) Support-vector-machine-based ranking significantly improves the effectiveness of similarity searching using 2D fingerprints and multiple reference compounds. *Journal of Chemical Information and Modeling*, **48** (4), 742–746.

24 Bemis, G.W. and Murcko, M.A. (1996) The properties of known drugs. 1. Molecular frameworks. *Journal of Medicinal Chemistry*, **39** (15), 2887–2893.

25 Peltason, L. and Bajorath, J. (2007) Molecular similarity analysis uncovers heterogeneous structure–activity relationships and variable activity landscapes. *Chemistry & Biology*, **14** (5), 489–497.

26 Maggiora, G.M. (2006) On outliers and activity cliffs: why QSAR often disappoints. *Journal of Chemical Information and Modeling*, **46** (4), 1535.

27 Wang, Y. and Bajorath, J. (2008) Balancing the influence of molecular complexity effects on fingerprint similarity searching. *Journal of Chemical Information and Modeling*, **48** (1), 75–84.

28 Flower, D.R. (1998) On the properties of bit string-based measures of chemical similarity. *Journal of Chemical Information and Computer Sciences*, **38** (3), 379–386.

29 Irwin, J.J. and Shoichet, B.K. (2005) ZINC: a free database of commercially available compounds for virtual screening. *Journal of Chemical Information and Modeling*, **45** (1), 177–182.

30 Lipinski, C.A., Lombardo, F., Dominy, B.W., and Feeney, P.J. (1997) Experimental and computational approaches to estimate solubility and permeability in drug discovery and development settings. *Advanced Drug Delivery Reviews*, **23** (1–3), 3–25.

31 Walters, W.P., Stahl, M.T., and Murcko, M.A. (1998) Virtual screening: an overview. *Drug Discovery Today*, **3** (17), 160–178.

32 Godden, J.W., Stahura, F.L., and Bajorath, J. (2004) POT-DMC: a virtual screening method for the identification of potent hits. *Journal of Medicinal Chemistry*, **47** (23), 5608–5611.

33 Peltason, L. and Bajorath, J. (2007) SAR index: quantifying the nature of structure–activity relationships. *Journal of Medicinal Chemistry*, **50** (23), 5571–5578.

34 Sheridan, R.P. and Kearsley, S.K. (2002) Why do we need so many chemical similarity search methods? *Drug Discovery Today*, **7** (17), 903–911.

35 McGaughey, G.B., Sheridan, R.P., Bayly, C.I., Culberson, J.C., Kreatsoulas, C., Lindsley, S., Maiorov, V., Truchon, J.F., and Cornell, W.D. (2007) Comparison of topological, shape, and docking methods in virtual screening. *Journal of Chemical Information and Modeling*, **47** (4), 1504–1519.

36 Eckert, H. and Bajorath, J. (2007) Molecular similarity analysis in virtual screening: foundations, limitations and novel approaches. *Drug Discovery Today*, **12** (5–6), 225–233.

37 Salim, N., Holliday, J., and Willett, P. (2003) Combination of fingerprint-based similarity coefficients using data fusion. *Journal of Chemical Information and Computer Sciences*, **43** (2), 435–442.

38 Eckert, H., Vogt, I., and Bajorath, J. (2006) Mapping algorithms for molecular similarity analysis and ligand-based virtual screening: design of DynaMAD and comparison with MAD and DMC. *Journal of Chemical Information and Modeling*, **46** (4), 1623–1634.

39 Bajorath, J. (2002) Integration of virtual and high-throughput screening. *Nature Reviews. Drug Discovery*, **1** (11), 882–894.

40 Parker, C.N., Shamu, C.E., Kraybill, B., Austin, C.P., and Bajorath, J. (2006) Measure, mine, model, and manipulate: the future for HTS and chemoinformatics? *Drug Discovery Today*, **11** (19–20), 863–865.

41 Engels, M.F. and Venkatarangan, P. (2001) Smart screening: approaches to efficient HTS. *Current Opinion in Drug Discovery & Development*, **4** (3), 275–283.

42 Shoda, M., Harada, T., Yano, K., Stahura, F.L., Himeno, T., Shiojiri, S., Kogami, Y., Kouji, H., and Bajorath, J. (2007) Virtual screening leads to the discovery of an effective antagonist of

lymphocyte function-associated antigen-1. *ChemMedChem*, **2** (4), 515–521.

43 Stumpfe, D., Frizler, M., Sisay, M.T., Batista, J., Vogt, I., Gütschow, M., and Bajorath, J. (2008) Hit expansion through selectivity searching. *ChemMedChem*, **4** (1), 52–54.

44 Martz, E. (1987) LFA-1 and other accessory molecules functioning in adhesions of T and B lymphocytes. *Human Immunology*, **18** (1), 3–37.

45 Randi, A.M. and Hogg, N.I. (1994) I domain of beta 2 integrin lymphocyte function-associated antigen-1 contains a binding site for ligand intercellular adhesion molecule-1. *The Journal Biological Chemistry*, **269** (17), 12395–12398.

46 Shimaoka, M., Xiao, T., Liu, J.H., Yang, Y., Dong, Y., Jun, C.D., McCormack, A., Zhang, R., Joachimiak, A., Takagi, J., Wang, J.H., and Springer, T.A. (2003) Structures of the alpha L I domain and its complex with ICAM-1 reveal a shape-shifting pathway for integrin regulation. *Cell*, **112** (1), 99–111.

47 Arkin, M.R. and Wells, J.A. (2004) Small-molecule inhibitors of protein–protein interactions: progressing towards the dream. *Nature Reviews. Drug Discovery*, **3** (4), 301–317.

48 Kallen, J., Welzenbach, K., Ramage, P., Geyl, D., Kriwacki, R., Legge, G., Cottens, S., Weitz-Schmidt, G., and Hommel, U. (1999) Structural basis for LFA-1 inhibition upon lovastatin binding to the CD11a I-domain. *Journal of Molecular Biology*, **292** (1), 1–9.

49 Gadek, T.R., Burdick, D.J., McDowell, R.S., Stanley, M.S., Marsters, J.C., Jr., Paris, K.J., Oare, D.A., Reynolds, M.E., Ladner, C., Zioncheck, K.A., Lee, W.P., Gribling, P., Dennis, M.S., Skelton, N.J., Tumas, D.B., Clark, K.R., Keating, S.M., Beresini, M.H., Tilley, J.W., Presta, L.G., and Bodary, S.C. (2002) Generation of an LFA-1 antagonist by the transfer of the ICAM-1 immunoregulatory epitope to a small molecule. *Science*, **295** (5557), 1086–1089.

50 Xue, L., Godden, J.W., and Bajorath, J. (2003) Mini-fingerprints for virtual screening: design principles and generation of novel prototypes based on information theory. *SAR and QSAR in Environmental Research*, **14** (1), 27–40.

51 Xue, L. and Bajorath, J. (2000) Molecular descriptors for effective classification of biologically active compounds based on principal component analysis identified by a genetic algorithm. *Journal of Chemical Information and Computer Sciences*, **40** (3), 801–809.

52 Spring, D.R. (2004) Chemical genetics to chemical genomics: small molecules offer big insights. *Chemical Society Reviews*, **34** (6), 472–482.

53 Bredel, M. and Jacoby, E. (2004) Chemogenomics: an emerging strategy for rapid target and drug discovery. *Nature Reviews. Genetics*, **5** (4), 262–275.

54 Stumpfe, D., Ahmed, H.E.A., Vogt, I., and Bajorath, J. (2007) Methods for computer-aided chemical biology. Part 1: design of a benchmark system for the evaluation of compound selectivity. *Chemical Biology & Drug Design*, **70** (3), 182–194.

55 Vogt, I., Stumpfe, D., Ahmed, H.E.A., and Bajorath, J. (2007) Methods for computer-aided chemical biology. Part 2: evaluation of compound selectivity using 2D fingerprints. *Chemical Biology & Drug Design*, **70** (3), 195–205.

56 Stumpfe, D., Geppert, H., and Bajorath, J. (2008) Methods for computer-aided chemical biology. Part 3: analysis of structure–selectivity relationships through single- or dual-step selectivity searching and Bayesian classification. *Chemical Biology & Drug Design*, **71** (6), 518–528.

57 Vogt, I., Ahmed, H.E.A., Auer, J., and Bajorath, J. (2008) Exploring structure–selectivity relationships of biogenic amine GPCR antagonists using similarity searching and dynamic compound mapping. *Molecular Diversity*, **12** (1), 25–40.

58 Wassermann, A.M., Geppert, H., and Bajorath, J. (2009) Searching for target-selective compounds using different combinations of multiclass support vector machine ranking methods, kernel functions, and fingerprint descriptors. *Journal of Chemical Information and Modeling*, **49** (3), 582–592.

59 Brömme., D. and Kaleta, J. (2002) Thiol-dependent cathepsins: pathophysiological implications and recent advances in inhibitor design. *Current Pharmaceutical Design*, **8** (18), 1639–1658.

60 Nägler, D.K. and Menard, R. (2003) Family C1 cysteine proteases: biological diversity or redundancy? *Biological Chemistry*, **384** (6), 837–843.

61 Batista, J. and Bajorath, J. (2008) Similarity searching using compound class-specific combinations of substructures found in randomly generated molecular fragment populations. *ChemMedChem*, **3** (1), 67–73.

62 Shoichet, B.K., (2004) Virtual screening of chemical libraries. *Nature*, **432** (7019), 862–865.

12
Applications and Success Stories in Virtual Screening

Hans Matter and Christoph Sotriffer

12.1
Introduction

To discover novel lead structures for pharmaceutical research, the focus is increasingly placed on technologies [1] complementing high-throughput screening (HTS) [2]. Today's lead finding strategies include knowledge from publications, patents, related projects, and protein 3D information as well as combinatorial chemistry and high-throughput screening. The combination of random and rational approaches into knowledge-driven lead identification covering a significant portion of the leadlike chemistry space is anticipated to deliver more new lead structures fulfilling quality criteria for drug discovery programs [2]. A clear process driven by relevant metrics for compound progression is required due to the implications that the identification of promising leads has for any discovery program [3].

Virtual screening represents an *in silico* approach to identify starting points complementary to other strategies [4, 5]. Several review articles have recently highlighted methods and applications [6–11], and many aspects of the virtual screening process are discussed in detail in this book. In virtual screening, compounds or libraries are selected from an existing pool with a certain probability to be active at the molecular target of interest. This selection is guided by predictive filters from data mining and computational models. One goal of virtual screening is the identification of novel chemotypes to enrich the basis for a project (*scaffold hopping*) or produce starting points for optimization. This search may be based on active ligands, protein–ligand crystal structures, or validated homology models. Alternatively, one would like to retrieve analogous compounds of privileged scaffolds, which have an increased probability for biological activity (*similarity searching*). Hence, the objective of a virtual screening influences the selection of algorithms, methods, models, and descriptors. Different starting points for virtual screening justify the development of novel descriptors, similarity and docking tools to explore targets and ligands from different perspectives.

This chapter summarizes selected prospective virtual screening applications from the medicinal chemistry literature of the last decade. It does not attempt to provide

Virtual Screening. Edited by C. Sotriffer

ISBN: 978-3-527-32636-5

an exhaustive discussion of all relevant studies, since application studies are also discussed in other chapters of this book, particularly in Part IV (in addition, pharmacophore-based virtual screening studies are summarized in Chapter 5; a detailed list of virtual screening applications based on homology models can be found in Chapter 14; and finally, a tabular listing of prospective virtual screening studies in Appendix B provides a quick reference to all application studies mentioned in the book). Here, individual case studies are grouped by structure- or ligand-based workflows and the target protein family. Particular emphasis is placed on workflow comparison. Interestingly, the chosen examples also suggest that ligand- and structure-based approaches are not competing, but could be combined to enhance hit rates.

12.2
Practical Considerations

Today there is no general process for ligand- or structure-based virtual screening. Every application requires a fundamental understanding of the problem, tuning of key parameters, and adjustment of components of the employed workflow. The first step is to analyze all information about the problem for generating validated models and defining workflows. The preparation of molecular screening databases requires particular care (cf. Chapters 1 and 2). It is important, for example, to consider the treatment of ionization and tautomers in the input structures [12, 13], as this significantly influences the quality of results for both ligand- and structure-based virtual screening. Although this is challenging, some software has emerged for corrections and adjustments in an automatic, yet reliable, fashion.

A useful discussion of practical aspects of virtual screening, including a workflow for a structure-based protocol, is provided by Lyne [14]. He pointed out that any successful virtual screening campaign should include a number of consecutive computational steps, from database filtering and preparation to target setup, predocking filters, docking, postdocking analysis, and prioritization of compounds for testing.

Individual tasks in virtual screening could be arranged into four steps based on the level of complexity [2]. Very simple one-dimensional filters could be used at early phases to significantly reduce the number of virtual candidates. This step should eliminate unwanted chemical compounds containing substructures or features that make it unlikely for these molecules to become drug candidates [15]. Such criteria include physicochemical properties of "druglike" molecules like "rule of five" [16] or related criteria [17], summarizing simple, intuitive parameters as alert for compounds that are unlikely to be orally absorbed. Other simple criteria for filtering include reactive, toxic, or otherwise undesirable fragments, potential metabolic liabilities, lead- or druglike property filters [18, 19], and others. In the past years, several virtual screening filters based on straightforward 2D descriptors have also been established to weed out compounds with a potentially undesirable side effect at an early stage before evaluating their capability to fit to the target. Such filters for liabilities might include the prediction of frequent hitters [20], hERG channel blocking [21–24], or CYP3A4 and CYP2D6 inhibition [25–27], among others.

Experience in medicinal chemistry suggests that successful drug discovery programs also depend on the nature of the molecular target. It has been suggested that certain organic compounds can modulate more readily some privileged protein target classes, which led to the development of target family-related approaches and a selection of tractable targets in addition to a careful selection following therapeutic requirements.

The second step encompasses similarity searching starting from known actives for a particular target using simple two-dimensional descriptors like fingerprints, topological descriptors like atom pair fingerprints, topological pharmacophores, or feature trees. While 3D pharmacophore searching can be classified as third step, it requires more knowledge about existing ligands for a molecular target of interest. The fourth and most complex step requires even more structural knowledge when potential candidate molecules are flexibly docked into binding sites of target protein structures and candidates for biological testing are then selected using scoring functions.

Each virtual screening run requires an analysis phase to minimize the number of false positives and propagate the true hits to the top of the lists. Techniques like consensus scoring or more demanding approaches involving electrostatics and desolvation could be applied. Furthermore, geometrical filtering by essential or undesirable protein–ligand interactions, shape complementarity, exposed hydrophobic parts of a ligand, and unrealistic conformations might be useful; such tasks are often efficiently accomplished by visual inspection of top-ranking compounds in the result list. Clearly, the application of virtual screening filters and methods depends on their stage in the virtual screening workflow. A sequential process should always be set up to focus on the compound set as much as possible for more time-consuming investigations (for example, flexible docking). Further details about various practical considerations are provided in many other chapters of this book, particularly in Chapters 1 and 3.

12.3
Successful Applications of Virtual Screening

The goal of virtual screening is to identify starting points for chemical optimization that have a potential for conversion into viable drug candidates. This goal, however, limits the number of reported successes in the medicinal chemistry literature, as early projects still require significant effort to propagate a hit into a promising clinical candidate. Furthermore, the results after optimization are unpredictable and the attrition rate is high. Another reason for rare reports on successful virtual screening applications could clearly be attributed to the proprietary nature of the identified molecules of potential interest.

Although an increasing number of prospective virtual screening outcomes are now reported, most studies are still retrospective with a focus on novel software or virtual screening strategies. However, it is of utmost importance for assessing the real value of any approach to separate retrospective studies from prospective applications. Consequently, the following discussion will focus on prospective applications of different virtual screening approaches.

The first section provides an overview of successful structure-based virtual screening applications, followed by some comments on structure-based library design. This is followed by a summary of recent ligand-based virtual screening examples. Within each section, examples are organized by target families to focus on successes and challenges in different areas relevant to medicinal chemistry.

12.3.1 Structure-Based Virtual Screening

12.3.1.1 Kinases

The discovery of a novel and selective kinase CK2 inhibitor by a high-throughput docking protocol was reported by Vangrevelinghe *et al.* [28]. The authors employed DOCK [29] in order to flexibly dock a large portion of the Novartis corporate database with ∼400 000 compounds into the ATP binding site of a human CK2α homology model. This homology model was constructed from the X-ray structure of *Zea mays* CK2α. The authors also described a multistep workflow that encompassed filter criteria on molecular weight, number of rotatable bonds, undesirable substructures prior to 3D conversion, and adjustment of protonation states using a rule-based method. The authors conclude that structure-based virtual screening is useful for lead identification, but only if postdocking filtering and other postprocessing procedures are applied to the raw hit lists after the flexible docking runs. To this end, the compounds with best DOCK scores were further pruned using a three-step postprocessing treatment. First, a filtering of the hit list by additionally available pharmacophore information, that is, hydrogen bonds to the kinase hinge region, was done, followed by ranking of acceptable compounds using the scoring function from Wang *et al.* [30] prior to a visual inspection of the best compounds. This process then resulted in a total of 12 compounds as candidates for biological testing. Visual inspection was seen as a critical step to discard compounds with unfavorable interactions in the kinase binding site or those with unrealistic conformations. The best inhibitor identified on a rigid molecular scaffold exhibited an IC_{50} value of 80 nM after biological testing (Figure 12.1a).

Peng *et al.* [31] described the identification of novel Bcr-Abl tyrosine kinase inhibitors from a database of 200 000 commercially available compounds using a related docking protocol on the basis of DOCK [29]. From 1000 candidate molecules having the best DOCK energy scores, 15 compounds were finally selected after clustering them in structurally diverse classes and applying druglikeness filters. Eight of them showed significant activity after biological testing with IC_{50} values between 10 and 200 μM. Other successful applications of DOCK have been reported for targets like HIV-1 protease [32], thymidylate synthase [33, 34], influenza hemagglutinin [35], parasitic proteases [36], PTP1b [37], Kinesin [38], and others.

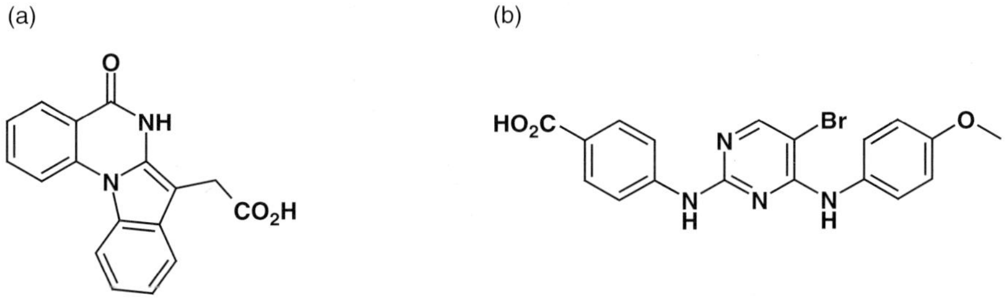

Figure 12.1 Structure-based virtual screening examples for kinases. (a) CK2 kinase inhibitor, IC_{50}: 80 nM. (b) Chk-1 kinase inhibitor, IC_{50}: 450 nM.

Another application of a structure-based virtual screening protocol to the kinase target checkpoint kinase-1 (Chk-1) was reported by Lyne *et al.* [39]. The authors applied a strategy involving filtering of the AstraZeneca collection using physicochemical properties and substructures followed by 3D pharmacophore searching to identify compounds with a potential to bind to the kinase hinge binding region. The remaining database of ~200 000 molecules was then docked with pharmacophore constraints using FlexX-Pharm [40] into the ATP binding site of Chk-1. After consensus scoring and visual inspection, 103 compounds were selected for biological testing. Thirty-six molecules representing four different chemical classes were Chk-1 inhibitors with IC_{50} values ranging from 0.11 to 68 μM, but structures were shown for only a few examples (Figure 12.1b).

Foloppe *et al.* [41] also used Chk-1 kinase as target for structure-based virtual screening. They employed X-ray structures of the human Chk-1 kinase for docking of a filtered subset of commercially available compounds. A total of ~700 000 molecules were used for docking into the X-ray structure of Chk-1 using the program rDock [42]. Docking combined with further filtering on the basis of scoring and visual inspection led to the selection of 1179 compounds for biological testing. This approach led to the discovery of nine novel Chk-1 kinase inhibitors on novel scaffolds with druglike properties and IC_{50} values between 15 and 32 μM. Moreover, the X-ray structures of four of these hits could be solved, which provided some medicinal chemistry rational toward optimization of these hits. Hence, this report is one of the nice and instructive examples, where the proposed binding mode from virtual screening is later validated, thus strongly supporting the rationale of the virtual screening experiment.

In an interesting study, Polgár *et al.* [43] compared experiment and theory to identify inhibitors of the serine/threonine kinase GSK-3β. Virtual screening was performed using FlexX [44], FlexE [45], and FlexX-Pharm [40] on a subset of ~16 000 compounds of the Gedeon Richter collection. In parallel a high-throughput screening of this collection was carried out. While HTS led to a hit rate of 0.55%, the virtual screen resulted in 12.9% hits. The authors concluded that a comparison of true and false positives and negatives revealed the complementarity of experimental and computational approaches. Direct comparison of hit lists and identified series revealed a certain degree of overlap. Furthermore, this study suggests that validated workflows might be transferable to structurally related protein binding sites.

12.3.1.2 **Proteases**

Ward *et al.* [46] reported a virtual screening to identify novel inhibitors for dipeptidyl peptidase IV (DPP-IV) to provide starting points for medicinal chemistry at AstraZeneca. This virtual screen was performed after analysis of an HTS with extremely low hit rates where the majority of actives were irreversible inhibitors. An internal database of ~800 000 compounds was used for a sequential protocol, which included initial filtering by physicochemical properties, followed by pharmacophore searches. At this point, the authors also noted that reasonable tautomers and protonation states plus unknown stereocenters were enumerated in order to provide an enhanced start for ligand- and structure-based investigations. Pharmacophore searching was then done using an in-house method against two DPP-IV-derived queries, also including a measure for the overlap with the DPP-IV active site volume. The resulting ~20 000 molecules were docked into the DPP-IV X-ray crystal structure using Glide [47]. Finally, the best 8000 compounds were clustered and a representative sample of 4000 compounds was selected for biological testing. This led to the identification of 51 active compounds, with the best activity of 81.9% inhibition at 30 μM concentration (Figure 12.2a). Although the corresponding hit rate and the activity were reported as low, these relatively small compounds provided more starting points for chemistry follow-up as the HTS campaign.

Li *et al.* [48] described a virtual screen on the SPECS database to identify inhibitors for the cysteine protease falcipain-2 as promising target for malaria treatment. Based on the available X-ray structure of falcipain-2, two different docking protocols based on Glide [47] and GAsDock [49] were employed to identify 28 nonpeptidic inhibitors. The best compound exhibited an IC_{50} value of 2.4 μM (Figure 12.2b). Further biochemical evaluations showed that the best inhibitor interacts noncovalently with the active site of this cysteine protease.

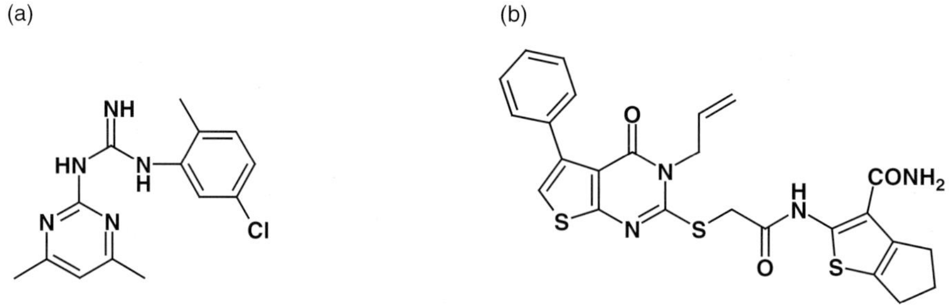

Figure 12.2 Structure-based virtual screening examples for proteases. (a) DPP-IV inhibitor, showing 81.9% inhibition at 30 μM. (b) Falcipain-2 inhibitor, IC_{50}: 2.4 μM.

12.3.1.3 **Nuclear Receptors**

Schapira *et al.* used structure-based virtual screening to identify novel nuclear hormone receptor antagonists [50]. As only X-ray structures of ligand binding domains of agonist-bound nuclear receptors with exception of the antagonist-bound estrogen receptor-α were available at the time of their study, the authors decided to construct an "inactive" conformational model for the human retinoic acid receptor-α using the estrogen receptor structure as template. This model then was successfully employed for structure-based virtual screening using the docking program ICM [51]. The compounds with the best rank after scoring were subjected to conformational postfiltering and visual inspection; 32 compounds were tested and led to 2 novel antagonists. The authors emphasize their approach to exclude any a priori privileged substructure and pharmacophore knowledge from their protocol in order to retrieve an unbiased set of candidates with potential interactions with the receptor. This success was attributed to the quality of the docking program in combination with its scoring function. It was also pointed out that some protein binding sites with particular characteristics in terms of hydrogen bonding and hydrophobicity favor different docking and scoring tools, as demonstrated in a comparative study of different binding pockets by Schulz-Gasch and Stahl [52]. Another comparison of automated docking programs for five different targets and 1000 compounds is reported by Cummings *et al.* [53]. Here the authors conclude that the ability to prioritize known ligands on the basis of docking poses that resemble known crystal structures depends on both the method and the corresponding biomolecular target protein. The results for the estrogen receptor binding site [51] suggest that steric complementarity and hydrophobic interactions are in fact determining the docking results into selected nuclear receptor binding sites.

A similar virtual screening approach led to the identification of thyroid hormone receptor antagonists [54]. This study was again based on a homology model for this receptor in its hypothetical antagonist-bound conformation. A total of 100 candidate molecules were finally selected using docking from a library of ~250 000 compounds. After subsequent biological testing, 14 out of 75 molecules were identified with IC_{50} values ranging from 1.5 to 30 μM. One of the best ligands from this study then served to design a follow-up virtual library. After a synthesis cycle, some second-generation antagonists were obtained with biological activities in the submicromolar range (Figure 12.3a). The diversity of these novel antagonists demonstrates that structure-based virtual screening is able to identify diverse scaffolds in agreement with structural rules for nuclear receptor antagonism.

The same group also demonstrated that significant enrichment rates could be obtained for a variety of other nuclear hormone receptors [55]. By docking 5000 structurally diverse compounds, including 78 known nuclear receptor ligands against a total of 18 nuclear receptor X-ray structures plus one homology model, they obtained significant results for all but 1 target. In their discussion, the authors point to the problem that receptor flexibility still remains to be fully included into the structure-based virtual screening protocol, at least for this target family. Consequently, the choice of the appropriate binding site geometry critically determines the virtual screening outcome. This finding again prompts for a careful validation of

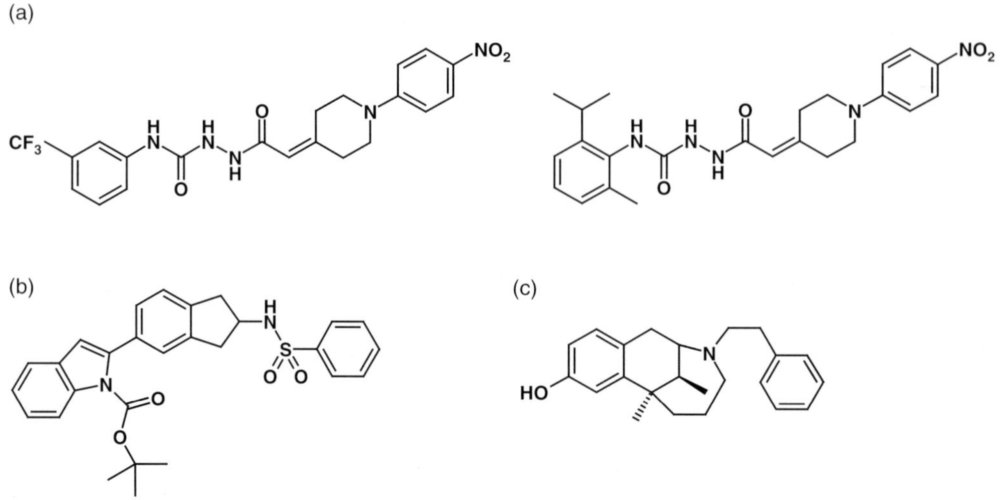

Figure 12.3 Structure-based virtual screening examples for nuclear receptors. (a) Two thyroid hormone receptor antagonists with IC_{50} values of 20 μM (left) and 0.75 μM (right). (b) Liver X receptor (LXR) agonist, EC_{50} 0.21 μM for LXRβ. (c) Liver X receptor (LXR) agonist.

any structural and pharmacophore model for novel targets prior to a virtual screening campaign.

Bakir *et al.* [56] reported the discovery of a structurally novel liver X receptor (LXR) agonist from the internal compound collection at Tanabe Research Laboratories. Virtual screening was performed using Glide and the X-ray structure of human LXRβ. Starting from 135 000 compounds evaluated, the 1290 compounds with the highest score were subjected to experimental testing by high-throughput genomic technology for gene expression profiling including several LXR target genes (HTG Inc.). The most promising compound showed an EC_{50} of 0.21 μM (Figure 12.3b) and was used as starting point for lead exploration to result in LXR agonists with low nanomolar activity employing minor structural changes. Another chemical series resulting from a virtual screen using Glide on the same nuclear receptor was disclosed by Cheng *et al.* in another publication from Tanabe [57]. One interesting series in particular was confirmed as potent LXR agonist by relevant function assays (Figure 12.3c).

Knox *et al.* [58] developed a four-step scoring and filtering approach to minimize the number of false positives arising from docking into the estrogen receptor α (ERα). This approach was applied to a virtual screening starting from the SPECS database with ~200 000 commercially available compounds. After docking using the program LIGIN [59], a postdocking filter was introduced, consisting of distance constraints to key protein residues. The remaining compounds were scored and selected after visual inspection. A total of seven molecules were experimentally tested; three molecules were found active as novel and selective ERα antagonists with IC_{50} values from 0.05 to 1.4 μM. In this example, the application of distance constraints as additional filter prior to scoring and analysis allowed focusing on relevant poses in structure-based virtual screening.

12.3.1.4 **Short-Chain Dehydrogenases**

Schuster *et al.* [60] first described the identification of 11β-hydroxysteroid dehydrogenase 1 (HSD1) inhibitors by pharmacophore-based virtual screening. At the time of their study, no X-ray structure of this short-chain dehydrogenase was available; hence, ligand-derived pharmacophore models for 11β-HSD1 and 11β-HSD2 were developed using Catalyst [61]. Both models were applied to 12 commercially available compound libraries. The resulting hit lists were filtered using topological and physicochemical filters in addition to a hERG potassium channel pharmacophore as undesirable antitarget. Thirty compounds found by either model were experimentally tested, which resulted in seven actives, although only two of them were not related to a steroid scaffold (Figure 12.4a).

In a following study from the same group [62], a combination of pharmacophore models and docking was used for virtual screening to identify nonsteroidal 17β-HSD1 inhibitors. The initial pharmacophore models were derived from 17β-HSD1 X-ray crystal structures with steroidal ligands using the program LigandScout [63]. The most promising pharmacophore model after validation of several candidate models was then employed for screening both the NCI and Specs databases with a total of 340 000 compounds. The resulting 1559 hits were subsequently docked using GOLD [64] into the pocket of 17β-HSD1. Fourteen compounds were tested after scoring and visual inspection, resulting in four hits with IC_{50} values $<50\,\mu M$, two of them having a nonsteroid scaffold. The best compound from a novel class of 17β-HSD1 inhibitors showed an IC_{50} of 5.7 μM (Figure 12.4b).

12.3.1.5 **G Protein-Coupled Receptors (GPCRs)**

The feasibility of GPCR homology models for structure-based virtual screening was initially demonstrated in a few retrospective [65, 66] and prospective applications [67, 68]. Varady *et al.* [69] reported on the discovery of novel and potent dopamine D3 ligands from a hybrid pharmacophore- and structure-based approach. Of the 20 tested compounds, 8 showed K_i values $<1\,\mu M$.

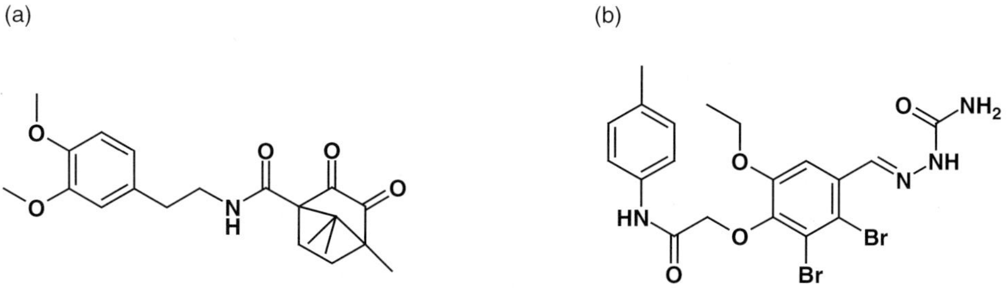

Figure 12.4 Structure-based virtual screening examples for short-chain dehydrogenases (SCDs). (a) 11β-HSD1 inhibitor, IC_{50}: 2.03 μM. (b) 17β-HSD1 inhibitor, IC_{50}: 5.7 μM.

Carefully validated homology models for structure-based virtual screening were used by Evers *et al.* to identify antagonists for the neurokinin-1 (NK1) [70, 71] and the α1A adrenergic (α1Aa) receptors [72]. The strategy to identify NK1 receptor antagonists started from a homology model derived using the MOBILE approach [73], which models proteins by homology with explicitly considering information on bound ligands as restraints to obtain more realistic ligand binding site geometries. This model (as well as many others) was derived from the X-ray structure of bovine rhodopsin [74], which provided a reasonable template before new GPCR X-ray structures emerged in 2008. From the NK1 model, a composite protein- and ligand-based pharmacophore model was derived for a stepwise screening procedure. A database of 827 000 commercial compounds was filtered by physicochemical and 2D topological criteria before the pharmacophore model was employed to restrict the number of compounds to ~11 000. Docking using FlexX [44] followed by postscoring resulted in 1000 hits, which were investigated by force field calculations. One out of seven compounds selected for testing showed an IC_{50} of 0.25 μM, thus underscoring the effectiveness of this approach (Figure 12.5a).

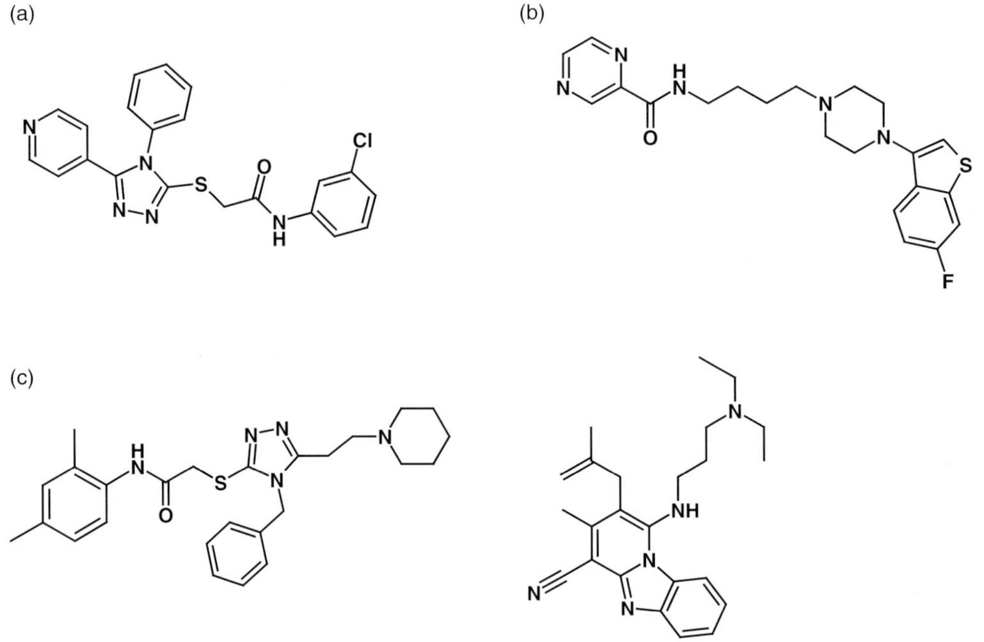

Figure 12.5 Structure-based virtual screening examples for GPCRs. (a) Neurokinin-1 receptor antagonist, IC_{50}: 251 nM. (b) α1A receptor antagonist, K_i: 1.4 nM. (c) Two chemokine receptor CCR5 agonists with EC_{50} values of 3.0 μM (left) and 1.9 μM (right). (d) Thyrotropin-releasing hormone receptor TRH-R1 antagonist, K_i: 0.29 μM. (e) β2-Adrenergic receptor inverse agonist, K_i: 9 nM. (f) Histamine H4 receptor ligands with 95.8% (left) and 92.6% (right) ^{3}H-histamine displacement at 5 μM concentration.

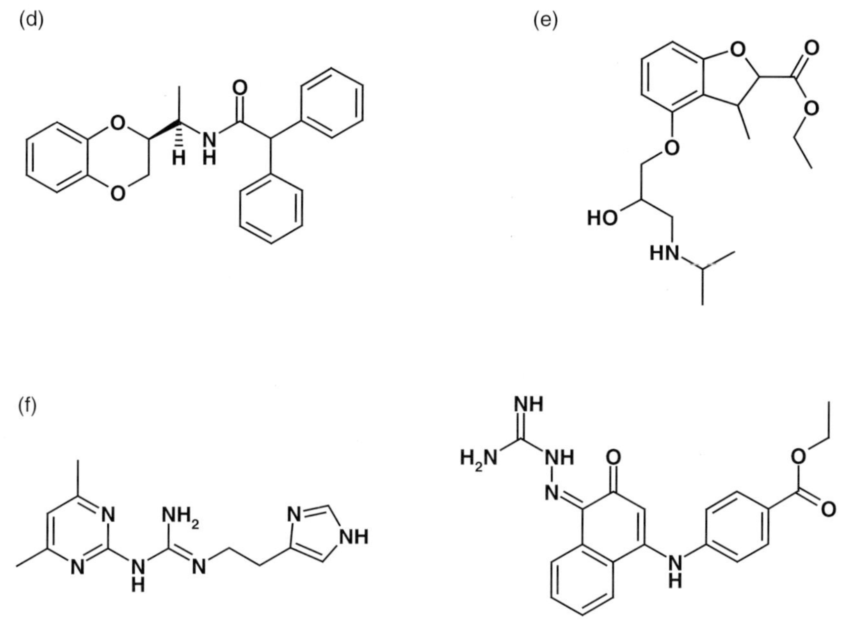

Figure 12.5 *(Continued)*.

A related approach was then used by Evers and Klabunde [72] to derive a homology model for the α1A adrenergic receptor (α1Aa) and apply this for virtual screening. The hierarchical virtual screening protocol including physicochemical filters and 3D pharmacophore models using Catalyst [61] was employed to search a compound library at Aventis. The remaining ~23 000 compounds were docked into the homology model using Gold [64]. After postscoring, 80 diverse compounds were selected and tested. Of these compounds, 37 revealed K_i values <1 μM; the most active compound binds with 1.4 nM to this receptor (Figure 12.5b). This study as well as subsequent reports clearly demonstrated that carefully validated GPCR homology models, often combined with ligand-based pharmacophore models as "prefilters," provide a relevant structural basis for structure-based virtual screening.

Triballeau *et al.* [75] described the development of a virtual screening workflow directed toward the identification of agonists for the metabotropic glutamate receptor subtype 4 (mGlu4R). The workflow was based on a subset of 1069 molecules, extracted by substructure-based filtering from ~720 000 commercially available compounds. This subset was docked with LigandFit [76] into an ensemble of receptor conformations. The development of the virtual screening protocol was based on an implementation of the "receiver operating characteristic" (ROC) curve method as objective method to evaluate the ability to discriminate between active and inactive molecules. Compounds with a score above a certain threshold using the preferred scoring function were subjected to visual inspection. A total of 38 compounds were selected and tested, of which 6 showed agonistic activity on mGlu4R.

Kellenberger et. al [77] described the identification of nonpeptidic CCR5 receptor agonists based on a homology model of this chemokine receptor. A library of 1.6 million commercially available compounds was filtered via a protocol including druglikeness, 2D pharmacophore model, 3D docking (Gold [64] and Surflex [78]), and scaffold clustering. Finally, 10 compounds out of 59 tested virtual hits were moderately active as agonists of the CCR5 receptor (Figure 12.5c). One of these molecules was also found active in secondary assays promoting efficient receptor internalization. The authors followed each of their active structures using 2D similarity search to enrich the motifs of each active compound and to establish early structure–activity relationships.

Engel *et al.* [79] reported a workflow combining pharmacophore searching using UNITY with docking using FlexE [45] into a homology model of the thyrotropin-releasing hormone receptor TRH-R1. The docking approach accounts for the inherent flexibility of the GPCR model. With this protocol, the authors screened 1 million druglike compounds from the ZINC database; 100 molecules were finally selected after application of scoring functions for testing, which resulted in the identification of 5 diverse antagonists of TRH-R1 and TRH-R2, with the most active compound having a K_i of 0.29 μM for TRH-R1 (Figure 12.5d).

Kiss *et al.* [80] described the discovery of novel histamine H4 receptor (H4R) ligands using a structure-based virtual screening protocol employing a recently built and validated H4R homology model and a nonfiltered collection of 8.7 million compounds from ZINC and various vendors representing 5 million unique structures. Docking was performed using FlexX [44] on a cluster production grid system in Hungary, and ranking of the compounds was done with ChemScore. The best 2000 compounds were visually inspected, while from another set of 45 000 compounds, a relevant subset for testing was chosen by criteria of protonation and diversity. Finally, a set of 255 available compounds were tested in a radioligand binding assay, and 16 of them on multiple scaffolds had significant biological activity. This is a remarkable success for a structure-based virtual screening with a GPCR homology model, especially since this model was built from the inactive crystal structure of bovine rhodopsin, where the second extracellular loop is considerably folded down to the transmembrane part, which typically results in shrinkage of the resulting homology models.

Kolb *et al.* [81] employed the recent X-ray structure of the β2-adrenergic receptor [82, 83] in structure-based virtual screening of novel ligands for this GPCR. This landmark X-ray structure was previously investigated with structure-based screening techniques by Sabio *et al.* [84] and de Graaf and Rognan [85]. After docking 1 million of available leadlike molecules using DOCK [29] against this experimental structure, 25 high-ranking compounds were experimentally tested, 6 were active with affinities <4 μM, with the best compound exhibiting a K_i of 9 nM. Five of these actives were shown to be GPCR inverse agonists, and the list of experimentally validated ligands contained some new scaffolds.

In an extensive comparative virtual screening study on GPCRs [86], it was concluded that ligand-based approaches outperform structure-based techniques on amine binding GPCRs, while there is no complete overlap of hits between these complementary approaches. Hence, these and other authors conclude that structure-based virtual screening is also useful for lead finding in this area, while effectiveness of the employed protocol clearly depends on the quality of the receptor model. These findings on successful applications in the area of GPCRs suggest the value of homology models as structural basis for virtual screening-based lead discovery in this particular target family.

12.3.1.6 **Antiinfectives**

Brenk *et al.* applied a sequential protocol to identify submicromolar lead structures for tRNA-guanine transglycosylase (TGT) [87–89]. Their virtual screening approach started with the analysis of an X-ray structure of a previously determined TGT complex with a small-molecule ligand. Three differing protein-based pharmacophore hypotheses were generated from a rather unexpected binding mode (cf. Chapter 10 for details about the role of a water molecule in this context) and employed for virtual screening, which led to the detection of a diverse set of candidates. The most acceptable compounds were docked into one of the two alternating TGT binding site conformers using FlexX [44], resulting in a final list of nine active molecules with significant biological affinity in the micromolar and submicromolar range (Figure 12.6).

Barreiro *et al.* [90] used virtual screening to identify nonnucleoside inhibitors of HIV-1 reverse transcriptase (NNRTIs). Virtual screening was performed using ~70 000 compounds from the Maybridge database. Approximately 2000 molecules that are most similar to the known active NNRTIs were then docked into the HIV-1 RT X-ray structure using Glide [47] and postscored with an MM–GB/SA (molecular mechanics–generalized Born/surface area) approach. Four compounds were tested, but none showed any significant activity in the biological assay. To follow up on this result, the proposed binding mode for the highest scoring molecule was analyzed to identify additional substituents to optimize protein–ligand interactions. After synthesis of a few derivatives, actives up to an EC_{50} of 0.31 μM for this target were identified. This interesting study demonstrated that it is possible to learn from unsuccessful virtual screening and evolve a false positive into a true active analogue after rational chemical modifications suggested by careful analysis of protein–ligand interactions.

Nicola *et al.* [91] reported the discovery of novel inhibitors of the enoylacyl carrier protein reductase (ENR) in *Plasmodium falciparum* by structure-based virtual screening based on the X-ray structure of this complex with triclosan. Virtual screening was done using ICM [51] and a library of 336 600 preferably druglike compounds from ChemBridge. The final selection of compounds with reasonable docking score was done by considering structural diversity and predicted ADMET properties. Sixteen compounds from a total of 169 tested in this assay showed a significant rate of inhibition, with three of them showing IC_{50} values between 5 and 25 μM (Figure 12.7a).

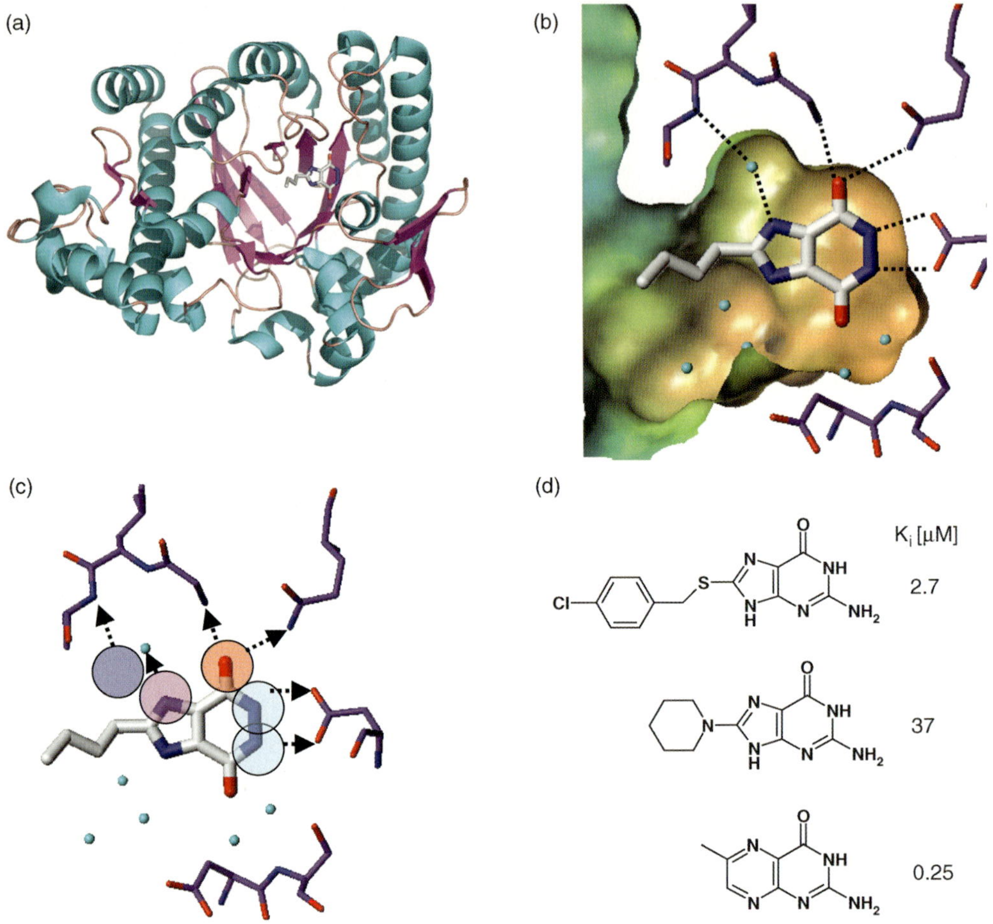

Figure 12.6 Example for successful structure-based virtual screening to identify submicromolar tRNA-guanine transglycosylase (TGT) inhibitors based on X-ray structures of weaker ligands. (a) X-ray structure of *Zymomonas mobilis* TGT at 2.1 Å resolution (PDB entry 1N2V). (b) Experimental binding mode for pyridazinedione scaffold (K_i: 83 μM) including structural water molecules from 1N2V. (c) Definition of structure-based pharmacophore model with ligand interactions as spheres (red – acceptor, light blue – donor, magenta – water) and protein-side interaction points indicated by arrows. An alternative ligand donor site (dark blue) was defined on the basis of an X-ray structure with a different ligand (not shown) where the backbone is flipped and the carbonyl group is oriented toward the binding pocket instead of the amide NH. (d) New TGT inhibitors discovered by virtual screening protocol.

Perez-Pineiro *et al.* [92] reported the implementation of a sequential computational approach for virtual screening to identify inhibitors of trypanothione reductase (TryR). Their workflow combines a 2D similarity-based virtual screening using a fragment-based Bayesian model with docking into the X-ray structure of TryR from *Trypanosoma cruzi* employing Autodock [93]. The 2D model significantly reduced

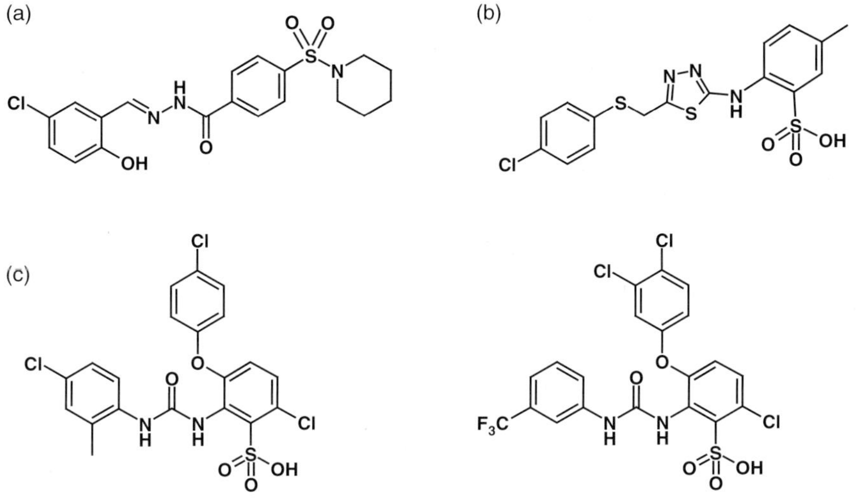

Figure 12.7 Structure-based virtual screening examples for antiinfective targets. (a) *Plasmodium falciparum* enoyl-acyl carrier protein reductase (ENR) inhibitor, IC_{50}: 6.0 μM. (b) *Streptococcus pneumoniae* penicillin binding protein (PBP2x) inhibitor, IC_{50} (5204-PBP2x strain): 219 μM. (c) *Streptococcus pneumoniae* penicillin binding protein (PBP2x) inhibitors, IC_{50} (5204-PBP2x strain): 71 μM (left), 72 μM (right).

the input ZINC database to 1312 molecules for docking. Of the 29 molecules tested, 10 were found as active with IC_{50} values between 20 and 90 μM for the target enzyme from *T. cruzi* or *T. brucei*, respectively.

Miguet *et al.* [94] reported on the discovery of new inhibitors of the resistant *Streptococcus pneumoniae* penicillin binding protein (PBP2x) by structure-based virtual screening. A hierarchical procedure using the NCI database on 260 000 compounds was followed, which started by developing and validating a homology model of spPBP2x from a highly resistant strain. Then a ligand-based pharmacophore model was developed using PHASE [95]. The identified ~6000 hits were subjected to docking into the homology model using FlexX-Pharm [40]. After experimental testing of 55 available virtual hits, 3 actives with IC_{50} values between 70 and 220 μM on 2 novel scaffolds were identified as inhibitors of the resistant strain 5204-spPBP2x (Figure 12.7b and c).

12.3.1.7 **Other Target Proteins**

The successful application of sequential virtual screening in search for novel inhibitors of human carbonic anhydrase II was reported by Grüneberg *et al.* [96, 97]. The authors applied a series of hierarchical filters to a database of ~100 000 compounds. A selection based on privileged functional groups from inspecting protein–ligand X-ray structures was followed by database searching using a protein-derived pharmacophore model. The similarity to known actives was used for ranking. Then 100 acceptable compounds were docked using FlexX [44] and 13 compounds were selected for testing. This resulted in remarkable affinities for most

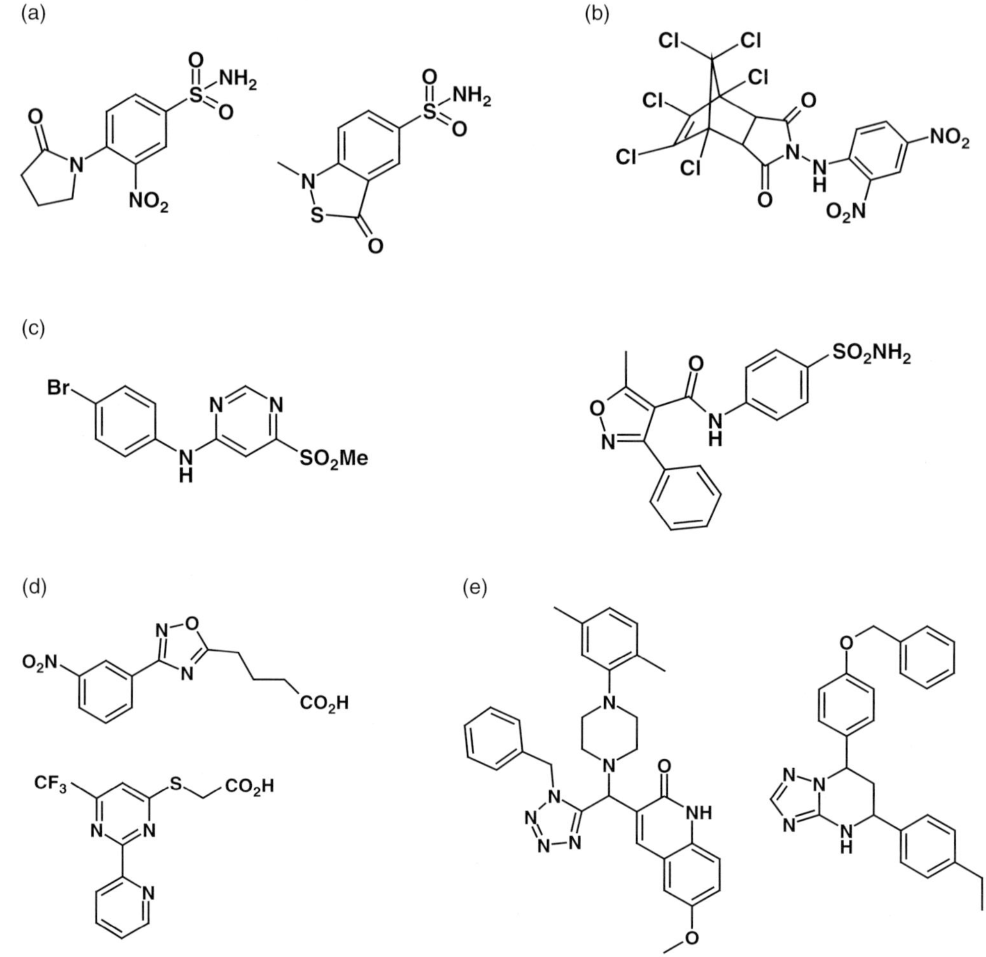

Figure 12.8 Structure-based virtual screening examples for miscellaneous targets. (a) Carbonic anhydrase II inhibitors, IC_{50}: 0.6 nM (left), 248 nM (right). (b) Farnesyltransferase inhibitor, IC_{50}: 25 μM. (c) COX-2 inhibitors with 60% (left) and 48% (right) inhibition at 1 μM concentration. (d) Aldose reductase inhibitors with IC_{50} values of 2.4 μM (upper panel) and 16.7 μM (lower panel). (e) DNA alkyltransferase MGMT inhibitors with IC_{50} values of 54 μM (left) and 24 μM (right).

of the tested structures, including three inhibitors with subnanomolar affinity on a new chemotype for this target. Most remarkably, the binding modes from docking could be validated by X-ray structure analysis of two inhibitors (Figure 12.8a).

Perola *et al.* successfully applied a structure-based virtual screening protocol to a database of ~220 000 commercially available compounds to identify farnesyltransferase (FT) inhibitors [98]. First, they applied a number of consecutive filters to remove undesirable structures from the database. The remaining compounds were subjected to a rigid docking protocol using the program EUDOC, developed in the same group. Again, the fundamental importance of protonation states and predocking filters on the quality of the results was emphasized. These parameters critically depend on the nature of the employed target structure. The final postdocking filtering included AMSOL solvation energies and visual inspection of docking modes. Interestingly enough, among 21 final candidates, 4 inhibited FT with IC_{50} values between 25 and 100 μM, while none of the 21 randomly selected compounds from the same starting database had an IC_{50} value lower than 100 μM (Figure 12.8b).

Enyedy *et al.* [99] described a structure-based virtual screening targeting a protein–protein interaction. They started from a homology model of Bcl-2 on the basis of the NMR-derived structure for Bcl-X_L in complex with the Bak BH3 peptide. The National Cancer Institute (NCI) database containing 207 000 compounds was then docked into the Bcl-2 binding site using DOCK [29]. Filtering of the top-scoring candidates resulted in 35 compounds, which were subjected to biological testing. Seven of these compounds had IC_{50} values <100 μM with a binding constant of 7 μM for the best Bcl-X_L ligand identified.

Mozziconacci *et al.* described the development and validation of a docking/scoring protocol in search for COX-2 inhibitors [100]. This virtual screening protocol was developed using known ligands and inactive molecules. The modification of docking parameters in DOCK [29] led to significant improvement of docking accuracy. The virtual hits were then subjected to consensus scoring. The application of this protocol to ~69 000 sulfonamides and sulfones of a library of 1.2 Mio compounds resulted in 12 candidates for biological testing. Four of these compounds were active with an inhibition >50% at 1 μM concentration (Figure 12.8c).

Structure-based virtual screening also led to the identification of inhibitors for human aldose reductase using a high-resolution X-ray crystal structure (0.66 Å), as reported by Krämer *et al.* [101]. Although the protein is known to exhibit significant flexibility in the region of its specificity pocket, only a single conformation was used and the binding pocket was treated as nonflexible. This allows the screening to be done in a fast and efficient manner, although it inherently limits the scope of this search. The application of a hierarchical filter protocol to the ACD as starting library involving 2D substructure searching, pharmacophore searching and docking led to the selection of nine compounds after visual inspection, of which six diverse hits showed IC_{50} values in the micromolar range with the best inhibitor having an IC_{50} value of 2.4 μM (Figure 12.8d).

The identification of a novel class of human and *E. coli* thymidine phosphorylase (TP) inhibitors by structure-based virtual screening was reported by McNally *et al.* [102]. The employed strategy involved a hierarchical computational screening of the NCI database of ~250 000 compounds using the program DOCK [29]. A series of nonnucleobase-derived inhibitors of human thymidine phosphorylase was identified as promising candidate for lead optimization. The docking studies were conducted using a previously built homology model of the human TP on the basis of the *E. coli* X-ray structure in an open cleft conformation. After further filtering, the final 444 top-scoring ligands were docked again including full ligand flexibility. All compounds from the final set of 13 acceptable compounds available from the NCI repository were found to be inhibitors of *E. coli* TP with 20 μM as best inhibition constant, while the 2 best molecules significantly inhibited human TP (77 μM).

Kenyon *et al.* [103] described the identification of novel inhibitors for human platelet-type 12 and reticulocyte 15-lipoxygenase-1 (12-hLO and 15-hLO) using structure-based virtual screening on homology models for both targets. A set of ∼50 000 commercially available druglike molecules from the ChemBridge "diversity set" was docked using Glide [47] into both homology models after validation of these structural binding site templates. The 20 best scoring molecules were selected after visual inspection and experimentally tested, which resulted in the identification of three inhibitors of either 12- or 15-hLO with IC_{50} values between 6 and 18 μM.

Ruiz *et al.* [104] described the identification of nonnucleosidic DNA alkyltransferase MGMT inhibitors by structure-based virtual screening. A total of 2.3 million compounds from the ZINC database were first docked using DOCK [29] into the X-ray structures of MGMT. The resulting 1662 molecules were then redocked using the program CDOCK [105] for a more exhaustive analysis of protein–ligand interactions, followed by a detailed postscoring approach involving the estimation of desolvation and electrostatic interactions. Seventeen molecules were tested after ranking and visual inspection of the poses, of which four compounds were shown to inactivate MGMT with IC_{50} values between 22 and 54 μM (Figure 12.8e). These structures can be classified into two distinct families, which are not related to the typical nucleoside-based pseudo-substrate analogues.

12.3.2
Structure-Based Library Design

The value of integrating combinatorial chemistry with structure-based library design and virtual screening has been highlighted in the literature [106, 107] and prompted for successful applications [108, 109]. The underlying idea is that relevant protein–ligand interactions coupled with a biased library approach result more rapidly in broader SAR information about directionality and physicochemical requirements of preferred building blocks. This concept is based on the availability of synthetically feasible scaffolds for exploring protein sites using parallel synthesis or a combinatorial approach.

Böhm described combinatorial docking [110] as extension of the program LUDI [111] based on generating ligands using geometrical constraints imposed by a structurally known protein site following a predefined chemical reaction scheme. First applications included amide formation and reductive amination in search for potent thrombin inhibitors. The most active compound from this study finally had a K_i value of 95 nM (Figure 12.9a). Furthermore, the authors confirmed the binding mode of this inhibitor by X-ray structure analysis [112].

Murray *et al.* described another combination of structure-based and focused combinatorial library design [113], starting with positioning synthetically accessible

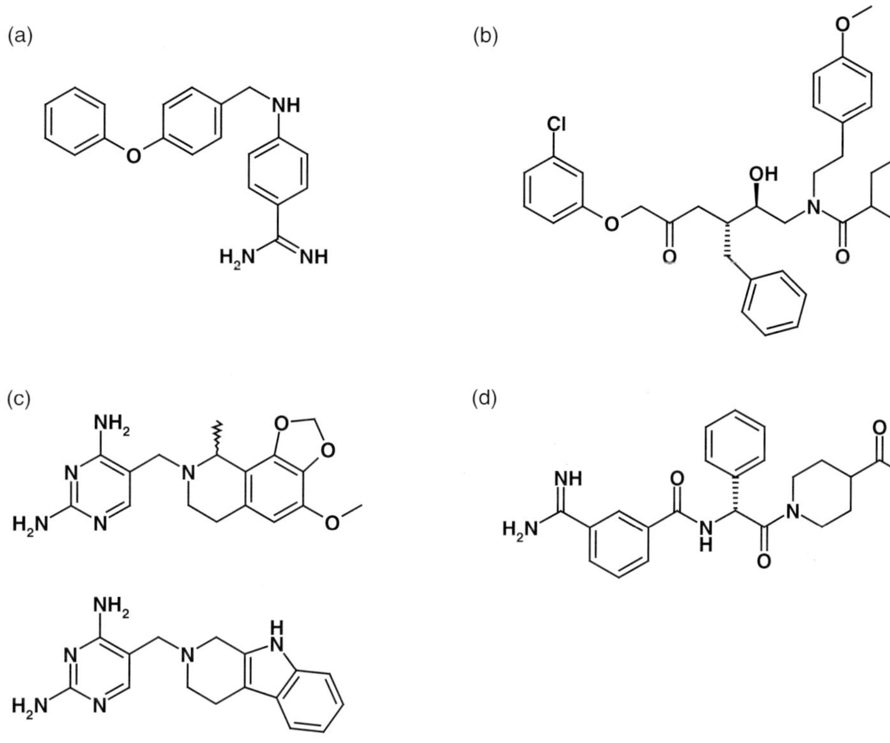

Figure 12.9 Successful applications of structure-based library design. (a) Thrombin inhibitor, K_i: 95 nM. (b) Plasmepsin II inhibitor, K_i: 2 nM. (c) Dihydrofolate reductase inhibitors. (d) Factor Xa inhibitor, K_i: 16 nM.

scaffolds within the protein site, followed by retrieval of reagents for attachment points that interact with the binding site. These building blocks have to be compatible with the synthetic scheme for library validation and production. Consequently, many filters are applied prior to optimizing and scoring to identify promising candidates for chemical synthesis. A similar approach using a preoriented template structure is realized in the program QXP [114] for virtual combinatorial library prioritization. First, preselected side chains at single attachment points are docked, followed by a combination of the best building blocks and conformations at different sites. The best molecules are subjected to a final annealing protocol and ranked using QXP interaction energy parameters. Jones *et al.* described a similar strategy [115] for GOLD. Here, fragments are individually docked into the binding site; subsequently, it is evaluated whether both fragments could potentially be connected by a linkage.

Similar strategies have been implemented for other docking programs. For example, the DOCK approach has been extended [116] by an efficient strategy for docking large virtual combinatorial libraries. For multiple scaffold orientations, all potential fragments are attached to the scaffold, their interactions with the receptor are individually scored, and factorial combinations of fragments are constructed and evaluated. In another study, an extended suite of programs for combinatorial docking and ligand evaluation based on efficient docking algorithms has been developed by the same group [117]. Both approaches were used for retrospective analyses and for design of novel enzyme inhibitors [118, 119]. In a prospective application, Haque *et al.* reported the design and synthesis of several potent low nanomolar plasmepsin II inhibitors [120], with the best inhibitor from a set of focused libraries showing a K_i value of 2 nM (Figure 12.9b).

Wyss *et al.* reported the discovery of novel dihydrofolate reductase inhibitors by structure-based library design based on a 5-(dialkylamino)-2,4-diaminopyrimidine scaffold [121]. From a virtual library of ~9000 compounds containing the diaminopyrimidine head group, 252 molecules were selected for synthesis by docking using FlexX [44]. This library led to 54 hits (21%) after biological testing (Figure 12.9c). In contrast, a second, low scoring library did only produce 4 hits (1%), while diversity-based selection resulted in 17 hits (3%). The authors concluded that compounds selected using structure-based virtual screening and library design resulted in a higher fraction of active molecules and lead compounds with higher activities than compounds selected on the basis of molecular diversity considerations.

Liebeschuetz *et al.* described the discovery of selective factor Xa inhibitors by structure-based virtual screening combined with array-based chemistry [122] as follow-up to a previous virtual screening study for factor Xa, thrombin and estrogen receptor ligands [123]. They applied the program PROSELECT for identification of virtual libraries for factor Xa. This led the authors to explore a small seed fragment in three iterations of library design, virtual screening, and rapid synthesis, which resulted in selective factor Xa inhibitors (Figure 12.9d).

Those examples show that the integration of structure-based design with combinatorial chemistry was accompanied with novel algorithms toward focused library design and subset selection using steric, electrostatic, and hydrophobic binding site constraints. The combinatorial nature of the problem often allows a very efficient implementation to build and rank only candidate molecules from previously ranked building block lists. These emerging techniques enable researchers to computationally build and screen virtual combinatorial libraries for binding site complementarity, while selection criteria might involve empirical scoring functions, diversity assessment, and synthetic feasibility.

12.3.3
Ligand-Based Virtual Screening

Ligand-based virtual screening approaches have been used for almost two decades to identify interesting molecules in 3D structure databases using hypotheses on ligand motifs linked to biological activity. It is clearly beyond the scope of this chapter to summarize all different methods and success stories from the literature (further details about ligand-based approaches can be found in Chapter 3, 11 and 13). In contrast, this section aims at illustrating the scope of ligand-based workflows using some instructive prospective virtual screening examples. We will focus in particular on 3D methods, including shape similarity and pharmacophore searching. Some examples for 2D similarity methods with a particular view on "scaffold hopping" will also be presented, while we will not cover the broader range of 2D similarity-based methods, which have recently been reviewed comprehensively [124].

12.3.3.1 **Ion Channels**

Schneider *et al.* [125] developed and applied CATS descriptors as topological pharmacophores for "scaffold hopping." This approach led to the prediction of novel cardiac T-type Ca^{2+} channel blocking agents using mibefradil as starting structure. From the highest ranking molecules, one interesting compound exhibited an IC_{50} value <1 μM (Figure 12.10a).

Pirard *et al.* reported the application of a protein-based pharmacophore model derived from a homology model in a study to identify novel inhibitors for the potassium channel Kv1.5 [126]. Two hundred and forty-four molecules were identified from searching their corporate database, and 19 molecules were found to be active for this target. Five of these compounds, belonging to five structurally different classes, revealed IC_{50} values <10 μM. In their study, the authors demonstrated that there is no overlap between hit lists from ligand- and structure-based virtual screening on this target, again underscoring the value of multiple approaches to address a problem.

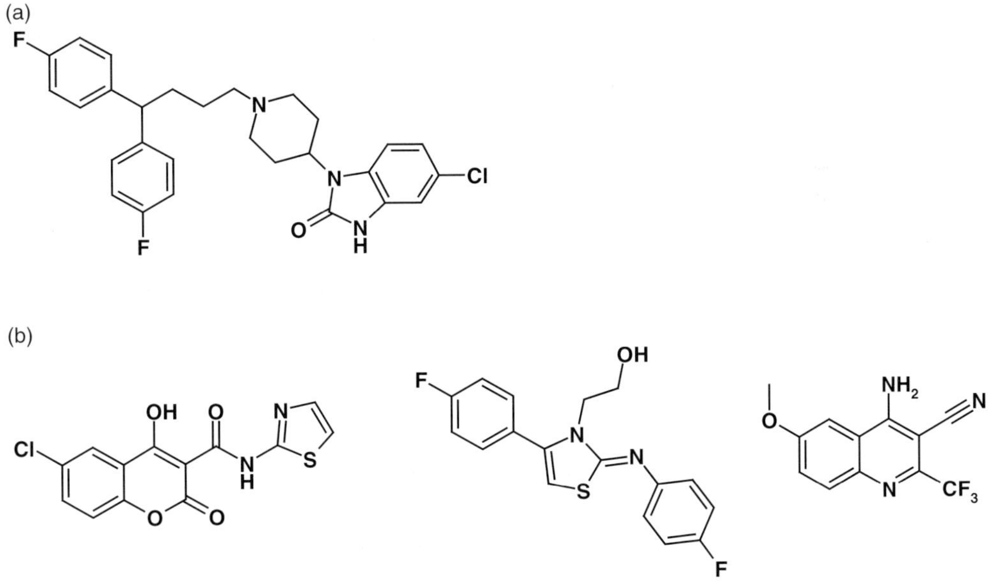

Figure 12.10 Ligand-based virtual screening examples for ion channels. (a) Calcium antagonist clopimozid from topological pharmacophore searching, $IC_{50} < 1$ μM. (b) Pancreatic K_{ATP} channel openers obtained from three different methods: EC_{50}: >30 μM (left), 21 μM (middle), 15 μM (right).

Carosati *et al.* [127] described an iterative ligand-based approach to search for novel structures as openers of the Kir6.2/SUR1 K_{ATP} ion channel. Starting from a set of ~65 000 commercially available structures from the ZINC database [128], pharmacokinetic filtering using VolSurf [129] reduced the data set to 1913 molecules. Six known K_{ATP} channel openers were then used as queries for 3D similarity searching using three approaches: GRIND [130], FLAP [131], and TOPP [131]. These molecular interaction field (MIF)-based methods encode structural information differently into pharmacophore models. From 32 virtual hits, a total of 3 hits resulted after testing with EC_{50} values from 15 to ~30 μM (Figure 12.10b). Interestingly, the authors observe that parallel application of different searching approaches improves hit detection, as none of the different pharmacophore methods was able to top rank all actives. Moreover, each hit was detected by a different computational approach, further underscoring the importance to apply different tools in parallel.

In another publication from the same group, a related methodology was applied to identify novel calcium channel antagonists [132] starting from a database of ~340 000 commercially available compounds. The database was first filtered by simple properties, followed by ligand-based virtual screening via 3D database searching using FLAP [131] starting from a known blocker as query. Twenty hits from the resulting hit list were experimentally tested and 12 reported actives showed promising behavior as L-type calcium entry blockers with negative inotropic EC_{50} values <1 μM.

12.3.3.2 **Kinases**

Naerum *et al.* [133] used topological pharmacophores to search for novel glycogen synthase kinase-3 inhibitors at Novo Nordisk. Using virtual screening based on the CATS descriptor, a novel chemotype with activity against GSK-3 was identified. After parallel synthesis around the identified motifs, interesting inhibitors with GSK-3 activity <1 μM were found (Figure 12.11a).

Chen *et al.* [134] described a successful sequential focused virtual screening in the Johnson & Johnson corporate chemical database for novel inhibitors of Janus kinase 3 (JAK3). Starting from a previous lead, the virtual screening was performed iteratively using ligand-based searching. Screening candidates at each round were selected based on the emerging structure–activity data from previous iterations. Initially, a 2D topological similarity search resulted in 40 analogues to establish a first SAR. A combination of 3D docking plus substructure and similarity searching then led to the identification of a diazaindazole scaffold (IC_{50}: 98 nM, Figure 12.11b, left). On the basis of its docking mode, a pair of four-point pharmacophore searching queries for Catalyst [61] were designed, resulting in novel motifs with best IC_{50} of 2.64 μM (Figure 12.11b, right). Biological testing of only 79 selected molecules led to the discovery of 19 compounds with IC_{50} values <20 μM, with 4 of them in the nanomolar range. In contrast, the parallel HTS resulted in a hit rate of less than 0.1%, while missing to identify the most active virtual screening hit. At least in this case, virtual screening outperformed HTS in terms of hit rate and quality. As the entire screening process is subdivided into

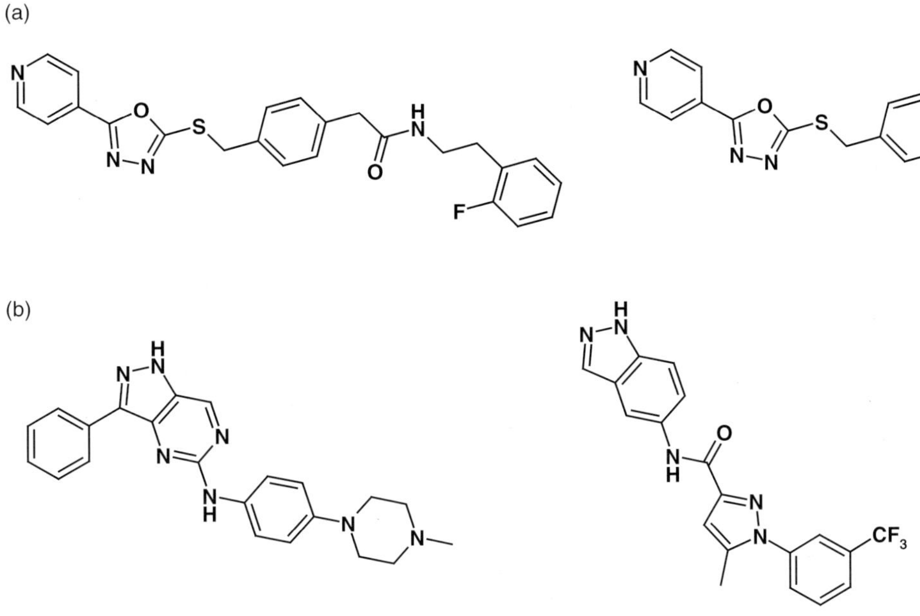

Figure 12.11 Ligand-based virtual screening examples for kinases. (a) GSK-3 inhibitors from topological pharmacophore searching with IC_{50}: 1.2 μM (left) and from subsequent lead optimization with IC_{50}: 0.39 μM (right). (b) Kinase JAK3 inhibitors, IC_{50}: 98 nM (left) and 2.6 μM (right), from sequential focused ligand-based virtual screening.

multiple rounds, different computational analysis and search techniques can be utilized at different stages. This introduces significant flexibility, allowing selecting the most appropriate computational and biological analysis approach based on the emerging SAR data for the protein target.

12.3.3.3 **Nuclear Hormone Receptors**

Markt *et al.* [135] applied virtual screening based on pharmacophore modeling, 3D shape, and electrostatic similarity screening to identify novel ligands for three PPAR subtypes α, γ, and δ. The structure-based pharmacophore approach from Ligand Scout was used to derive models from different PPAR agonist X-ray structures in the PDB database. Moreover, ligand-based pharmacophore models were derived using Catalyst [61]. The resulting models were carefully validated using a test database. The successful application of a protein-derived pharmacophore model was previously reported by Greenidge *et al.* for thyroid hormone receptor ligands [136]. The most selective four pharmacophore models were then used for virtual screening of a total of ~1 Mio vendor compounds. The resulting 14 311 hits were first filtered by physicochemical properties of known PPAR ligands before using 3D shape and electrostatic similarity to selected known PPAR ligands as additional selection step using ROCS and EON (ROCS and EON available from Openeye Scientific Software

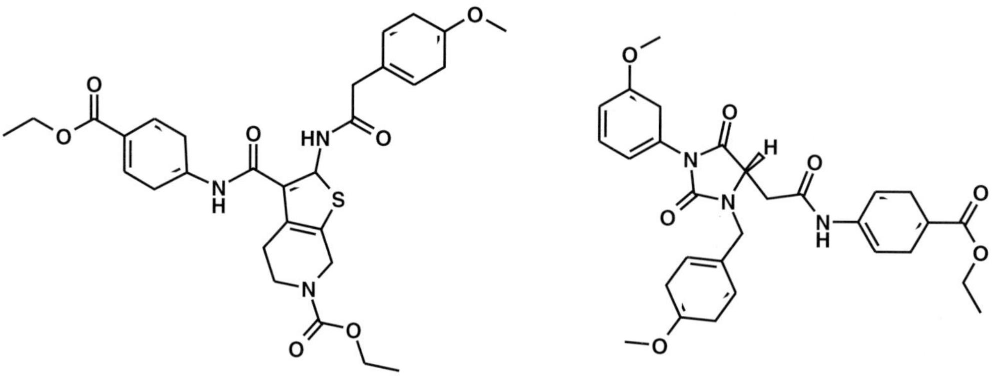

Figure 12.12 Nuclear receptor ligands from ligand-based virtual screening with IC_{50} values of 1.5 μM for PPARα (a) and 13 μM for PPARγ (b), obtained from pharmacophore-based searching.

Inc., Santa Fe, NM, 2007). From the resulting 10 virtual screening hits, 5 were active in PPAR ligand binding domain transactivation assays on either one or two of these subtypes (Figure 12.12).

12.3.3.4 **G Protein-Coupled Receptors (GPCRs)**

The CATS descriptor was also successful for selective purinergic receptor (A2A) antagonists [137]. To this end, a procedure based on this topological pharmacophore similarity metric was used to optimize combinatorial products as P1 purinergic receptor antagonists. Using an initial structure–activity relationship derived from self-organizing neural networks, a virtual library was projected onto this network. Selection, synthesis, and testing of 17 combinatorial products yielded threefold lower binding affinities and 3.5-fold higher selectivity than the initial library. The most selective antagonist revealed a 121-fold relative selectivity for A2A with K_i (A2A) = 2.4 nM and K_i (A1) = 292 nM.

A prospective study using 3D topomeric fields for angiotensin II antagonists was done using the ChemSpace technology [138]. The authors showed that the most similar compounds to known antagonists are those with highest activity suggesting that this descriptor is also useful to capture bioisosteres. This study was complemented by validations to quantify the ability of topomer shape similarity for forecasting a broad variety of biological affinities [139]. The biological testing of 308 selected compounds for 13 biological targets in a prospective trial of this descriptor led to the identification of 11 active compounds.

Guba *et al.* reported the identification of novel nonpeptidic NPY5 receptor antagonists using pharmacophore-based virtual screening [140]. The authors have chosen a hybrid approach starting from three reference compounds and combining their features into a Catalyst [61] virtual screening query containing 3D pharmacophoric information plus topological elements. A total of 632 molecules were selected for biological testing; 31 molecules showed an IC_{50} value <10 μM. The best compound on an aminothiazole scaffold showed an IC_{50} value of 40 nM. The

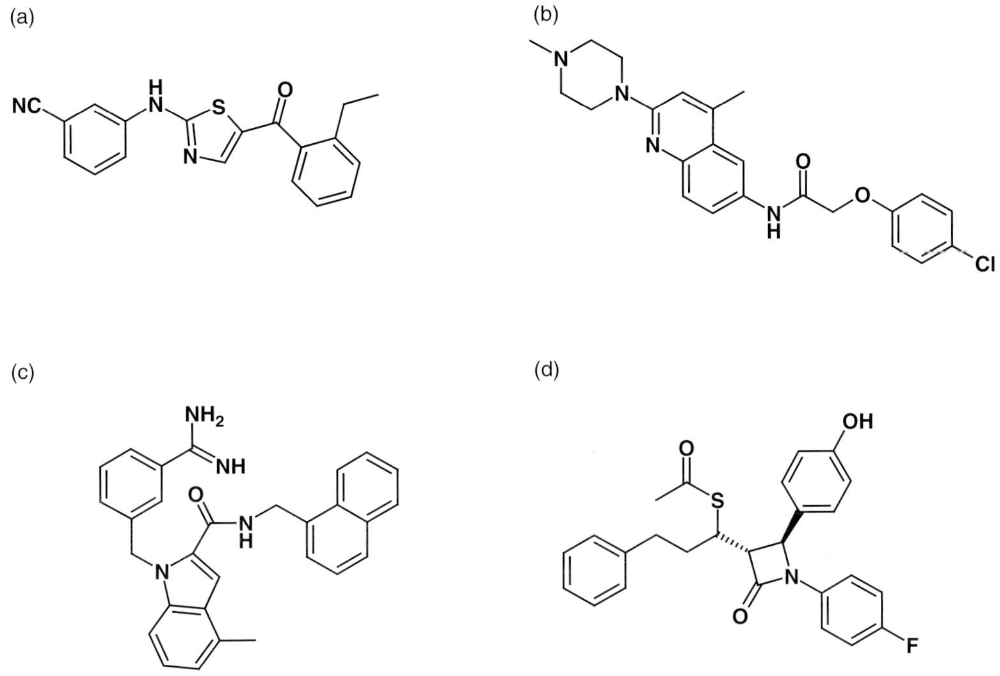

Figure 12.13 Ligand-based virtual screening examples for GPCRs. (a) NPY5 receptor antagonist from 3D pharmacophore searching and chemical optimization, IC_{50}: 2.8 nM. (b) MCH-1R antagonist from ligand-based virtual screening, IC_{50}: 55 nM. (c) Urotensin II antagonist from 3D pharmacophore searching, IC_{50}: 400 nM. (d) Cannabinoid CB1 receptor antagonist, K_i: 52.8 nM.

resulting novel and potent hit class was optimized using only two cycles of iterative chemistry optimization to result in a much broader understanding of essential factors driving the structure–activity relationship against this important GPCR target and in a lead compound with an IC_{50} value of 2.8 nM binding affinity (Figure 12.13a).

Clark *et al.* [141] used virtual screening to identify antagonists of the melanin-concentrating hormone 1 receptor (MCH-1). Multiple series were discovered using a variety of virtual screening techniques. This agrees with previous reports showing that different searching techniques typically result in different set of hits [142]. Based on 11 literature-known compounds active for this GPCR, multiple searches were conducted within a subset of about 615 000 commercially available compounds compiled from applications of numerous filter steps. Each compound served as query in multiple 2D substructure- and similarity-, as well as 3D substructure- and similarity-based virtual screening approaches. In addition, some molecules were docked into an MCH-1 homology model and structure-guided pharmacophore searches were carried out on the basis of these binding modes. A total of 3015 hits after combining all results were processed, yielding 795 diverse molecules, which were purchased and subjected to biological testing. Sixty-two actives were identified with the most potent compound having an IC_{50} value of 55 nM and thus providing a valuable starting point for further chemical optimization (Figure 12.13b).

The identification of muscarinic (M3) antagonists by pharmacophore searching was described by Marriott *et al.* [143]. Three out of 177 hits were found to be potent antagonists of the GPCR, although structurally dissimilar from previous antagonists. In search for novel angiotensin II receptor antagonists, Kiyama *et al.* applied a three-feature pharmacophore model to search the MDDR database [144]. The resulting 139 hits led to the identification of a novel lead series with activities in the nanomolar range. A sequential database searching strategy, including 2D substructure searching, followed by pharmacophore searching was described by Leysen and Kelder to discover selective 5-HT2c ligands [145].

Flohr *et al.* [146] reported a similar pharmacophore-based virtual screening in search for nonpeptidic urotensin II receptor antagonists. In addition to focused screening of the internal GPCR biased library, a rational approach by gathering structure–activity information through an alanine scan and by NMR studies on urotensin II was employed. The minimal sequence Trp7–Lys8–Tyr9 and an NMR-derived solution structure of the Urotensin II peptide were employed to model a hypothetical receptor-bound conformation and derive a three-point pharmacophore model. This pharmacophore model contained two hydrophobic features from the aromatic moieties of tryptophan and tyrosine and a positive ionizable center from the terminal amino group of lysine. In addition, the shape of the peptide sequence was considered for searching. The virtual screen returned six scaffold classes, with the most active antagonist exhibiting an IC_{50} value of 400 nM (Figure 12.13c). Again, relevant information about the original peptide could be converted into nonpeptide structures as starting point for a drug discovery program using a carefully chosen bioactive conformation followed by a pharmacophore-based virtual screening approach.

Bologa *et al.* [147] described the identification of selective agonists for the estrogen binding GPCR GPR30. They started from a library of ~10 000 compounds, pre-optimized for GPCR binding by appropriate privileged motifs, and employed a combination of 2D similarity searching combined with 3D shape searching using ROCS and GRIND descriptors to identify a potent and selective GPR30 agonist. The top-ranked 100 molecules were chosen for testing; only 1 molecule was confirmed to bind with GPR30 and further profiled.

Wang *et al.* [148] at Schering-Plough reported the identification of a new series of azetidinone cannabinoid CB1 receptor antagonists using a pharmacophore-based virtual screening approach. First, a Catalyst [61] HipHop pharmacophore model was developed from known CB1 antagonists. The resulting five-point model was then employed to identify hits in ~500 000 internal compounds at Schering-Plough, resulting in ~23 000 compounds as start for further filtering using availability, physicochemical properties, and a Bayesian model for CB1 activity. Finally 420 molecules were experimentally tested, resulting in 5 compounds from 1 chemical series with K_i values $<1\,\mu M$ for CB1 (Figure 12.13d).

12.3.3.5 **Other Protein Targets**

Wang *et al.* reported the application of an X-ray structure-derived pharmacophore model to identify novel HIV-1 protease inhibitors. After searching the NCI database (206 000 molecules), testing of 50 molecules resulted in submicromolar activity for the best 2 compounds [149]. In a search for HIV-1 integrase inhibitors, a protein-derived pharmacophore model produced 340 hits from 10 different classes. Four compounds were shown to have affinities $<30\,\mu M$ [150] against this enzyme.

Kaminski *et al.* described 3D database searching for farnesyltransferase inhibitors [151]. They constructed a pharmacophore model and used this motif to identify candidates matching this pattern within the Schering-Plough corporate database. From 718 hits after 3D database searching, the 5 best compounds after biological testing had IC_{50} values $<5\,\mu M$. This led to the identification of a novel series of dihydrobenzothiophenes.

Singh *et al.* [152] applied Catalyst [61] to search for integrin $\alpha 4\beta 1$ antagonists. Potent inhibitors of $\alpha 4\beta 1$ were discovered using a pharmacophore-based virtual screening approach by replacing the peptide region of a known peptide inhibitor from fibronectin. The search query was constructed from the X-ray conformation of the peptide-related integrin binding region of the vascular cell adhesion molecule-1 (VCAM-1). The following virtual screening identified 12 promising hits from a virtual library of 8624 candidates. All subsequently synthesized molecules were found to inhibit the interaction between $\alpha 4\beta 1$ and VCAM-1, with the most potent candidate showing an IC_{50} value of 1 nM (Figure 12.14a), comparable to the starting compound. Hence, the authors were able to demonstrate that pharmacophore searches led to the identification of nonpeptidic structures using peptide information as starting point.

Shoda *et al.* [153] used a combination of ligand-based virtual screening and analogue design to identify novel antagonists of the lymphocyte function-associated antigen-1 (LFA-1) to its intracellular adhesion molecule-1 (ICAM-1). Known antagonists of this LFA-1/ICAM-1 protein–protein interaction were then used to search a library of ~2.5 million commercially available compounds by similarity methods. To this end, the authors used a compact 2D MiniFingerPrint (MFP) [154] plus cell partitioning on different 1D and 2D descriptors to identify interesting molecules. Experimental evaluation of only 25 compounds resulted in 1 compound with moderate activity (IC_{50}: $70\,\mu M$). This structure was used for further searching to result in a structure–activity relationship for this series with the most active compound showing an IC_{50} value of $4.3\,\mu M$.

Tervo *et al.* [155] described a successful virtual screening experiment for the class III histone deacylase sirtuin type 2 (SIRT2). Using two databases of commercially available compounds plus a receptor-based pharmacophore query, 4 out of 11 tested molecules showed weak to moderate inhibitory activity. The two most active inhibitors with IC_{50} values of 51 and $91\,\mu M$ had new scaffolds (Figure 12.14b).

Franke *et al.* [156] reported on a study to identify natural product-derived compounds as potential novel 5-lipoxygenase (5-LO) inhibitors using a two-step ligand-based virtual screening approach. In the first step, natural products and natural

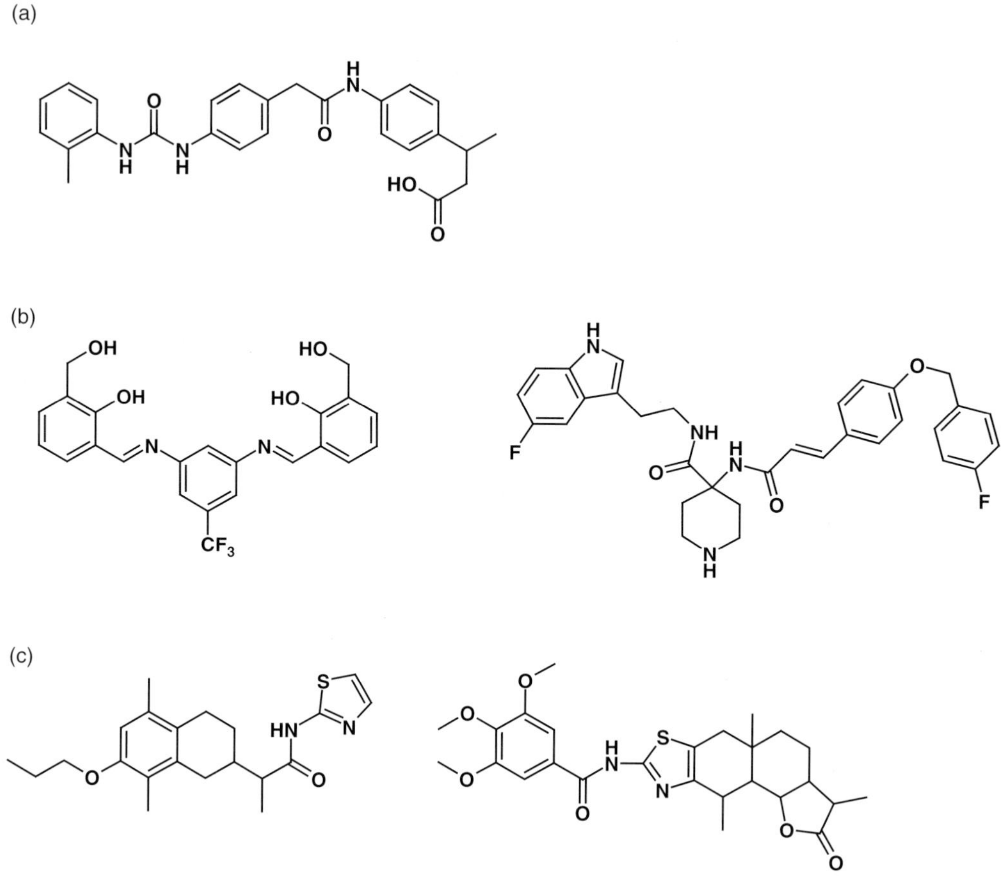

Figure 12.14 Ligand-based virtual screening examples for miscellaneous targets. (a) α4β1 (VLA-4) antagonist from pharmacophore searching, IC_{50}: 1 nM. (b) Class III histone deacylase sirtuin type 2 (SIRT2) inhibitors with IC_{50} values of 91 μM (left) and 51 μM (right). (c) 5-lipoxygenase (5-LO) inhibitors with IC_{50} values of 0.8 μM (left) and 0.9 μM (right).

product-derived combinatorial compounds from the AnalytiCon Discovery collections were virtually screened with 43 query molecules known to be active on this target using the CATS topological pharmacophore pair descriptor [125]. For each reference, the most similar compounds were retrieved and filtered and then a set of 18 molecules were selected for the first round of experimental testing. Two novel 5-LO inhibitors on structurally different classes were identified with IC_{50} values <1 μM; these were used as queries for a second round of ligand-based searching employing three CATS variations and MACCS 2D substructure keys. The best molecules from this second, more focused set of ligands were again shown to be experimentally active in the same affinity range and represent a novel class of 5-LO inhibitors (Figure 12.14c).

12.4 Conclusion

Over the past years, information-guided lead finding by virtual screening has emerged as potential alternative to high-throughput screening in some areas. Many reports in the literature have convincingly shown that novel chemical structures can be retrieved from chemical databases by this approach. As demonstrated in this section, the amount of information in a project often determines the choice of computational approaches, while a combination of complementary strategies with hierarchical filter protocols is effective to identify novel compound classes on many targets from different gene families.

Due to the proprietary nature of new molecules, not all successful virtual screens in the past years have been published. Hence, there is a strong bias toward case studies from academia in the literature. This chapter aimed to compile a representative collection of recent success stories covering multiple approaches on diverse protein targets. The examples show that a remarkable collection of studies already exists, documenting the success of lead generation by virtual screening. Nevertheless, it should be mentioned that only positive results are usually published, which makes it difficult to estimate the true success rate of this approach.

Two general conclusions can be drawn from these examples and the experiences gained today, as stated by Köppen in a recent review [11]: (1) There is no virtual screening method that is clearly superior to others. (2) The success of virtual screening depends in an unpredictable manner on the combination of the screen method, the target, and the chemical space that is virtually screened. Numerous comparative studies also led to some general trends [10]: 2D similarity methods are often as effective as 3D ligand-derived descriptors and frequently outperform them; 3D methods appear to allow more efficiently the “scaffold hopping”; and the ligand-based methods are reported to be as effective as the structure-based methods. Problems, challenges, and caveats of the various approaches are discussed in more detail in other chapters of this book.

These conclusions are also supported by the presented examples, but some additional trends should be pointed out. Effective virtual screening today includes a multitude of approaches, often applied in a sequential manner or integrated within a flexible workflow. There is no unique protocol for every virtual screening task – every problem is unique and requires careful validation, filtering, and parameterization in the beginning to result in a protocol with the potential to yield valuable hit lists after productive application to large databases. Extensive validation based on sample databases of known actives and decoy molecules is essential.

In structure-based virtual screening, docking and scoring are usually decoupled from each other. The importance of high-quality conformations and binding poses is often pointed out; accordingly, postdocking filters and advanced scoring protocols are developed and applied, but some fundamental problems of correctly capturing the underlying principles of molecular recognition still remain. Another area of active research is the consideration of receptor flexibility, which is included only to very limited extent in most current applications and standard docking protocols (a detailed discussion of protein flexibility approaches already available for docking and virtual screening is given in Chapters 8 and 9).

The practical use of homology models for structure-based virtual screening has been debated in the scientific literature, but numerous successful applications presented in this chapter – in particular for the GPCR target family – underscore the value of this approach in the absence of high-resolution X-ray structures. Again, validation of the employed models is a critical aspect for successful application. In a recent study by Fan *et al.* [157], similar enrichment rates were obtained on average in retrospective virtual screens employing crystal structures or homology models for 38 targets. Chapter 14 provides further examples and a detailed discussion of virtual screening based on homology models.

Ligand-based virtual screening can rapidly search large databases. Hence, it is often applied as prefilter before employing more complex tools. Many applications are reported for pharmacophore- and shape-based searching, while the use of the multitude of 2D descriptors is straightforward and tightly integrated in today's workflows.

A very important trend is to rapidly explore new virtual screening hits by a second round of analogue searching to establish early structure–activity relationships. Initial actives are valuable as queries for a second screening iteration to explore the available chemical space using experimentally validated information. In many cases, the selection of analogues might allow to rapidly evaluate a particular series and to put this into perspective with the docking or pharmacophore model.

Different virtual screening techniques applied to a single target might result in differences in the enrichment of active compounds and in complementary hit lists. As it cannot be estimated in advance which approach might perform best, it is strongly recommended to apply more than one approach in combination for prospective settings, thus increasing the likelihood of identifying active molecules.

Thus, although many scientific questions for virtual screening tools still need to be addressed, this technique deserves the increasing attention as alternative lead finding approach. Since the first reports in the field more than a decade ago, a more mature technique integrating multiple tools and model has emerged, which has proven to be valuable for drug discovery efforts.

References

1 Hillisch, A. and Hilgenfeld, R. (2003) *Modern Methods of Drug Discovery*, Birkhäuser, Basel.

2 Bleicher, K.H., Böhm, H.-J., Müller, K., and Alanine, A.I. (2003) Hit and lead generation: beyond high throughput screening. *Nature Reviews. Drug Discovery*, **2**, 369–378.

3 Alanine, A., Nettekoven, M., Roberts, E., and Thoma, A.W. (2003) Lead generation: enhancing the success of drug discovery by investing in the hit to lead process. *Combinatorial Chemistry & High Throughput Screening*, **6**, 51–66.

4 Böhm, H.-J. and Schneider, G. (eds) (2000) *Virtual Screening for Bioactive Molecules*, Wiley-VCH Verlag GmbH, Weinheim.

5 Bajorath, J. (2002) Integration of virtual and high throughput screening.

Nature Reviews. Drug Discovery, **1**, 882–894.

6 Oprea, T.I. and Matter, H. (2004) Integrating virtual screening in lead discovery. *Current Opinion in Chemical Biology*, **8**, 349–358.

7 Klebe, G. (2006) Virtual ligand screening: strategies, perspectives and limitations. *Drug Discovery Today*, **11**, 580–594.

8 Seifert, M.H.J., Kraus, J., and Kramer, B. (2007) Virtual high-throughput screening of molecular databases. *Current Opinion in Drug Discovery & Development*, **11**, 298–307.

9 Rester, U. (2008) From virtuality to reality: virtual screening in lead discovery and lead optimization – a medicinal chemistry perspective. *Current Opinion in Drug Discovery & Development*, **11**, 559–568.

10 Green, D.V.S. (2008) Virtual screening of chemical libraries for drug discovery. *Expert Opinion on Drug Discovery*, **3**, 1011–1026.

11 Köppen, H. (2009) Virtual screening: what does it give us? *Current Opinion in Drug Discovery & Development*, **12**, 397–407.

12 Pospisil, P., Ballmer, P., Scapozza, L., and Folkers, G. (2003) Tautomerism in computer-aided drug design. *Journal of Receptor and Signal Transduction Research*, **23**, 361–371.

13 Milletti, F., Storchi, L., Sforna, G., Cross, S., and Cruciani, G. (2009) Tautomer enumeration and stability prediction for virtual screening on large chemical databases. *Journal of Chemical Information and Modeling*, **49**, 68–75.

14 Lyne, P.D. (2002) Structure-based virtual screening: an overview. *Drug Discovery Today*, **7**, 1047–1055.

15 Matter, H., Baringhaus, K.H., Naumann, T., Klabunde, T., and Pirard, B. (2001) Computational approaches towards the rational design of drug-like compound libraries. *Combinatorial Chemistry & High Throughput Screening*, **4**, 453–475.

16 Lipinski, C.A., Lombardo, F., Dominy, B.W., and Feeney, P.J. (1997) Experimental and computational approaches to estimate solubility and permeability in drug discovery and development settings. *Advanced Drug Delivery Reviews*, **23**, 3–25.

17 Veber, D.F., Johnson, S.R., Cheng, H.Y., Smith, B.R., Ward, K.W., and Kopple, K.D. (2002) Molecular properties that influence the oral bioavailability of drug candidates. *Journal of Medicinal Chemistry*, **12**, 2615–2623.

18 Oprea, T.I., Davis, A.M., Teague, S.J., and Leeson, P.D. (2001) Is there a difference between leads and drugs? A historical perspective. *Journal of Chemical Information and Computer Sciences*, **41**, 1308–1315.

19 Teague, S.J., Davis, A.M., Leeson, P.D., and Oprea, T. (1999) The design of leadlike combinatorial libraries. *Angewandte Chemie, International Edition*, **38**, 3743–3748.

20 Roche, O., Schneider, P., Zuegge, J., Guba, W., Kansy, M., Alanine, A., Bleicher, K., Danel, F., Gutknecht, E.M., Rogers-Evans, M., Neidhart, W., Stalder, H., Dillon, M., Sjoegren, E., Fotouhi, N., Gillespie, P., Goodnow, R., Harris, W., Jones, P., Taniguchi, M., Tsujii, S., von Saal, W., Zimmermann, G., and Schneider, G. (2002) Development of a virtual screening method for identification of "Frequent Hitters" in compound libraries. *Journal of Medicinal Chemistry*, **45**, 137–142.

21 Roche, O., Trube, G., Zuegge, J., Pflimlin, P., Alanine, A., and Schneider, G. (2002) A virtual screening method for prediction of the hERG potassium channel liability of compound libraries. *ChemBioChem*, **3**, 455–459.

22 Pearlstein, R., Vaz, R., and Rampe, D. (2003) Understanding the structure–activity relationship of the human ether-a-go-go-related gene cardiac K+ channel. A model for bad behavior. *Journal of Medicinal Chemistry*, **46**, 2017–2022.

23 Aronov, A.M. and Goldman, B.B. (2004) A model for identifying HERG K+ channel blockers. *Bioorganic & Medicinal Chemistry Letters*, **12**, 2307–2315.

24 Aronov, A.M. (2005) Predictive *in silico* modeling for hERG channel blockers. *Drug Discovery Today*, **10**, 149–155.

25 Zuegge, J., Fechner, U., Roche, O., Parrott, N., Engkvist, O., and Schneider, G. (2002) A fast virtual screening filter for cytochrome P450 3A4 inhibition liability of compound libraries. *Quantitative Structure–Activity Relationships*, **21**, 249–256.

26 Ekins, S., Berbaum, J., and Harrison, R.K. (2003) Generation and validation of rapid computational filters for CYP2D6 and CYP3A4. *Drug Metabolism and Disposition: The Biological Fate of Chemicals*, **31**, 1077–1080.

27 Kriegl, J.M., Eriksson, L., Arnhold, T., Beck, B., Johansson, E., and Fox, T. (2005) Multivariate modeling of cytochrome P450 3A4 inhibition. *European Journal of Pharmaceutical Sciences*, **24**, 451–463.

28 Vangrevelinghe, E., Zimmermann, K., Schoepfer, J., Portmann, R., Fabbro, D., and Furet, P. (2003) Discovery of a potent and selective protein kinase CK2 inhibitor by high-throughput docking. *Journal of Medicinal Chemistry*, **46**, 2656–2662.

29 Ewing, T.J.A., Makino, S., Skillman, A.G., and Kuntz, I.D. (2001) DOCK 4.0: search strategies for automated molecular docking of flexible molecule databases. *Journal of Computer-Aided Molecular Design*, **15**, 411–428.

30 Wang, R., Liu, L., Lai, L., and Tang, Y. (1998) SCORE: a new empirical method for estimating the binding affinity of a protein–ligand complex. *Journal of Molecular Modeling*, **4**, 379–394.

31 Peng, H., Huang, N., Qi, J., Xie, P., Xu, C., Wang, J., and Yang, C. (2003) Identification of novel inhibitors of BCR-ABL tyrosine kinase via virtual screening. *Bioorganic & Medicinal Chemistry Letters*, **13**, 3693–3699.

32 Filikov, A.V. and James, T.L. (1998) Structure-based design of ligands for protein basic domains: application to the HIV-1 Tat protein. *Journal of Computer-Aided Molecular Design*, **12**, 229–240.

33 Shoichet, B.K., Stroud, R.M., Santi, D.V., Kuntz, I.D., and Perry, K.M. (1993) Structure-based discovery of inhibitors of thymidylate synthase. *Science*, **259**, 1445–1450.

34 Tondi, D., Slomczynska, U., Costi, M.P., Watterson, D.M., Ghelli, S., and Shoichet, B.K. (1999) Structure-based discovery and in-parallel optimization of novel competitive inhibitors of thymidylate synthase. *Chemistry & Biology*, **6**, 319–331.

35 Bodian, D.L., Yamasaki, R.B., Buswell, R.L., Stearns, J.F., White, J.M., and Kuntz, I.D. (1993) Inhibition of the fusion-inducing conformational change of influenza hemagglutinin by benzoquinones and hydroquinones. *Biochemistry*, **32**, 2967–2978.

36 Ring, C.S., Sun, E., McKerrow, J.H., Lee, G.K., Rosenthal, P.J., Kuntz, I.D., and Cohen, F.E. (1993) Structure-based inhibitor design by using protein models for the development of antiparasitic agents. *Proceedings of the National Academy of Sciences of the United States of America*, **90**, 3583–3587.

37 Doman, T.N., McGovern, S.L., Witherbee, B.J., Kasten, T.P., Kurumbail, R., Stallings, W.C., Connolly, D.T., and Shoichet, B.K. (2002) Molecular docking and high-throughput screening for novel inhibitors of protein tyrosine phosphatase-1B. *Journal of Medicinal Chemistry*, **45**, 2213–2221.

38 Hopkins, S.C., Vale, R.D., and Kuntz, I.D. (2000) Inhibitors of kinesin activity from structure-based computer screening. *Biochemistry*, **39**, 2805–2814.

39 Lyne, P.D., Kenny, P.W., Cosgrove, D.A., Deng, C., Zabludoff, S., Wendoloski, J.J., and Ashwell, S. (2004) Identification of compounds with nanomolar binding affinity for checkpoint kinase-1 using knowledge-based virtual screening. *Journal of Medicinal Chemistry*, **47**, 1962–1968.

40 Hindle, S.A., Rarey, M., Buning, C., and Lengauer, T. (2002) Flexible docking under pharmacophore constraints. *Journal of Computer-Aided Molecular Design*, **16**, 129–149.

41 Foloppe, N., Fisher, L.M., Howes, R., Potter, A., Robertson, A.G.S., and Surgenor, A.S. (2006) Identification of chemically diverse Chk1 inhibitors by receptor-based virtual screening. *Bioorganic & Medicinal Chemistry*, **14**, 4792–4802.

42 Morley, S.D. and Afshar, M. (2004) Validation of an empirical RNA-ligand scoring function for fast flexible docking using RiboDock. *Journal of Computer-Aided Molecular Design*, **18**, 189–208.

43 Polgár, T., Baki, A., Szendrei, G.I., and Keresü, G.M. (2005) Comparative virtual and experimental high-throughput screening for glycogen synthase kinase-3β inhibitors. *Journal of Medicinal Chemistry*, **48**, 7946–7959.

44 Rarey, M., Kramer, B., Lengauer, T., and Klebe, G. (1996) A fast flexible docking method using an incremental construction algorithm. *Journal of Molecular Biology*, **261**, 470–489.

45 Claussen, H., Buning, C., Rarey, M., and Lengauer, T. (2001) FlexE: efficient molecular docking considering protein structure variations. *Journal of Molecular Biology*, **308**, 377–395.

46 Ward, R.A., Perkins, T.D.J., and Stafford, J. (2005) Structure-based virtual screening for low molecular weight chemical starting points for dipeptidyl peptidase IV inhibitors. *Journal of Medicinal Chemistry*, **48**, 6991–6996.

47 Friesner, R.A., Banks, J.L., Murphy, R.B., Halgren, T.A., Klicic, J.J., Mainz, D.T., Repasky, M.P., Knoll, E.H., Shelley, M., Perry, J.K., Shaw, D.E., Francis, P., and Shenkin, P.S. (2004) Glide: a new approach for rapid, accurate docking and scoring. 1. Methods and assessment of docking accuracy. *Journal of Medicinal Chemistry*, **47**, 1739–1749.

48 Li, H., Huang, J., Chen, L., Liu, X., Chen, T., Zhu, J., Lu, W., Shen, X., Li, J., Hilgenfeld, R., and Jiang, H. (2009) Identification of novel falcipain-2 inhibitors as potential antimalarial agents through structure-based virtual screening. *Journal of Medicinal Chemistry*, **52**, 4936–4940.

49 Li, H., Li, C., Gui, C., Luo, X., Chen, K., Shen, J., Wang, X., and Jiang, H. (2004) GAsDock: a new approach for rapid flexible docking based on an improved multipopulation genetic algorithm. *Bioorganic & Medicinal Chemistry Letters*, **14**, 4671–4676.

50 Schapira, M., Raaka, B.M., Samuels, H.H., and Abagyan, R. (2000) Rational discovery of novel nuclear hormone receptor antagonists. *Proceedings of the National Academy of Sciences of the United States of America*, **97**, 1008–1013.

51 Totrov, M. and Abagyan, R. (1997) Flexible protein–ligand docking by global energy optimization in internal coordinates. *Proteins*, **29** (Suppl. 1), 215–220.

52 Schulz-Gasch, T. and Stahl, M. (2003) Binding site characteristics in structure-based virtual screening: evaluation of current docking tools. *Journal of Molecular Modeling*, **9**, 47–57.

53 Cummings, M.D., DesJarlais, R.L., Gibbs, A.C., Mohan, V., and Jaeger, E.P. (2005) Comparison of automated docking programs as virtual screening tools. *Journal of Medicinal Chemistry*, **48**, 962–976.

54 Schapira, M., Raaka, B.M., Das, S., Fan, L., Totrov, M., Zhou, Z., Wilson, S.R., Abagyan, R., and Samuels, H.H. (2003) Discovery of diverse thyroid hormone receptor antagonists by high-throughput docking. *Proceedings of the National Academy of Sciences of the United States of America*, **100**, 7354–7359.

55 Schapira, M., Abagyan, R., and Totrov, M. (2003) Nuclear hormone receptor targeted virtual screening. *Journal of Medicinal Chemistry*, **46**, 3045–3059.

56 Bakir, F., Kher, S., Pannala, M., Wilson, N., Nguyen, T., Sircar, I., Takedomi, K., Fukushima, C., Zapf, J., Xu, K., Zhang, S.-H., Liu, J., Morera, L., Schneider, L., Sakurai, N., Jack, R., and Cheng, J.-F. (2007) Discovery and structure–activity relationship studies of indole derivatives as liver X receptor (LXR) agonists. *Bioorganic & Medicinal Chemistry Letters*, **17**, 3473–3479.

57 Cheng, J.-F., Zapf, J., Takedomi, K., Fukushima, C., Ogiku, T., Zhag, S.-H., Yang, G., Sakurai, N., Barbosa, M., Jack, R., and Xu, K. (2008) Combination of virtual screening and high throughput gene profiling for identification of novel liver X receptor modulators. *Journal of Medicinal Chemistry*, **51**, 2057–2061.

58 Knox, A.J.S., Meegan, M.J., Sobolev, V., Frost, D., Zisterer, D.M., Williams, D.C., and Lloyd, D.G. (2007) Target specific

virtual screening: optimization of an estrogen receptor screening platform. *Journal of Medicinal Chemistry*, **50**, 5301–5310.

59 Sobolev, V., Moallem, T.M., Wade, R.C., Vriend, G., and Edelman, M. (1997) CASP2 molecular docking prediction with the LIGIN software. *Proteins*, **29** (Suppl. 1), 210–214.

60 Schuster, D., Maurer, E.M., Laggner, C., Nashev, L.G., Wilckens, T., Langer, T., and Odermatt, A. (2006) The discovery of new 11β-hydroxysteroid dehydrogenase type 1 inhibitors by common feature pharmacophore modeling and virtual screening. *Journal of Medicinal Chemistry*, **49**, 3454–3466.

61 Greene, J., Kahn, S., Savoj, H., Sprague, S., and Teig, S. (1994) Chemical function queries for 3D database search. *Journal of Chemical Information and Computer Sciences*, **34**, 1297–1308.

62 Schuster, D., Nashev, L.G., Kirchmair, J., Laggner, C., Wolber, G., Langer, T., and Odermatt, A. (2008) Discovery of nonsteroidal 17β-hydroxysteroid dehydrogenase 1 inhibitors by pharmacophore-based screening of virtual compound libraries. *Journal of Medicinal Chemistry*, **51**, 4188–4199.

63 Wolber, G. and Langer, T. (2005) LigandScout: 3-D pharmacophores derived from protein-bound ligands and their use as virtual screening filters. *Journal of Chemical Information and Computer Sciences*, **45**, 160–169.

64 Jones, G., Willett, P., Glen, R.C., Leach, A.R., and Taylor, R. (1997) Development and validation of a genetic algorithm for flexible docking. *Journal of Molecular Biology*, **267**, 727–748.

65 Bissantz, C., Bernard, P., Hibert, M., and Rognan, D. (2003) Protein-based virtual screening of chemical databases. II. Are homology models of G-protein coupled receptors suitable targets? *Proteins*, **50**, 5–25.

66 Becker, O.M., Shacham, S., Marantz, Y., and Nioman, S. (2003) Modeling the 3D structure of GPCRs: advances and application to drug discovery. *Current Opinion in Drug Discovery & Development*, **6**, 353–361.

67 Becker, O.M., Marantz, Y., Shacham, S., Inbal, B., Heifetz, A., Kalid, O., and Bar-Heim, S. (2004) G-protein-coupled receptors: *in silico* drug discovery in 3D. *Proceedings of the National Academy of Sciences of the United States of America*, **101**, 11304–11309.

68 Bissantz, C., Logean, A., and Rognan, D. (2004) High-throughput modeling of human G-protein coupled receptors: amino acid sequence alignment, three-dimensional model building, and receptor library screening. *Journal of Chemical Information and Computer Sciences*, **44**, 1162–1176.

69 Varady, J., Wu, X., Fang, X., Min, J., Hu, Z., Levant, B., and Wang, S. (2003) Molecular modeling of the three-dimensional structure of dopamine 3 (D3) subtype receptor: discovery of novel and potent D3 ligands through a hybrid pharmacophore and structure-based database searching approach. *Journal of Medicinal Chemistry*, **46**, 4377–4392.

70 Evers, A. and Klebe, G. (2004) Ligand-supported homology modeling of G-protein-coupled receptor sites: models sufficient for successful virtual screening. *Angewandte Chemie, International Edition*, **43**, 248–251.

71 Evers, A. and Klebe, G. (2004) Successful virtual screening for a submicromolar antagonist of the neurokinin-1 receptor based on a ligand-supported homology model. *Journal of Medicinal Chemistry*, **47**, 5381–5392.

72 Evers, A. and Klabunde, T. (2005) Structure-based drug discovery using GPCR homology modeling: successful virtual screening for antagonists of the Alpha1A adrenergic receptor. *Journal of Medicinal Chemistry*, **48**, 1088–1097.

73 Evers, A., Gohlke, H., and Klebe, G. (2003) Ligand-supported homology modelling of protein binding-sites using knowledge-based potentials. *Journal of Molecular Biology*, **334**, 327–345.

74 Palczewski, K., Kumasaka, T., Hori, T., Behnke, C.A., Motoshima, H., Fox, B.A., Trong, I.L., Teller, D.C., Okada, T., Stenkamp, R.E., Yamamoto, M., and Miyano, M. (2000) Crystal structure of

rhodopsin: a G protein-coupled receptor. *Science*, **289**, 739–745.

75 Triballeau, N., Acher, F., Brabet, I., Pin, J.-P., and Bertrand, H.-O. (2005) Virtual screening workflow development guided by the "receiver operating characteristic" curve approach. Application to high-throughput docking on metabotropic glutamate receptor subtype 4. *Journal of Medicinal Chemistry*, **48**, 2534–2547.

76 Venkatachalam, C.M., Jiang, X., Oldfield, T., and Waldman, M. (2003) LigandFit: a novel method for shape-directed rapid docking of ligands to protein active sites. *Journal of Molecular Graphics & Modelling*, **21**, 289–307.

77 Kellenberger, E., Springael, J.-Y., Parmentier, M., Hachet-Haas, M., Galzi, J.-L., and Rognan, D. (2007) Identification of nonpeptide CCR5 receptor agonists by structure-based virtual screening. *Journal of Medicinal Chemistry*, **50**, 1294–1303.

78 Jain, A.N. (2003) Surflex: fully automatic flexible molecular docking using a molecular similarity-based search engine. *Journal of Medicinal Chemistry*, **46**, 499–511.

79 Engel, S., Skoumbourdis, A.P., Childress, J., Neumann, S., Deschamps, J.R., Thomas, C.J., Colson, A.-O., Costanzi, S., and Gershengorn, M.C. (2008) A virtual screen for diverse ligands: discovery of selective G protein-coupled receptor antagonists. *Journal of the American Chemical Society*, **130**, 5115–5123.

80 Kiss, R., Kiss, B., Könczöl, À., Szalai, F., Jelinek, I., László, V., Noszál, B., Falus, A., and Keresü, G.M. (2008) Discovery of novel human histamine H4 receptor ligands by large-scale structure-based virtual screening. *Journal of Medicinal Chemistry*, **51**, 3145–3153.

81 Kolb, P., Rosenbaum, D.M., Irwin, J.J., Fung, J.J., Kobilka, B.K., and Shoichet, B.K. (2009) Structure-based discovery of β2-adrenergic receptor ligands. *Proceedings of the National Academy of Sciences of the United States of America*, **106**, 6843–6848.

82 Rosenbaum, D.M., Cherezov, V., Hanson, M.A., Rasmussen, S.G.F., Thian, F.S., Kobilka, T.S., Choi, H.-J., Yao, X.-J., Weis, W.I., Stevens, R.C., and Kobilka, B.K. (2007) GPCR engineering yields high-resolution structural insights into β2-adrenergic receptor function. *Science*, **318**, 1266–1273.

83 Cherezov, V., Rosenbaum, D.M., Hanson, M.A., Rasmussen, S.G.F., Thian, F.S., Kobilka, T.S., Choi, H.-J., Kuhn, P., Weis, W.I., Kobilka, B.K., and Stevens, R.C. (2007) High-resolution crystal structure of an engineered human β2-adrenergic G protein-coupled receptor. *Science*, **318**, 1258–1265.

84 Sabio, M., Jones, K., and Topiol, S. (2008) Use of the X-ray structure of the β2-adrenergic receptor for drug discovery. Part 2: identification of active compounds. *Bioorganic & Medicinal Chemistry Letters*, **18**, 5391–5395.

85 de Graaf, C. and Rognan, D. (2008) Selective structure-based virtual screening for full and partial agonists of the β2 adrenergic receptor. *Journal of Medicinal Chemistry*, **51**, 4978–4985.

86 Evers, A., Hessler, G., Matter, H., and Klabunde, T. (2005) Virtual screening of biogenic amine–amine binding G-protein coupled receptors: comparative evaluation of protein- and ligand-based virtual screening protocols. *Journal of Medicinal Chemistry*, **48**, 5448–5465.

87 Brenk, R., Naerum, L., Graedler, U., Gerber, H.-D., Garcia, G.A., Reuter, K., Stubbs, M.T., and Klebe, G. (2003) Virtual screening for submicromolar leads of tRNA-guanine transglycosylase based on a new unexpected binding mode detected by crystal structure analysis. *Journal of Medicinal Chemistry*, **46**, 1133–1143.

88 Brenk, R., Gerber, H.-D., Kittendorf, J.D., Garcia, G.A., Reuter, K., and Klebe, G. (2003) From hit to lead: *de novo* design based on virtual screening hits of inhibitors of tRNA-guanine transglycosylase, a putative target of shigellosis therapy. *Helvetica Chimica Acta*, **86**, 1435–1452.

89 Brenk, R., Meyer, E., Reuter, K., Stubbs, M.T., Garcia, G.A., Diederich, F., and Klebe, G. (2004) Crystallographic study of inhibitors of tRNA-guanine

transglycosylase suggests a new structure-based pharmacophore for virtual screening. *Journal of Molecular Biology*, **338**, 55–75.

90 Barreiro, G., Kim, J.T., Guimarães, C.R.W., Bailey, C.M., Domaoal, R.A., Wang, L., Anderson, K.S., and Jorgensen, W.L. (2007) From docking false-positive to active anti-HIV agent. *Journal of Medicinal Chemistry*, **50**, 5324–5329.

91 Nicola, G., Smith, C.A., Lucumi, E., Kuo, M.R., Karagyozov, K., Fidock, D.A., Sacchettini, J.C., and Abagyan, R. (2007) Discovery of novel inhibitors targeting enoyl-acyl-carrier protein reductase in *Plasmodium falciparum* by structure-based virtual screening. *Biochemical and Biophysical Research Communications*, **358**, 686–691.

92 Perez-Pineiro, R., Burgos, A., Jones, D.C., Andrew, L.C., Rodriguez, H., Suarez, M., Fairlamb, A.H., and Wishart, D.S. (2009) Development of a novel virtual screening cascade protocol to identify potential trypanothione reductase inhibitors. *Journal of Medicinal Chemistry*, **52**, 1670–1680.

93 Morris, G.M., Goodsell, D.S., Halliday, R.S., Huey, R., Hart, W.E., Belew, R.K., and Olson, A.J. (1998) Automated docking using a Lamarckian genetic algorithm and an empirical binding free energy function. *Journal of Computational Chemistry*, **19**, 1639–1662.

94 Miguet, L., Tervosen, A., Gerards, T., Pasha, F.A., Luxen, A., Disteche-Nguyen, M., and Thomas, A. (2009) Discovery of new inhibitors of resistant *streptococcus pneumoniae* penicillin binding protein (PBP) 2x by structure-based virtual screening. *Journal of Medicinal Chemistry*, **52**, 5926–5936.

95 Dixon, S.L., Smondyrev, A.M., and Rao, S.N. (2006) PHASE: a novel approach to pharmacophore modeling and 3D database searching. *Chemical Biology and Drug Design*, **67**, 370–372.

96 Grüneberg, S., Stubbs, M.T., and Klebe, G. (2002) Successful virtual screening for novel inhibitors of human carbonic anhydrase: strategy and experimental confirmation. *Journal of Medicinal Chemistry*, **45**, 3588–3602.

97 Grüneberg, S., Wendt, B., and Klebe, G. (2001) Subnanomolar inhibitors from computer screening: a model study using human carbonic anhydrase II. *Angewandte Chemie, International Edition*, **40**, 389–393.

98 Perola, E., Xu, K., Kollmeyer, T.M., Kaufmann, S.H., Prendergast, F.G., and Pang, Y.-P. (2000) Successful virtual screening of a chemical database for farnesyltransferase inhibitor leads. *Journal of Medicinal Chemistry*, **43**, 401–408.

99 Enyedy, I.J., Ling, Y., Nacro, K., Tomita, Y., Wu, X., Cao, Y., Guo, R., Li, B., Zhu, X., Huang, Y., Long, Y., Roller, P., Yang, D., and Wang, S. (2001) Discovery of small-molecule inhibitors of Bcl-2 through structure-based computer screening. *Journal of Medicinal Chemistry*, **44**, 4313–4324.

100 Mozziconacci, J.-C., Arnoult, E., Pernard, P., Do, Q.T., Marot, C., and Morin-Allory, L. (2005) Optimization and validation of a docking-scoring protocol: application to virtual screening of COX-2 inhibitors. *Journal of Medicinal Chemistry*, **48**, 1055–1068.

101 Krämer, O., Hazemann, I., Podjarny, A.D., and Klebe, G. (2004) Virtual screening for inhibitors of human aldose reductase. *Proteins*, **55**, 814–823.

102 McNally, V.A., Gbaj, A., Douglas, K.T., Stratford, I.J., Jaffar, M., Freeman, S., and Bryce, R.A. (2003) Identification of a novel class of inhibitor of human and *Escherischia coli* thymidine phosphorylase by *in silico* screening. *Bioorganic & Medicinal Chemistry Letters*, **13**, 3705–3709.

103 Kenyon, V., Chorny, I., Carvajal, W.J., Holman, T.R., and Jacobson, M.P. (2006) Novel human lipoxygenase inhibitors discovered using virtual screening with homology models. *Journal of Medicinal Chemistry*, **49**, 1356–1363.

104 Ruiz, F.M., Gil-Redondo, R., Morreale, A., Ortiz, A.R., Fábrega, C., and Bravo, J. (2008) Structure-based discovery of novel non-nucleosidic DNA alkyltransferase inhibitors: virtual screening and *in vitro* and *in vivo* activities. *Journal of Chemical Information and Modeling*, **48**, 844–854.

105 Perez, C. and Ortiz, A.R. (2001) Evaluation of docking functions for protein–ligand docking. *Journal of Medicinal Chemistry*, **44**, 3768–3785.

106 Antel, J. (1999) Integration of combinatorial chemistry and structure-based drug design. *Current Opinion in Drug Discovery & Development*, **2**, 224–233.

107 Salemme, F.R., Spurlino, J., and Bone, R. (1997) Serendipity meets precision: the integration of structure-based drug design and combinatorial chemistry for efficient drug discovery. *Structure (London, England: 1993)*, **5**, 319–324.

108 Illig, C., Eisennagel, S., Bone, R., Radzicka, A., Murphy, L., Randle, T., Spurlino, J., Jaeger, E., and Salemme, F.R. (1998) Expanding the envelope of structure-based drug design using chemical libraries: application to small-molecule inhibitors of thrombin. *Medicinal Chemistry Research*, **8**, 244–260.

109 Brady, S.F., Stauffer, K.J., Lumma, W.C., Smith, G.M., Ramjit, H.G., Lewis, S.D., Lucas, B.J., Gardell, S.J., Lyle, E.A., Appleby, S.D., Cook, J.J., Holahan, M.A., Stranieri, M.T., Lynch, Y.J., Lin, J.H., Chen, I.W., Vastag, K., Naylor-Olsen, A.M., and Vacca, J.P. (1998) Discovery and development of the novel potent orally active thrombin inhibitor *N*-(9-hydroxy-9-fluorenecarboxy)-prolyl *trans*-4-aminocyclohexylmethyl amide (L-372,460): coapplication of structure-based design and rapid multiple analog synthesis on solid support. *Journal of Medicinal Chemistry*, **41**, 401–406.

110 Böhm, H.-J. (1997) Combinatorial docking, in *Computer-Assisted Lead Finding and Optimization: Current Tools for Medicinal Chemistry* (eds H. Van de Waterbeemd, B. Testa, and G. Folkers), Wiley-VCH Verlag GmbH, Weinheim, pp. 125–133.

111 Böhm, H.-J. (1992) The computer program LUDI: a new method for the *de novo* design of enzyme inhibitors. *Journal of Computer-Aided Molecular Design*, **6**, 61–78.

112 Böhm, H.-J., Banner, D.W., and Weber, L. (1999) Combinatorial docking and combinatorial chemistry: design of potent non-peptide thrombin inhibitors. *Journal of Computer-Aided Molecular Design*, **13**, 51–56.

113 Murray, C.W., Clark, D.E., Auton, T.R., Firth, M.A., Li, J., Sykes, R.A., Waszkowycz, B., Westhead, D.R., and Young, S.C. (1997) PRO_SELECT: combining structure-based drug design and combinatorial chemistry for rapid lead discovery. 1. Technology. *Journal of Computer-Aided Molecular Design*, **11**, 193–207.

114 McMartin, C. and Bohacek, R.S. (1997) QXP: powerful, rapid computer algorithms for structure-based drug design. *Journal of Computer-Aided Molecular Design*, **11**, 333–344.

115 Jones, G., Willett, P., Glen, R.C., Leach, A.R., and Taylor, R. (1999) Further development of a genetic algorithm for ligand docking and its application to screening combinatorial libraries. *ACS Symposium Series*, **19**, 271–291.

116 Sun, Y., Ewing, T.J.A., Skillman, A.G., and Kuntz, I.D. (1998) CombiDOCK: structure-based combinatorial docking and library design. *Journal of Computer-Aided Molecular Design*, **12**, 597–604.

117 Makino, S., Ewing, T.J.A., and Kuntz, I.D. (1999) DREAM++: flexible docking program for virtual combinatorial libraries. *Journal of Computer-Aided Molecular Design*, **13**, 513–532.

118 Aronov, A.M., Munagala, N.R., Ortiz de Montellano, P.R., Kuntz, I.D., and Wang, C.C. (2000) Rational design of selective submicromolar inhibitors of *Tritrichomonas foetus* hypoxanthine-guanine-xanthine phosphoribosyltransferase. *Biochemistry*, **39**, 4684–4691.

119 Bi, X., Haque, T.S., Zhou, J., Skillman, A.G., Lin, B., Lee, C.E., Kuntz, I.D., Ellman, J.A., and Lynch, G. (2000) Novel cathepsin D inhibitors block the formation of hyperphosphorylated tau fragments in hippocampus. *Journal of Neurochemistry*, **74**, 1469–1477.

120 Haque, T.S., Skillman, A.G., Lee, C.E., Habashita, H., Gluzman, I.Y., Ewing, T.J.A., Goldberg, D.E., Kuntz, I.D., and Ellman, J.A. (1999) Potent, low-molecular-weight non-peptide inhibitors of malarial aspartyl protease plasmepsin

II. *Journal of Medicinal Chemistry*, **42**, 1428–1440.

121 Wyss, P.C., Gerber, P., Hartman, P.G., Hubschwerlen, C., Locher, H., Marty, H.-P., and Stahl, M. (2003) Novel dihydrofolate reductase inhibitors. Structure-based versus diversity-based library design and high-throughput synthesis and screening. *Journal of Medicinal Chemistry*, **46**, 2304–2312.

122 Liebeschuetz, J.W., Jones, S.D., Morgan, P.J., Murray, C.W., Rimmer, A.D., Roscoe, J.M.E., Waszkowycz, B., Welsh, P.M., Wylie, W.A., Young, S.C., Martin, H., Mahler, J., Brady, L., and Wilkinson, K. (2002) PROSELECT: combining structure-based drug design and array-based chemistry for rapid lead discovery. 2. The development of a series of highly potent and selective factor Xa inhibitors. *Journal of Medicinal Chemistry*, **45**, 1221–1232.

123 Baxter, C.A., Murray, C.W., Waszkowycz, B., Li, J., Sykes, R.A., Bone, R.G.A., Perkins, T.D.J., and Wylie, W. (2000) New approach to molecular docking and its application to virtual screening of chemical databases. *Journal of Chemical Information and Computer Sciences*, **40**, 254–262.

124 Willett, P. (2006) Similarity-based virtual screening using 2D fingerprints. *Drug Discovery Today*, **11**, 1046–1053.

125 Schneider, G., Neidhart, W., Giller, T., and Schmidt, G. (1999) "Scaffold-hopping" by topological pharmacophore search: a contribution to virtual screening. *Angewandte Chemie, International Edition*, **111**, 3068–3070.

126 Pirard, B., Brendel, J., and Peukert, S. (2005) The discovery of Kv1.5 blockers as a case study for the application of virtual screening approaches. *Journal of Chemical Information and Computer Sciences*, **45**, 477–485.

127 Carosati, E., Mannhold, R., Wahl, P., Hansen, J.B., Fremming, T., Zamora, I., Cianchetta, G., and Baroni, M. (2007) Virtual screening for novel openers of pancreatic K_{ATP} channels. *Journal of Medicinal Chemistry*, **50**, 2117–2126.

128 (a) Irwin, J.J. and Shoichet, B.K. (2005) ZINC: a free database of commercially available compounds for virtual screening. *Journal of Chemical Information and Modeling*, **45**, 177–182 (b) http://zinc.docking.org.

129 Cruciani, G., Meniconi, M., Carosati, E., Zamora, I., and Mannhold, R. (2003) VolSurf: a tool for drug ADME properties prediction, in *Drug Bioavailability. Estimation of Solubility, Permeability, Absorption and Bioavailability* (eds H. van de Waterbeemd, H. Lennernaes, and P. Artursson), Wiley-VCH Verlag GmbH, Weinheim.

130 Pastor, M., Cruciani, G., McLay, I., Pickett, S., and Clementi, S. (2000) GRid-INdependent descriptors (GRIND): a novel class of alignment-independent three-dimensional molecular descriptors. *Journal of Medicinal Chemistry*, **43**, 3233–3243.

131 Baroni, M., Cruciani, G., Sciabola, S., Perruccio, F., and Mason, J.S. (2007) A common reference framework for analyzing/comparing proteins and ligands: FLAP theory and application. *Journal of Chemical Information and Modeling*, **47**, 279–294.

132 Carosati, E., Cruciani, G., Chiarini, A., Budriesi, R., Ioan, P., Spisani, R., Spinelli, D., Cosimelli, B., Fusi, F., Frosini, M., Matucci, R., Gasparrini, F., Ciogli, A., Stephens, P.J., and Devlin, F.J. (2006) Calcium channel antagonists discovered by a multidisciplinary approach. *Journal of Medicinal Chemistry*, **49**, 5206–5216.

133 Naerum, L., Norskov-Lauritsen, L., and Olesen, P.H. (2002) Scaffold hopping and optimization towards libraries of glycogen synthase kinase-3 inhibitors. *Bioorganic & Medicinal Chemistry Letters*, **12**, 1525–1528.

134 Chen, X., Wilson, L.J., Malaviya, R., Argentieri, R.L., and Yang, S.-M. (2008) Virtual screening to successfully identify novel Janus kinase 3 inhibitors: a sequential focused screening approach. *Journal of Medicinal Chemistry*, **51**, 7015–7019.

135 Markt, P., Petersen, R.K., Flindt, E.N., Kristiansen, K., Kirchmair, J., Spitzer, G., Distinto, S., Schuster, S., Wolber, G., Laggner, C., and Langer, T. (2008)

Discovery of novel PPAR ligands by a virtual screening approach based on pharmacophore modelling, 3D shape, and electrostatic similarity screening. *Journal of Medicinal Chemistry*, **51**, 6303–6317.

136 Greenidge, P.A., Carlsson, B., Bladh, L.G., and Gillner, M. (1998) Pharmacophores incorporating numerous excluded volumes defined by X-ray crystallographic structure in three-dimensional database searching: application to the thyroid hormone receptor. *Journal of Medicinal Chemistry*, **41**, 2503–2512.

137 Schneider, G. and Nettekoven, M. (2003) Ligand-based combinatorial design of selective purinergic receptor (A2A) antagonists using self-organizing maps. *Journal of Combinatorial Chemistry*, **5**, 233–237.

138 Cramer, R.D., Poss, M.A., Hermsmeier, M.A., Caulfield, T.J., Kowala, M.C., and Valentine, M.T. (1999) Prospective identification of biologically active structures by topomer shape similarity searching. *Journal of Medicinal Chemistry*, **42**, 3919–3933.

139 Cramer, R.D., Jilek, R.J., Guessregen, S., Clark, S.J., Wendt, B., and Clark, R.D. (2004) "Lead hopping": Validation of topomer similarity as a superior predictor of similar biological activities. *Journal of Medicinal Chemistry*, **47**, 6777–6791.

140 Guba, W., Neidhart, W., and Nettekoven, M. (2005) Novel and potent NPY5 receptor antagonists derived from virtual screening and iterative parallel chemistry design. *Bioorganic & Medicinal Chemistry Letters*, **15**, 1599–1603.

141 Clark, D.E., Higgs, C., Wren, S.P., Dyke, H.J., Wong, M., Norman, D., Lockey, P.M., and Roach, A.G. (2004) A virtual screening approach to finding novel and potent antagonists at the melanin-concentrating hormone 1 receptor. *Journal of Medicinal Chemistry*, **47**, 3962–3971.

142 Sheridan, R.P. and Kearsley, S.K. (2002) Why do we need so many chemical similarity search methods? *Drug Discovery Today*, **7**, 903–911.

143 Marriott, D.P., Dougall, I.G., Meghani, P., Liu, Y.J., and Flower, D.R. (1999) Lead generation using pharmacophore mapping and three-dimensional database searching: application to muscarinic M3 receptor antagonists. *Journal of Medicinal Chemistry*, **42**, 3210–3216.

144 Kiyama, R., Honma, T., Hayashi, K., Ogawa, M., Hara, M., Fujimoto, M., and Fujishita, T. (1995) Novel angiotensin II receptor antagonists. Design, synthesis, and *in vitro* evaluation of dibenzo[*a*, *d*] cycloheptene and dibenzo[*b*, *f*]oxepin derivatives. Searching for bioisosteres of biphenyltetrazole using a three-dimensional search technique. *Journal of Medicinal Chemistry*, **38**, 2728–2741.

145 Leysen, D. and Kelder, J. (1998) Ligands for the 5-HT2C receptor as potential antidepressants and anxiolytics. *Pharmacochemistry Library*, **29**, 49–61.

146 Flohr, S., Kurz, M., Kostenis, E., Brkovich, A., Fournier, A., and Klabunde, T. (2002) Identification of nonpeptidic urotensin II receptor antagonists by virtual screening based on a pharmacophore model derived from structure–activity relationships and nuclear magnetic resonance studies on urotensin II. *Journal of Medicinal Chemistry*, **45**, 1799–1805.

147 Bologa, C.G., Revankar, C.M., Young, S.M., Edwards, B.S., Arterburn, J.B., Hiselyov, A.S., Parker, M.A., Tkachenko, S.E., Savchuck, N.P., Sklar, L.A., Oprea, T.I., and Prossnitz, E.R. (2006) Virtual and biomolecular screening converge on a selective agonist for GPR30. *Nature Chemical Biology*, **2**, 207–212.

148 Wang, H., Duffy, R.A., Boykow, G.C., Chackalamannil, S., and Madison, V.S. (2008) Identification of novel cannabinoid CB1 receptor antagonists by using virtual screening with a pharmacophore model. *Journal of Medicinal Chemistry*, **51**, 2439–2446.

149 Wang, S., Milne, G.W.A., Yan, X., Posey, I., Nicklaus, M.C., Graham, L., and Rice, W.G. (1996) Discovery of novel, non-peptide HIV-1 protease inhibitors by pharmacophore searching. *Journal of Medicinal Chemistry*, **39**, 2047–2054.

150 Hong, H., Neamati, N., Wang, S., Nicklaus, M.C., Mazumder, A., Zhao, H.,

Burke, T.R., Pommier, Y., and Milne, G.W.A. (1997) Discovery of HIV-1 integrase inhibitors by pharmacophore searching. *Journal of Medicinal Chemistry*, **40**, 930–936.

151 Kaminski, J.J., Rane, D.F., Snow, M.E., Weber, L., Rothofsky, M.L., Anderson, S.D., Lin, S., and Stanley, L.L. (1997) Identification of novel farnesyl protein transferase inhibitors using three-dimensional database searching methods. *Journal of Medicinal Chemistry*, **40**, 4103–4112.

152 Singh, J., van Vlijmen, H., Liao, Y., Lee, W.-C., Cornebise, M., Harris, M., Shu, I., Gill, A., Cuervo, J.H., Abraham, W.M., and Adams, S.P. (2002) Identification of potent and novel a4b1 antagonists using *in silico* screening. *Journal of Medicinal Chemistry*, **45**, 2988–2993.

153 Shoda, M., Harada, T., Yano, K., Stahura, F.L., Himeno, T., Shiojiri, S., Kogami, Y., Kouji, H., and Bajorath, J. (2007) Virtual screening leads to the discovery of an effective antagonist of lymphocyte function-associated antigen-1. *ChemMedChem*, **2**, 515–521.

154 Xue, L., Godden, J.W., and Bajorath, J. (2003) Mini-fingerprints for virtual screening: design principles and generation of novel prototypes based on information theory. *SAR and QSAR in Environmental Research*, **14**, 27–40.

155 Tervo, A.J., Suuronen, T., Lyrylenko, S., Kuusisto, E., Kiviranta, P.H., Salminen, A., Leppänen, J., and Poso, A. (2006) Discovering inhibitors of human sirtuin type 2: novel structural scaffolds. *Journal of Medicinal Chemistry*, **49**, 7239–7241.

156 Franke, L., Schwarz, O., Müller-Kuhrt, L., Hoernig, C., Fischer, L., George, S., Tanrikulu, Y., Schneider, P., Werz, O., Steinhilber, D., and Schneider, G. (2007) Identification of natural-product-derived inhibitors of 5-lipoxygenase activity by ligand-based virtual screening. *Journal of Medicinal Chemistry*, **50**, 2640–2646.

157 Fan, H., Irwin, J.J., Webb, B.M., Klebe, G., Shoichet, B.K., and Sali, A. (2009) Molecular docking screens using comparative models of proteins. *Journal of Chemical Information and Modeling*, **49**, 2512–2527.

Part Four
Scenarios and Case Studies: Routes to Success

Virtual Screening. Edited by C. Sotriffer

ISBN: 978-3-527-32636-5

13
Scenarios and Case Studies: Examples for Ligand-Based Virtual Screening

Trevor Howe, Daniele Bemporad, and Gary Tresadern

13.1
Introduction

The popularity of ligand-based virtual screening has largely stemmed from a demand to make maximal informed use of the corporate collections of large pharma and chemical vendors [1–3]. The basic theoretical assumption underlying the methods is that some level of chemical similarity between an active molecule and a putative replacement molecule will confer biological activity in a similar way on a similar target. This gross assumption has many subtexts, but for practical purpose is simply broken down into two problems: (i) defining the molecule and (ii) defining the measure of similarity.

The description of the template query, the ligand against which similarity is measured in the virtual screen, is usually determined by the number of compounds one wishes to sample against. If an exhaustive similarity search against a large database (many hundreds of thousands of compounds) is envisaged, then a 2D method of description is often chosen. This is usually a variation on molecular fingerprint keys with a Tanimoto-like scoring system. Such a search might be executed against a large pharma corporate compound library to extract a limited number of similar compounds for alternative hit identification. For a more complex task, or a search using some form of pharmacophore to define biological activity, 3D descriptors can used. In such cases, the conformational problem applies and an understanding of a "bioactive conformation" is assumed. Unless unlimited CPU time is available, there are limitations to the size of the archive that can be explored. In a 3D search, there are two basic strategies: searching with a fixed conformation against a fixed set of archived conformations in translational space or allow a rotatable bond flexible fit of the archived structures against a fixed conformation or number of conformations of the query molecule.

The basic assumption that chemical similarity gives rise to equivalent biological responses is a very approximate concept. The descriptors are reductions of molecular complexity created to enable rapid assessment of chemical similarity, that these descriptors then continue to contain measures of biological activity by capturing the

Virtual Screening. Edited by C. Sotriffer

ISBN: 978-3-527-32636-5

chemical–biological space is an approximation. There is no precise definition in the descriptors of the components that confer *in vitro* biological response. This concept of descriptors associated with activity can be captured using Bayesian methods [4] where there is a concomitant statistical correlation of descriptors with biological response, but this is at the cost of an almost complete loss of understanding of the chemical space.

It is important to realize that in most ligand-based virtual screens there is no understanding of which components of the molecule constitute the major contributors to the pharmacodynamic response, the property most often under investigation. There is nothing in the encoding of the descriptors that would inherently address this. It is sometimes argued that within congeneric series noncovalent interactions can be treated as additive, but this is a misleading assumption [5] since interactions can be mutually reinforcing and/or destabilizing. Protein–ligand binding as seen in classical GPCR antagonists or transition-state binding in enzymes is a dynamic process of the freezing of motions in the protein and the ligand [6]. Such complex thermodynamic and entropy enthalpy compensation effects are simply not accounted for in similarity-based virtual screening approaches.

It is easy to see then that there are many approximations in the methods and even the choice of mathematical similarity calculation (though most practitioners have settled on Tanimoto) can give highly variable results on identical data sets. No one would pretend virtual screening gives exact and perfect results, but it can give starting points. At best, the output should be treated as a collective of data enriched in more than likely similar molecules. The mode of binding cannot be readily inferred from the output and the depth of the similarity should be manually judged.

13.2
1D Ligand-Based Virtual Screening

Reviews of ligand-based virtual screening that include 1D methods have been published recently [1, 7]. 1D ligand-based virtual screening (1DLBVS) considers bulk molecular properties, disregarding the 2D atomic connectivity or the 3D conformations. The most common descriptors used to compare molecules include molecular weight, polar surface area, number of rotatable bonds, number of H-bond donors/acceptors, and calculated log$P$ (octanol/water partition coefficient). Molecules are often compared by Euclidean distance in their descriptor space. Some descriptors are highly correlated, for example, molecular weight and log$P$. Therefore, the molecular property they describe, such as hydrophobicity, is overrepresented compared to the other properties. Principal component analysis (PCA) is a technique that eliminates descriptor correlation. The descriptors are projected onto a smaller number of perpendicular vectors (principal components, PC) that describe the value variability. The molecules are then compared in the PC space instead of that of the original descriptors.

The most widely used 1DLBVS is Lipinski's rule of five [8]. In this case, the virtual screening is used to identify molecules with physicochemical properties favorable for oral bioavailability: number of H-bond donors ≤ 5, number of H-bond acceptors ≤ 10, molecular weight ≤ 500, and calculated $\log P \leq 5$. Such filters are often used to define "druglike" compounds. Alternative 1DLBVS filters have been suggested for leadlike molecules, or compounds able to cross the blood–brain barrier [9], or compounds that are suitable for *in vitro* fragment screening [10].

In general 1DLBVS is unsuitable for focused design where the aim is to identify compounds that bind to specific molecular targets. In these cases, 2D and 3D methods are more appropriate.

13.3 2D Ligand-Based Virtual Screening

Principles and methods used in 2D ligand-based virtual screening (2DLBVS) have also been reviewed in detail [1–3, 7, 11, 12]. In 2DLBVS, a compound collection is compared to one or more reference compounds, or queries, by describing the molecules as lists of atoms and covalent bonds. Despite lacking the information on how the atoms are oriented in space, 2D methods have the advantage of being able to successfully retrieve analogues at very low computational cost. Published retrospective studies comparing 2D and 3D methods suggest that the 2D information is often sufficient to produce accurate results and can also identify novel scaffolds.

13.3.1 Examples from the Literature

Among recent works, Franke *et al.* [13] and Schwarz *et al.* [14] at AnalytiCon Discovery identified novel inhibitors of the 5-lipoxygenase (5-LO) pathway using 2DLBVS on their in-house compound collection. The queries constituted a list of 43 chemically diverse known inhibitors compiled from published data. Queries and in-house compounds were represented using the CATS descriptors and the MACCS keys. CATS descriptors are generated by considering each atom in a molecule as one of the 5 types (H-bond donor, D; H-bond acceptor, A; positively charged, P; negatively charged, N; or lipophilic node, L) and producing a histogram of the number of occurences of each of the 15 possible pairs of atom types as a function of the number of covalent bonds between the two atoms in the pair up to ten bonds. This is shown in Figure 13.1. The molecules are thus represented as 150-dimensional vectors containing the number of all possible two-point pharmacophores. The molecular similarity is quantified by the Euclidian distance in this 150-dimensional space. MACCS keys, explained in Figure 13.2, are an example of 2D molecular fingerprints. A fingerprint is a sequence of bits associated with structural features. A bit is set to 1 if the associated feature is present in the molecule or to 0 if absent. Each feature corresponds to a predefined molecular substructure listed in a dictionary. Therefore, the molecules are described as N-dimensional vectors indicating whether the N substructures listed in the MACCS dictionary are present or not. In this

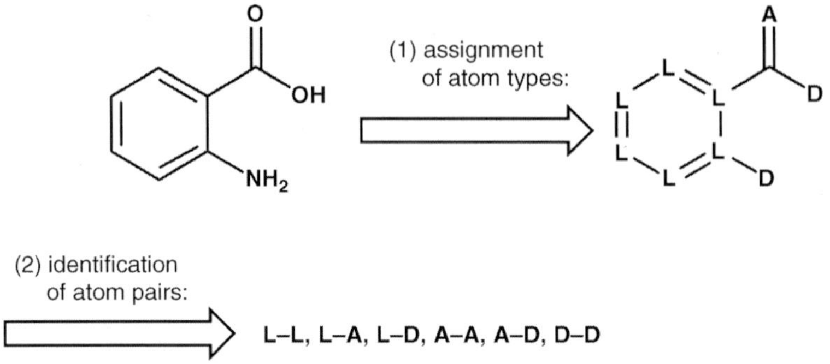

(3) count of occurrences as a function of bond distance:

pair	1 bond	2 bonds	3 bonds	4 bonds	5 bonds	6 bonds	7 bonds	8 bonds	9 bonds	10 bonds
L-L	6	6	6	6	6	0	0	0	0	0
L-A	0	1	2	2	1	0	0	0	0	0
L-D	1	3	4	3	1	0	0	0	0	0
A-A	0	0	0	0	0	0	0	0	0	0
A-D	0	1	0	1	0	0	0	0	0	0
D-D	0	0	0	1	0	0	0	0	0	0

Figure 13.1 Generation of CATS descriptors. See text for explanation.

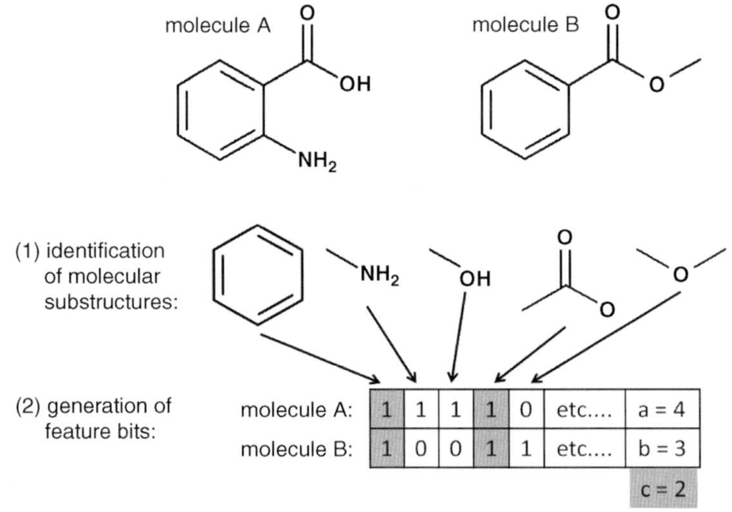

(3) Tanimoto similarity:

$$T = \frac{c}{a+b-c} = \frac{2}{4+3-2} = 0.4$$

Figure 13.2 MACS keys are 2D molecular fingerprints, that is, sequences of bits whose value is 1 if the molecular substructure they represent is present in the molecule or 0 if the substructure is absent. Eventually, the similarity between two molecules is quantified with the Tanimoto coefficient *T*, based on the number of substructures in common *c*.

case, the similarity between any two molecules is calculated with the Tanimoto coefficient *T*:

$$T = \frac{c}{a + b - c},$$

where a is the number of MACCS substructures present in molecule A, b is the number of substructures present in molecule B, and c is the number of substructures present in both molecules. The Tanimoto coefficient is 1 if two molecules are identical and share all substructures, 0 if the two molecules are completely different and have no substructure in common.

From the compounds with the highest similarity to the 43 queries, 18 were screened in cellular and cell-free assays for inhibition of the synthesis of 5-LO products. Two were found to be sufficiently active. These two hits were in turn used as queries for a second round of virtual screening on the same in-house compound collection. None of the further 55 analogues screened showed higher potency, but nevertheless the 2 original hits represented novel chemotypes of inhibitors of the 5-LO pathway.

2DLBVS was also used by Noeske *et al.* [15] at Merz Pharmaceuticals to successfully identify a new negative allosteric modulator (NAM) of the metabotropic glutamate receptor 1 (mGluR1). They used the CATS descriptors to cluster in-house and publicly available compounds with known pharmacological activity and identified two clusters with high density of mGluR1 NAMs. They selected 28 diverse compounds belonging to those 2 clusters and had no data on mGluR1. One of them was found particularly active in binding and functional assays. Subsequently, they docked this compound into a homology model of mGluR1, derived a 3D binding mode able to explain the observed activity, and used it to guide the synthesis of analogues. This was an example of optimal use of virtual screening techniques: first a fast 2D method is applied on a large data set and then a more computationally expensive 3D method is used on a smaller set of focused compounds.

An identical approach was used by Branca *et al.* [16] at Merck and led to the identifcation of a novel inhibitor of poly(ADP-ribose) polymerase-1 (PARP1). The 2D descriptors were similar to the CATS: all the two-point pharmacophores in each molecule were derived from all possible atom pairs and described in terms of atom types, number of π electrons, number of heavy atoms attached, and number of covalent bonds separating the two atoms along the shortest path. Known PARP1 inhibitors were collected from patents, publications, and publicly available databases and used to train a support vector machine (SVM) classifier. A SVM constructs the plane that best separates active and inactive compounds in the multidimensional space defined by the molecular descriptors. The results of the SVM were used to classify the compounds in the Merck collection and those predicted to be active were screened. One compound was particularly potent and was chosen as the starting point for a structure–activity relationship (SAR) exploration of this chemical class. Docking studies on the PARP1 crystal structure were used to guide the synthetic efforts.

13.3.2
Applications at J&JPRD Europe

At Johnson & Johnson Pharmaceutical Research and Development (J&JPRD) in Europe 2DLBVS is routinely applied in conjunction with *in vitro*high-throughput screening (HTS). Some of the common scenarios are as follows:

1) **Preparation of a focused compound library**: The collection of chemically diverse compounds normally tested in an HTS (a few hundred thousands) can be replaced or complemented with analogues of known ligands, if these are known in-house or are available from public sources. The analogues are identified in the corporate collection by using the known ligands as queries in 2DLBVS.
2) **Analogue search**: After a first round of screening at single concentration, the primary HTS hits are used as queries in 2DLBVS to extract their analogues from the rest of the in-house collection that was not submitted to the HTS. The primary hits and their analogues are then tested at various doses in a second screening round to generate EC_{50} or IC_{50} values. This approach helps both to retrieve additional hits and to derive a preliminary SAR of the active chemical series before one or some of them are chosen as starting points for hit-to-lead chemistry efforts.
3) **Outlier detection**: 2DLBVS is also used to identify close analogues of the hits among the compounds that were not active in the primary single-dose *in vitro* screening. Following the 2DLBVS assumption that chemically similar molecules are likely to exhibit similar biological activity, it is possible that close analogues of hits that appear inactive may be false negatives due to experimental errors. Once identified, they can be rescued by a repeat screen.

Virtual screening used in conjunction with HTS should yield a higher hit rate than the default HTS. The latter can be considered to comprise a random selection, for the most part, of drug-like compounds.

In all the above scenarios, the most common descriptors used at J&JPRD Europe for 2DLBVS are atom-type extended connectivity fingerprints (ECFP) and functional-class extended connectivity fingerprints (FCFP) computed in Pipeline Pilot [4, 17]. These, like all molecular fingerprints, are sequences of bits representing structural features: a bit is set to 1 if the feature it represents is present in the molecule or to 0 if that feature is absent. In constrast to MACCS keys, the structural features represented in ECFP and FCFP are not those in a predefined list, but rather they correspond to all the possible structural units that can be identified in the set of compounds under study. The advantage is the possibility to describe any set of molecules, not only those with predefined structural features. The structural units are extracted from the compounds as depicted in Figure 13.3, by taking each atom and all its neighbours up to a desired number of covalent bonds away. At iteration 0, the fingerprint contains information only about the atom itself, at iteration 1 it contains information about the atom and the atoms directly bonded to it, at iteration 2 it contains information about the atom, its first covalently bonded neighbours, and the atoms covalently bonded to the first neighbours, and so on until the desired number

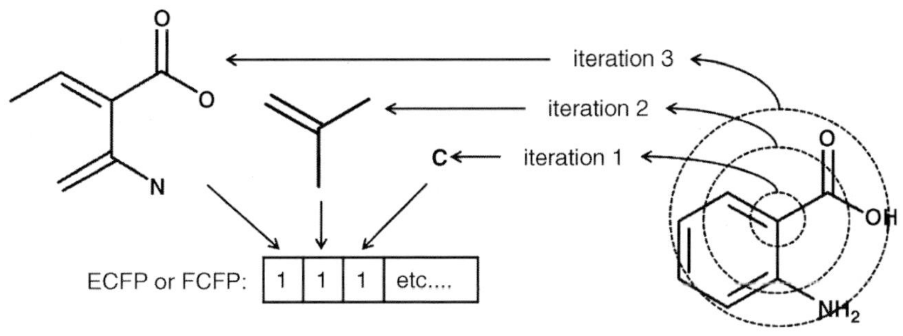

Figure 13.3 The molecular substructures for the FCFP and ECFP fingerprints in Pipeline Pilot are generated by extracting every atom and its neighbors up to a number of covalent bonds away in an iterative fashion.

of iterations is reached. Normally, this number is 2 or 3. In FCFP, the atoms are generalized to a limited list of types including H-bond donors and acceptors, positively and negatively charged atoms, halogens, and aromatic atoms. In ECFP, the types are generated considering the number of covalent bonds, the element, the charge, and the mass of each atom. The molecules are therefore described by vectors whose dimensionality equals the number of unique structural features extracted from the compound set.

In all of the three scenarios at J&JPRD Europe, there are two common methods for 2DLBVS. The first consists in calculating the fingerprint similarity between the queries and the compound set using the Tanimoto coefficient, that is, counting the number of structural features in common. The compounds with the highest similarity are ranked at the top.

The second method makes use of the Bayesian statistics implemented in Pipeline Pilot [4]. This identifies the fingerprints that best distinguish active from inactive molecules. The ratio of actives (A) and inactives (I) in the entire set, A/I, is compared with the ratio between the number of occurrences of the fingerprint in the actives (NA) and the number of occurrences in the inactives (NI), NA/NI. If NA/NI > A/I, the fingerprint is associated with active compounds more often than expected and therefore its presence is assumed to give a higher likelihood of activity. This is used to associate a probability of activity with each fingerprint, and the overall likelihood of a compound to be active is computed by summing all the probabilities. The Bayesian classifier is trained using both active and inactive reference compounds, which are the known ligands from the literature when building a focused library, or the results of the HTS primary screen in analogue search and outlier detection. The compounds from the corporate collection with the highest Bayesian probability to be active are ranked at the top.

The highest ranking compounds from Tanimoto and Bayesian methods are combined and submitted to biological screening. This type of data fusion is preferred to the consensus scoring, where the scores or ranks from the two methods are somehow summed to generate a new score or rank. When building a focused library, if 2DLBVS is to be used to entirely rerank the compounds for HTS, the total number of compounds for screening can be as large as 150 000. In analogue search and outlier detection, this number is always <10 000. In recent years the number of additional hits delivered by such 2DLBVS has been extremely variable: across the three scenarios, in some cases the hits were <1% of the screened compounds, 0.2% in the worst case, >50% in other cases, and 73.96% in the best case. There are several reasons for this high variability. The main reason is probably the different overlap between chemical and biological space: for some targets, the biological space has been more widely explored than for others in the company history and therefore 2DLBVS retrieves more hits for closely related targets. However, the compound collection for HTS is not always the same, it slowly changes with stock availability and with the replacement of the old compounds with those from the latest chemistry programs and newly bought chemical libraries. Some *in vitro* assays are less stable than others and therefore measured activities can vary in different batches. For some targets, there are many more known diverse ligands or primary hits than for other targets and this affects dramatically the list of compounds retrieved by 2DLBVS. Some public sources, especially patents, do not report activity explicitely and there are doubts if the query used in 2DLBVS is truly active. There are also limitations intrinsic to all 2DLBVS methods: the 3D structure of targets and ligands is not considered and the descriptors applied may not be appropriate for some systems. The methods described here have additional limitations. They do not take into account the extent of activity of the reference compounds and do not predict potency. When comparing compounds, all fingerprints are given equal importance; there is no accounting for which contribute most to the activity.

2DLBVS can also be used for the opposite purpose, that is, to identify compounds with undesired biological activities; such compounds are then removed from the screening collection. Another application is the estimation of activity on additional targets beside that of interest: this helps to prioritize compounds with the desired selectivity spectrum. For both applications, at J&JPRD Europe we use in-house data to build Bayesian classifiers of all screened targets, including those related to ADME-Tox, such as cytochrome inhibition, blood–brain barrier penetration and HERG binding. This type of 2DLBVS is also called at J&JPRD Europe virtual compound profiling. It is used both to assess the quality of the HTS hits and to prioritize synthetic chemistry efforts in later hit-to-lead or lead optimization phases.

13.4 3D Ligand-Based Virtual Screening

Three-dimensional ligand-based virtual screening (3DLBVS) approaches use molecular descriptors calculated from at least one 3D conformation of a query molecule. A similarity calculation is performed to rank an entire collection of commercial or in-house available molecules to the query and thereby identify the closest hits. Studying biological response with molecular shape descriptors can be traced back to work performed by Amoore *et al.* who in 1969 used silhouette photographs of molecular models as descriptors for scanning with a pattern recognition machine [18]. They identified correlation between shape and ant alarm pheromone activity. By 1980 the work of Carbo [19] and Hopfinger [20] had moved to more sophisticated computational representations of 3D structure. Methodological advancements mean such approaches can now be applied to databases of millions of compounds; however, the underlying theory is little changed and most of the methods discussed are now mature in development.

At first consideration, 3D molecular representation seems closer to the reality of the ligand–receptor binding process. Despite this it is known from published comparisons that 3D methods do not necessarily outperform 2D approaches in terms of retrieving actives [21–23]. There may be many explanations for this, including subtle deficiencies in the quality of the descriptors and noise associated with incomplete conformational sampling. Also, 3D coordinates may not offer additional information beyond that implicit in the 2D connectivity. Typical lead optimization programs deliver series of actives with similar covalent connectivity and therefore the data sets used in retrospective enrichment studies are biased toward this 2D view of chemical space. Nevertheless, characteristics such as shape, electrostatics, or pharmacophore features have been shown to perform better than 2DLBVS at scaffold hopping [24]. This is the process of identifying active molecules with alternative chemotype. Scaffold hopping can be a desirable outcome for many reasons such as intellectual property, ADME problems with a lead series, or simply the need to find a new scaffold once exploration of a first has been exhausted. Here, we do not review all approaches for 3DLBVS; instead, we focus on methods used in J&JPRD and selected applications from the literature and in-house.

The 3DLBVS methods we apply can be categorized in two ways: those using a single query to perform 3D shape and field searches, and those using hypothesis-derived pharmacophores using the 3D arrangement of identified important features. In the former case, the user decides on the conformation to use for the search query. Options include the lowest energy conformation, the bioactive conformation if known from X-ray crystallography, or a supposed bioactive conformation based on alignment with other actives. These choices are unlikely to have a large impact on the success of the VS [25]. The database being searched is often a prebuilt multiconformer compound collection. Consideration is paid to the parameters used to generate conformations such as the allowed energy window and the maximum number of conformations per molecule. When conformations for query and database are available the searches are performed and 3D similarity returned. In the case of pharmacophore methods, the approach is somewhat different [26]. A pharmacophore hypothesis is derived via the overlap of multiple active and inactive compounds that form the training set. The overlays facilitate the identification of shared pharmacophore features. Combinations of features yield alternative hypotheses that are submitted to statistical test on the training set. The best pharmacophore hypothesis is used as a query to search over a multiconformer compound collection. Hits with the same features are found and can be recommended for biological testing. The generated pharmacophore can often provide additional benefit and understanding to an ongoing medicinal chemistry program, helping to identify the crucial features for activity.

13.4.1
Methods

Rapid Overlay of Chemical Structure (ROCS) [27, 28] from OpenEye Scientific Software is based on superposition method that optimizes the overlap between molecules. In ROCS volume, overlap is calculated using Gaussian distributions to make the problem computationally tractable. ROCS aligns each conformation of the target molecule to each of the query and then keeps the alignment with the highest shape overlap. The ROCS shape Tanimoto similarity is given by the following equation:

$$\text{Shape Tanimoto} = \frac{V_{\mathrm{C}}}{V_{\mathrm{A}} + V_{\mathrm{B}} - V_{\mathrm{C}}}$$

where V_{C} is the volume in common between the two molecules, V_{A} is the total volume of the query molecule, and V_{B} is the total volume of the target molecule. The coefficient ranges from 0, no shape overlap, to 1, identical shape. In addition, a color force field is used to measure chemical complementarity and the 3D overlap is refined on the basis of the matching of simple pharmacophoric features, which include H-bond acceptor and donor, hydrophobes, anions, cations, and rings. The color force field determines the atom centers and functional groups that can be attributed to the pharmacophoric features. Interactions between features of the same time are always attractive, thereby favoring the process of overlaying similar features. The force field is parameterized for this purpose and includes terms to weight the strength and range of the interactions. The color force field and shape Tanimoto similarity can be combined to yield the so-called ROCS combo-score that is effectively the sum of the shape Tanimoto and color score.

In Topomers (dbtop) [29, 30] from Tripos query and data set, molecules are fragmented across all acyclic bonds, the open valence is capped, and one single 3D conformation of each fragment is generated with the CONCORD program. The fragments are first oriented according to the open valence bond and then the rest is oriented using a rule-based scheme. Spatially aligned fragments can then be compared on the basis of their 3D steric field generated in a similar way to CoMFA using an sp^3 carbon probe on a 2 Å lattice around the fragment. The absence of pharmacophoric features in 3D space yields a penalty to the similarity between two fragments. The features include aromatic, positive, negative, H-bond donor, and acceptor. The total Topomer similarity between two molecules is calculated in a geometric fashion as $(A^2 + B^2)^{1/2}$, where A and B denote the similarity between two constituent fragments. The Topomer approach benefits from being rule based and not requiring multiconformer databases. As such, it is extremely fast and can be applied to the very largest databases. At J&JPRD, it is used for screening our collection of ~10 million commercially available compounds.

Similarly to ROCS, the Cresset FieldScreen approach [31, 32] considers multiple 3D conformations. These are generated with a force field based on nonatom-centered extended electron distribution charges (XED). From the interaction energy with molecular probes, four 3D field properties are then calculated: steric, hydrophobic, positively, and negatively charged. All fields are simplified to their maxima and minima and stored for each conformer for the similarity calculation. The Cresset FieldScreen method combines a stepwise approach to database searching using increasingly sophisticated processes. In the first step, the most dissimilar compounds are discarded on the basis of a fast comparison of the 1D encoded field prints. The field prints are calculated from the distance matrix of field points for each conformer. The remaining top ranking ~50% of the database is then subjected to similarity assessment via 3D field points, the so-called clique refinement. In the last step, the top ranking ~20% from the clique refinement are reranked via an optimized alignment.

In EON [33], also from OpenEye Scientific Software, the Poisson–Boltzmann equation is solved to calculate the electrostatic potential on the nodes of a 3D grid constructed around a molecule. The molecule has MMFF94 nuclei-centered charges assigned. The OpenEye Electrostatic Tanimoto (OEET) similarity is given by

$$\text{Electrostatic Tanimoto} = \frac{A \times B}{A \times A + B \times B - A \times B}$$

where A is the electrostatic potential around the query molecule and B is the electrostatic potential around the target molecule. The coefficient ranges between $-1/3$, when the two molecules have equal but opposite potentials, and 1, when the two molecules have identical potentials. EON does not generate new alignments to maximize the electrostatic Tanimoto; it only scores the alignments generated from the ROCS shape overlap.

Pharmacophore methods have been developed and applied since the early 1990s and several programs, such as Unity (Tripos) [34] and Catalyst (Accelrys) [35], are still in use today albeit in updated versions [26, 36]. Pharmacophore searching first requires the identification of a plausible query hypothesis. Within the molecular operating environment (MOE, Chemical Computing Group) used in J&JPRD, this is handled via the Pharmacophore Elucidator tool. Multiple conformations of input molecules are generated and pharmacophore queries identified that provide good overlay of active molecules and separate actives from inactives. To ensure the process is computationally tractable, all two point pharmacophores of active molecules are generated. From these, subsequent three- and then four-point pharmacophores are identified yielding fewer yet more detailed hypotheses. Further manual modification is often applied using the MOE Pharmacophore Query Editor. Statistical performance of the pharmacophore can sometimes be improved with excluded or included volumes that are otherwise not identified via the automatic procedure. Additional modifications can be tested at this stage such as feature partial matching that is effectively specifying features as present but nonessential or combining features at the same point in space. In practice, this flexibility helps to differentiate pharmacophore searching from other 3DLBVS approaches. Also, pharmacophore approaches can overcome one of the drawbacks of shape-based VS methods. Shape-based VS actives with different shape are usually classified as false negatives; that is to say, they have a low ranking. With pharmacophores there is often no restriction on the overall shape or size of the hits.

13.4.2
3DLBVS Examples

13.4.2.1 CRF1 Antagonists

We recently described both retrospective and prospective applications of 3DLBVS methods to identify corticotropin releasing factor 1 (CRF1) antagonists [24]. This was part of a larger internal study we performed across multiple projects evaluating 2D and 3DLBVS methods. In the retrospective study, the ability of different methods to distinguish known actives from inactives was investigated. Subsequently, we applied a selection of the methods to recommend new compounds for screening and identify several novel CRF1 antagonists.

With a data set of 1261 active and ~175 000 inactive CRF1 antagonists, four different molecules were used as queries with various LBVS approaches and their ability to correctly identify the actives was examined. For three of the four query molecules, similar performance was observed. Figure 13.4 shows the enrichment plots for two of the search queries used. Query 02 is representative of the three queries that yielded similar performance for the different methods. In those cases, the OpenEye Shape Tanimoto (OEST) and OpenEye ComboScore (OECS) marginally outperformed Topomers. Together, these three methods were much better than other techniques including the more sophisticated electrostatic methods Cresset FieldScreen and OpenEye Electrostatic Tanimoto. It was shown that Alog *P* ranking of the data set could deliver up to approximately threefold enrichment compared to random at 1% of database retrieval (Table 13.1). Methods that favored shape above electrostatics performed well on this CRF1 data set. Using Query 01 with the same methods produced some differences in performance. In this case, the Fingerprints, ECFP6, performed relatively better, Topomers worse, while OEST and OECS methods still performed well. In brief, the query was smaller than the majority of the actives that

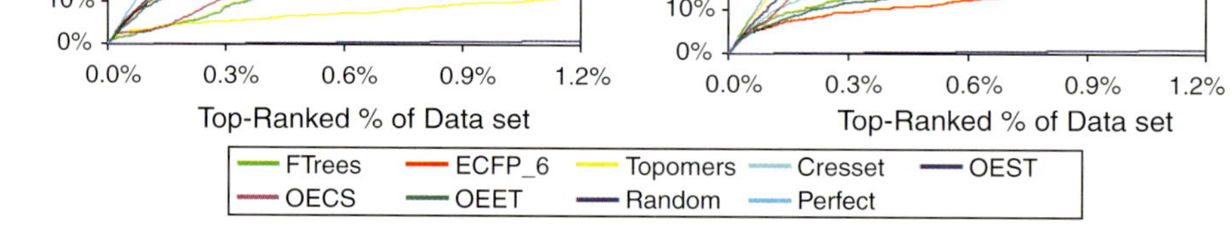

Figure 13.4 Enrichment plots showing the retrieval of actives versus % of database searched for each method with the four query molecules. The top ranked 1.2% of samples corresponded to ~2100 compounds. OEST refers to OpenEye Shape Tanimoto, OECS to OpenEye ComboScore, and OEET to OpenEye Electrostatic Tanimoto.

Table 13.1 Enrichment factors at 1% of database retrieval compared to random.

	Query molecule	
	01	02
ECFP6	33.9	14.4
FTrees	25.1	22.5
Topomers	10.2	46.3
OEST	40.1	51.9
OECS	41.2	55.2
OEET	32.8	20.7
Cresset	24.3	27.1
Alog *P*	2.6	1.9
MW	0.2	1.7
Surf area[a)]	1.0	2.5
PSA[a)]	1.5	1.2
Vol[a)]	0.3	1.9
Element counts	1.3	1.0

a) Descriptors calculated in Pipeline Pilot using a 2D method [17].
OEST refers to OpenEye Shape Tanimoto, OECS to OpenEye ComboScore, and OEET to OpenEye Electrostatic Tanimoto.

presented difficulties for some methods. Enrichment at 1% of database retrieval ranking by MW and Vol descriptors was worse than random, 0.2 and 0.3, respectively (Table 13.1). It was of interest to note that this was an example where 3DLBVS methods outperformed 2DLBVS. Finally, it was shown that within the top ranked 200 identified actives, the electrostatic methods Cresset FieldScreen and OEET retrieved more chemical scaffolds (Figure 13.5). These results along with further studies of the

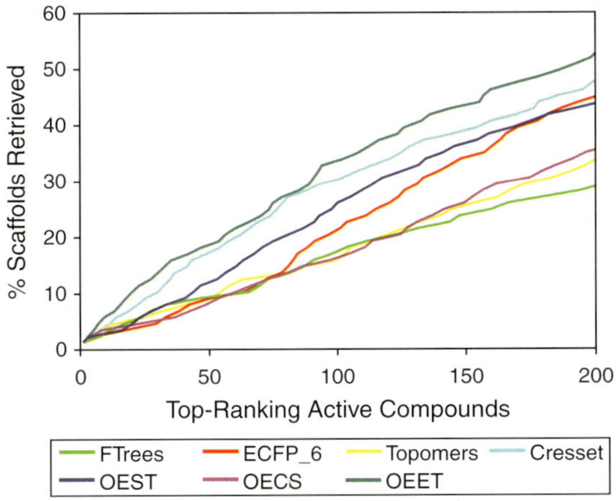

Figure 13.5 Plots of average retrieval rates of active scaffolds among only the top ranking 200 confirmed active hits for each query molecule with the different virtual screening methods.

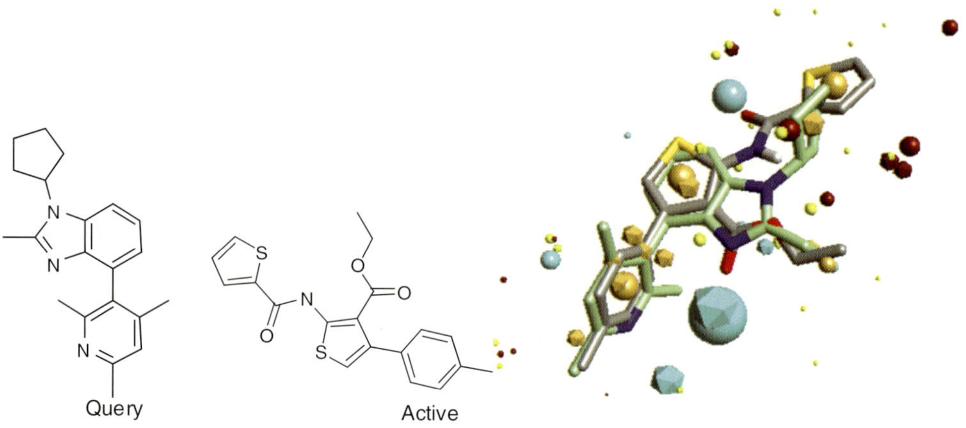

Figure 13.6 Query and active molecules from the prospective CRF1 VS work and Cresset FieldScreen overlay between query (green carbons) and active (gray carbons) molecules. Field points for query and active are shown as icosahedra and spheres, respectively. Negative field is blue, positive red, steric yellow, and hydrophobic orange.

2D fingerprint Tanimoto similarity of the hits confirmed that the field-based approaches were better at scaffold hopping and delivered more diverse hits.

For the prospective part of the same study, the OEST, OECS, Topomer, and Cresset FieldScreen methods were used to identify top ranking compounds for biological testing. We departed from a process of how we would normally apply such methods within a project in order to ensure a fair evaluation. First, there was no human intervention by members of the project team and second, we did not apply any data fusion or look for overlapping hits between the methods. From a total of 655 compounds recommended for screening, 10 molecules displayed greater than 20% inhibition at 10 μM concentration. This was actually a favorable hit rate compared to a later HTS. Overall Topomers ranked the actives highly but other methods were also successful at identifying new CRF1 antagonists. The structure of one active is shown in Figure 13.6. Of particular interest was the difference in 2D structure with the query. Also, the molecule was a departure from the conventional pharmacophore. The active was highly ranked by the Cresset FieldScreen method and the predicted overlay with the query is given in Figure 13.6. The new active replaces the scaffold acceptor by the carbonyl of the ester. The ester and amide groups pendant from the central thiophene have a restricted conformation due to interaction between amide NH and alkoxy oxygen of the ester. These groups and their intramolecular interaction replace the scaffold center present in the pharmacophore. Although the pendant aryl ring does not contain the usual *ortho* substitution, twisted conformations were nevertheless identified. The two molecules have similar size and good overall steric overlap. The distal thiophene group provides small hydrophobic and positive charge regions that match well with similar field points from the cyclopentane of the query. The relatively good overlap of the hydrophobic fields can be seen by the close location of the orange field points at the center of the cyclopentane and thiophene rings. An aromatic hydrogen of the thiophene ring and the NH of the amide in the same molecule together present a single positive charge field point (red sphere) that overlaps well with positive charge field points from the cyclopentane of the query. Overall, the active represented an interesting modification to known CRF1 compounds.

13.4.2.2 **Ion Channel Antagonism**

In a recent lead optimization program on an ion channel target at J&JPRD Europe, the main chemical series derived from an HTS hit displayed insurmountable ADME problems that could not be corrected while maintaining the activity. Therefore, it was decided to run a 3DLBVS to find a new and different hit among the in-house compounds that were not included in the initial HTS. A few hundred known chemically diverse binders of the target under study were retrieved from public sources. Their cross similarities were calculated with ROCS ComboScore and the similarity values were used as descriptors to cluster the known ligands into 18 clusters. The reason for using ROCS ComboScore to cluster the known ligands was because this descriptor was also used later for the virtual screening. The 18 cluster centers were representative of the range of shapes and pharmacophores among these compounds and were used as queries for the 3DLBVS. The entire J&J compound collection was used, after removing compounds already tested, no longer in stock or with undesired physicochemical properties, such as not satisfying the Lipinski's rule of five. For each compound, 18 scores were generated, one for each reference, but only the highest was retained. This type of data fusion was chosen because it was not important to distinguish to which specific query the compounds were most similar, compounds were likely to show activity as long as they were similar to any of the queries, assuming that the virtual screening assumption held. Of the 9162 compounds with the highest ROCS ComboScore screened *in vitro* at 10 μM, 248 showed an effect $> 50\%$ at this concentration and 9 had a $pIC_{50} > 5$. Among these, one was chosen as the starting point for chemistry efforts on a backup series.

13.4.2.3 **Metabotropic Glutamate Receptor**

We were recently targeting allosteric modulation of a member of the metabotropic glutamate receptor (mGluR) family with few known ligands. At the early stage, we had no in-house hits and only one reported reference compound. We applied different LBVS approaches that suited the different needs of the project at that time.

In the first instance, we wanted to find close analogues of the reported hit. Such compounds would probably not make ideal chemical starting points because they are too close to the intellectual property space of the reference compound. In this case, it was of value to understand the SAR of a new target and provide active compounds to help with assay validation. To perform these searches, we used 2D fingerprints complemented with substructure searches. The substructure search is still a valuable tool in this regard as it ensures all available compounds with the specific scaffold or chemotype are identified and screened. This satisfies the medicinal chemistry aim of mapping the SAR around chemotypes.

A second objective of the virtual screening was to identify hits with alternative chemotypes, scaffold hopping. Searches were performed with ROCS ComboScore

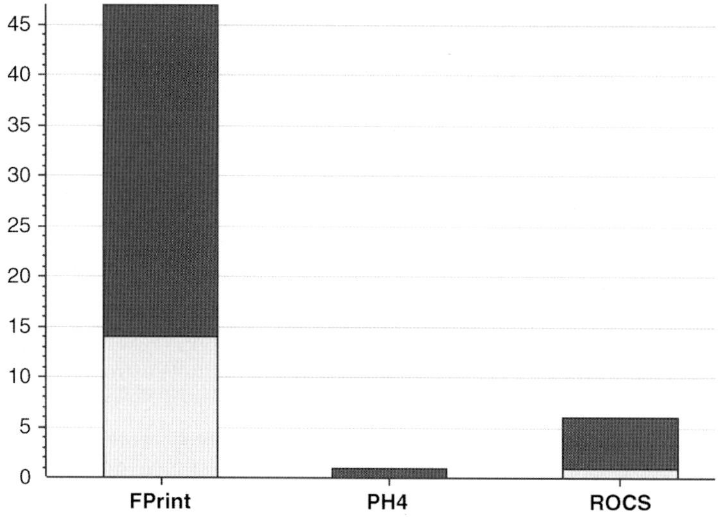

Figure 13.7 Histogram displaying how the actives ($pIC_{50} > 5$) identified via VS for mGluR ligands were split between the different methods. Yellow highlight represents actives with $pIC_{50} > 6$. PH4: pharmacophore; FPrint: 2D fingerprints; ROCS: ROCS ComboScore.

and a feature-based pharmacophore query. Although we did not have a training set to derive a rigorous pharmacophore, the features were manually edited to provide an alternative to the ComboScore approach. To specify that certain features must be matched is a powerful tool and, combined with an overall molecular volume filter, helps to limit the total number of returned hits.

We were restricted by the low throughput of the assay and only 179 compounds were recommended for screening from all methods. However, the results were very promising. In total, 54 compounds displayed a $pIC_{50} > 5$. The reference compound had a $pIC_{50} = 7.0$ and $E_{max} = 92\%$ in the same assay. Although none of the VS hits were more active, there were 15 compounds within one log unit of activity containing different chemotypes. Overall, the majority of actives came from the 2D fingerprints (see Figure 13.7), 47 of the total 54. This is not a surprise, as in most cases they were close analogues of the query and because fingerprint suggestions formed 45% of the original screening request. Potentially, one of the most interesting hits was from the ROCS search and had $pIC50 = 6.1$ and $E_{max} = 50\%$. The ROCS searches delivered fewer actives, 6 out of 54, despite forming 40% of the screened set. Finally, the pharmacophore search retrieved just one active but fewer compounds were requested for screening based on this approach, only 9% of the initial set.

13.5 Summary

In practice ligand-based virtual screening is contributing active molecules to pharmaceutical research projects. The brief results presented here show how different methods are applied according to the stage of development and needs of the project. We have shown how hit rates are often quite low, but it only takes one interesting hit identified at the right time to spark a new chemical exploration within a project. It is difficult to evaluate this impact.

It is now well understood and accepted that different LBVS methods capture different information of molecular structure. Many comparative studies highlight that alternative methods perform better on different data sets. In general, some approaches appear more consistent than others, but as Sheridan and Kearsley said in 2002, trying to identify the optimal method for searching databases is a "futile exercise" [37]. Instead, research is focusing on what may be the preferred combination to use or how the ranked hit lists should be combined, whether by data fusion [38], parallel selection of individual rankings [39], machine learning and weighting applied to data fusion [40], or application of Belief Theory to data fusion [41]. As this new avenue is being explored, we should be aware that in practice the application of LBVS methods strongly depends on the aim of a given project at a certain time and overly complex and parameterized fusion approaches may not be needed. Instead, a good understanding of the strengths and weaknesses and therefore the suitability of one approach may often suffice. Finally, we hope that investigations on fundamentals of electrostatic interactions may offer promise and improvement for future virtual screening methods [42].

References

1 Reddy, A., Pati, S., Kumar, P., Pradeep, H., and Sastry, G. (2007) Virtual screening in drug discovery: a computational perspective. *Current Protein and Peptide Science*, **8** (4), 329–351.

2 Good, A. (2006) Virtual screening. *Comprehensive Medicinal Chemistry II*, **4**, 459–494.

3 Hristozov, D., Oprea, T., and Gasteiger, J. (2007) Virtual screening applications: a study of ligand-based methods and different structure representations in four different scenarios. *Journal of Computer-Aided Molecular Design*, **21** (10–11), 617–640.

4 Hassan, M., Brown, R.D., Varma-O'Brien, S., and Rogers, D. (2006) Cheminformatics analysis and learning in a data pipelining environment. *Molecular Diversity*, **10** (3), 283–299.

5 Yogendra, P., Gillet, V., Howe, T., Pastor, J., Oyarzabal, J., and Willett, P. (2008) Assessment of additive/nonadditive effects in structure–activity relationships for iterative drug design. *Journal of Medicinal Chemistry*, **51** (23), 7552–7562.

6 Lee, G.M. and Craik, C.S. (2009) Trapping moving targets with small molecules. *Science*, **324**, 213–215.

7 Pozzan, A. (2006) Molecular descriptors and methods for ligand based virtual high throughput screening in drug discovery. *Current Pharmaceutical Design*, **12** (17), 2099–2110.

8 Lipinski, C.A., Lombardo, F., Dominy, B.W., and Feeney, P.J. (2001) Experimental and computational approaches to estimate solubility and permeability in drug discovery and development settings. *Advanced Drug Delivery Reviews*, **46** (1–3), 3–26.

9 Hou, T., Wang, J., Zhang, W., Wang, W., and Xu, X. (2006) Recent advances in computational prediction of drug absorption and permeability in drug discovery. *Current Medicinal Chemistry*, **13** (22), 2653–2667.

10 Miles, C., Robin, C., Chris, M., and Harren, J. (2003) A "rule of three" for

fragment-based lead discovery? *Drug discovery today*, **8** (19), 876–877.

11 Auer, J. and Bajorath, J. (2008) Molecular similarity concepts and search calculations. *Methods in Molecular Biology*, **453** (Bioinformatics, vol. 2), 327–347.

12 Douguet, D. (2008) Ligand-based approaches in virtual screening. *Current Computer-Aided Drug Design*, **4** (3), 180–190.

13 Franke, L., Schwarz, O., Mueller-Kuhrt, L., Hoernig, C., Fischer, L., George, S., Tanrikulu, Y., Schneider, P., Werz, O., Steinhilber, D., and Schneider, G. (2007) Identification of natural-product-derived inhibitors of 5-lipoxygenase activity by ligand-based virtual screening. *Journal of Medicinal Chemistry*, **50** (11), 2640–2646.

14 Schwarz, O., Jakupovic, S., Ambrosi, H.-D., Haustedt, L.O., Mang, C., and Mueller-Kuhrt, L. (2007) Natural products in parallel chemistry: novel 5-lipoxygenase inhibitors from BIOS-based libraries starting from alpha-santonin. *Journal of Combinatorial Chemistry*, **9** (6), 1104–1113.

15 Noeske, T., Trifanova, D., Kauss, V., Renner, S., Parsons, C., Schneider, G., and Weil, T. (2009) Synergism of virtual screening and medicinal chemistry: identification and optimization of allosteric antagonists of metabotropic glutamate receptor 1. *Bioorganic and Medicinal Chemistry*, **17** (15), 5708–5715.

16 Branca, D., Cerretani, M., Jones, P., Koch, U., Orvieto, F., Palumbi, M.C., Rowley, M., Toniatti, C., and Muraglia, E. (2009) Identification of aminoethyl pyrrolo dihydroisoquinolinones as novel poly (ADP-ribose) polymerase-1 inhibitors. *Bioorganic and Medicinal Chemistry Letters*, **19**, 4042–4045.

17 Stevenson, J.M. and Mulready, P.D. (2003) Pipeline Pilot 2.1, by SciTegic. *Journal of the American Chemical Society*, **125** (5), 1437–1438.

18 Amoore, J.E., Palmieri, G., Wanke, E., and Blum, M.S. (1969) Ant alarm pheromone activity: correlation with molecular shape by scanning computer. *Science*, **165**, 1266–1269.

19 Carbo, R., Leyda, L., and Arnau, M. (1980) An electron density measure of the similarity between two compounds. *International Journal of Quantum Chemistry*, **17**, 1185–1189.

20 Hopfinger, A.J. (1980) QSAR investigation of DHFR inhibition by Baker Triazines based upon molecular shape analysis. *Journal of the American Chemical Society*, **102**, 7196–7206.

21 Brown, R.D. and Martin, Y.C. (1996) Use of structure–activity data to compare structure-based clustering methods and desriptors for use in compound selection. *Journal of Chemical Information and Computer Sciences*, **36**, 572–584.

22 Matter, H. and Pötter, T. (1999) Comparing 3D pharmacophore triplets and 2D fingerprints for selecting diverse compound subsets. *Journal of Chemical Information and Modeling*, **39**, 1211–1225.

23 Schuffenhauer, A., Gillet, V.J., and Willett, P. (2000) Similarity searching in files of three-dimensional chemical structures: analysis of the BIOSTER database using two-dimensional fingerprints and molecular field descriptors. *Journal of Chemical Information and Computer Sciences*, **40**, 295–307.

24 Tresadern, G., Bemporad, D., and Howe, T. (2009) A Comparison of ligand based virtual screening methods and application to corticotropin releasing factor 1 receptor. *Journal of Molecular Graphics and Modelling*, **27**, 860–870.

25 Hawkins, P.C.D., Skillman, A.G., and Nicholls, A. (2007) Comparison of shape-matching and docking as virtual screening tools. *Journal of Medicinal Chemistry*, **50**, 74–82. And http://www.eyesopen.com/about/events/presentations/talks/2007/MedChem_USA_07.pdf.

26 Güner, O.F. (2002) History and evolution of the pharmacophore concept in computer-aided drug design. *Current Topics in Medicinal Chemistry*, **2**, 1321–1332.

27 Grant, J.A., Gallardo, M.A., and Pickup, B.T. (1996) A fast method of molecular shape comparison: a simple application of Gaussian description of molecular shape. *Journal of Computational Chemistry*, **17**, 1653–1666.

28 Rush, T.S., Grant, J.A., Mosyak, L., and Nicholls, A. (2005) A shape-based 3D scaffold hopping method and its

application to a bacterial protein–protein interaction. *Journal of Medicinal Chemistry*, **48**, 1489–1495.

29 Cramer, R.D., Jilek, R.J., and Andrews, K.M. (2002) dbtop: Topomer similarity searching of conventional structure databases. *Journal of Molecular Graphics and Modelling*, **20**, 447–462.

30 Jilek, R.J. and Cramer, R.D. (2004) Topomers: a validated protocol for their self-consistent generation. *Journal of Chemical Information and Computer Sciences*, **44**, 1221–1227.

31 Vinter, J.G. and Trollope, K.I. (1995) Multiconformational composite molecular-potential fields in the analysis of drug-action. 1. Methodology and first evaluation using 5-HT and histamine action as examples. *Journal of Computer-Aided Molecular Design*, **9**, 297–307.

32 Cheeseright, T., Mackey, M., Rose, S., and Vinter, A. (2006) Molecular field extrema as descriptors of biological activity: definition and validation. *Journal of Chemical Information and Modeling*, **46** (2), 665–676.

33 Nicholls, A., MacCuish, N.E., and MacCuish, J.D. (2004) Variable selection and model validation of 2D and 3D molecular descriptors. *Journal of Computer-Aided Molecular Design*, **18**, 451–474.

34 Hurst, T.J. (1994) Flexible 3D searching: the directed tweak technique. *Journal of Chemical Information and Computer Sciences*, **34**, 190–196.

35 Sprague, P.W. (1995) Automated chemical hypothesis generation and database searching with catalyst, in *De Novo Design* (ed K. Muller) ESCOM Science Publishers, Leiden, pp. 1–20.

36 Khedkar, F.S.A., Alpeshkumar, K.M., Countinho, E.C., and Srivastava, S. (2007) Pharmacophore modeling in drug discovery and development: an overview. *Medicinal Chemistry*, **3**, 187–197.

37 Sheridan, R.P. and Kearsley, S.K. (2002) Why do we need so many chemical similarity search methods? *Drug Discovery Today*, **7** (17), 903–911.

38 Willett, P. (2006) Enhancing the effectiveness of ligand-based virtual screening using data fusion. *QSAR and Combinatorial Science*, **25** (12), 1143–1152.

39 Tan, L., Geppert, H., Sisay, M.T., Gutschow, M., and Bajorath, J. (2008) Integrating structure and ligand-based virtual screening: comparison of individual, parallel, and fused molecular docking and similarity search calculations on multiple targets. *ChemMedChem*, **3**, 1566–1571.

40 Chen, J., Holliday, J., and Bradshaw, J. (2009) A machine learning approach to weighting schemes in the data fusion of similarity coefficients. *Journal of Chemical Information and Modeling*, **49** (2), 185–194.

41 Muchmore, S.W., Debe, D.A., Metz, J.T., Brown, S.P., Martin, Y.C., and Hajduk, P.J. (2008) Application of belief theory to similarity data fusion for use in analog searching and lead hopping. *Journal of Chemical Information and Modeling*, **48** (5), 941–948.

42 Truchon, J.-F., Nicholls, A., Roux, B., Iftimie, R.I., and Bayly, C.I. (2009) Integrated continuum dielectric approaches to treat molecular polarizability and the condensed phase: refractive index and implicit solvation. *Journal of Chemical Theory and Computation*, **5** (7), 1785–1802.

14
Virtual Screening on Homology Models

Róbert Kiss and György M. Keserű

14.1
Introduction

Setting up a structure-based virtual screen requires three basic steps. In addition to the optimization and selection of the docking and scoring protocol, it needs a preconditioned database of screening compounds and the three-dimensional structure of the target. Although the first two requirements could be fulfilled in virtually all discovery programs, the availability of an atomic resolution structure of the target would be a limiting factor. Virtual screening applications typically utilize structures obtained by experimental and theoretical methods. The present practice prefers X-ray structures to theoretical models; however, X-ray crystallography also has some limitations. Crystallization and X-ray crystallography of membrane proteins are very challenging tasks. The Protein Data Bank (PDB) consists of 551 coordinate sets for 202 unique membrane proteins including proteins of same type from different species (http://blanco.biomol.uci.edu/Membrane_Proteins_xtal.html (August 22, 2009)). Recent years have seen significant achievements in crystallization and structure determination of several pharmacologically important targets and antitargets. A couple of G-protein-coupled receptor (GPCR) structures have been published [1], the structure of amino acid transporters (e.g., [2]) and ion channels (e.g., [3]) have been revealed, mammalian cytochrome P450 structures have been investigated experimentally [4], and, more recently, the atomic resolution structure of the Pgp transporter became available [5]. Despite the exponential increase in the number of unique structures during the past 10 years, membrane protein structures represent only about 1% of the PDB. The overall quality of X-ray structures should also limit their applications in virtual screening. Davis *et al.* demonstrated [6] that high-resolution structures (<1.5 Å) are 95% based on observed data; however, structures with resolution lower than 2.5 Å are rather subjective. Very recently, Nielsen and coworkers also concluded that structural artifacts such as crystal contacts and water-mediated contacts in protein–ligand complexes influence the performance of scoring functions and consequently the outcome of virtual screening [7].

In the lack of X-ray structures, homology models are typically used for virtual screening. Homology models are obtained by comparative modeling using structural

Virtual Screening. Edited by C. Sotriffer

ISBN: 978-3-527-32636-5

information obtained for proteins sharing sequence homology with the target [8]. A recent review estimated that since 2000 almost 25% of structure-based virtual screening applications were performed against homology models [9]. Homology modeling has been extensively used for the structure prediction of important drug targets such as GPCRs, kinases, proteases, ion channels, and transporters. These models were subsequently used for structure-based virtual screening with variable performance. Table 14.1 shows a collection of homology model-based virtual screening applications including both retrospective and prospective studies. Entries reported in this table are identified by Scopus using the keywords "homology model" and "virtual screening."

14.2
Homology Models versus Crystal Structures: Comparative Evaluation of Screening Performance

The performance of homology models depends on multiple factors that were thoroughly analyzed comparing the results with those obtained using X-ray structures [10]. In most cases, the performance of virtual screening was measured calculating enrichment factors. Enrichment factors (EFs) assess the quality of the rankings:

$$\mathrm{EF}(\%) = \frac{\left(N_{\mathrm{active}(\%)}/N_{(\%)}\right)}{\left(N_{\mathrm{active}}/N_{\mathrm{all}}\right)}$$

where EF(%) is given at the top (%) percentage of the ranked database, $N_{\mathrm{active}(\%)}$ is the number of active compounds in a selected subset of the ranked database, $N_{(\%)}$ is the number of compounds in the subset, and N_{active} and N_{all} are the number of active molecules and the number of compounds in the screening database, respectively. Larger EF means better performance.

14.2.1
Soluble Proteins

One of the first studies was reported by Schafferhans and Klebe [45] identifying experimental binding modes for ligands by docking into homology models. These authors concluded that homology models constructed from templates sharing at least 40% of sequence identity with the target gave comparable binding modes compared to X-ray structures. This result fits well to previous findings suggesting that above 30% of sequence identity, comparative modeling correctly predicts the overall fold. Below this cutoff, the quality of homology models varies widely [46]. Comparative evaluation of X-ray structures and homology models in virtual screening situation was first reported by Grootenhuis and coworkers [47]. The authors built several homology models for CDK2 and factor VIIa, using templates with different sequence identity, and investigated the enrichment achieved on screening data sets. The CDK2 screening set consisted of approximately 17 000 compounds while they screened

Table 14.1 Successful structure-based virtual screening studies on homology models.

Target	Seq. id. (%)	Software		Screening data					Reference
		Protein modeling	Docking	Screening database	*A*	Hit rate (%)	EF(%)	Best compound	
mGluR5 negative allosteric modulator	26.7	NA	FlexX-Pharm	1951 NCI, diverse, druglike	159	—	23.5 (1)	—	[11]
c-ME malic enzyme inhibitor	92.6	NA	FlexX	10 000 fragment-based virtual library, diverse, druglike	6	60	—	$IC_{50} = 0.15\,\mu M$	[12]
11β-Hydroxy steroid dehydrogenase inhibitor	17.4	Whatif	Gold/Glide	114 000 natural products	15	13.3	—	$IC_{50} = 10\,\mu M$	[13]
Dopamine D3 antagonist	16.3	Sybyl Biopol. + Loop search	Dock	990 ACD, MW filtered, random	10	0	0 (15)	—	[14]
			FlexX			19	70 (15)		
			Gold			30	—		
Muscarinic M1 antagonist	16	Sybyl Biopol. + Loop search	Dock	990 ACD, MW filtered, random	10	5	—	—	[14]
			FlexX			10	50 (25)		
			Gold			5	—		

(*Continued*)

Table 14.1 (*Continued*)

Target	Seq. id. (%)	Software		Screening data					Reference
		Protein modeling	Docking	Screening database	*A*	Hit rate (%)	EF(%)	Best compound	
Vasopressin V1a antagonist	16.7	Sybyl Biopol. + Loop search	Dock	990 ACD, MW filtered, random	10	0	—	—	[14]
			FlexX			38	50 (15)		
			Gold			27	—		
Dopamine D3 agonist	16	Sybyl Biopol. + Loop search	Dock	990 ACD, MW filtered, random	10	25	70 (15)	—	[14]
			FlexX			32	60 (15)		
Adrenergic β2 agonist	17.1	Sybyl Biopol. + Loop search	Dock	990 ACD, MW filtered, random	10	7	50 (15)	—	[14]
			FlexX			27	70 (15)		
δ Opioid agonist	19.9	Sybyl Biopol. + Loop search	Dock	990 ACD, MW filtered, random	10	15	60 (20)	—	[14]
			FlexX			26	90 (20)		
Autotaxin ATX (NPP2) inhibitor	30	MOE	MOE	500 Chembridge H2L library, focused by similarity	19	20.1	—	91% inhib. at 10 μM	[15]
Histamine H4 modulator	13.7	Modeller	FlexX	5 million ZINC + selected vendors	16	6.3		$K_i = 85$ nM	[16]

Histone Arg-Me transferase PRMT1 inhibitor	47	MOE	Gold	6.232 Chembridge MW, TPSA, and pharmacophore filtered	9	44.4	16.7 (30)	$IC_{50} = 12.7\,\mu M$	[17]
Farnesyl pyropho-sphatase synthase inhibitor	63	Modeller	Gold	1009 diverse, druglike	14	—	60(1)	—	[18]
MCHR1 antagonist	19	Modeller ligand refined	ICM	5508 diverse, druglike	11	—	39(1)	$K_i = 7.5\,\mu M$	[19]
				187 084 from 37 vendors	6	4.6	11.8(1)		
Photoactivated rhodopsin–G-protein interaction inhibitor	—	—	Autodock	1990 NCI diverse	2	22.2	—	$EC_{50} = 45\,\mu M$	[20]
IKKβ kinase inhibitor	31	Modeller	FlexX Pharm	26 953 ChemDiv diverse	6	8	6.2(10)	$IC_{50} = 1.76\,\mu M$	[21]
Cdc25 phosphatase inhibitor	76.5	Modeller	Autodock	85 000 InterBioScreen diverse	16	8.8	—	$IC_{50} = 0.82\,\mu M$	[22]
Ribosomal S6 kinase (RSK2) inhibitor	27	Modeller ligand refined	Accelrys	837 NCI, volume and pharmacophore filtered	2	10.5	—	$IC_{50} = 1\,\mu M$	[23]
Chemokine receptor CXCR4 antagonist	20.7	Modeller	Autodock	4944 Maybridge diverse	248	—	4(1)	—	[24]
			Gold				7(1)		
			Fred				7(1)		
			Hex				5(1)		

(Continued)

Table 14.1 (*Continued*)

Target	Seq. id. (%)	Software		Screening data					Reference
		Protein modeling	Docking	Screening database	*A*	Hit rate (%)	EF(%)	Best compound	
Chemokine receptor CCR5 antagonist	19.7	Modeller	Autodock	5050 Maybridge diverse	354	—	12(1)	—	[24]
			Gold				7(1)		
			Fred				7(1)		
			Hex				4(1)		
Serotonin 5HT2c agonist	13	Modeller	FlexX	530 ChemDiv GPCR library, MW and pharmacophore filtered	5	12.8	—	$IC_{50} = 20.1$ nM	[25]
α-Glucosidase inhibitor	38.5	Modeller	Autodock	85 000 InterBioScreen, druglike	13	6.9	—	71.4 % inhib. at 50 μM	[26]
mGluR4 agonist	43.2	MD, ligand refined	Ligandfit	1069 multivendor, druglike	6	15.8	—	280-fold increase of IP formation at 100 μM	[27]
Neurokinin NK1 antagonist	21	Modeller MOBILE	FlexX Pharm	11 109 leadlike, pharmacophore filtered	1	14.3	—	$K_i = 251$ nM	[28]
Casein kinase 2 (CK2) inhibitor	72	Whatif	Dock	400 000 Novartis in-house	4	33.3	—	$IC_{50} = 80$ nM	[29]

SARS 3C-like proteinase inhibitor	32	Modeller + multicanonical MD	Dock	630 000 diverse NCI, ACD, MDDR	3	7.5	—	$IC_{50} = 61\,\mu M$	[30]
PDGFR β kinase inhibitor	55	Modeller	LibDock	32 161 diverse	161	—	6.9 (1)	—	[31]
VEGFR1 kinase inhibitor	77	Modeller	LibDock	32 046 diverse	46	—	7.5 (1)	—	[31]
Adenosine A1A antagonist	15.8	Modeller MOBILE	Gold	1000 diverse MDDR	50	60	12(1)	—	[32]
Serotonin 5HT2a antagonist	16.7	Modeller MOBILE	Gold	1000 diverse MDDR	50	60	12(1)	—	[32]
Dopamine D2 antagonist	17.7	Modeller MOBILE	Gold	1000 diverse MDDR	50	20	4(1)	—	[32]
Muscarinic M1 antagonist	16	Modeller MOBILE	Gold	1000 diverse MDDR	50	60	12(1)	—	[32]
Type 12 lipoxygenase inhibitor	61	PLOP	Glide	50 000 diverse, druglike	2	10	—	$IC_{50} = 12.3\,\mu M$	[33]
Type 15 lipoxygenase inhibitor	80	PLOP	Glide	50 000 diverse, druglike	3	15	—	$IC_{50} = 6.8\,\mu M$	[33]
Chemokine receptor CCR5 agonist	17.7	Modeller + MD refined	Glide	44 524 druglike multivendor, pharmacophore focused	10	16.9	60(5)	$IC_{50} = 17\,\mu M$, $EC_{50} = 3\,\mu M$	[34]
			Surflex				52(5)		

(Continued)

Table 14.1 (*Continued*)

Target	Seq. id. (%)	Software		Screening data					Reference
		Protein modeling	Docking	Screening database	*A*	Hit rate (%)	EF(%)	Best compound	
Falcipain 2 and 3 protease inhibitor	40	NA	Gold	60 000 druglike ChemBridge	12	14.3	—	FP2 $IC_{50} = 1\,\mu M$, FP3 $IC_{50} = 4.9\,\mu M$	[35]
Falcipain 2 protease inhibitor	40	NA	Gold	80 000 druglike ACD	18	18	—	$IC_{50} = 1.4\,\mu M$	[36]
Cannabinoid receptor CB2 agonist	18.5	Insight + Gromacs refined	Gold	10.340 druglike Maybridge, pharmacophore filtered	1	1.2	—	$pEC_{50} = 5.3$	[37]
CRFR1 antagonist	11	NA	Gold	1000 diverse	13	—	69(1)	—	[38]
Glucagon receptor antagonist	27.1	NA	Gold	144 000 diverse, druglike	6	24	—	—	[38]
Fatty acid receptor agonist	20.3	NA	Glide	70 477 diverse, druglike, pharmacophore filtered	1	10	—	$EC_{50} = 3.6\,\mu M$	[39]
Cannabinoid receptor CB2 agonist	18.5	Ligand refined MD	FlexX Pharm	1000 diverse, druglike NCI	33	—	11(10)	—	[40]

Dopamine D3 antagonist	16.3	MD + NOE restrains	Ligandfit	6727 pharmacophore focused NCI	11	55	—	$IC_{50} = 11$ nM	[41]
Adenosine A1A antagonist	15.8	Modeller MOBILE	Gold	22 950 Aventis in-house, MW and rot. bond filtered, pharmacophore focused	38	47.5	—	$K_i \leq 10$ μM	[42]
Jak2 kinase inhibitor	36	ProModII	Dock	6451 NCI	1	14.3	—	$IC_{50} \sim 1$ μM	[43]
Jak2 kinase inhibitor	62	Modeller	FlexX	223 481 NCI (from ZINC)	5	12.8	—	$IC_{50} = 60$ nM	[44]

Number of actives is given as A. Enrichment factors are calculated at the given percentage of the ranked database. Abbreviations: sequence identity (seq. id.), data not available (NA), molecular weight (MW), topological polar surface area (TPSA), number of actives confirmed experimentally (*A*). Hit rate (given in %) was defined as the ratio of *A* to the number of compounds tested experimentally.

Table 14.2 Effect of sequence identity on enrichments obtained by homology model based virtual screening.

Target protein	Enrichment factors					Reference
	Experimental		Homology models			
	At %	X-ray	At %	High identity (%)	Low identity (%)	
Factor VIIa	0.5	5.7	0.5	6.6 (77)	1.2 (37)	[47]
CDK2	0.6	4.5	0.6	3.1 (60)	3.5 (43)	[47]
EGFR	1.0	6.0	1.0	—	3.9 (31)	[31]
FGFR1	1.0	1.0	1.0	1.0 (38)	—	[31]
P38	1.0	11.5	1.0	1.5 (49)	—	[31]
SRC	1.0	5.3	1.0	10.8 (66)	—	[31]
DHFR	0.4	28	4.9	—	3 (34)	[48]
PNP	0.1	57	0.1	57 (50)	—	[48]
PARP	3.8	10	35.5	2 (87)	—	[48]
Thrombin	0.1	19	0.1	20 (85)	—	[48]
GART	0.1	159	9.4	—	4 (28)	[48]
SAHH	0.2	29	4.8	3 (61)	—	[48]
AR	2.6	9	3.3	4 (69)	—	[48]
AChE	0.5	28	0.3	—	4 (36)	[48]
TS	0.1	38	0.4	16 (66)	—	[48]

Sequence identities are in parentheses. Enrichment factors are calculated at (%) percentage of the ranked database. Enrichment factors obtained by holo structures were used from Ref. [48].

21 000 compounds against factor VIIa. All compounds were investigated experimentally and the enrichment of actives achieved by virtual screening was analyzed. Enrichments obtained with homology models of different quality were compared to that realized using the X-ray structure of the target. Their results showed that models generated at larger than 50% of sequence identity near the binding site yielded fivefold enrichment relative to random that was comparable to docking into crystal structures (Table 14.2). In the case of factor VIIa, the enrichment dropped significantly with decreasing sequence identity. On the other hand, CDK2 enrichments seem to be independent of the sequence identity that was rationalized by possible induced fit effects. Diller and Li investigated the performance of virtual screening against different protein kinases and compared the enrichment with that obtained by the corresponding crystal structure [31]. By docking a database of random decoys and known inhibitors into homology models, they found that except for FGFR1 actives were enriched 2.6–38.6-fold in the top 5% of the ranked compounds (Table 14.2). Using the crystal structure of apo-EGFR, results were comparable to those obtained by the homology model. For P38, the homology model performed significantly weaker than the X-ray structure. Since known P38 inhibitors used in this enrichment study are structurally similar to the cocrystallized SB203 580, selection of this crystal

structure might represent some bias for X-ray structure-based screening. In the case of SRC kinase, homology model outperformed the crystal structure. Since there are many factors influencing the performance of homology models [49], it is not obvious whether the success of homology models is always due to the correctly predicted binding site and binding mode. On the other hand, the closed binding site of the SRC structure used in this study might explain the moderate performance of the crystal structure. Virtual screening against FGFR1 was unsuccessful irrespective of the source of the target structure. The authors hypothesized that the small cocrystallized inhibitor resulted in a small-volume binding site unable to recognize the majority of FGFR1 inhibitors. The homology model was also too closed for accommodating actives. It should be noted, however, that enrichments achieved using homology models were significantly better than random in all other cases. On the basis of the overall performance of kinase homology models, it can be concluded that homology models are useful for identifying actives from large data sets in the absence of experimental structures.

McGovern and Shoichet performed a detailed comparative study using both apo and holo crystal structures and homology models of nine enzymes [48]. In general, they found that best results were obtained with the holo crystal structure (Table 14.2). For dihydrofolate reductase (DHFR), poly(ADP-ribose) polymerase (PARP), glycinamide ribonucleotide transformylase (GART), *S*-adenosylhomocysteine hydrolase (SAHH), aldose reductase (AR), acetylcholinesterase (AChE), and thymidylate synthase (TS) holo crystal structures outperformed homology models. On the other hand, in the case of purine nucleoside phosphorylase (PNP) and thrombin, homology models gave comparable enrichment to that obtained by the corresponding crystal structures. These cases were rationalized as exceptions when the holo structure is overspecialized and homology models may provide improved discrimination between true ligands and decoys. Considering the fact that homology models provided significantly better enrichments than random, this study also suggests the usefulness of homology models in virtual screening when no X-ray structure of the target is available. The authors noted that the moderate performance of homology models in a number of cases was due to small structural errors such as inappropriate side-chain conformations. This observation is in line with the findings of the Critical Assessment of Techniques for Protein Structure Prediction (CASP) challenge [50, 51] demonstrating that side-chain conformations are primarily responsible for incorrect protein–ligand contacts found in most of the homology models (see Section 14.3.3 for more details).

Gilson and coworkers built homology models for carboxypeptidase A, factor Xa [52], peroxisome proliferator-activated receptor PPARα, CDK2 kinase, and AChE [49] using multiple templates with varying sequence identity to the targets and used these models for virtual screening. In contrast to others, these authors used average ranks as the measure of screening performance. The average rank, as a percentage, is calculated as

$$\langle r \rangle = (100\%/(N_{\mathrm{bind}} \times N_{\mathrm{tot}})) \times \sum r_i$$

Table 14.3 Effect of sequence identity (given in parentheses) on the average ranks obtained by homology model-based virtual screening [49, 52].

Target protein	Average ranks		
	X-ray	High identity (%)	Low identity (%)
Carboxypeptidase A	9.8	17.3 (67)	12.9 [30]
Factor Xa	2.6	2.1 (44)	2.8 [34]
PPARα	11.7	9.5 (62)	10.4 [28]
CDK2	22.0	39.0 (48)	43.0 [27]
AChE	16.7	19.0 (53)	25.4 [30]

where r_i is the rank of ligand i and N_{bind} and N_{tot} are the number of known ligands and the number of known ligands and decoys, respectively. Note that lower average rank indicates better enrichment of actives. A random selection of compounds from the mixture of binders and decoys should yield an average rank of 50%.

They found that in the case of factor Xa, PPARα, and AChE, homology models performed comparable to X-ray structures. For carboxypeptidase A and CDK2, however, crystal structures outperformed the models (Table 14.3). Similar to the results of previous studies, these authors found poor correlation between the sequence identity and enrichments obtained. It was suggested that this effect might be due to multiple factors. First, they concluded that considering the rigid docking used in most virtual screening applications, the crystal structure is not optimal for all of the ligands. Consequently, the improved similarity to the crystal structure is not a guarantee for increased enrichment when screening with homology models. Second, the hard Lennard-Jones term used in scoring functions causes a large penalty for small changes in the binding site. Therefore, even if the overall sequence identity between the target and the templates is acceptable, minor differences in the binding site would result in very different ranking. The uncertainties of side-chain conformation in homology models might be partially overcome by using less strict scoring functions (e.g., ROTA [53]) during virtual screening. These are recommended especially for homology models generated by using rotamer libraries without subsequent energy minimization.

14.2.2
Membrane Proteins

Limited availability of crystal structures prevented such detailed, comparative analysis for homology models of membrane proteins. Nevertheless, the performance of GPCR homology models was investigated in virtual screening situations. Until recently, the only high-resolution GPCR structure was bovine rhodopsin (BR) that was used as template for most of the GPCR homology models.

Archer *et al.* constructed the BR-based homology model of the peptidergic cholecystokinin receptor CCK1 [54] and compared its structure with the template.

In addition to several similarities including the conserved (E)DRY box and NPXXY motifs, marked structural differences were observed. One group of these alterations is related to helical packing of transmembrane helices (TM1, TM3, and TM7) of the CCK1 receptor. These changes resulted in different orientation of binding site residues that should have significant impact on ligand recognition. Docking cholecystokinin (CCK) to the binding site revealed several problems. In addition to the disfavored orientation of the binding site residues, the conformation of the second extracellular loop (ECL2) prevented this motif interacting with CCK. Furthermore, similar to the previous findings these authors also underlined that inappropriate side-chain conformation could also be responsible for incorrect protein–ligand interactions.

BR-based homology models of three human GPCRs including dopamine D3, muscarinic M1, and vasopressin V1a receptors were investigated by Rognan and coworkers [14]. The active site of these receptors was refined using an antagonist. These authors found homology models suitable for the discrimination of known antagonists from random decoys (Table 14.1). On the other hand, BR-based models were unable to recognize known agonists, which was not improved by refining the binding site with different agonists. Since BR was crystallized in an inactive conformation, this finding was not unexpected. BR-based homology models were therefore subjected to a pharmacophore-based approach stimulating agonist like conformational changes. Modified structures were found to be suitable for the identification of agonists (Table 14.1).

The high-resolution X-ray structure of the β2 adrenoreceptor (β2AR) [55] can be considered a real breakthrough of the structural biology of GPCRs. Topiol and Sabio investigated the usefulness of the X-ray structure of β2AR in virtual screening applications [56]. First, they docked the cocrystallized ligand carazolol to the active site and found that the binding mode produced by the docking tools overlapped with that identified by crystallography. Next, it was demonstrated that binding modes of further six beta blockers (propranolol, timolol, butoxamine, dichloroisoprenaline, celiprolol, and carvediol) are all reasonable. Finally, the authors performed an enrichment study by virtual screening of 400 000 compounds against the crystal structure of β2AR. Carazolol and carvediol were found in the top 30 (0.008%) of the ranked database and furthermore the top 100 (0.025%) contained 11 known beta blockers or very closely related structures. These results demonstrated that the β2AR structure is useful in exploring novel chemical series of β2 inhibitors.

A comparative study on the docking performance of β2AR homology models and crystal structure was performed by Costanzi [57]. In this work, the author docked carazolol at two BR-based homology models of the β2AR. The two models were distinguished by the conformation of the second extracellular loop (ECL2). One has a BR-like conformation, while the other has a *de novo* built loop. The latter model with an adjusted side-chain at the binding site performed significantly better than that with the BR-like loop. This might be explained by the fact that BR has a deeply buried ECL2 that creates hurdles to the correct positioning of several ligands. *De novo* design of ECL2 resulted in a less buried ECL2 being more favorable for ligand binding. The conformation of ECL2 in both models was, however, still significantly different from that found in the β2AR crystal structures. As a result, neither model was able to capture all of the protein–ligand interactions identified in the crystal structure. This observation is in line with those reported for human adenosine A2A recently [58].

GPCR Dock 2008 was a community-wide assessment of GPCR modeling and ligand docking. Twenty-nine groups submitted 206 models of human adenosine A2A with ZM241 385 ligands docked to the binding site that were compared with the corresponding crystal structure. Although the best model submitted by Costanzi showed RMSD values for the ligand, the binding site, transmembrane helices, ECL2 Cα atoms, and protein Cα atoms all around 3 Å, it missed more than half the protein–ligand interactions found experimentally. Other models predicted the contacts less accurately with large errors in ECL2 Cα positions.

The availability of multiple GPCR crystal structures prompted Filizola and coworkers to investigate which structural template to use for homology modeling a GPCR target [59]. Considering the crystal structures of β2AR, β1AR [60], and A2A [61], these authors concluded that these structures are suitable templates for 16%, 18%, and 12% of class A GPCRs, respectively, while the BR template can be considered only for 1–2% of them. Comparing BR-based homology models with the corresponding crystal structures, they failed to predict appropriate binding modes. However, they found that lacking loops in β2AR did not prevent them from finding the correct binding mode of carazolol. This finding suggests that omitting loops might yield better performance in virtual screening applications than considering all the loops in inappropriate conformations. This study underlined the crucial importance of side-chain orientation. Carazolol was correctly docked only in those cases when highly similar templates such as β1AR were used. Docking to models constructed from templates with sequence identity lower than 35% showed significantly weaker performance.

Comparative virtual screening studies against crystal structures and homology models revealed that homology models could be considered viable alternatives. In addition to enrichment studies mimicking the real-life screening situation, there are a number of examples for successful prospective screening. Homology model-based virtual screening contributed to the discovery of new chemotypes in several cases (Table 14.1). In the last section of this chapter, we describe the details of two case studies of this type.

14.3
Challenges of Homology Model-Based Virtual Screening

Uncertainties of homology models could be attributed to multiple factors including side-chain packing, main-chain shifts in aligned and incorrect loop conformations in unaligned regions, and the use of misaligned or irrelevant templates [62]. On the basis of these pitfalls of comparative modeling and our personal experience, most important specific challenges associated with homology model-based virtual screening are summarized in the following sections. All of these have significant impact on the accuracy of binding mode predictions and consequently on the performance shown in virtual screening applications.

14.3.1
Level of Sequence Identity

Homology modeling is fundamentally based on the evolution theory of proteins. It assumes that the degree of identity shared by two proteins correlates with their phylogenetic similarity and the probability of comprising similar structural folds. It has been shown that the level of sequence identity of two protein structures directly correlates with the deviation of the Cα atoms of their common core [63]. In fact, homology models built on highly similar templates generally performed better than low similarity counterparts in virtual screens. On the other hand, sequence identity neither for the overall protein nor at the binding site strongly correlates with the performance. This is probably due to the fact that the efficiency of virtual screening depends on several other key factors, for example, ligand preparation, docking and scoring algorithm, and protein flexibility. Besides its direct effect on the quality of homology models, low sequence identity makes the sequence alignment of the template and target more complicated. In this case, additional information should be used to guide the alignment process. Alignment with the highest similarity is not necessarily the correct one when the overall sequence identity is low. Therefore, preliminary sequence alignment generated by dynamic programming based on sequence homology should be followed by manual adjustments. Experimental data, such as site-directed mutagenesis may be applied to identify crucial residues for ligand binding and/or functioning of the target protein. Since residues participating, for example, in ligand binding should face the interior of the binding site, several false alignments can be easily excluded by analyzing the orientation of these residues in the resulting models. Another possibility to improve sequence alignment is applying secondary structure prediction tools, such as PSIPRED [64]. It was also demonstrated that aligning multiple sequences or even profiles [65, 66] instead of single sequences usually improves the quality of the alignment [67]. Application of profile alignment tools makes it possible to identify proteins with similar folds possessing low sequence identity [68]. Besides the generally similar fold, target-template pairs with low sequence identity also have significant structural differences that cannot be handled simply by homology modeling. This problem might be overcome by applying thorough refinement techniques for short sequences, but at the moment there is little possibility to see complete refolding of longer chains even by applying reasonably long simulations. On the other hand, there is a continuous progress in molecular simulation techniques and hardware development [69, 70] that might provide the conditions to fix smaller misfolded parts of homology models in near future.

It is generally considered that a sequence identity below 30% is insufficient to build a useful homology model. Success stories of GPCR homology modeling based on the BR template somewhat contradict this rule of thumb. BR that shares only low sequence identity with therapeutically relevant targets (typically 15–20%) was the only template for GPCR homology modeling until the end of 2007. However, BR-based templates were successfully used for the analysis of mutational data [71–74], for mapping ligand binding sites, for docking known ligands [75–78], and even for structure-based virtual screening (Table 14.1). This can be explained by the conserved structure of GPCRs. The cell membrane stabilizes the α-helical secondary structure of the TM domain resulting in a conserved fold with only smaller individual alterations among the different GPCRs. Therefore, the main-chain atoms of GPCRs can be effectively predicted by homology modeling [79].

14.3.2 Main-Chain Flexibility

One of the basic assumptions of homology modeling is that the main-chain is primarily responsible for maintaining the similar fold of the target and the template proteins. Therefore preliminary homology models usually adopt the main-chain coordinates found in the template. Sometimes, even the subsequent relaxation steps leave the main-chain conformation unchanged. However, it should be noted that even the main-chain of the target proteins diverges from that of the template to some extent. Our results from the human H4 receptor homology model suggested that freezing the backbone atoms during optimization can result in serious steric clashes, while these can be relaxed by allowing the backbone to move freely [80]. The general fold and structural characteristics can be still maintained by optimizing the whole structure. A frequently applied technique is to start the optimization with relaxing the side-chains first and allow more and more parts of the protein to move. In the final stage, the whole protein including the main-chain can freely rotate.

The significant differences found in the backbone of BR and that of the recently solved GPCRs also underline the importance of main-chain relaxation. This can also be achieved by MD simulations with explicit membrane and water molecules. In this method, however, it is difficult to decide which frame of the simulation to use for further investigations and, furthermore, it is difficult to judge whether the system reached the global minimum.

14.3.3 Side-Chain Conformation: Induced Fit Effects of Ligands

Side-chains are generally believed to play an important role in assigning the uniqueness of the individual binding sites. Therefore, the conformation of the side-chains is typically less conserved and its prediction is a big challenge in homology modeling. Side-chain modeling programs based on rotamer libraries with preferred torsional angles are available [81]. It was demonstrated that backbone conformation has an effect on the frequency of the specific rotamers; therefore, a backbone-dependent rotamer library is often used in side-chain modeling [68, 82, 83]. Molecular simulations can also be suitable to optimize the side-chain conformations. If the main-chain was correctly modeled, side-chain relaxation can be accomplished in a reasonable time of simulation. This process might be facilitated by incorporating ligand information into the modeling of the binding site and use ligand–side-chain interactions to guide this optimization procedure. On the other hand, extensive optimizations in the absence of ligands might result in the shrinkage of the binding site that makes them unsuitable for virtual screening [80].

Ligand information can be incorporated into the model in different ways. We recently demonstrated that docking of known ligands and subsequent optimization of the receptor–ligand complexes can result in homology models suitable for virtual screens [80]. Evers *et al.* recently described a straightforward method for Modeling Binding sites Including Ligand information Explicitly (MOBILE) [84]. The MOBILE process starts with the generation of some crude homology models. Next, previously placed ligands are considered explicitly by defining restraints between protein and ligand atoms. These restraints are expressed in terms of knowledge-based distance-dependent pair potentials. Subsequently, the most favorable models are selected by ranking the interactions between the ligands and the generated pockets using these potentials. Final models are obtained by selecting the best-ranked side-chain conformers from various models, followed by an energy optimization of the entire complex using a common force field.

Another alternative, ligand-steered homology modeling was recently introduced by Cavasotto *et al.* [19]. This method includes an extensive sampling of possible ligand orientations and conformations and side-chain conformations at the binding site. All these studies suggest that ligand information can significantly improve the efficiency of homology models in virtual screening. However, it should be noted that incorporation of too specific ligand information might result in a binding site that is unable to recognize other active chemotypes that makes it unsuitable for virtual screening. Some authors demonstrated that proper side-chain orientation induced by the different ligands has a large impact on the applicability of the protein structures for virtual screening. Rockey and Elcock found that in some cases the cocrystallized ligand has a larger effect on the docking results than the source of the protein (i.e. crystal structure of the target or homology model based on another kinase template) [85]. Explicit ligand information might also facilitate the active/inactive transformation of proteins [86]. Although nanosecond scale simulations are usually not sufficient to obtain a fully activated protein model starting with the inactive conformation, these models may be more effective to identify agonists rather than antagonists by virtual screening.

14.3.4
Loop Modeling

Structural similarity between the target and the template is considered to be the lowest in loop regions. These are usually less conserved parts of the protein, which makes their prediction extremely challenging [87]. Some loops are proved to play a role in ligand binding and/or in receptor activation. For example, ECL2 adopts significantly different conformations in the available GPCR crystal structures. In BR, this loop forms direct interactions with the ligand retinal. On the other hand, in the recently solved GPCR structures, ECL2 is oriented toward the extracellular milieu leaving more space for the ligands at the binding site. It is also important to mention that even the human A2AR and β2AR structures have different ECL2 loops suggesting that this loop cannot be modeled simply by using a closely related GPCR as a template.

Loop modeling in general can be considered a problem similar to modeling a whole protein structure. Therefore, the methods that can be used are also similar. One might apply an *ab initio* (*de novo*) method, where the conformational search algorithm is based on general physical principles and involves the generation of a large number of randomly chosen conformations. Some of these methods utilize the available information derived from known loop structures, such as the main-chain Phi/Psi, or side-chain torsion angle distributions [68]. Alternatively, a knowledge-based approach can be used, where the search algorithm is seeking a suitable loop template in a database of experimentally determined three-dimensional structures. The disadvantage of *ab initio* methods is that the conformational sampling cannot effectively explore the potential energy surface, while the latter method might fail for shorter sequences where no conserved 3D structure can be assigned to the given sequence. Since the number of crystal structures in the PDB is continuously increasing, rotamer libraries used by knowledge-based methods might be significantly improved in future. On the other hand, the speed of these methods will be decreased in parallel. The loop modeling algorithm of Modeller [88] can be classified as an *ab initio* method [89]. It uses an energy function based on statistical preferences of atoms for different geometries as obtained from a nonredundant database of known protein structures and energy terms from the CHARMM22 force field [90]. The COILS software is an example of methods using a knowledge-based rotamer library [91]. It can be used to calculate the probability that a query sequence will adopt a coiled-coil conformation. This is realized by comparing a query sequence to a database of known parallel two-stranded coiled-coils. By comparing the calculated similarity score to the distribution of scores in globular and coiled-coil proteins, the program then calculates the probability. CODA [92] is another loop modeling approach utilizing a knowledge-based filtering algorithm (FREAD) combined with an *ab initio* method (PETRA) [93]. FREAD uses four rule-based filters: (i) the difference between anchor Cα separations of the target and the prediction; (ii) the RMSD between the backbone atoms of the anchor region of the target and the prediction; (iii) the energy of the predicted fragment in the target structure; and (iv) an environmentally constrained substitution score. These tools might be used effectively to predict reasonable loop conformations. On the other hand, the conformation of loops near the binding site highly depends on ligand binding. It is difficult or even impossible to generate a singe loop conformation favorable for docking different ligands. This suggests that protein flexibility should be considered during docking even in the case of virtual screens ideally by molecular simulations.

14.4
Case Studies

14.4.1
Virtual Screening on the Homology Model of Histamine H4 Receptor [16]

The human histamine H4 receptor (hH4R) is a member of the GPCR superfamily. It is the most recently discovered histamine receptor that is primarily expressed in cells of the hematopoietic lineage (e.g., eosinophils, basophils, dendritic cells, natural killer cells, CD8 + Tcells, and mast cells [94, 95]). Several preclinical studies suggest that H4R is a promising drug target for the treatment of inflammatory diseases [96]. The first potent and selective H4 antagonist (JNJ7 777 120) was identified by an in-house high-throughput screening (HTS) assay by researchers at Johnson & Johnson [97]. JNJ7 777 120 was widely used for the analysis of hH4R *in vitro* and *in vivo* [94]. Several other pharma companies demonstrated serious efforts to identify novel H4 ligands that could be suitable chemical starting points to develop potent and selective H4 antagonists [98]. Interestingly, at least eight companies (Bayer, Johnson & Johnson, Argenta, Pfizer, UCB Pharma, Cellzome, Abbott, and Palau) patented amino-pyrimidines as H4 modulators by making this scaffold the other large group of H4 antagonists besides the analogues of JNJ7 777 120. This suggests that the amino-pyrimidine scaffold was part of the compound library of all the above-mentioned companies and after identifying its significant H4 activity, they all exhibited serious efforts to develop potent and selective H4 antagonists based on this scaffold. However, starting the optimization from the same scaffold resulted in an extremely high competition. This highlights the limitations of HTS approaches that require existing chemical libraries biased by the accessible compounds of large vendor companies. On the contrary, computational tools can be used to screen several orders of magnitude more compounds virtually.

In 2004, our group initiated a research project to identify novel H4 ligands by virtual screening. As the available ligand information was limited at that time, we decided to apply a structure-based virtual screening approach. A homology model of hH4R was built using the high-resolution crystal structure of BR as template. The overall sequence identity between BR and hH4R is low (13.7%). However, the conserved structural domains and sequence motifs can effectively guide the sequence alignment. First, we built six preliminary homology models by Modeller [88]. We used the site-directed mutagenesis data available on the histamine binding site to distinguish between the models, and found that one of the six models possessed a favorable binding site for histamine to form interactions with the crucial residues Asp94 (3.32) and Glu182 (5.46), simultaneously. We further tested the quality of this model by Procheck [99], Whatif [100], and Harmony [101] validation tests. In the next step, we incorporated some ligand information into the model, that is, after docking the ligands to the binding site, the side chain, and in some cases even the backbone conformation was refined to accommodate the ligands more favorably. We found that rotation of a single torsion angle results in more favorable docking of known H4 ligands including histamine. Consequently, we used this model for setting up a large-scale virtual screen. We collected more than 8.7 million 3D structures representing commercially or academically available compounds. A reasonable amount of the molecules was derived from the ZINC database [102], where ligands are already in a "ready to dock" format. Other molecules were prepared for docking in two steps. First, we generated the physiologically relevant protonation state of the compounds by the "washing" module of MOE (MOE, version 2005.06, Chemical Computing Group Inc., Montreal, Canada). Then, Concord 4.0 (TriposAssociates, St. Louis, MO, USA) was applied to generate 3D coordinates. This compound database was screened on the hH4R homology model by docking to the binding site. We applied FlexX [103] to generate reasonable binding poses that were scored by the best scoring function combination found previously by enrichment tests (i.e., the docked poses for the individual compounds were ranked by ChemScore (CScore package) (TriposAssociates, St. Louis, MO, USA), and the best poses for all the compounds were ranked by FlexX-Score). Since docking can be effectively parallelized, we ran FlexX on several hundred CPUs. After the virtual screening, we selected compounds for *in vitro* testing by two different methodologies. The first method was primarily based on the analysis of the binding mode of the 2000 top scored compounds. Several false positives, such as low-probability tautomers and protomers and compounds with unacceptable binding mode were excluded and finally 128 compounds were suggested for *in vitro* testing. Sixty-six out of these were available from the vendors. Previous enrichment results showed that highest enrichment can be achieved in the top 0.5% of the database. Consequently, in the second selection method, we analyzed the top 45 000 compounds, applied a pharmacophore postfiltering step and a subsequent Unity 2D fingerprint-based dissimilarity selection (TriposAssociates, St. Louis, MO, USA) (Tanimoto coefficient < 0.7). This resulted in 229 virtual hits, from among which 166 were available from the vendors. Twenty-three additional close analogues of unavailable compounds were also ordered.

In summary, 255 compounds arrived at our lab and we tested them in a radioligand binding assay on hH4R overexpressing SK-N-MC cells [104] by using [^{3}H]histamine as a radioligand. Sixteen of these compounds showed significant H4 affinity to a [^{3}H]histamine displacement above 20% at 5 μM (hit rate: 6.3%). Seven compounds composed two groups and the others were singletons. Representative compounds of the two groups and the singletons are shown in Figure 14.1.

H4 affinity of the best compounds varied between 85 nM and 1.48 μM. We did not apply any druglike or leadlike prefiltering on the screened database; therefore, some of the identified compounds possessed nondruglike properties. On the other hand, the druglikeness of these compounds can be improved during the hit-to-lead and lead optimization processes. For example, the frequently occurring aminoguanidine functionality might be exchanged by a more druglike piperazine group. Interestingly, some of the identified compounds showed remarkable similarity to previously described known H4 ligands. For example, we identified a rotationally less constrained analogue of JNJ7 777 120 (see compound **5** in Figure 14.1). Furthermore, two compounds containing the 2-aminopyrimidine scaffold were also discovered (see compounds **1** and **9** in Figure 14.1). On the other hand, these novel H4 ligands comprise a reasonably diverse set of molecules that can be considered suitable

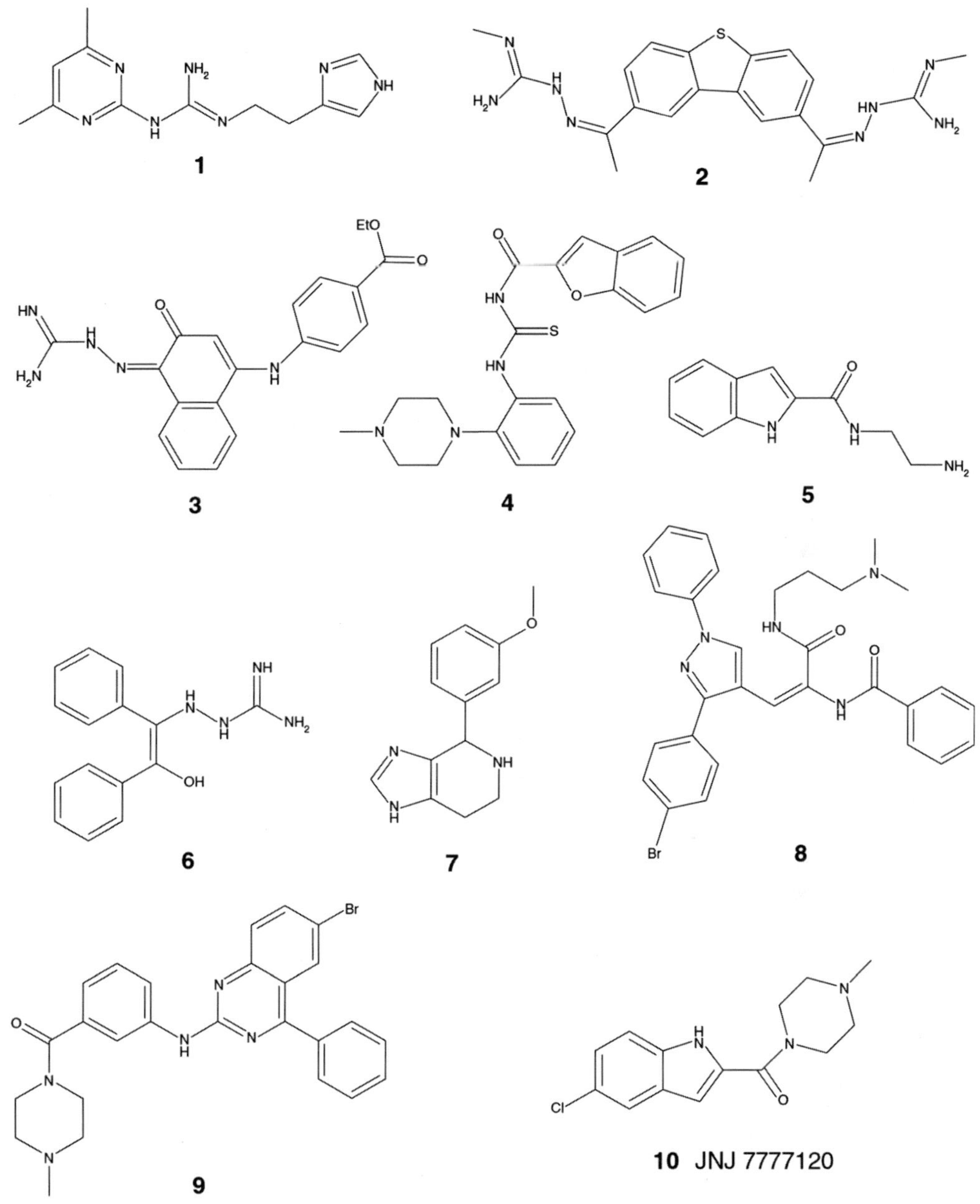

Figure 14.1 Representative *in vitro* hits (**1**–**9**) of the hH4R virtual screen and JNJ7 777 120 (**10**). Reprinted with permission from ref. [16], copyright 2008 American Chemical Society.

starting points for further optimization. This suggests that structure-based virtual screening should be applied when applicable in parallel with HTS to identify as many chemical starting points as possible. This is important to avoid narrowing the chemical space by ground flouring a project on the optimization of a single scaffold. Our results also demonstrate that homology models may be successfully utilized for virtual screening in the absence of experimental protein structures.

14.4.2
Virtual Screening on the Homology Model of Janus Kinase 2 [44]

Janus kinase 2 (JAK2) belongs to the JAK kinase family [105]. Similarly to other JAK family members, it contains seven conserved Janus homology (JH) domains: a tyrosine kinase domain at the C-terminus (JH1), a pseudokinase domain (JH2), and five more domains believed to interact with regulatory proteins or cytokine receptors (JH3–JH7). JAK2 plays a role in the pathomechanism of myeloproliferative disorders and hematologic malignancies. In particular, a constitutively active mutant (Val617Phe in the JH2 domain) occurs in 98% of patients with polycythemia vera and 50% of patients with essential thrombocythemia and primary myelofibrosis [106]. This suggests that potent JAK2 kinase inhibitors might have benefits in these pathological conditions. We therefore initiated a structure-based virtual screening project to identify novel JAK2 inhibitors.

Experimentally determined JAK2 structures were not available at the start of our JAK2 project. On the other hand, the crystal structure of JAK3 in complex with staurosporine was already published [107]. This crystal structure provided us a suitable template (with 62% overall sequence identity) for building a mouse JAK2 homology model. We generated 100 preliminary homology models by Modeller [88]. The best model indicated by the Modeller objective function was chosen for further investigations. There are two phosphotyrosine residues in the JAK3 crystal structure (pTyr980 and pTyr981). Since Modeller does not have a template for phosphotyrosine residues by default, the corresponding residues in JAK2 were considered as dephosphorylated tyrosines (Tyr1007 and Tyr1008) during the model building. Tyrosine residues (Tyr1007 and Tyr1008) were phosphorylated back to phosphotyrosines and the 5 Å environment of the two residues were subjected to energy minimization. Next, we carried out enrichment tests to find the optimal docking settings and scoring functions for virtual screening. We used FlexX for generating reliable docking poses and scored them both by the own score of FlexX and by the available scoring functions in CScore. We collected a diverse set of random decoys from the World Drug Index (WDI) to reduce artificial enrichment by excluding nondruglike compounds. Since the low number of available JAK2 inhibitors did not make it possible to build up a reliable enrichment test system, we followed the guideline of Lyne *et al.* [108] who showed that enrichment results are transferable between phylogenetically close kinase analogues. Accordingly, we performed the enrichment tests with 51 diverse JAK3 actives on the JAK3 crystal structure (PDB ID: 1YVJ). We also analyzed the influence of the application of pharmacophore constraints. In this case, ligands had to form an H-bond with either the backbone oxygen of Glu930 or the backbone nitrogen of Leu932 – in line with the interactions found in the JAK3 crystal structure. The results showed that with optimal settings (pharmacophore constraint, FlexX-Score for pose extraction and ChemScore for ranking) a 12-fold enrichment of actives in the top 1% can be achieved. We applied these settings to screen the whole NCI database (http://dtp.nci.nih.gov/docs/misc/available_samples/dtp_indsamples.html. Accessed 13 Sept. 2009) on our JAK2 homology model. We previously found that the NCI database is reasonably diverse probably due to the fact that its samples are provided by many individual research groups. In all 26 589 out of the 223 481 NCI compounds fulfilled the pharmacophore criterion. In line with the enrichment studies, the top scored 2235 compounds (top 1%) were selected for further investigations. Next, a diverse subset of 245 compounds (Tanimoto coefficient < 0.61) was considered for *in vitro* testing. The top scored 60 compounds of this set were ordered and 39 of these arrived at our laboratory. We tested these compounds in a human erythroleukemia (HEL) cell growth inhibition assay at 25 μM. This cell line contains the JAK2-Val617Phe mutation on both alleles and therefore the observed effect of the compounds is indicative of both their JAK2 inhibition and their therapeutical potential. We identified 5 out of the 39 tested compounds with an inhibition above 50%. The most potent compound, **G6**, possessed an IC_{50} of 60 nM (see Figure 14.2).

G6 was subjected to a series of biological tests to evaluate its JAK2 inhibitory potential and selectivity. Besides its remarkable *in vitro* potency, **G6** effectively inhibited the growth of polycythemia vera patient cells in an *ex vivo* study. These studies suggest that **G6** identified by virtual screening on our JAK2 homology model is a promising candidate for further optimizations.

On the basis of the docking calculations, we found that **G6** forms a strong salt bridge with Asp994 at the active site of JAK2 (Figure 14.2). This residue does not form any interaction with the previously published, cocrystallized JAK2 ligands. We

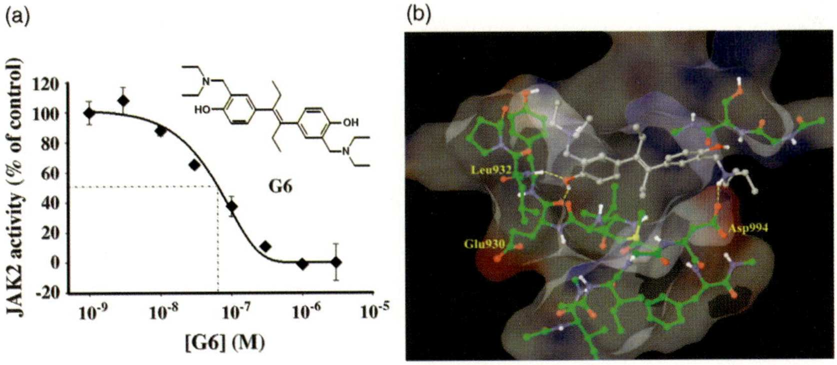

Figure 14.2 Inhibition of JAK2 Val617Phe kinase activity by **G6** ($IC_{50} = 60 \pm 4.5$ nM) (a). Binding mode of **G6** (gray) at the JAK2 binding site (green) (b). Van der Waals surfaces of the most important residues are shown and colored by their electrostatic potential. Picture was generated with Maestro (Version 8.5, Schrodinger, New York). Reprinted with permission from Ref. [44], copyright 2009 Elsevier.

suggest that this salt bridge might be responsible for the high JAK2 affinity of this compound.

In conclusion, the growing number of successful virtual screens on homology models suggests that in the absence of experimental 3D structure, high quality models can be used to identify suitable chemical starting points for drug discovery programs. Despite the recent progress of homology modeling tools and computational resources, the efficiency of homology model-based virtual screens significantly varies. The probability of success depends on multiple factors that should be considered to build up a reliable model and a predictive screening system. In this review, we summarized the most crucial factors to be addressed during the model building process and collected the recently reported success stories of the field.

References

1 Topiol, S. and Sabio, M. (2009) X-ray structure breakthroughs in the GPCR transmembrane region. *Biochemical Pharmacology*, **78** (1), 11–20.

2 Singh, S.K., Piscitelli, C.L., Yamashita, A., and Gouaux, E. (2009) A competitive inhibitor traps LeuT in an open-to-out conformation. *Science*, **322** (5908), 1655–1661.

3 Kawate, T., Michel, J.C., Birdsong, W.T., and Gouaux, E. (2009) Crystal structure of the ATP-gated P2X4 ion channel in the closed state. *Nature*, **460** (7255), 592–598.

4 Denisov, I.G., Makris, T.M., Sligar, S.G., and Schlichting, I. (2005) Structure and chemistry of cytochrome P450. *Chemical Reviews*, **105** (6), 2253–2277.

5 Aller, S.G., Yu, J., Ward, A., Weng, Y., Chittaboina, S., Zhuo, R., Harrell, P.M., Trinh, Y.T., Zhang, Q., Urbatsch, I.L., and Chang, G. (2009) Structure of P-glycoprotein reveals a molecular basis for poly-specific drug binding. *Science*, **323** (5922), 1718–1722.

6 Davis, A.M., Teague, S.J., and Kleywegt, G.J. (2003) Application and limitations of X-ray crystallographic data in structure-based ligand and drug design. *Angewandte Chemie – International Edition in English*, **42** (24), 2718–2736.

7 Søndergaard, C.R., Garrett, A.E., Carstensen, T., Pollastri, G., and Nielsen, J.E. (2009) Structural artifacts in protein–ligand X-ray structures: implications for the development of docking scoring functions. *Journal of Medicinal Chemistry*. Epub ahead of print. doi: 10.1021/jm8016464

8 Kryshtafovych, A. and Fidelis, K. (2009) Protein structure prediction and model quality assessment. *Drug Discovery Today*, **14** (7–8), 386–393.

9 Tuccinardi, T. (2009) Docking-based virtual screening: recent developments. *Combinatorial Chemistry & High Throughput Screening*, **12** (3), 303–314.

10 Fan, H., Irwin, J.J., Webb, B.M., Klebe, G., Shoichet, B.K., and Sali, A. (2009) Molecular docking screens using comparative models of proteins. *Journal of Chemical Information and Modeling*, **49**, 2512–2527 and references therein.

11 Radestock, S., Weil, T., and Renner, S. (2008) Homology model-based virtual screening for GPCR ligands using docking and target-biased scoring. *Journal of Chemical Information and Modeling*, **48** (5), 1104–1117.

12 Zhang, Y.J., Wang, Z., Sprous, D., and Nabioullin, R. (2006) In *silico* design and synthesis of piperazine-1-pyrrolidine-2,5-dione scaffold-based novel malic enzyme inhibitors. *Bioorganic & Medicinal Chemistry Letters*, **16** (3), 525–528.

13 Miguet, L., Zhang, Z., Barbier, M., and Grigorov, M.G. (2006) Comparison of a homology model and the crystallographic structure of human 11β-hydroxysteroid dehydrogenase type 1 (11βHSD1) in a structure-based identification of

inhibitors. *Journal of Computer-Aided Molecular Design*, **20** (2), 67–81.

14 Bissantz, C., Bernard, P., Hibert, M., and Rognan, D. (2003) Protein-based virtual screening of chemical databases. II. Are homology models of G-protein coupled receptors suitable targets? *Proteins*, **50** (1), 5–25.

15 Parrill, A.L., Echols, U., Nguyen, T., Pham, T.C., Hoeglund, A., and Baker, D.L. (2008) Virtual screening approaches for the identification of non-lipid autotaxin inhibitors. *Bioorganic and Medicinal Chemistry*, **16** (4), 1784–1795.

16 Kiss, R., Kiss, B., Könczöl, Á., Szalai, F., Jelinek, I., László, V., Noszál, B., Falus, A., and Keserű, G.M. (2008) Discovery of novel human histamine H4 receptor ligands by large-scale structure-based virtual screening. *Journal of Medicinal Chemistry*, **51** (11), 3145–3153.

17 Heinke, R., Spannhoff, A., Meier, R., Trojer, P., Bauer, I., Jung, M., and Sippl, W. (2009) Virtual screening and biological characterization of novel histone arginine methyltransferase PRMT1 inhibitors. *ChemMedChem*, **4** (1), 69–77.

18 Mukherjee, P., Desai, P.V., Srivastava, A., Tekwani, B.L., and Avery, M.A. (2008) Probing the structures of leishmanial farnesyl pyrophosphate synthases: homology modeling and docking studies. *Journal of Chemical Information and Modeling*, **48** (5), 1026–1040.

19 Cavasotto, C.N., Orry, A.J.W., Murgolo, N.J., Czarniecki, M.F., Kocsi, S.A., Hawes, B.E., O'Neill, K.A., Hine, H., Burton, M.S., Voigt, J.H., Abagyan, R.A., Bayne, M.L., and Monsma, F.J., Jr. (2008) Discovery of novel chemotypes to a G-protein-coupled receptor through ligand-steered homology modeling and structure-based virtual screening. *Journal of Medicinal Chemistry*, **51** (3), 581–588.

20 Taylor, C.M., Barda, Y., Kisselev, O.G., and Marshall, G.R. (2008) Modulating G-protein coupled receptor/G-protein signal transduction by small molecules suggested by virtual screening. *Journal of Medicinal Chemistry*, **51** (17), 5297–5303.

21 Nagarajan, S., Doddareddy, M., Choo, H., Cho, Y.S., Oh, K.S., Lee, B.H., and Pae, P.A. (2009) IKKb inhibitors identification part I: homology model assisted structure based virtual screening. *Bioorganic and Medicinal Chemistry*, **17** (7), 2759–2766.

22 Park, H., Bahn, Y.J., Jung, S.K., Jeong, D.G., Lee, S.H., Seo, I., Yoon, T.S., Kim, S.J., and Ryu, S.E. (2008) Discovery of novel Cdc25 phosphatase inhibitors with micromolar activity based on the structure-based virtual screening. *Journal of Medicinal Chemistry*, **51** (18), 5533–5541.

23 Nguyen, T.L., Gussio, R., Smith, J.A., Lannigan, D.A., Hecht, S.M., Scudiero, D.A., Shoemaker, R.H., and Zaharevitz, D.W. (2006) Homology model of RSK2 N-terminal kinase domain, structure based identification of novel RSK2 inhibitors, and preliminary common pharmacophore. *Bioorganic and Medicinal Chemistry*, **14** (17), 6097–6105.

24 Pérez-Nueno, V.I., Ritchie, D.W., Rabal, O., Pascual, R., Borrell, J.I., and Teixidó, J. (2008) Comparison of ligand-based and receptor-based virtual screening of HIV entry inhibitors for the CXCR4 and CCR5 receptors using 3D ligand shape matching and ligand-receptor docking. *Journal of Chemical Information and Modeling*, **48** (3), 509–533.

25 Ahmed, A., Choo, H., Cho, Y.S., Park, W.K., and Pae, A.N. (2009) Identification of novel serotonin 2C receptor ligands by sequential virtual screening. *Bioorganic and Medicinal Chemistry*, **17** (13), 4559–4568.

26 Park, H., Hwang, K.Y., Oh, K.H., Kim, Y.H., Lee, J.Y., and Kim., K. (2008) Discovery of novel α-glucosidase inhibitors based on the virtual screening with the homology-modeled protein structure. *Bioorganic and Medicinal Chemistry*, **16** (1), 284–292.

27 Triballeau, N., Acher, F., Brabet, I., Pin, J.P., and Bertrand, H.O. (2005) Virtual screening workflow development guided by the "receiver operating characteristic" curve approach. Application to high-throughput docking on metabotropic glutamate receptor subtype 4. *Journal of Medicinal Chemistry*, **48** (7), 2534–2547.

28 Evers, A. and Klebe, G. (2004) Ligand-supported homology modeling of G-protein-coupled receptor sites: models sufficient for successful virtual screening. *Angewandte Chemie – International Edition in English*, **43** (2), 248–251.

29 Vangrevelinghe, E., Zimmermann, K., Schoepfer, J., Portmann, R., Fabbro, D., and Furet, P. (2003) Discovery of a potent and selective protein kinase CK2 inhibitor by high-throughput docking. *Journal of Medicinal Chemistry*, **46** (13), 2656–2662.

30 Liu, Z., Huang, C., Fan, K., Wei, P., Chen, H., Liu, S., Pei, J., Shi, L., Li, B., Yang, K., Liu, Y., and Lai, L. (2005) Virtual screening of novel noncovalent inhibitors for SARS-CoV 3C-like proteinase. *Journal of Chemical Information and Modeling*, **45** (1), 10–17.

31 Diller, D.J. and Li, R. (2003) Kinases, homology models, and high throughput docking. *Journal of Medicinal Chemistry*, **46** (22), 4638–4647.

32 Evers, A., Hessler, G., Matter, H., and Klabunde, T. (2005) Virtual screening of biogenic amine-binding G-protein coupled receptors: comparative evaluation of protein- and ligand-based virtual screening protocols. *Journal of Medicinal Chemistry*, **48** (17), 5448–5465.

33 Kenyon, V., Chorny, I., Carvajal, W.J., Holman, T.R., and Jacobson, M.P. (2006) Novel human lipoxygenase inhibitors discovered using virtual screening with homology models. *Journal of Medicinal Chemistry*, **49** (4), 1356–1363.

34 Kellenberger, E., Springael, J.Y., Parmentier, M., Hachet-Haas, M., Galzi, J.L., and Rognan, D. (2007) Identification of nonpeptide CCR5 receptor agonists by structure-based virtual screening. *Journal of Medicinal Chemistry*, **50** (6), 1294–1303.

35 Desai, P.V., Patny, A., Sabnis, Y., Tekwani, B., Gut, J., Rosenthal, P., Srivastava, A., and Avery, M. (2004) Identification of novel parasitic cysteine protease inhibitors using virtual screening. 1. The ChemBridge database. *Journal of Medicinal Chemistry*, **47** (26), 6609–6615.

36 Desai, P.V., Patny, A., Gut, J., Rosenthal, P.J., Tekwani, B., Srivastava, A., and Avery, M. (2006) Identification of novel parasitic cysteine protease inhibitors by use of virtual screening. 2. The available chemical directory. *Journal of Medicinal Chemistry*, **49** (5), 1576–1584.

37 Salo, O.M., Raitio, K.H., Savinainen, J.R., Nevalainen, T., Lahtela-Kakkonen, M., Laitinen, J.T., Järvinen, T., and Poso, A. (2005) Virtual screening of novel CB2 ligands using a comparative model of the human cannabinoid CB2 receptor. *Journal of Medicinal Chemistry*, **48** (23), 7166–7171.

38 de Graaf, C., Giordanetto, F., Abbas, G., Unson, C.G., and Rognan, D. (2008) Class B G-protein coupled receptors as targets for protein-based virtual screening. The 236th American Chemical Society National Meeting, MEDI-409, Aug 17–21, Philadelphia, PA, USA.

39 Tikhonova, I.G., Sum, C.S., Neumann, S., Engel, S., Raaka, B.M., Costanzi, S., and Gershengorn, M.C. (2008) Discovery of novel agonists and antagonists of the free fatty acid receptor 1 (FFAR1) using virtual screening. *Journal of Medicinal Chemistry*, **51** (3), 625–633.

40 Chen, J.Z., Wang, J., and Xie, X.Q. (2007) GPCR structure-based virtual screening approach for CB2 antagonist search. *Journal of Chemical Information and Modeling*, **47** (4), 1626–1637.

41 Varady, J., Wu, X., Fang, X., Min, J., Hu, Z., Levant, B., and Wang, S. (2003) Molecular modeling of the three-dimensional structure of dopamine 3 (D3) subtype receptor: discovery of novel and potent D3 ligands through a hybrid pharmacophore- and structure-based database searching approach. *Journal of Medicinal Chemistry*, **46** (21), 4377–4392.

42 Klabunde, T. and Evers, A. (2005) GPCR antitarget modeling: pharmacophore models for biogenic amine binding GPCRs to avoid GPCR-mediated side effects. *Chembiochem: A European Journal of Chemical Biology*, **6** (5), 876–889.

43 Sandberg, E.M., Ma, X., He, K., Frank, S.J., Ostrov, D.A., and Sayeski, P.P. (2005) Identification of 1,2,3,4,5,6-hexabromocyclohexane as a small molecule inhibitor of Jak2 tyrosine kinase

autophosphorylation. *Journal of Medicinal Chemistry*, **48** (7), 2526–2533.

44 Kiss, R., Polgár, T., Kirabo, A., Sayyah, J., Figueroa, N.C., List, A.F., Sokol, L., Zuckerman, K.S., Gali, M., Bisht, K.S., Sayeski, P.P., and Keserű, G.M. (2009) Identification of a novel inhibitor of JAK2 tyrosine kinase by structure-based virtual screening. *Bioorganic & Medicinal Chemistry Letters*, **19** (13), 3598–3601.

45 Schafferhans, A. and Klebe, G. (2001) Docking ligands onto binding site representations derived from proteins. *Journal of Molecular Biology*, **307** (1), 407–427.

46 Sternberg, M.J.E. (1996) Protein structure prediction: principles and approaches, in *Protein Structure Prediction*, Oxford University Press, Oxford, pp. 1–30.

47 Oshiro, C., Bradley, E.K., Eksterowicz, J., Evensen, E., Lamb, M.L., Lanctot, J.K., Putta, S., Stanton, R., and Grootenhuis, P.D.J. (2004) Performance of 3D-database molecular docking studies into homology models. *Journal of Medicinal Chemistry*, **47** (3), 764–767.

48 McGovern, S.L. and Shoichet, B.K. (2003) Information decay in molecular docking screens against holo, apo, and modeled conformations of enzymes. *Journal of Medicinal Chemistry*, **46** (14), 2895–2907.

49 Fernandes, M.X., Kairys, V., and Gilson, M.K. (2004) Comparing ligand interactions with multiple receptors via serial docking. *Journal of Chemical Information and Computer Sciences*, **44** (6), 1961–1970.

50 Moult, J., Fidelis, K., Zemla, A., and Hubbard, T. (2003) Critical assessment of methods of protein structure prediction (CASP): round V. *Proteins*, **53** (Suppl. 6), 334–339.

51 DeWeese-Scott, C. and Moult, J. (2004) Molecular modeling of protein function regions. *Proteins*, **55** (4), 942–961.

52 Kairys, V., Fernandes, M.X., and Gilson, M.K. (2006) Screening drug-like compounds by docking to homology models: a systematic study. *Journal of Chemical Information and Modeling*, **46** (1), 365–379.

53 Hartmann, C., Antes, I., and Lengauer, T. (2009) Docking and scoring with alternative side-chain conformations. *Proteins*, **74** (3), 712–726.

54 Archer, E., Maigret, B., Escrieut, C., Pradayrol, L., and Fourmy, D. (2003) Rhodopsin crystal: new template yielding realistic models of G-protein-coupled receptors? *Trends in Pharmacological Sciences*, **24** (1), 36–40.

55 Cerezov, V., Rosenbaum, D.M., Hanson, M.A., Rasmussen, S.G.F., Thian, F.S., Kobilka, T.S., Choi, H.J., Kuhn, P., Weis, W.I., Kobilka, B.K., and Stevens, R.C. (2007) High-resolution crystal structure of an engineered human beta2-adrenergic G protein-coupled receptor. *Science*, **318** (5854), 1258–1265.

56 Topiol, S. and Sabio, M. (2008) Use of the X-ray structure of the beta2-adrenergic receptor for drug discovery. *Bioorganic & Medicinal Chemistry Letters*, **18** (5), 1598–1602.

57 Costanzi, S. (2008) On the applicability of GPCR homology models to computer-aided drug discovery: a comparison between *in silico* and crystal structures of the beta2-adrenergic receptor. *Journal of Medicinal Chemistry*, **51** (10), 2907–2914.

58 Michino, M., Abola, E.(GPCR Dock 2008 participants), Brooks, C.L. 3rd, Dixon, J.S., Moult, J., and Stevens, R.C. (2009) Community-wide assessment of GPCR structure modelling and ligand docking: GPCR Dock 2008. *Nature Reviews. Drug Discovery*, **8** (6), 455–463.

59 Mobarec, J.C., Sanchez, R., and Filizola, M. (2009) Modern homology modeling of G-protein coupled receptors: which structural template to use? *Journal of Medicinal Chemistry*, **52** (16), 5207–5216.

60 Warne, T., Serrano-Vega, M.J., Baker, J.G., Moukhametzianov, R., Edwards, P.C., Henderson, R., Leslie, A.G., Tate, C.G., and Schertler, G.F. (2008) Structure of a beta1-adrenergic G-protein-coupled receptor. *Nature*, **454** (7203), 486–491.

61 Jaakola, V.P., Griffith, M.T., Hanson, M.A., Cherezov, V., Chien, E.Y., Lane, J.R., Ijzerman, A.P., and Stevens, R.C. (2008) The 2.6 angstrom crystal structure of a human A2A adenosine receptor bound to an antagonist. *Science*, **322** (5905), 1211–1217.

62 Martí-Renom, M.A., Stuart, A.C., Fiser, A., Sánchez, R., Melo, F., and Sali, A. (2000) Comparative protein structure modeling of genes and genomes. *Annual Review of Biophysics and Biomolecular Structure*, **29**, 291–325.

63 Chothia, C. and Lesk, A.M. (1986) The relation between the divergence of sequence and structure in proteins. *The EMBO Journal*, **5** (4), 823–826.

64 Jones, D.T. (1999) Protein secondary structure prediction based on position-specific scoring matrices. *Journal of Molecular Biology*, **292** (2), 195–202.

65 Altschul, S., Madden, T.L., Schaffer, A.A., Zhang, J., Zhang, Z., Miller, W., and Lipman, D.J. (1997) Gapped BLAST and PSI-BLAST: a new generation of protein database search programs. *Nucleic Acids Research*, **25** (17), 3389–3402.

66 Krogh, A., Brown, M., Mian, I., Sjolander, K., and Haussler, D. (1994) Hidden Markov models in computational biology. Applications to protein modeling. *Journal of Molecular Biology*, **235** (5), 1501–1531.

67 Edgar, R.C. and Sjölander, K. (2004) A comparison of scoring functions for protein sequence profile alignment. *Bioinformatics (Oxford, England)*, **20** (8), 1301–1308.

68 Xiang, Z. (2006) Advances in homology protein structure modeling. *Current Protein & Peptide Science*, **7** (3), 217–227.

69 Bowers, K.J., Chow, E., Xu, H., Dror, R.O., Eastwood, M.P., Gregersen, B.A., Klepeis, J.L., Kolossvary, I., Moraes, M.A., Sacerdoti, F.D., Salmon, J.K., Shan, Y., and Shaw, D.E. (2006) Scalable algorithms for molecular dynamics simulations on commodity clusters. Conference on High Performance Networking and Computing archive, Proceedings of the 2006 ACM/IEEE Conference on Supercomputing, November 2006, Tampa, FL, USA.

70 Shaw, D.E., Deneroff, M.M., Dror, R.O., Kuskin, J.S., Larson, R.H., Salmon, J.K., Young, C., Batson, B., Bowers, K.J., Chao, J.C., Eastwood, M.P., Gagliardo, J., Grossman, J.P., Ho, C.R., Ierardi, D.J., Kolossváry, I., Klepeis, J.L., Layman, T., McLeavey, C., Moraes, M.A., Mueller, R., Priest, E.C., Shan, Y., Spengler, J., Theobald, M., Towles, B., and Wang, S.C. (2008) Anton, a special-purpose machine for molecular dynamics simulation. *Communications of the ACM*, **51** (7), 91–97.

71 Furse, K.E. and Lybrand, T.P. (2003) Three-dimensional models for beta-adrenergic receptor complexes with agonists and antagonists. *Journal of Medicinal Chemistry*, **46** (21), 4450–4462.

72 Costanzi, S., Mamedova, L., Gao, Z.G., and Jacobson, K.A. (2004) Architecture of P2Y nucleotide receptors: structural comparison based on sequence analysis, mutagenesis, and homology modeling. *Journal of Medicinal Chemistry*, **47** (22), 5393–5404.

73 Clark, D.E., Higgs, C., Wren, S.P., Dyke, H.J., Wong, M., Norman, D., Lockey, P.M., and Roach, A.G. (2004) A virtual screening approach to finding novel and potent antagonists at the melanin-concentrating hormone 1 receptor. *Journal of Medicinal Chemistry*, **47** (16), 3962–3971.

74 Salo, O.M., Lahtela-Kakkonen, M., Gynther, J., Jarvinen, T., and Poso, A. (2004) Development of a 3D model for the human cannabinoid CB1 receptor. *Journal of Medicinal Chemistry*, **47** (12), 3048–3057.

75 Onuffer, J., McCarrick, M.A., Dunning, L., Liang, M., Rosser, M., Wei, G.P., Ng, H., and Horuk, R. (2003) Structure function differences in nonpeptide CCR1 antagonists for human and mouse CCR1. *Journal of Immunology (Baltimore, MD: 1950)*, **170** (4), 1910–1916.

76 ter Laak, A.M., Timmerman, H., Leurs, R., Nederkoorn, P.H., Smit, M.J., and Donne-Op den Kelder, G.M. (1995) Modelling and mutation studies on the histamine H1-receptor agonist binding site reveal different binding modes for H1-agonists: Asp116 (TM3) has a constitutive role in receptor stimulation. *Journal of Computer-Aided Molecular Design*, **9** (4), 319–330.

77 Mouillac, B., Chini, B., Balestre, M.N., Elands, J., Trumpp-Kallmeyer, S., Hoflack, J., Hibert, M., Jard, S., and

Barberis, C. (1995) The binding site of neuropeptide vasopressin V1a receptor. Evidence for a major localization within transmembrane regions. *Journal of Biological Chemistry*, **270** (43), 25771–25777.
78 Hibert, M.F., Trumpp-Kallmeyer, S., Bruinvels, A., and Hoflack, J. (1991) Three-dimensional models of neurotransmitter G-binding protein-coupled receptors. *Molecular Pharmacology*, **40** (1), 8–15.
79 Punta, M., Forrest, L.R., Bigelow, H., Kernytsky, A., Liu, J., and Rost, B. (2007) Membrane protein prediction methods. *Methods (San Diego, CA)*, **41** (4), 460–474.
80 Kiss, R., Noszál, B., Rácz, A., Falus, A., Erős, D., and Keserű, G.M. (2008) Binding mode analysis and enrichment studies on homology models of the human histamine H4 receptor. *European Journal of Medicinal Chemistry*, **43** (5), 1059–1070.
81 Ponder, J.W. and Richard, F.M. (1987) Tertiary templates for proteins. Use of packing criteria in the enumeration of allowed sequences for different structural classes. *Journal of Molecular Biology*, **193** (4), 775–791.
82 Dunbrack, R.L., Jr., and Karplus, M. (1993) Backbone-dependent rotamer library for proteins. Application to side-chain prediction. *Journal of Molecular Biology*, **230** (2), 543–574.
83 Canutescu, A.A., Shelenkov, A.A., and Dunbrack, R.L., Jr. (2003) A graph-theory algorithm for rapid protein side-chain prediction. *Protein Science: A Publication of the Protein Society*, **12** (9), 2001–2014.
84 Evers, A., Gohlke, H., and Klebe, G. (2003) Ligand-supported homology modelling of protein binding-sites using knowledge-based potentials. *Journal of Molecular Biology*, **334** (2), 327–345.
85 Rockey, W.M. and Elcock, A.H. (2006) Structure selection for protein kinase docking and virtual screening: homology models or crystal structures? *Current Protein & Peptide Science*, **7** (5), 437–457.
86 Jójárt, B., Kiss, R., Viskolcz, B., and Keserű, G.M. (2008) Activation mechanism of the human histamine H4 receptor: an explicit membrane molecular dynamics simulation study. *Journal of Chemical Information and Modeling*, **48** (6), 1199–1210.
87 Osmani, S.A., Bak, S., and Møller, B.L. (2009) Substrate specificity of plant UDP-dependent glycosyltransferases predicted from crystal structures and homology modeling. *Phytochemistry*, **70** (3), 325–347.
88 Sali, A. and Blundell, T.L. (1993) Comparative protein modelling by satisfaction of spatial restraints. *Journal of Molecular Biology*, **234** (3), 779–815.
89 Fiser, A., Do, R.K., and Sali, A. (2000) Modeling of loops in protein structures. *Protein Science: A Publication of the Protein Society*, **9** (9), 1753–1773.
90 Brooks, B.R., Bruccoleri, R.E., Olafson, B.D., States, D.J., Swaminathan, S., and Karplus, M. (1983) CHARMM: a program for macromolecular energy, minimization, and dynamics calculations. *Journal of Computational Chemistry*, **4**, 187–217.
91 Lupas, A., Van Dyke, M., and Stock, J. (1991) Predicting coiled coils from protein sequences. *Science*, **252** (5009), 1162–1164.
92 Deane, C.M. and Blundell, T.L. (2001) CODA: a combined algorithm for predicting the structurally variable regions of protein models. *Protein Science: A Publication of the Protein Society*, **10** (3), 599–612.
93 Deane, C.M. and Blundell, T.L. (2000) A novel exhaustive search algorithm for predicting the conformation of polypeptide segments in proteins. *Proteins*, **40** (1), 135–144.
94 Zhang, M., Thurmond, R.L., and Dunford, P.J. (2007) The histamine H4 receptor: a novel modulator of inflammatory and immune disorders. *Pharmacology & Therapeutics*, **113** (3), 594–606.
95 Zhu, Y., Michalovich, D., Wu, H., Tan, K.B., Dytko, G.M., Mannan, I.J., Boyce, R., Alston, J., Tierney, L.A., Li, X., Herrity, N.C., Vawter, L., Sarau, H.M., Ames, R.S., Davenport, C.M., Hieble, J.P., Wilson, S., Bergsma, D.J., and Fitzgerald, L.R. (2001) Cloning, expression, and

pharmacological characterization of a novel human histamine receptor. *Molecular Pharmacology*, **59** (3), 434–441.

96 de Esch, I.J., Thurmond, R.L., Jongejan, A., and Leurs, R. (2005) The histamine H4 receptor as a new therapeutic target for inflammation. *Trends in Pharmacological Sciences*, **26** (9), 462–469.

97 Jablonowski, J.A., Grice, C.A., Chai, W., Dvorak, C.A., Venable, J.D., Kwok, A.K., Ly, K.S., Wei, J., Baker, S.M., Desai, P.J., Jiang, W., Wilson, S.J., Thurmond, R.L., Karlsson, L., Edwards, J.P., Lovenberg, T.W., and Carruthers, N.I. (2003) The first potent and selective non-imidazole human histamine H4 receptor antagonists. *Journal of Medicinal Chemistry*, **46** (19), 3957–3960.

98 Kiss, R. and Keserű, G.M. (2009) Histamine H4 receptor ligands and their potential therapeutic applications. *Expert Opinion on Therapeutic Patents*, **19** (2), 119–135.

99 Laskowski, R.A., MacArthur, M.W., Moss, D.S., and Thorton, J.M. (1993) PROCHECK: a program to check the stereochemical quality of protein structures. *Journal of Applied Crystallography*, **26** (2), 283–291.

100 Vriend, G. and Sander, C. (1993) Quality control of protein models: Directional atomic contact analysis. *Journal of Applied Crystallography*, **26** (1), 47–60.

101 Pugalenthi, G., Shameer, K., Srinivasan, N., and Sowdhamini, R. (2006) HARMONY: a server for the assessment of protein structures. *Nucleic Acids Research*, **34**, W231–W234.

102 Irwin, J.J. and Shoichet, B.K. (2005) ZINC: a free database of commercially available compounds for virtual screening. *Journal of Chemical Information and Modeling*, **45** (1), 177–182.

103 Rarey, M., Kramer, B., Lengauer, T., and Klebe, G. (1996) A fast flexible docking method using an incremental construction algorithm. *Journal of Molecular Biology*, **261** (3), 470–489.

104 Liu, C., Ma, X., Jiang, X., Wilson, S.J., Hofstra, C.L., Blevitt, J., Pyati, J., Li, X., Chai, X., Carruthers, N., and Lovenberg, T.W. (2001) Cloning and pharmacological characterization of a fourth histamine receptor (H(4)) expressed in bone marrow. *Molecular Pharmacology*, **59** (3), 420–426.

105 Leonard, W.J. and O'Shea, J.J. (1998) Jaks and STATs: biological implications. *Annual Review of Immunology*, **16**, 293–322.

106 Levine, R.L., Wadleigh, M., Cools, J., Ebert, B.L., Wernig, G., Huntly, B.J., Boggon, T.J., Wlodarska, I., Clark, J.J., Moore, S., Adelsperger, J., Koo, S., Lee, J.C., Gabriel, S., Mercher, T., D'Andrea, A., Fröhling, S., Döhner, K., Marynen, P., Vandenberghe, P., Mesa, R.A., Tefferi, A., Griffin, J.D., Eck, M.J., Sellers, W.R., Meyerson, M., Golub, T.R., Lee, S.J., and Gilliland, D.G. (2005) Activating mutation in the tyrosine kinase JAK2 in polycythemia vera, essential thrombocythemia, and myeloid metaplasia with myelofibrosis. *Cancer Cell*, **7** (4), 387–397.

107 Boggon, T.J., Li, Y., Manley, P.W., and Eck, M.J. (2005) Crystal structure of the Jak3 kinase domain in complex with a staurosporine analog. *Blood*, **106** (3), 996–1002.

108 Lyne, P.D., Kenny, P.W., Cosgrove, D.A., Deng, C., Zabludoff, S., Wendoloski, J.J., and Ashwell, S. (2004) Identification of compounds with nanomolar binding affinity for checkpoint kinase-1 using knowledge-based virtual screening. *Journal of Medicinal Chemistry*, **47** (8), 1962–1968.

15
Target-Based Virtual Screening on Small-Molecule Protein Binding Sites

Ralf Heinke, Urszula Uciechowska, Manfred Jung, and Wolfgang Sippl

15.1
Introduction

It has become common sense in drug discovery to use computer-based *in silico* design techniques to identify and optimize novel molecules with a desired biological activity [1–5]. As a practical matter, computer-based methods are frequently split into disciplines that focus on either structure-based or ligand-based approaches. If the 3D structure of a target protein is known, it is possible to apply structure-based methods. New candidate molecules may be docked into a particular binding pocket in order to study if they can interact optimally with the protein. In an ideal situation, the target protein has already been crystallized in complex with a first lead structure. But in particular for novel targets, structural information is frequently not available at the time of the first experiments (e.g., high-throughput screening). When no 3D structure is available, although a sufficient number of active analogues have already been synthesized, pharmacophore-based methods can be applied to identify novel molecules that fit a particular pharmacophore model [1, 2]. It may seem straightforward to develop new molecules for known proteins by applying structure-based approaches, but there are significant problems that can emerge. Protein flexibility, multiple ligand binding modes, solvation, or entropic effects are some of the problems that must be solved to attain reliable models. Earlier studies demonstrate the efficiency of ligand- and structure-based approaches in direct comparison [2], as well as synergies obtained by using both approaches in combination [3]. As the costs for computational power are steadily decreasing and parallel computing is now available, it is no longer a problem to apply *in silico* modeling techniques to large databases comprising millions of compounds [4]. In general, *in silico* methods gained influence on the validation of targets, hit finding, hit to lead expansion, lead optimization, and also the prediction of suitable ADMET and off-target activity profiles (for review, see Ref. [5]).

Virtual Screening. Edited by C. Sotriffer

ISBN: 978-3-527-32636-5

15.1.1 Pharmacophore-Based Methods

The term pharmacophore is originally defined by the IUPAC working party that states, "A pharmacophore is the ensemble of steric and electronic features that is necessary to ensure the optimal supramolecular interaction with a specific biological target structure and to trigger (or block) its biological response." Thus, in other words, a pharmacophore is a three-dimensional (3D) representation of the crucial molecular features responsible for the binding of a set of ligands to a macromolecular target. A pharmacophoric element (also called feature) is generally defined as an atom or a group of atoms (e.g., a hydrogen bond donor atom or an aromatic ring system) common to active compounds with respect to a target protein and essential for the activity. However, not all scientists use the term pharmacophore in the same way. Computational chemists often use the term pharmacophore in a relatively abstract way. Influenced by the structural representation of molecules, a set of topological connections is used to define the properties and dimension of a molecule in only two dimensions (2D). Here, the spatial and topological distribution of pharmacophoric features is converted to a lower dimensional representation, for example, vectors. Such vectors that represent pharmacophore descriptors are referred to as "fingerprints," "keys," "bit strings," or "correlation vectors," depending on the type of information stored. The pharmacophore descriptors or fingerprints can be regarded as a transformed molecular representation instead of an explicit 3D structure [6]. The main advantage of the 2D approaches is that they are easy to calculate and can be applied for fast database screening. However, due to the simplification, 2D models are not as accurate as 3D pharmacophores in discriminating active compounds from inactive decoys. For more information about both strategies, the reader is referred to a recently published review [7].

15.1.2 Ligand Docking

The increase of available structural data of protein–ligand complexes has accelerated the development of structure-based methods. Today, protein–ligand docking is considered the most important tool for structure-based drug design. The docking process can be divided into two major parts: (1) the placement of a molecule in a protein binding pocket and (2) the prediction of ligand affinities by a so-called scoring function [2]. Considering the complexity of the underlying thermodynamics of the ligand binding process, this evidently is a challenging task. After more than 20 years of development, a large number of docking programs and even more scoring functions are available (see also chapter 7 in this book). In contrast to pharmacophore screening approaches, the performance of docking methods is a trade-off between computational demand and accuracy. A major problem of many docking programs is that they do not take into account protein flexibility or do not consider protein/ligand desolvation processes. Only recently, docking programs were developed (e.g., AutoDock4 [8], GOLD4 (GOLD Cambridge Crystallographic Data Centre, Cambridge, UK. Available at http://www.ccdc.cam.ac.uk), Glide (Glide Schrödinger, Portland, OR. Available at http://www.schroedinger.com), or FlexE (FlexE BiosolveIT, St. Augustin, Germany. Available at http://biosolveit.de)) that consider protein flexibility to some extent (see also chapter 8 in this book). Another problem that often occurs in ligand docking is the correct placement and treatment of water molecules within the binding site, which represent putative ligand binding partners. Structure-based approaches are able to provide important information about the interaction between a ligand and a macromolecule, but the accurate prediction of the binding affinity is still an unsolved problem [9]. A detailed discussion of the limitations of docking and scoring programs can be found in recently published reviews [9, 10] and in chapter 6 of this book.

15.1.3 Virtual Screening

High-throughput screening of chemical libraries is a well-established method for finding new lead structures in early drug discovery. However, the increasing number of purchasable compounds makes fast and reliable prefiltering methods necessary to reduce the number of compounds selected for experimental testing. In contrast to high-throughput screening, virtual screening (VS) compounds are selected on the basis of computer-based prediction. In this way, VS approaches try to select the most promising compounds from supplier/in-house databases for biological testing. VS can be carried out by applying different approaches: by searching databases for molecules with chemical similarity to a set of known actives [7], by identifying compounds that match a given pharmacophore [11], or by fitting molecules into the three-dimensional structure of a macromolecular target [12]. In addition, prescreening filters are usually applied that filter out compounds with potentially poor pharmacokinetic properties or unwanted chemical reactivity. The secret to success in VS lies in the choice of an appropriate combination of methods [4, 9].

To evaluate the performance of a given VS technique, validation studies are usually carried out. For this purpose, known binders are pooled with a set of randomly selected compounds (called decoys) to assess how well the known binders "enrich" during the course of the screening process. There is a big debate as to how similar the decoys should be to the active molecules and what the ratio of actives and decoys should be [13–16]. Such considerations are relevant for the development of new methods; however, in actual drug discovery projects, at the end of the day, a newly discovered chemotype or a druglike lead structure represents the ultimate goal. Impressive enrichment rates of known actives will not be convincing when it is easy to separate them from the decoys solely on simple 1D descriptors such as molecular weight or protonation state [9]. For that purpose, some guidelines are given in the literature on how to assemble a right decoy set [14]. Since the early VS attempts, a plethora of application studies has been performed and the list of success stories is steadily growing. Despite the fact that VS is still a developing discipline, it has been reviewed frequently [5, 10, 12, 17], most recently in comprehensive overviews [4, 9, 18].

15.1.4
Binding Free Energy Calculations

Accurate prediction of binding affinities for a diverse set of ligands using scoring functions turns out to be genuinely difficult [12]. In general, this is a problem of subtraction of large numbers, inaccurately calculated, to arrive at a small number. The large numbers are the protein–ligand interaction energy on the one hand and the cost of bringing protein and ligand out of solvent and into a complex on the other hand. The result of this subtraction is the free energy of binding, the small number we want to know. As long as full protein–ligand flexibility and the complexity of protein–ligand–water interaction are not covered in docking and scoring, an accurate affinity prediction cannot be expected. Of course, more accurate methods may be considered. Among the most accurate today are thermodynamic integration/free energy calculation methods, which can sometimes calculate the differences in affinities between related molecules within 1.0 kcal/mol [19]. The problem with these methods is that they demand so much computation time as to be infeasible for a large compound selection usually studied in VS. Recent reports suggest that progress is being made in calculating absolute binding affinities, but these methods too remain very slow for docking screens, though they may be useful in rescoring docking hit lists [20–22].

To illustrate how structure-based VS in combination with pharmacophore searches can be applied successfully to the discovery of novel bioactive molecules, we have chosen two examples with experimental validation from our own work [23–27]. The selection of the two examples was made since they represent two common situations in early drug discovery programs. In the first example, we focus on the discovery of inhibitors for a new target – the histone arginine methyltransferase PRMT1 – for which the 3D structure was available but no potent druglike inhibitors were known. So, the challenging aspect here was to see whether target-based approaches are able to provide first bioactive molecules for further optimization. In the second example, we focus on an already validated drug target – the histamine H_3 receptor – for which several series of active antagonists were available. However, as for many other G-protein-coupled receptors (GPCR), the crystal structure of the histamine H_3 receptor has not been published yet. Thus, the main purpose of the applied computer-based approach was to see whether a combination of pharmacophore-based virtual screening and docking into a homology model is successful in identifying novel antagonists with yet unknown scaffolds.

15.2
Structure-Based VS for Histone Arginine Methyltransferase PRMT1 Inhibitors

Histones are subject to a whole set of different posttranslational modifications that set a pattern of molecular signals for the access of transcription factors toward DNA, the so-called histone code [28]. The histone N-termini, which are rich in arginine and lysine residues, protrude out of the histone octamers and undergo various types of posttranslational modifications such as acetylation, methylation, phosphorylation, ubiquitinylation, or sumoylation (for review, see Ref. [29]). The extent of chromatin condensation is regulated in part through these modifications, which have an impact on gene transcription and the maintenance of altered transcription after cell division. Today, histone acetylation and DNA methylation are epigenetic modifications that have been linked closely to the pathology of human cancers [30]. Since connections between histone methylation patterns and cancer progression have been recognized, histone methyltransferases constitute promising targets for future cancer treatment. Besides cofactor analogues like sinefungin, there are only a few nondruglike inhibitors of arginine methyltransferases available.

Since the X-ray structure of human PRMT1 was not available, we considered the homologous rat PRMT1 (sequence identity 95.1%) and PRMT3 (sequence identity 47.2%) to generate a 3D structure of the human enzyme [23, 31]. The rat PRMT1 X-ray structure [32] does not represent suitable target structure for VS. The crystal structure of rat PRMT1 was obtained at a nonphysiological pH value (pH 4.7; maximum enzymatic activity at pH 8.5). In addition, not all residues of the substrate binding site were resolved in the PRMT1 crystal structure. The N-terminal region (residue 1–40), including a helical section (helix αX) near to the binding pocket, is missing in the PRMT1 structure (disordered structure), but was resolved for the PRMT3 protein [33]. Therefore, the PRMT1 model was generated using the coordinates of the rat PRMT3 enzyme and subsequently minimized. The derived model was first validated by docking the substrate and cofactor into the binding pocket and by comparing the predicted binding mode with the experimental one. Since we found that the docking program GOLD was able to reproduce the correct position of the cocrystallized ligands (cosubstrate analogue *S*-adenosylhomocysteine (SAH) cocrystallized with PRMT3 (1F3L.pdb) and with PRMT1 (1OR8.pdb) and the arginine side chain of the substrate cocrystallized with PRMT1 (1OR8.pdb)) with RMSD values below 1.5 Å, we used the same approach for docking the ligands into the homology model of human PRMT1. We observed the same binding mode in the crystal structures and in the homology model for both the cofactor and the arginine side chain.

15.2.1 Structure-Based VS of the NCI Diversity Set

The PRMT1 model was used in a first step to virtually screen the NCI Diversity Set comprising 1990 structurally diverse molecules [23]. The 1990 compounds were derived from around 140 000 compounds submitted to the NCI from a range of sources worldwide. In using this diverse subset of molecules as a compound source, we were able to virtually screen a wide range of chemical structures for binding to PRMT1 in short time. The use of different molecular descriptors excluded compounds that seemed to have undesirable pharmacokinetic properties. The following limits were applied: molecular weight >150 Da and <500 Da, topological surface area (TPSA) <150 Å^2, and log$P$ < 7. In addition, compounds bearing metal ions were omitted from the data set. The remaining 1630 compounds were docked into the PMRT1 binding pocket using the program GOLD (default docking parameters). During the docking run, the substrate analogue *S*-adenosyl-homocysteine (SAH)

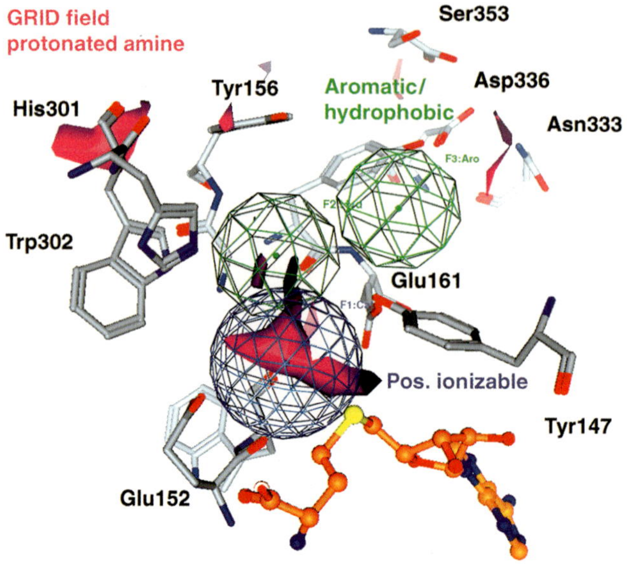

Figure 15.1 GRID-based pharmacophore model of PRMT1 inhibitors targeting the substrate binding site. The three pharmacophoric features are shown as colored spheres (positive ionizable: blue, hydrophobic: dark gray, aromatic: green). The calculated GRID field for a protonated amino group is shown in magenta and the bound cofactor analogue SAH is colored orange.

remained in the binding pocket and was regarded as a part of the protein. This was necessary to ensure that the VS identified substrate-competitive inhibitors and not compounds blocking the SAM binding site, which is present in many methyltransferases.

To analyze the thousands of docking poses, we generated a simple pharmacophore model derived from calculated GRID interaction fields [34]. A detailed map showing favorable areas of interaction within the binding pocket for a positively charged amino probe and an aromatic carbon probe was obtained and transformed into a pharmacophore model. The derived pharmacophore model, which consists of a cationic or hydrogen bond donor feature and two aromatic/hydrophobic features (Figure 15.1), was subsequently used to filter the GOLD docking results. Only docking poses that matched the pharmacophore model were selected. The selected 36 compounds were tested afterward in *in vitro* assays for their ability to inhibit PRMT1. For seven compounds (**1–7**, Figure 15.2), we could determine IC_{50} values in the range between 1.7 and 80 μM. For two compounds allantodapsone (IC_{50} 1.7 μM) and stilbamidine (IC_{50} 56 μM) (Figure 15.2), we could show a competition with the histone substrate and the inhibition of PRMT1 *in vivo*. The interaction of allantodapsone with the human PRMT1 substrate binding site is shown in Figure 15.3. A common feature of the active inhibitors is the interaction (hydrogen bond) of a basic or polar group with the acidic residue Glu152 that mimics the interaction of the Arg-guanidine group of the substrate peptide.

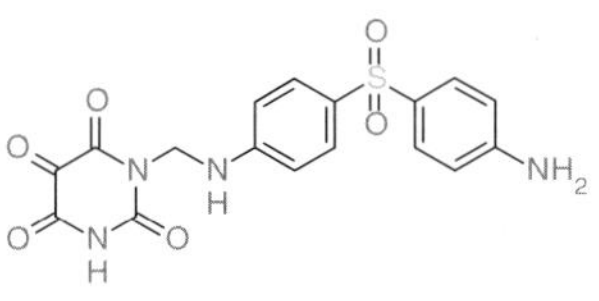

1
Allantodapsone

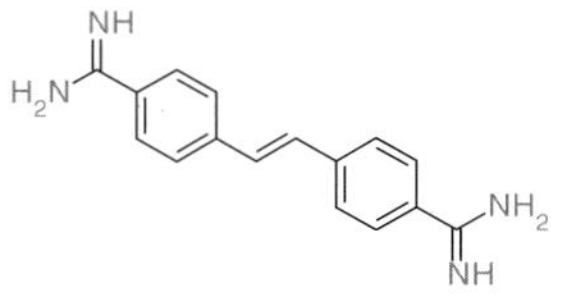

2
Stilbamidine

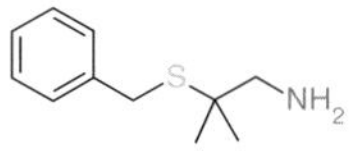

3

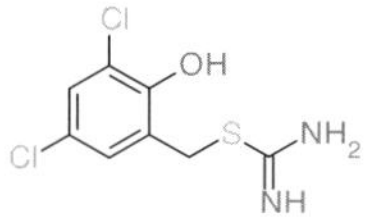

4

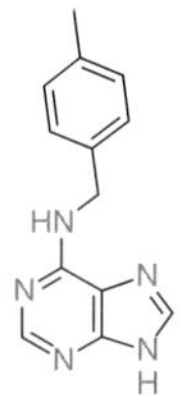

5

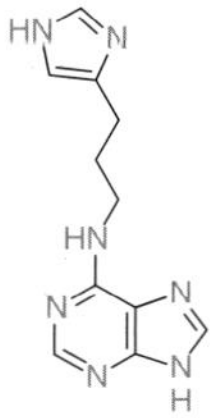

6

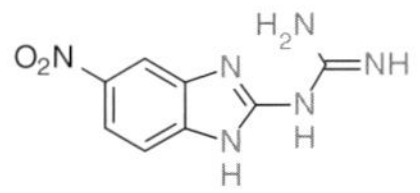

7

Figure 15.2 Structures of selected and experimentally tested PRMT1 VS hits.

15.2.2
Pharmacophore-Based VS

Based on the successful VS of the diversity subset of the NCI, we expanded our search for novel PRMT inhibitors to larger compound collections. Therefore, the Chembridge database containing 328 000 molecules [24] was screened. Since we were interested in novel leadlike PRMT inhibitors, we filtered the Chembridge database for molecules with a molecular weight below 400 Da, a TPSA below 150 $Å^2$, and containing at least one nitrogen atom. This resulted in 189 000 molecules that were converted into a multiconformer library comprising 19 million conformations. This library was first virtually screened using a structure-based pharmacophore model. We used the LigandScout software (Inteligand, Vienna, Austria) to derive the pharmacophore from the PRMT1–allantodapsone complex. LigandScout is a program for developing structure-based pharmacophore models based on a given protein–ligand complex [35]. The derived pharmacophore model, shown in Figure 15.4, contains one hydrogen bond donor (interaction with side chain carboxylate of Glu152 and backbone CO of Glu152) and one hydrogen bond acceptor function (interaction with side chain OH of Tyr156), as well as two hydrophobic/aromatic features. In addition, we used 1 included volume and 23 excluded volumes on the basis of allantodapsone structure and the surrounding amino acid residues.

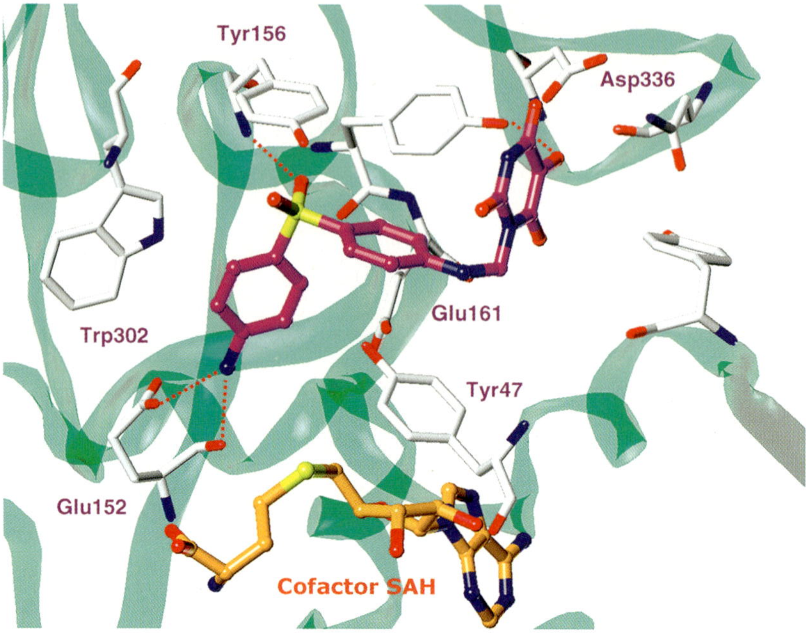

Figure 15.3 Interaction of the inhibitor allantodapsone (colored magenta) with the PRMT1 substrate binding site. Hydrogen bonds are shown as red dashed lines. The cofactor analogue SAH is colored orange and the protein backbone is shown as cyan ribbon.

LigandScout generates the excluded volumes on the basis of the Cα atoms of amino acids defining the binding pocket.

In the subsequent pharmacophore search, the screened compounds were required to match at least four out of the five essential pharmacophoric features. The screening resulted in 6232 compounds (3.3%) that passed the LigandScout pharmacophore model. Since it was likely that not all the 6232 hits were PRMT1 inhibitors, we further filtered the compound selection by carrying out a docking study.

The 6232 compounds were docked subsequently into the substrate binding pocket of PRMT1 containing the SAH molecule as described before. Due to the fact that docking scores are not good discriminators between true actives and false positives, we not only focused on the derived GoldScores but also used additional filters for selecting potential candidates for the biological testing. Using the SVL script language within MOE (MOE 2008.10, Chemical Computing Group, Toronto, Canada. Available at http://www.chemcomp.com), we filtered the docking output for appropriate poses that showed a similar binding mode as the known PRMT1 inhibitors allantodapsone and stilbamidine. We calculated the distances to amino acids of the binding pocket that were already identified as essential binding partners (i.e., Glu152 and Tyr156). These two distance constraints reduced the number of potential hits down to 370. Among the top-ranked 100 docking poses that fulfilled the distance constraints (hydrogen bond with distance <3.5 Å to Glu152 and

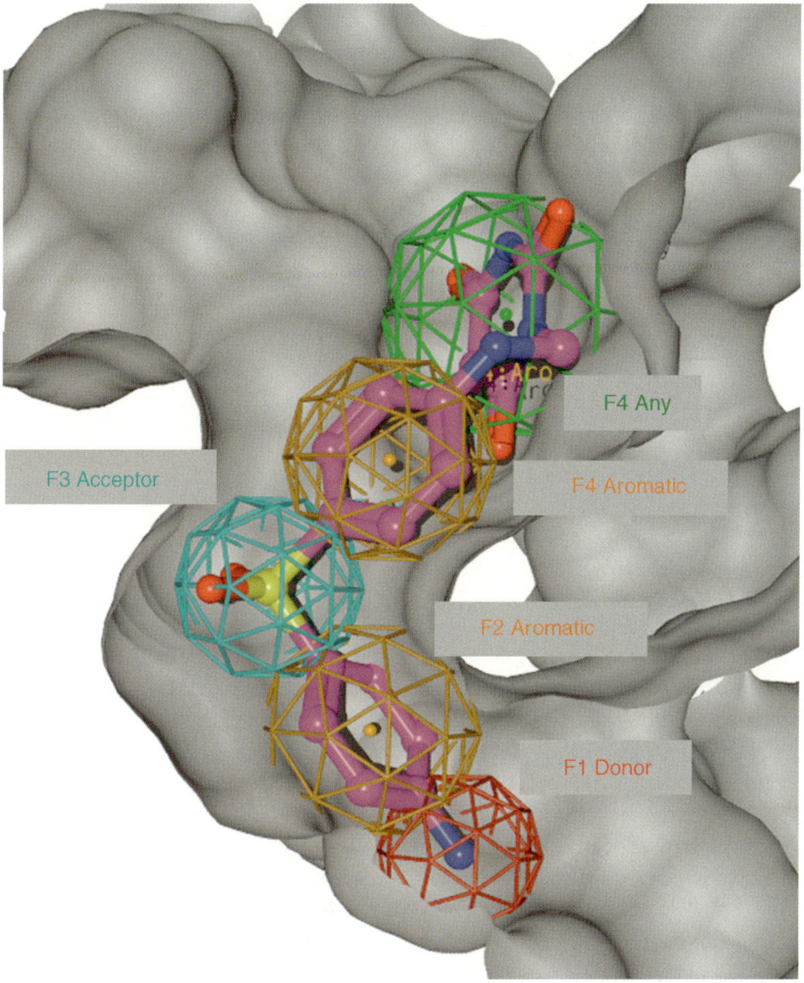

Figure 15.4 Structure-based pharmacophore model derived from allantodapsone docked to the PRMT1 substrate binding pocket. The individual features are annotated.

Tyr156), we selected manually nine compounds from clusters of similar molecules (**8–16**, Figure 15.5). The selection was not done automatically, but all 100 protein–inhibitor complexes were analyzed visually. Thus, the derived docking poses were checked whether they show specific interactions with the enzyme (hydrogen bonds, charge–charge interactions) or just van der Waals interactions that often lead to high docking scores but usually not to high biological activity. Also, compounds that contain larger parts that are not completely buried in the binding pocket but rather face out of it were removed from the hit list. This careful inspection resulted in nine compounds that were tested afterward in an *in vitro* assay for their ability to inhibit hPRMT1. All nine selected compounds showed IC_{50} values in the low micromolar range (Table 15.1).

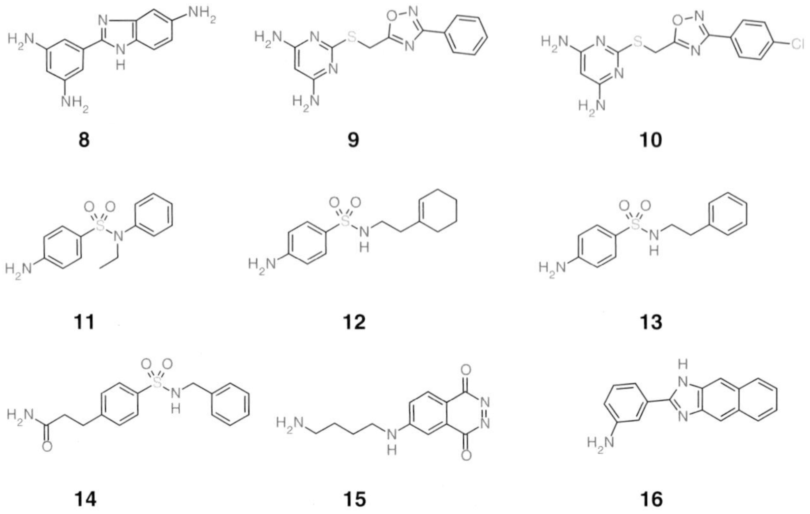

Figure 15.5 Chemical structures of nine selected and experimentally tested PRMT1 hits from the pharmacophore-based screening.

Of the nine compounds assayed, the aniline derivative **6** is the most potent hPRMT1 inhibitor (Table 15.1). The docking results show that the *p*-aminobenzenesulfonamide fragment of **4–6** adopts a similar orientation in the binding pocket as the corresponding element in the allantodapsone structure (Figure 15.4). The dapsone fragment of allantodapsone as well as the *p*-aminobenzenesulfonamide group of the novel inhibitors show two hydrogen bonds to the side chain and the

Table 15.1 Inhibition of hPRMT1 and structural similarity between the novel inhibitors and the reference compound allantodapsone.

Compound	$IC_{50} \pm SE$ (μM) hPRMT1	Tanimoto coefficient MACCS keys	Tanimoto coefficient graph-3-point pharmacophore	Actual docking rank GOLD
6000016 (**8**)	34 ± 17	0.28	0.33	45
7112201 (**9**)	37 ± 11	0.47	0.32	276
7155176 (**10**)	22 ± 2	0.45	0.30	311
7736382 (**11**)	30 ± 2	0.54	0.36	28
6689772 (**12**)	17 ± 3	0.48	0.27	158
7280948 (**13**)	13 ± 3	0.54	0.27	77
7789734 (**14**)	15 ± 5	0.57	0.37	12
5784982 (**15**)	34 ± 8	0.43	0.29	439
5756663 (**16**)	14 ± 1	0.25	0.27	42

The Tanimoto similarity indices are calculated on the basis of MACCS keys and graph-3-point pharmacophore fingerprints. The actual docking rank from the docking of the 6236 Chembridge compounds is indicated.

backbone of Glu152. In case of the more potent inhibitors **5** and **6**, the alkylbenzene and alkylcyclohexene rings interact with aromatic residues at the binding pocket (Tyr147 and Tyr160), whereas the less potent and smaller analogue **4** is not able to interact with these aromatic residues. Interestingly, the sulfonamide substructure was also identified as a binding motif in the structurally diverse amide **7**. However, the sulfonamide group of **7** is not involved in a hydrogen bond as observed for the inhibitors **5** and **6**. In case of the aromatic amine derivatives (**1**, **2**, **3**, and **9**), compound **9** with a single amino group in *meta*-position of the aromatic ring shows the most potent inhibitory activity. The aromatic nitrogen atom donates hydrogen bonds to the side chain and backbone CO of Glu152 as observed for allantodapsone. Compound **9** also forms van der Waals interactions with the two aromatic residues Tyr147 and Tyr160 as detected for the other potent inhibitors. Thus, besides the hydrogen bond to Glu152, van der Waals interaction also with the two aromatic residues seems to be a prerequisite for high inhibitory activity. It is interesting to see that the guanidine group of the Arg substrate can be mimicked not only by basic amino groups but also by an amide representing an appropriate binding motif. Based on the obtained docking poses, a qualitative interpretation of the structure–activity relationships was possible, whereas no significant correlation was obtained between docking scores and activity data.

In order to analyze the structural similarity between the retrieved Chembridge compounds and the known inhibitor allantodapsone used for the pharmacophore generation, we calculated similarity indices on the basis of MACCS keys and graph-3-point pharmacophore fingerprints. In Table 15.1, the Tanimoto similarity coefficients are listed for the nine novel inhibitors. Using the MACCS keys, the Tanimoto coefficients are all below 0.60 (graph-3-point pharmacophore <0.4), indicating the low structural similarity between the nine novel inhibitors and allantodapsone. Thus, although we applied a clearly defined pharmacophore for the VS, the identified hits represent different chemotypes.

In order to estimate the enrichment rate of the VS, we carried out two experiments. First, we randomly selected a subset of 500 compounds from the NCI Diversity Set and used it as set of decoys for the VS. We docked the randomly selected compounds and the nine identified active inhibitors into the hPRMT1 model using GOLD and the same settings as described before. All nine inhibitors were identified among the top 30% of the data set resulting in an enrichment rate of 16.7. Ligand enrichment among top-ranking hits is a key metric of VS. To assess an exact hit rate and enrichment factor, a biological testing of all compounds would be necessary. However, since we only had a limited amount of hPRMT1 protein available, it was not possible to screen a large number of compounds. Nonetheless, in order to determine whether the results we obtained would be different from those that would be attained from simply randomly sampling, five compounds (for structures, see Ref. [24]) were chosen at random, and their ability to inhibit hPRMT1 was also tested. None of the randomly chosen compounds from the NCI Diversity Set showed any inhibiting effect at 40 μM, whereas all nine compounds chosen by VS did exhibit an inhibition below 35 μM suggesting that a significant enrichment had occurred. When analyzing the obtained docking ranks (Table 15.2) and the interaction of the five inactive NCI

Table 15.2 Docking rank of the five inactive compounds of the NCI Diversity Set (500 selected compounds) observed in the PRMT1 VS.

Compound from NCI Diversity Set	VS rank
NSC 25141	104
NSC 143099	224
NSC 97845	231
NSC 134754	248
NSC 118176	473

For molecular structures, see Ref. [24].

compounds (not shown), we observed that none of the compounds is among the top 20% (top 100) of the NCI Diversity Set ranking list and that most of the molecules did not show an interaction with the active site residue Glu152.

In general, the VS on PRMT1 was successful. Both the selected compounds identified as virtual hits and the randomly selected NCI compounds predicted to be inactive were correctly classified. Of course, the limited number of compounds tested cannot be used to make a final judgment of the performance and accuracy of the applied VS approach. However, from the point of view of a medicinal chemist, it is more important to obtain biologically active compounds or ideas for further analogues out of a VS campaign than producing overfitted models based on retrospecitve studies.

15.3 Identification of Nanomolar Histamine H_3 Receptor Antagonists by Structure- and Pharmacophore-Based VS

The human histamine H_3 receptor (hH_3R) [36] is a G-protein-coupled receptor that modulates the release of various neurotransmitters in the central and peripheral nervous system, and therefore is a potential target in the therapy of numerous diseases, including several neurodegenerative disorders. Although ligands addressing this receptor are already known, the discovery of alternative lead structures still represents a challenge (for review, see Ref. [37]). In order to find new hH_3R ligands, initially the derivatives of the intrinsic ligand histamine were generated, leading to the class of imidazole-containing compounds. Due to several potential drawbacks of the imidazole moiety (interaction with P450 enzymes and low CNS penetration), great effort was put into the replacement of this moiety, resulting in the nowadays heterogeneous class of nonimidazole ligands containing mostly piperidine, pyrrolidine, or structurally related groups. [38].

We applied two well-established tools for *in silico* screening, namely, molecular docking into a hH_3R homology model and a pharmacophore-based search, to search for novel lead structures. The hH_3R ligand data set is extremely challenging in this respect as the ligands are in most cases highly flexible and different antagonist classes interact with different sets of receptor site points (Figure 15.6). Furthermore, the low number of mutational studies published for the hH_3R merely indicated the approximate position of the ligands in the hH_3R model rather than giving a detailed view on the amino acid side chains involved in ligand binding. Still, the existence of a large data set of experimentally tested hH_3R antagonists aided the validation of various VS techniques.

15.3.1
Generation of Homology Model of the hH_3R and hH_3R Antagonist Complexes

A model of the human histamine H_3 receptor was generated based on the crystal structure of bovine rhodopsin (PDB code 1HZX) as described in detail [27]. The main difficulty during the model building was the generation of a ligand-compatible binding site geometry, which was complicated due to the relatively low number of mutation data and the fact that at several sites small residues in the rhodopsin reference structure had been mutated to more voluminous amino acids in the hH_3R protein. Thus, after initial model generation, the binding site was blocked by amino acid side chains and did not allow the automated docking of hH_3R antagonists. In order to still allow an objective generation of ligand–receptor complexes, ligand information was included in the placement of amino acids in an "inverse docking" approach, which resulted in a binding site geometry capable of accommodating sterically demanding inverse hH_3R agonists. Different from a "normal" docking approach where a binding pocket conformation is used as a filter in screening structure databases for compatible ligands, here a ligand was used for retrieving the most suitable binding site. Antagonist **17** is a high-affinity ligand with a pK_i value of 10.04 (Figure 15.6) [39]. Consequently, a good fit between the ligand and the binding site can be expected. Based on this assumption, **17** was flexibly docked into alternative binding site geometries, which varied in the placement of amino acid side chains, for which clashes between the initially placed ligand and the receptor have been observed after adding side chains using the program SCWRL [40]. In total, we generated ~40 000 different binding site models that we considered for the ligand docking

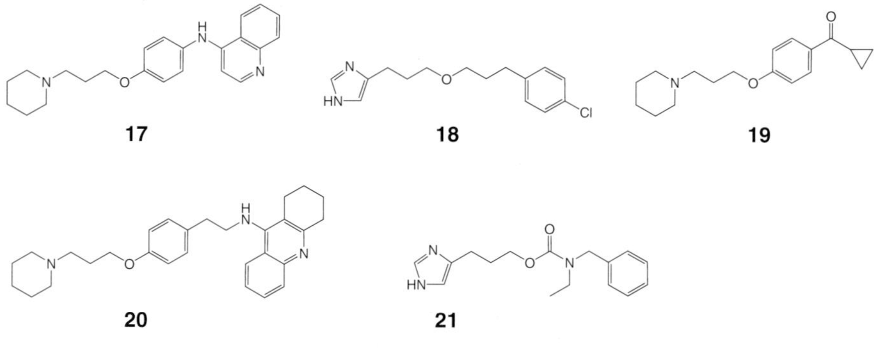

Figure 15.6 Structures of hH_3R antagonists mentioned in the text.

study using the GOLD program. The approximate position of antagonists in the hH_3R binding pocket was thereby known from mutational studies that showed that D3.32 in TM3 and E5.46 in TM5 were the major sites of interaction [41]. During docking compound **17** into all alternative binding sites, a distance constraint between the piperidyl nitrogen of antagonist **17** and D3.32 in TM3 was applied. D3.32 is the conserved aspartate residue in aminergic GPCR that is known as interaction site for agonists and antagonists containing an amino function. The resulting complexes were then ranked according to the obtained GoldScore. The binding site geometry for which **17** obtained the highest docking score was considered to be the most likely geometry and thus further used in subsequent MD simulation to refine the hH_3R–ligand complex.

The incorporation of ligand information into the generation of the binding site has also been discussed recently by Evers and Klebe for the NK1 receptor and was shown to significantly improve the quality of the obtained binding site [42]. Similar to the approach described here, Evers and Klebe generated 100 preliminary homology models and used a docking approach to choose a suitable binding site geometry. The approach herein described differs in that a flexible docking of the antagonist was carried out and that the ranking of the obtained complexes was based solely on the docking scores rather than the establishment of required contacts known from mutational studies. Although computationally more demanding, this strategy was given preference as no detailed mutational data were available to a priori exclude or favor any receptor–ligand complex.

15.3.2 Validation of the Homology Model by Docking Known Antagonists into the hH_3R Binding Site

For validating the hH_3R binding site obtained from the simulation of the compound **17**/hH_3R complex, a screening procedure was additionally carried out against a focused library, as several recently carried out VS studies showed [14, 15] that VS by protein–ligand docking can result in an artificial enrichment when screening against a random nonfocused library [43]. As a more robust alternative, a validation strategy is suggested in which docking scores of actives were compared to the scores obtained when docking a focused library comprising molecules with properties, similar to the actives. As active molecules, we used a focused in-house data set of 418 experimentally tested hH_3R antagonists with a pK_i range from 5.29 to 10.04.

For screening the World Drug Index (WDI) and the Maybridge Database (MDB) (in total ~116 000 compounds), in a first step ligands comprising an imidazole, a secondary or tertiary amine moiety, were selected (compounds comprising primary amines were excluded due to their unfavorable physicochemical properties) and a molecular weight cutoff of 600 Da was applied resulting in 13 524 compounds. In the next step, the distances $D(i, j)$ between all pairs of 138 active hH_3R antagonists with a binding affinity of $pK_i \geq 8$ were calculated using formula (15.1), which takes into account the 1D properties, (i) number of hydrogen bond donors (N_D), (ii) number of hydrogen bond acceptors (N_A), and (iii) number of nonpolar atoms (N_{NP}):

$$D(i,j) = \sqrt{(N_D(i)-N_D(j))^2 + (N_A(i)-N_A(j))^2 + (N_{NP}(i)-N_{NP}(j))^2} \qquad (15.1)$$

Then, the average distance D_{min} was calculated as an average of the individual distances $D(i,j)$ over all active compounds, which resulted in $D_{min} = 0.55$ for the set of 138 hH_3R antagonists. A focused library was then generated by choosing ligands from the WDI and MDB that were found within the distance D_{min} to at least one of the 138 highly active hH_3R compounds and – as a further constraint – contained a secondary or tertiary amine moiety or an imidazole group. A total of 3298 compounds fulfilled these requirements and were selected as decoy set.

The results of screening against a nonfocused library (11.4% WDI compounds ranking among the 80% top-ranked hH_3R antagonists) yielded a significantly better enrichment compared to the results obtained when screening against a focused library (23% WDI compounds ranking among the 80% top-ranked hH_3R antagonists), as can be recognized in the calculated ROC curves (Figure 15.7). This can be explained by the differences in chemical space spanned by the hH_3R antagonists and randomly chosen WDI compounds. Only 11% of the randomly chosen compounds fulfilled the criterion required for a compound to be part of the focused library. Preselected WDI compounds with properties (e.g., hydrogen bond acceptors, hydrogen bond donors, and $\log P$) resembling those of active hH_3R compounds have *per se* an increased likelihood of representing a hit. Exemplary ligand placement obtained during this docking procedure for a potent imidazole- and piperidine-containing hH_3R antagonist is shown in Figure 15.8 ((a) **18** and (b) **19**, respectively).

15.3.3 Pharmacophore-Based VS

Three pharmacophore models were defined based on the template molecules **17** (pK_i 10.04), **20** (pK_i 9.48), and **21** (pK_i 7.19) (Figure 15.6) [39] in their supposedly bioactive conformation, derived from the docking study. The choice of chemical moieties was thereby based on chemical functionalities observed in validated hH_3R antagonists and inspection of the hH_3R binding pocket. The linker moiety and the adjacent hydrophobic/π-electron rich system were placed in a cleft between TM 3, 6, and 7 of the hH_3R model. In order to decrease the number of false positives obtained from the application of the pharmacophore model, the shape of the molecules and forbidden volumes defined on the amino acid side chains of the receptor model (using the same approach as described for the PRMT1 pharmacophore model in Section 15.2.2) were included into the pharmacophore model of compound **17** (Figure 15.9).

The pharmacophore model was then used to screen MDB and WDI compounds for which conformational models had been generated, using the program Catalyst (Accelrys Inc., San Diego, CA, 2002). For validation purposes, again the database of 418 active hH_3R antagonists was simultaneously processed in order to assess the quality of the pharmacophore models in terms of retrieving known active hH_3R ligands. Application of the combined pharmacophore models retrieved 369 of 398 (93%) hH_3R ligands with a $pK_i > 7$. When applying the combined pharmacophore

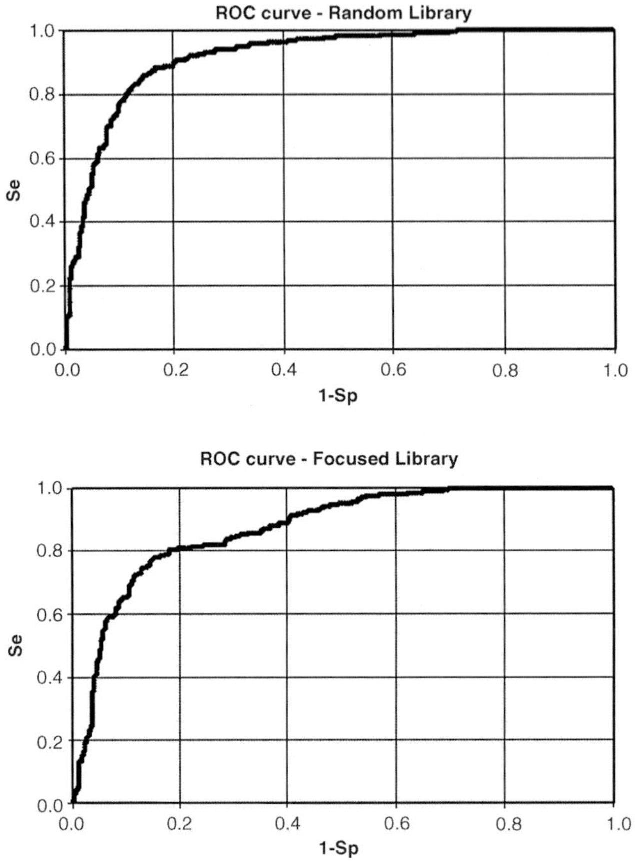

Figure 15.7 *Top*: ROC curve obtained when carrying out GOLD docking of hH_3R actives against a library of randomly selected compounds from the WDI and MDB. ROC curves are obtained by plotting the sensitivity (Se) versus the specificity (Sp) of a VS experiment. Sensitivity is the percentage of truly active compounds selected from the VS workflow and is calculated by dividing the number of true positives by the sum of true positives and false negatives. Specificity, on the other hand, is the percentage of truly inactive compounds being correctly identified by the VS experiment. It is calculated by dividing the number of true negative results by the sum of true negatives and false positives. Thus, in ROC curves, the activity signal (i.e., % actives) is plotted versus the detected noise (% inactives) at all possible detection thresholds. *Bottom*: ROC curve obtained when carrying our docking of 418 hH_3R actives against a focused library of MDB/WDI compounds.

model in screening WDI and MDB, 2668 compounds (2.5% of the entire databases) were identified.

In a second screening run, the application of a leave-one-out (LOO) filter comprising more pharmacophoric features was applied to favor the retrieval of compounds that would better fit the physicochemical properties of the hH_3R binding site, which should ensure receptor selectivity. Further screening of the 2668 WDI and MDB compounds with the leave-one-out filter reduced the number of hits to 320.

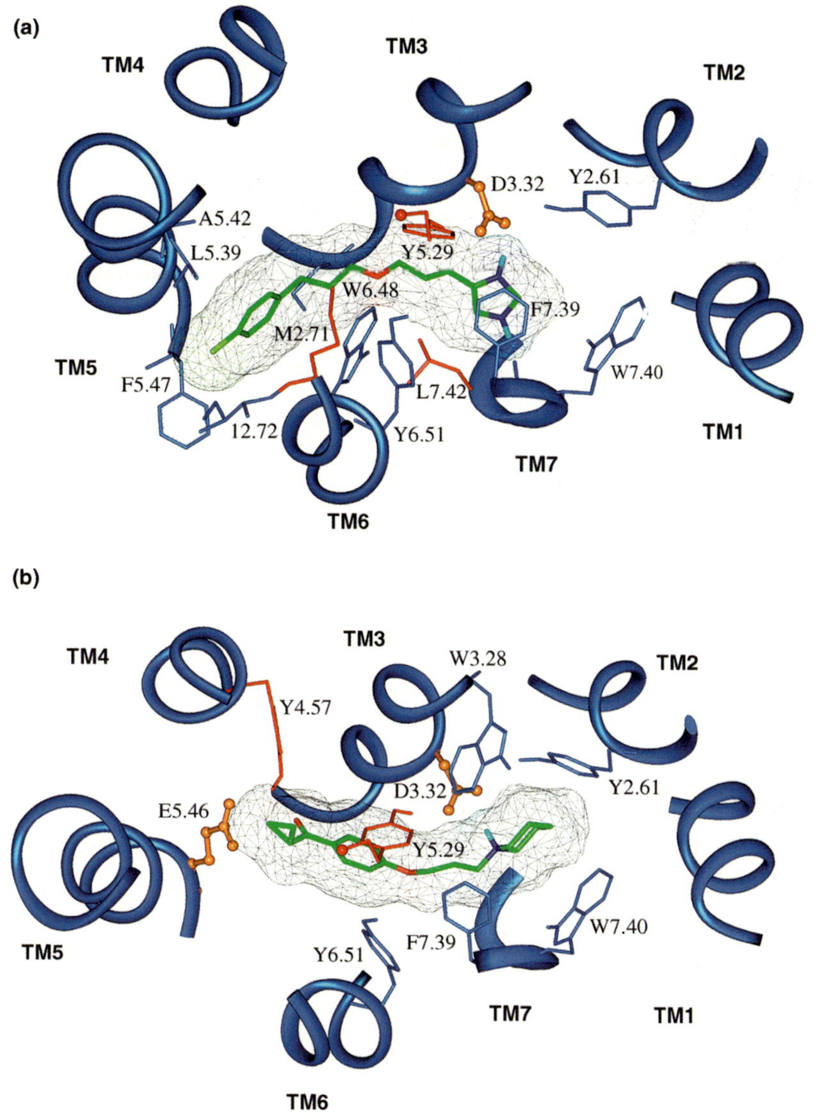

Figure 15.8 (a) Antagonist **18** (pK_i 8.00) in the hH_3R binding site. (b) Antagonist **19** (pK_i 8) in the hH_3R binding site. Both antagonists are participating in hydrogen bonds to D3.32 in TM3. The molecular volume of the antagonists is displayed by lines. Transmembrane domains (TM) are shown as blue ribbon, connecting loop regions are not displayed.

When screening the database of 418 hH_3R antagonists, only 25% could be retrieved by the LOO filter, although the filter was capable of filtering out 96% of the inactive (p$K_i < 6$) and 84% of the moderately active hH_3R antagonists ($6 < pK_i < 7$). In order to ensure that compounds selected by the pharmacophore-based screening could be accommodated into the hH_3R binding site, the 320 hits were docked into the hH_3R

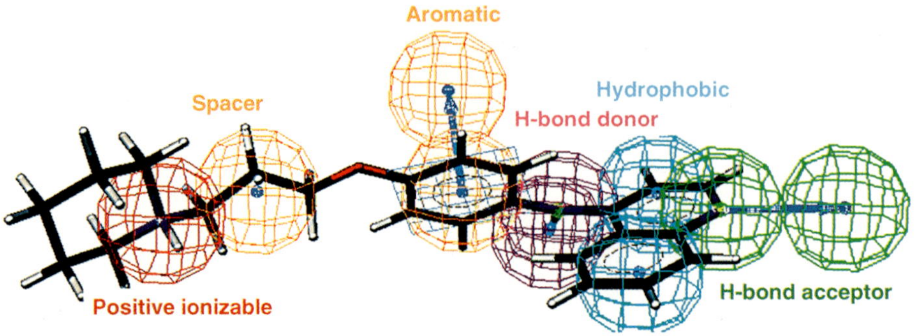

Figure 15.9 Features in antagonist **17** used for the definition of a leave-one-out pharmacophore model. While the positive ionizable moiety/imidazole group and the spacer moiety were required in all models, all other features were allowed to be missed in a combinatorial way resulting in a leave-one-out filter embracing five individual filters.

binding site and ranked according to their GoldScore. From the complexes that scored among the top 100, 7 compounds showing a different scaffold were manually selected and submitted to experimental testing. This limitation was made due to restrictions concerning the throughput of the biological assay.

In order to assess whether all these compounds selected were also compatible with the hH_3R binding site, the compounds selected via the pharmacophore search were additionally docked using GOLD. After ranking and clustering the molecules, the candidate compounds and validated hH_3R antagonists interestingly showed the same maximum GoldScores as observed in the docking described in Section 15.3.2 indicating that the prescreening with Catalyst was successful in selecting compounds that later resulted in a high docking score. By visual inspection we manually selected seven structurally diverse top-ranked compounds from the MDB fulfilling the pharmacophore requirements for experimental testing (Figure 15.10).

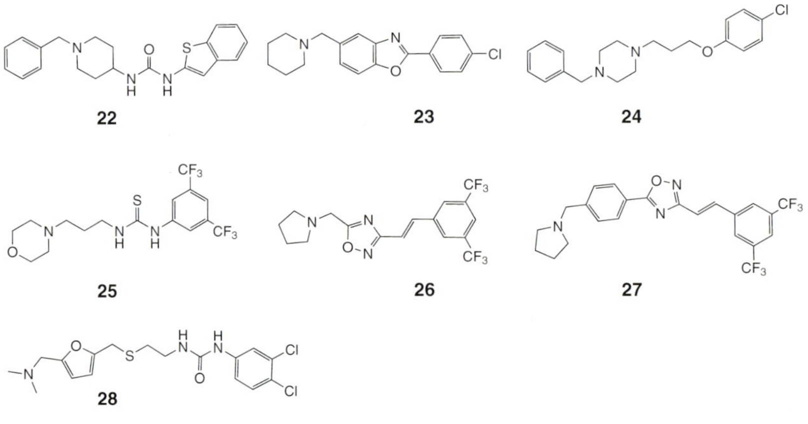

Figure 15.10 Selected hits when screening the MDB with the derived pharmacophore model and subsequently docking the compounds into the hH_3R model.

Table 15.3 Biological data and structural similarities of H_3 receptor VS hits.

Compound	K_i (μM)	Tanimoto coefficient graph-3-point pharmacophore	Tanimoto coefficient MACCS keys	Docking rank GOLD/GoldScore
HTS-07217 (**22**)	2.5	0.45	0.65	39 (72.89)
PD-00043 (**23**)	1.0	0.55	0.73	18 (79.21)
RJC-03033 (**24**)	0.38	0.59	0.83	9 (81.10)
BTB-12683 (**25**)	3.7	0.51	0.73	56 (65.97)
CD-04850 (**26**)	6.3	0.47	0.60	79 (60.13)
CD-06177 (**27**)	2.9	0.56	0.63	5 (82.21)
BTB-08079 (**28**)	0.08	0.45	0.57	1 (87.89)

Tanimoto coefficients between the seven hit structures and the most similar analogues were calculated on the basis of MACCS keys and graph-3-point pharmacophore fingerprints. The actual docking rank from the docking of the 320 Maybridge compounds that passed the pharmacophore model is indicated.

15.3.4 Experimental Testing of the Identified Hits

The seven compounds depicted in Figure 15.10 were purchased from Maybridge and experimentally tested for binding to the hH_3R in a competition binding experiment. All seven compounds are active in the range between 0.08 and 6.3 μM (Table 15.3). Two compounds BTB-08 079 (**28**) and RJC-03 033 (**24**) are highly potent and active in the nanomolar range [27]. In order to determine the structural similarity between the seven retrieved Maybridge compounds and the 418 hH_3R ligands, we calculated similarity indices on the basis of MACCS keys and graph-3-point pharmacophore fingerprints. Using the graph-3-point pharmacophore fingerprint, the similarity cutoffs are all below 0.60 indicating the low structural similarity between the seven hits and the original hH_3R ligand structures (Table 15.3) Using the MACCS key, we found several piperidine derivatives in the original data set as analogues of RJC-03 033 (**24**). Interestingly, for the most potent hit BTB-08 079 (**28**, 79 nM), the lowest similarity with the original hH3R ligand structures was observed (Figure 15.11). The dimethylaminofuran fragment, which is already known from the potent histamine H_2 receptor antagonist ranitidine, had not been reported before as structural element of potent H_3R antagonists.

15.3.5 Discussion of the Applied VS Strategies

Compared to the receptor-based VS by docking, application of the pharmacophore-based search resulted in significantly improved results. While in the docking approach 66.6% of the hH_3R ligands were retrieved, though limiting the number of WDI and MDB compounds to approximately 1720 structures (1.6%), application of a pharmacophore-based search allowed retrieval of 93% of active compounds, while

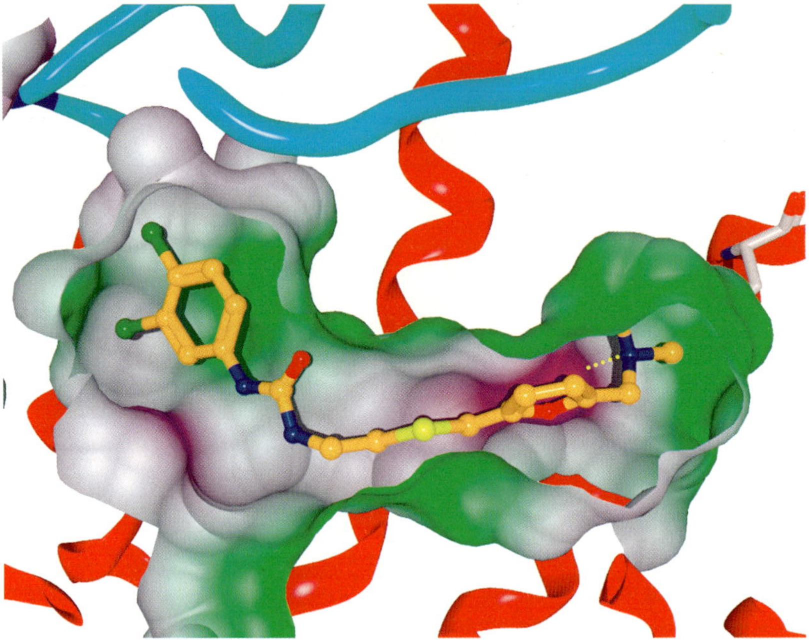

Figure 15.11 Docked BTB-08 079 (**28**) (orange) in the hH_3R binding site. The hydrogen bond to the key amino acid D3.32 is shown as yellow dashed line. The molecular surface of the binding pocket is colored according to the hydrophobicity (green: hydrophobic, magenta: hydrophilic).

reducing the number of WDI and MDB structures to 2668 compounds (2.5%). The ideal strategy for the flexible hH_3R ligand data set appeared to be a combined approach comprising a prescreening of commercial databases with relatively loose pharmacophore models that mainly reflect the available volume in the binding site (e.g., by considering shape queries of sterically demanding ligands and forbidden volumes derived from ligand superposition) and some essential requirements for binding such as the protonated head group. This way, the number of compounds for the subsequent docking was already significantly reduced to 320, which allowed the application of docking settings with better discriminatory properties (e.g., larger number of calculated poses, better sampling rate). Although the number of selected hits for testing was low (seven Maybridge compounds), the high success rate that we observed supports the chosen strategy and shows the possibility of identifying highly active compounds with a novel scaffold.

In an ideal situation, VS is carried out using a high-resolution structure of a ligand-bound protein. However, very often the crystal structure of the protein of interest is not available, or shows a low resolution, or has not been crystallized in the ligand-bound form. In such cases, structural protein models can be generated to get a detailed representation of the binding site. It is somehow surprising that homology models often provide significant enrichment of actives against a background of decoys. A variety of successful VS studies based on protein models have been published in the last few years [44–46]. In a retrospective study, Gilson and coworkers [47] analyzed five drug targets for which the crystal structure was available. The VS study showed that some homology models (based on a template with a sequence identity above 30%) yielded enrichment equal to or even greater than that obtained with the crystal structure of the target. They also observed that there is no smooth correlation between enrichment rate and sequence identity of the template. In general, it is difficult to predict a priori whether docking into a homology model yields reliable or misleading geometries. However, by critical validation of homology models and combination with pharmacophore-based screening, the accuracy and success of VS campaigns can be achieved.

15.4 Summary

Despite many technical challenges, structure-based VS plays an important role in drug discovery. Ligand docking and scoring technologies have steadily improved and the importance of the adequate validation of pragmatic VS protocols is now well recognized. While both ligand- and structure-based approaches have already demonstrated their value in the identification of novel lead compounds for a variety of targets, there is still the challenge to improve the predictive accuracy of scoring functions, particularly to enable scoring-based methods to have a greater impact in guiding lead optimization.

Another point to address is protein flexibility. The problem for structure-based approaches is that for a flexible target it is not known in advance which conformation the target will adopt in response to the binding of a particular ligand [48]. The most accurate scoring function is useless if the protein undergoes a conformational shift during ligand binding. Flexible fit phenomena are usually not captured in current virtual screening campaigns. However, several strategies have been developed recently that might help to overcome the current limitations [49–51].

First and foremost, as stated in a recent perspective by Schneider [52], we cannot expect that *in silico* screening studies yield perfect results, simply because no model is perfect. To demand a perfect biological response profile for a given screening compound is unrealistic and bears the risk of leading to overtrained models. Still, a combination of different methods and the application of intelligent filtering strategies might help to avoid false positives and rescue false negatives in VS. And, last but not least, since the chemical space is only partially covered by current compound libraries, it is very unlikely to identify hits with nanomolar affinity for any protein target.

Acknowledgment

Financial Support from the Deutsche Krebshilfe for the work on PRMT inhibitors is kindly acknowledged.

References

1 Hawkins, P.C.D., Skillman, A.G., and Nicholls, A. (2006) Comparison of shape-matching and docking as virtual screening tools. *Journal of Medicinal Chemistry*, **50**, 74–82.

2 Evers, A., Hessler, G., Matter, H., and Klabunde, T. (2005) Virtual screening of biogenic amine-binding G-protein coupled receptors: comparative evaluation of protein- and ligand-based virtual screening protocols. *Journal of Medicinal Chemistry*, **48**, 5448–5465.

3 Kirchmair, J., Laggner, C., Wolber, G., and Langer, T. (2005) Comparative analysis of protein-bound ligand conformations with respect to catalyst's conformational space subsampling algorithms. *Journal of Chemical Information and Modeling*, **45**, 422–430.

4 Waszkowycz, B. (2008) Towards improving compound selection in structure-based virtual screening. *Drug Discovery Today*, **13**, 219–226.

5 Stahl, M., Guba, W., and Kansy, M. (2006) Integrating molecular design resources within modern drug discovery research: the Roche experience. *Drug Discovery Today*, **11**, 326–333.

6 Ahlstrom, M.M., Ridderstrom, M., Luthman, K., and Zamora, I. (2005) Virtual screening and scaffold hopping based on GRID molecular interaction fields. *Journal of Chemical Information and Modeling*, **45**, 1313–1323.

7 Stahura, F.L. and Bajorath, J. (2005) New methodologies for ligand-based virtual screening. *Current Pharmaceutical Design*, **11**, 1189–1202.

8 Österberg, F., Morris, G.M., Sanner, G.M., Olson, A.J., and Goodsell, D.S. (2002) Automated docking to multiple target structures: incorporation of protein mobility and structural water heterogeneity in AutoDock. *Proteins: Structure, Function, and Genetics*, **46**, 34–40.

9 Klebe, G. (2006) Virtual ligand screening: strategies, perspectives and limitations. *Drug Discovery Today*, **11**, 580–594.

10 Tame, J. (2005) Scoring functions: the first 100 years. *Journal of Computer-Aided Molecular Design*, **19**, 445–451.

11 Kirchmair, J., Distinto, S., Schuster, D., Spitzer, G., Langer, T., and Wolber, G. (2008) Enhancing drug discovery through *in silico* screening: strategies to increase true positives retrieval rates. *Current Medicinal Chemistry*, **15**, 2040–2053.

12 Leach, A., Shoichet, B., and Peishoff, C. (2006) Prediction of protein–ligand interactions. Docking and scoring: successes and gaps. *Journal of Medicinal Chemistry*, **49**, 5851–5855.

13 Liebeschuetz, J. (2008) Evaluating docking programs: keeping the playing field level. *Journal of Computer-Aided Molecular Design*, **22**, 229–238.

14 Irwin, J.J. (2008) Community benchmarks for virtual screening. *Journal of Computer-Aided Molecular Design*, **22**, 193–199.

15 Good, A. and Oprea, T. (2008) Optimization of CAMD techniques 3. Virtual screening enrichment studies: a help or hindrance in tool selection? *Journal of Computer-Aided Molecular Design*, **22**, 169–178.

16 Cross, J., Thompson, D., Rai, B., Baber, C., Fan, K., Hu, Y., and Humblet, C. (2009) Comparison of several molecular docking programs: pose prediction and virtual screening accuracy. *Journal of Chemical Information and Modeling*, **49**, 1455–1474.

17 Kitchen, D.B., Decornez, H., Furr, J.R., and Bajorath, J. (2004) Docking and scoring in virtual screening for drug discovery: methods and applications. *Nature Reviews. Drug Discovery*, **3**, 935–949.

18 Hawkins, P., Warren, G., Skillman, A., and Nicholls, A. (2008) How to do an evaluation: pitfalls and traps. *Journal of Computer-Aided Molecular Design*, **22**, 179–190.

19 Pearlman, D.A. (2005) Evaluating the molecular mechanics Poisson–Boltzmann surface area free energy method using a congeneric series of ligands to p38 MAP kinase. *Journal of Medicinal Chemistry*, **48**, 7796–7807.

20 Chang, C.E. and Gilson, M.K. (2004) Free energy, entropy, and induced fit in host–guest recognition: calculations with the second-generation mining minima

algorithm. *Journal of the American Chemical Society*, **126**, 13156–13164.

21 Deng, Y. and Roux, B. (2006) Calculation of standard binding free energies: aromatic molecules in the T4 lysozyme L99A mutant. *Journal of Chemical Theory and Computation*, **2**, 1255–1273.

22 Jorgensen, W. (2009) Efficient drug lead discovery and optimization. *Accounts of Chemical Research*, **42**, 724–733.

23 Spannhoff, A., Heinke, R., Bauer, I., Trojer, P., Metzger, E., Gust, R., Schüle, R., Brosch, G., Sippl, W., and Jung, M. (2007) Target-based approach to inhibitors of histone arginine methyltransferases. *Journal of Medicinal Chemistry*, **50**, 2319–2325.

24 Heinke, R., Spannhoff, A., Meier, R., Trojer, P., Bauer, I., Jung, M., and Sippl, W. (2009) Virtual screening and biological characterization of novel histone arginine methyltransferase PRMT1 inhibitors. *ChemMedChem*, **4**, 69–77.

25 Uciechowska, U., Schemies, J., Neugebauer, R.C., Huda, E.-M., Schmitt, M.L., Meier, R., Verdin, E., Jung, M., and Sippl, W. (2008) Thiobarbiturates as sirtuin inhibitors: virtual screening, free-energy calculations, and biological testing. *ChemMedChem*, **3** 1965–1976.

26 Küblbeck, J., Jyrkkärinne, J., Poso, A., Turpeinen, M., Sippl, W., Honkakoski, P., and Windshügel, B. (2008) Discovery of substituted sulfonamides and thiazolidin-4-one derivatives as agonists of human constitutive androstane receptor. *Biochemical Pharmacology*, **76**, 1288–1297.

27 Schlegel, B., Laggner, C., Meier, R., Langer, T., Schnell, D., Seifert, R., Stark, H., Höltje, H.-D., and Sippl, W. (2007) Generation of a homology model of the human histamine H_3 receptor for ligand docking and pharmacophore-based screening. *Journal of Computer-Aided Molecular Design*, **21**, 437–453.

28 Jenuwein, T. and Allis, C.D. (2001) Translating the histone code. *Science*, **293**, 1074–1080.

29 Biel, M., Wascholowski, V., and Giannis, A. (2005) Epigenetics – an epicenter of gene regulation: histones and histone-modifying enzymes. *Angewandte Chemie, International Edition*, **44**, 3186–3216.

30 Schäfer, S. and Jung, M. (2005) Chromatin modifications as targets for new anticancer drugs. *Archiv der Pharmazie*, **338**, 347–357.

31 Bhaumik, S.R., Smith, E., and Shilatifard, A. (2007) Covalent modifications of histones during development and disease pathogenesis. *Nature Structural & Molecular Biology*, **14**, 1008–1016.

32 Zhang, X. and Cheng, X. (2003) Structure of the predominant protein arginine methyltransferase PRMT1 and analysis of its binding to substrate peptides. *Structure*, **11**, 509–520.

33 Zhang, X., Zhou, L., and Cheng, X. (2000) Crystal structure of the conserved core of protein arginine methyltransferase PRMT3. *EMBO Journal*, **19**, 3509–3519.

34 Goodford, P.J. (1985) A computational procedure for determining energetically favorable binding sites on biologically important macromolecules. *Journal of Medicinal Chemistry*, **28**, 849–857.

35 Wolber, G. and Langer, T. (2004) LigandScout: 3-D pharmacophores derived from protein-bound ligands and their use as virtual screening filters. *Journal of Chemical Information and Modeling*, **45**, 160–169.

36 Arrang, J.-M., Garbarg, M., and Schwartz, J.-C. (1983) Auto-inhibition of brain histamine release mediated by a novel class (H_3) of histamine receptor. *Nature*, **302**, 832–837.

37 Stark, H., Kathmann, M., Schlicker, E., Schunack, W., Schlegel, B., and Sippl, W. (2004) Medicinal chemical and pharmacological aspects of imidazole-containing histamine H_3 receptor antagonists. *Mini Reviews in Medicinal Chemistry*, **4**, 965–977.

38 Hancock, A.A. (2006) The challenge of drug discovery of a GPCR target: analysis of preclinical pharmacology of histamine H_3 antagonists/inverse agonists. *Biochemical Pharmacology*, **71**, 1103–1113.

39 Stark, H., Purand, K., Ligneau, X., Rouleau, A., Arrang, J.-M., Garbarg, M., Schwartz, J.-C., and Schunack, W. (1996) Novel carbamates as potent histamine H_3 receptor antagonists with high *in vitro* and oral *in vivo* activity. *Journal of Medicinal Chemistry*, **39**, 1157–1163.

40 Wang, Q., Canutescu, A.A., and Dunbrack, R.L. (2008) SCWRL and MolIDE: computer programs for side-chain conformation prediction and homology modeling. *Nature Protocols*, **3**, 1832–1847.

41 Ligneau, X., Morisset, S., Tardivel-Lacombe, J., Gbahou, F., Ganellin, C.R., Stark, H., Schunack, W., Schwartz, J.C., and Arrang, J.M. (2000) Distinct pharmacology of rat and human histamine H_3 receptors: role of two amino acids in the third transmembrane domain. *British Journal of Pharmacology*, **131**, 1247–1250.

42 Evers, A. and Klebe, G. (2004) Successful virtual screening for a submicromolar antagonist of the neurokinin-1 receptor based on a ligand-supported homology model. *Journal of Medicinal Chemistry*, **47**, 5381–5392.

43 Verdonk, M.L., Berdini, V., Hartshorn, M.J., Mooij, W.T., Murray, C.W., Taylor, R.D., and Watson, P. (2004) Virtual screening using protein–ligand docking: avoiding artificial enrichment. *Journal of Chemical Information and Computer Science*, **44**, 793–806.

44 Noeske, T., Jirgensons, A., Starchenkovs, I., Renner, S., Jaunzeme, I., Trifanova, D., Hechenberger, M., Bauer, T., Kauss, V., Parsons, C.G., Schneider, G., and Weil, T. (2007) Virtual screening for selective allosteric mGluR1 antagonists and structure–activity relationship investigations for coumarine derivatives. *ChemMedChem*, **2**, 1763–1773.

45 Parrill, A.L., Echols, U., Nguyen, T., Pham, T.C.T., Hoeglund, A., and Baker, D.L. (2008) Virtual screening approaches for the identification of non-lipid autotaxin inhibitors. *Bioorganic & Medicinal Chemistry*, **16**, 1784–1795.

46 Kellenberger, E., Springael, J.-Y., Parmentier, M., Hachet-Haas, M., Galzi, J.-L., and Rognan, D. (2007) Identification of nonpeptide CCR5 receptor agonists by structure-based virtual screening. *Journal of Medicinal Chemistry*, **50**, 1294–1303.

47 Kairys, V., Fernandes, M.X., and Gilson, M.K. (2006) Screening drug-like compounds by docking to homology models: a systematic study. *Journal of Chemical Information and Modeling*, **46**, 365–379.

48 Cozzini, P., Kellogg, G., Spyrakis, F., Abraham, D., Costantino, G., Emerson, A., Fanelli, F., Gohlke, H., Kuhn, L., Morris, G., Orozco, M., Pertinhez, T., Rizzi, M., and Sotriffer, C. (2008) Target flexibility: an emerging consideration in drug discovery and design. *Journal of Medicinal Chemistry*, **51**, 6237–6255.

49 Kazemi, S., Krüger, D., Sirockin, F., and Gohlke, H. (2009) Elastic potential grids: accurate and efficient representation of intermolecular interactions for fully flexible docking. *ChemMedChem*, **4**, 1264–1268.

50 May, A. and Zacharias, M. (2008) Protein–ligand docking accounting for receptor side chain and global flexibility in normal modes: evaluation on kinase inhibitor cross docking. *Journal of Medicinal Chemistry*, **51**, 3499–3506.

51 Totrov, M. and Abagyan, R. (2008) Flexible ligand docking to multiple receptor conformations: a practical alternative. *Current Opinion in Structural Biology*, **18**, 178–184.

52 Schneider, G. (2009) Virtual screening: what are we missing? *MedChemWatch*, **7**, 3–4, http://www.efmc.info/medchemwatch-2009-2.

16
Target-Based Virtual Screening to Address Protein–Protein Interfaces

Olivier Sperandio, Maria A. Miteva, and Bruno O. Villoutreix

16.1
Introduction

Protein–protein interactions (PPIs) are essential for almost all cellular processes and, therefore, one of the goals of postgenomic research is to understand and chart these interactions. Furthermore, aberrant PPIs contribute to most disease states, and as such PPIs represent a highly populated class of essentially untouched potential targets for drug discovery. The human genome contains about 35 000 protein-coding genes and the body should produce at least 100 000 proteins leading to an estimated number of about 650 000 protein–protein interactions [1, 2]. These numbers illustrate the magnitude of the challenge ahead and the situation gets even more overwhelming as PPIs in other organisms are also critical to assess (see, for instance, Ref. [3]). Indeed, for the time being, it is estimated that only 5–10% of all pairwise interactions have been charted in humans [4]. It is thus of major importance to use and develop new technologies to facilitate the discovery of PPI modulators (PPIMs) [5–7].

At present, small chemical compounds represent the majority of the active ingredients of drugs that are approved for human use by the FDA. Recent investigations indicate that cell surface receptors and enzymes represent more than 80% of the targets being drugged [8–10]. Additional major families of drug targets include nuclear receptors, ion channels, and transporters [11]. Present drug discovery research focuses on only a few protein classes (10–15% of all human proteins) indicating the tremendous potential of PPIs. The expansion of the target spectrum of small molecules to PPIs would also be highly beneficial for basic research because PPIMs are excellent tools for the analysis of protein function in genetically unmodified systems and can provide additional information compared to peptides or antibodies [12, 13]. However, identifying PPIMs is generally challenging and, in order to reduce the costs, it will be important to find new strategies and new public–private partnerships to capitalize on genomics investments and maintain a continuous stream of innovative drugs and molecular probes [14–17].

Virtual Screening. Edited by C. Sotriffer

ISBN: 978-3-527-32636-5

At present, three main classes of PPIMs are known, antibodies, peptides, and small chemical compounds, although nucleic acids and sugar molecules can also play that role. Focusing on the main classes, therapeutic antibodies are experiencing a considerably heightened interest due to their high specificity for their molecular targets and their stability in human serum. However, they are not cell-permeable and show a lack of oral bioavailability, at least given our knowledge about formulation. The cost and monitoring of antibodies (i.e., they have to be injected) is also very high and it would thus be highly desirable to replace them, whenever possible, with an oral pill [18, 19]. Peptides can also be applied as dimerization/interaction inhibitors [20–22]. Yet, they usually suffer from poor metabolic stability, low bioavailability and can induce immune reactions (*nota bene*: small drug-like compounds can also induce immune reactions). Some peptides are used as drugs in certain pathological conditions such as cancer or when the administration route is inhalation. In many situations, peptides can be used as a proof of concept to probe difficult targets prior to expensive screening campaigns [23, 24]. From a medicinal chemistry and drug development perspective, far more amenable to drug development is the third class: the so-called small-molecule PPIMs. These compounds are also very valuable as chemical probes to assess PPI networks. However, identification of PPIMs remains a formidable challenge in many cases, plagued with technical hurdles. When protein–protein interactions are suspected, various assays are used to identify competitive inhibitors (ELISA, FRET, BRET, SPR, NMR, X-ray, etc.) [18, 25–33]. Unfortunately, assays to investigate PPIs are usually difficult to develop for experimental low/medium or high-throughput screening. Thus, structure-based drug design, *in silico* screening, and chemoinformatics strategies will have to be developed, applied, and combined with appropriate experimental techniques in order to facilitate the development of PPIMs [7, 34–36].

One may wonder why protein–protein interfaces are usually difficult to modulate with a drug-like compound? Oral drugs usually have a molecular weight (MW) below 500 Da. Compounds with such property are well suited to fit into a small catalytic pocket, but, in contrast, protein–protein interfaces tend to be large and relatively flat and they usually have not evolved to bind small molecules. However, in spite of these observations, the discovery of hot spots within PPI interfaces has been critical to reconsider the feasibility of developing PPIMs [37]. Since protein–protein interfaces can be flexible, binding pockets at or close to the interface could be essentially invisible on the isolated protein partners or even in the presence of the experimental structure of the macromolecular complex [38–40]. Thus, the absence of preformed pockets makes the search of PPIMs complicated. The adaptive nature of protein surfaces implies that a single crystal structure may not reveal potential binding modes for small molecules, implying that several complementary tools have to be used to help designing PPIMs. In addition, while numerous efforts have been dedicated to the design of compound collections targeting enzymes, GPCR, and some other therapeutic targets, basically no strategies have been clearly devised for the development of dedicated PPIM collections so far [7]. Furthermore, essential structural and physicochemical properties required to design a good oral drug and the corresponding still ill-defined chemical space [41–44] have been empirically assessed during the development of enzyme/GPCR/ion channel/nuclear receptor inhibitors, but it is not known if this space fully or partially overlaps with the chemical space required for the successful design of PPIMs. Clearly, the absorption, distribution, metabolism, excretion, and toxicity (ADME/Tox) problem is less acute when the screening campaign aims at finding small chemical probes able to interfere with protein–protein association or dissociation, although frequent hitters and reactive molecules are usually not welcome in such studies. Another difficulty could be the optimization of PPIMs. Usually, because the hit rates are low, scientists tend to carry out initial screenings at relatively high concentration so as to find initial hits, even if they have low potency. It is thus unclear if it will be relatively easy to optimize low micromolar hits toward low nanomolar compounds using conventional medicinal chemistry programs, as the lead optimization funnel for PPIMs is likely to be shallower compared to regular therapeutic targets [18]. Although difficult, the rational design of PPIMs seems possible as discussed in some recent reviews [20, 45–56].

In this chapter, we briefly introduce challenges and opportunities pertaining to the field of PPIMs, key concepts, difficulties, and some recent success stories with a clear emphasis on structure-based virtual screening approaches. Protein–protein interfaces, notion of chemical space, binding pockets, and *in silico* methods are commented upon. We then focus on representative case studies using both structure-based *in silico* screening procedures and experimental screening. The PPIMs analyzed here involve a stabilizer of the superoxide dismutase-type 1 and some PPI inhibitors of the T-cell tyrosine kinase (Lck) protein. Allosteric inhibitors of PPIs are described in the case of antitrypsin polymerization, although such types of inhibitors can be considered as borderline with a clear PPIM. Obviously, space limitation does not allow an exhaustive review of the literature, but we hope that this chapter summarizes recent work in the field and provides practical examples to carry out structure-based screening of protein–protein interactions while anticipating future developments.

16.2 Some Recent PPIM Success Stories

Several recent comprehensive reviews reporting successful modulation of PPIs have been reported such as [20, 45–56]. The therapeutic potential of PPIMs is vast and includes, among others, cancers, infectious diseases, inflammation, central nervous system, cardiovascular diseases, protein misfolding, and aggregation (biostructural pathology) diseases. While the complexity of designing PPIMs has been considered insurmountable in the past, recently several protein complexes have been successfully probed with small nonpeptide compounds using experimental screening or a combination of experimental/biophysical and *in silico* approaches. The macromolecular complexes investigated involve, for instance, integrins [47], interleukin-2-interleukin receptor [47, 57], the Z-interacting protein–FtsZ complex [47], the MDM2-p53 complex [48, 49, 58], the Bcl-2 family [47, 58, 59], XIAP-caspase system [58, 60], the serine/threonine kinase polo-like kinase 1 [58], PDZ domains [58], the runx1 and CBFβ-SMMHC complex [58], iNOS dimerization [58], the JNK-JIP system [61]), PDK-1 [61], HSP90 [61], Calcineurin/NFAT [61], the HIV-1 Nef protein [62], SYK kinase [19], tubulin [63], Stat3 [64], and CXL12-CXCR4 [65].

16.3 Protein–Protein Interfaces

Protein–protein interfaces have been extensively analyzed over the years and several outstanding reviews have been reported on this topic, for instance, [66–73]. Proteins are usually involved in interactions with an estimated average of 5–10 protein partners. The binding site(s) with these partners may or may not overlap, illustrating the complexity of identifying, understanding, and predicting protein interaction networks. There are different types of protein–protein interactions, ranging from homo- and heterooligomeric complexes to obligate and nonobligate complexes (i.e., if two proteins of a complex can survive in their native state when separated). A related "nomenclature" classifies complexes as transient or permanent (i.e., notion of lifetimes of the complexes). Well-known examples can be, for a permanent complex, the interleukin 8 homodimer (PDB code 1il8), and for a nonobligate complex, the cytochrome *c* peroxidase associated with cytochrome *c* (PDB code 2pcb). The major points to consider with regard to drug design and PPIs are nature/size of the interface, geometry/shape, hot spots, cavities, plasticity/flexibility, energetics, and the role of water molecules. Depending on the types of complexes (permanent, transient, etc.), the nature of the interface usually differs, from somewhat hydrophobic/aromatic to a mixture of hydrophobic/aromatic and polar properties, but in most cases, an interface can be described as consisting of a network of usually unconnected hot spots (Table 16.1). Interfaces tend to be enriched in aliphatic and aromatic residues, but some charges can also be present, often to favor the formation of the encounter complex rather than acting on the stability of the complex [74]. The average size of the interfaces and the geometry also differ depending on the type of complexes [49, 66]. Different concepts have been extensively described in recent reviews, and, for example, it has been noted that regions important for the interactions tend to be formed by a conserved core enriched in hydrophobic and aromatic residues surrounded by a rim that has properties similar to the rest of the protein surface. The notion of dry and wet surfaces, of hot spot zones

Table 16.1 Key structural features of strong and weak transient dimers [76].

Parameters	Transient dimers (strong)	Transient dimers (weak)
Interface area (mean)	1152 Å^2	693 Å^2
Number of residues (mean)	31	17
% nonpolar residues in interface (mean)	39.5	42.8
Planarity index (mean)	3.46 Å	2.80 Å

The table reports only some mean values of some interface parameters.

being much smaller than the interface area, and the limited number of accessible rotameric states of some surface residues possibly pointing to zones of importance for PPIs have all been discussed and will not be commented upon further here (see, for instance, Ref. [75]).

The planarity index, assessing whether a protein–protein interface is flat or curved, is one important parameter to consider [77]. The planarity of the surfaces between two components of a complex is analyzed by calculating the root mean square deviation of all the interface atoms from the least squares plane through the atoms. If all atoms would exactly fit a plane, the planarity index would be zero. The average value of the planarity is around 3.5 for homodimers and 2.8 for heterocomplexes. When computing the planarity index via the PROTORP server [76] for the catalytic pocket of two enzymes, barnase and thrombin, and the planarity of some protein complexes that have been targeted by a small drug-like compound (e.g., MDM2, Bcl-xl, and interleukin 2 (IL-2), it is noted that the values tend to be similar to or even higher for PPIs (e.g., 2.7 Å for barnase and 3.6 Å for Bcl-xl). This seems to be the case for many protein–protein interfaces modulated thus far by a druglike compound but for the XIAP system (see Figure 16.1). This suggests that the PPIs that have been targeted so far might be in the more druggable end of the PPI difficulty spectrum.

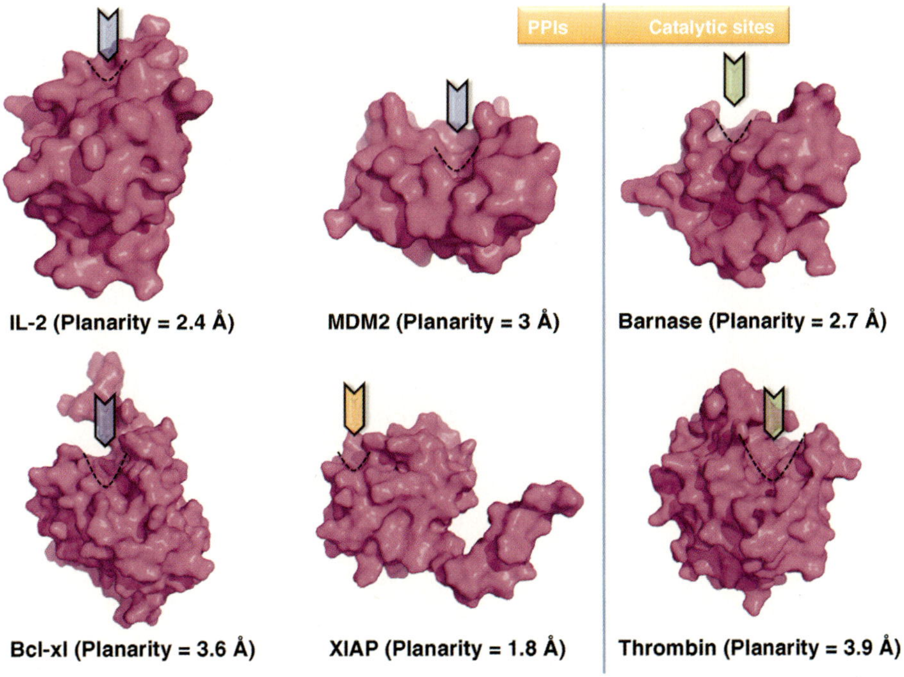

Figure 16.1 Planarity of some screened PPIs versus planarity values for two enzymes. The blue arrows indicate somewhat visible and curved pockets at the protein–protein interfaces, the orange arrow highlights a flat interface, and the green arrows point to catalytic sites. The figure was generated with PyMol.

Water molecules are usually present in abundance at the interfaces and play a major role in stabilizing the complexes. When two polypeptide chains interact with each other to form a stable specific complex, bulk solvent is excluded from the interface, creating a favorable hydrophobic effect. In spite of this phenomenon, structural biologists often report water molecules in X-ray structures, which are bound to interfaces between polypeptide chains. These solvent molecules are supposed to contribute to stability of the quaternary structure by forming extensive hydrogen-bonding networks with amino acid residues on both sides of the interface.

16.3.1 Interface Pockets, Flexibility, and Hot Spots

As mentioned above, a major problem with some targets is the flexibility (or plasticity or malleability) of the interface. Indeed, with regard to protein–protein complexes, only about one third can be docked without considerations of induced conformational changes [78], further highlighting the need of addressing this issue. Conformational variability leads to an ensemble of substates around the native protein structure. The distribution of populations of these conformational substates depends on binding or other physical influences [38, 39, 75, 79–85]. One direct consequence of plasticity is that PPIMs can induce conformational changes leading to grooves or pockets that are not visible in the unbound structure and that can differ from the interface geometry of a receptor bound to its natural protein partner. Structural evidence of such type of plasticity has been found upon binding of a small molecule to interleukin 2 (Figure 16.2) [86]. The small compound impedes the binding of the

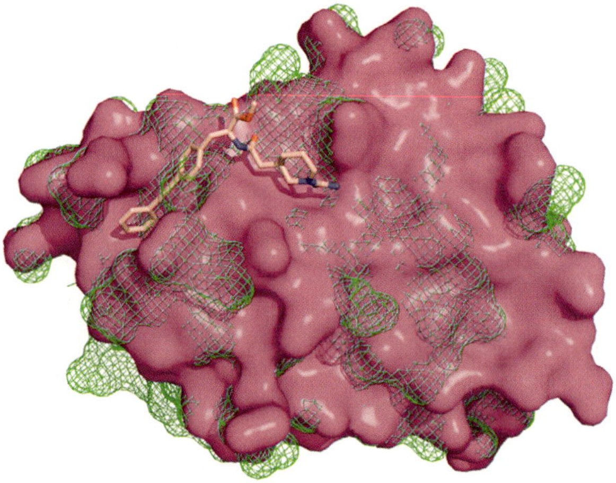

Figure 16.2 Interface plasticity. The molecular surface of a cocrystal structure of IL-2 in complex with a small compound (stick representation) is shown in magenta. The surface structure of the apo IL-2 experimental structure is presented as a green mesh. It is seen that the small compound could not fit into the apo IL-2 structure indicating structural adaptation of surface residues not only in the hot spot region but also in some remote areas. The figure was generated with PyMol.

cytokine IL-2 to its receptor. The structure of the IL-2-small molecule complex shows that side-chain rearrangements occur upon binding of the compound creating small cavities. The binding site for the small compound falls within the hot spot region of IL-2 for binding its receptor, but the surface structure of the IL-2-druglike molecule and the IL-2–IL-2 receptor differs and both are somewhat different from the IL-2 apo structure. Structural and thermodynamic studies further demonstrated that this portion of IL-2 is inherently flexible, and as such, one can expect that ligand binding captured a low-energy protein conformation instead of inducing a high-energy one. It would thus seem that small molecules can induce the formation of small binding pockets not seen in the unligated proteins and that the absence of preformed clefts does not mean that they cannot form [6, 18]. In principle, it should be possible to detect these potential binding sites in the unbound state by computational means, which may give a hint as to the druggability of these interfaces [87, 88]. Above all, appropriately taking into account protein flexibility and plasticity in the process of small-molecule PPIM discovery is mandatory. These challenges imposed by the structural and dynamical properties of interfaces also exist to some extent in the case of "classical" targets and starts to be addressed. For instance, recent molecular dynamics studies investigating transient pockets on protein surfaces directly located at the interfaces have been reported [89, 90]. The authors investigated Bcl-xL, IL-2, and MDM2 and proposed a new pocket detection protocol. They observed that the native inhibitor binding pocket was partly present in the unbound proteins. They performed 10 ns molecular dynamics simulations and scanned, on many structural snapshots collected along the trajectory, the surface of the proteins, in search of transient or more permanent cavities. They noticed that some cavities were opening up within 2.5 ps and that most of them appeared multiple times during the simulation. In the druggable region, they noticed that pockets of similar size compared to the experimental structures in complex with the ligand could be generated. Docking was successfully performed into these transient pockets, suggesting that this protocol is viable to study protein interfaces with the goal of designing antagonists and possibly stabilizers. Comparisons of catalytic pockets and interface pockets confirm some key concepts: regular binding pockets use fewer, larger cavities whereas PPI inhibitors use a greater number of smaller pockets. Interestingly, PPIs and regular pockets seem to be similar in size [91]. A point noted by Luque and Freire about catalytic sites is that these regions appear to have a dual nature characterized by regions of high stability and regions of high flexibility [92]. Analysis of pockets at the interfaces or near the interfaces is required to confirm this observation for PPIs. Taken together, these observations point to the need of developing tools that could predict the druggability index of protein–protein interfaces.

While the problem of flexibility and transient pockets is challenging, there are indications that in some cases PPIs can be targeted with small compounds. First, analyses of protein–protein complexes versus protein–peptide complexes show very similar thermodynamic behavior, despite considerable differences in the interface sizes [75]. Similarly, the stability of macromolecular complexes is somewhat independent of the interface size. Along these lines, extensive "alanine scanning" mutagenesis experiments in PPI revealed that only a small subset of amino acids ("hot spots") within the overall interface contributes significantly to the binding affinity [37]. These observations have far-reaching consequences for the discovery of PPIMs suggesting that many PPIs could be drugged or at least modulated by small compounds.

16.3.2 Databases and Tools to Analyze Interfaces

In order to analyze and rationalize protein–protein interfaces, several ingredients have to be available, such as nonredundant databases of real experimental structures of complexes together with the right computer tools to compute descriptors and parameters describing these interfaces and carry out relevant statistical analysis. Therefore, different *in silico* methods, web servers, and databases have been developed both to analyze the geometry, energetic (e.g., prediction of hot spots), and chemical nature of the protein–protein interfaces and to dock protein molecules. Numerous such approaches are described in recent reviews/papers [66, 75, 83, 85, 93–96] and we will provide here only some of the available tools.

First, experimental structures and PPI databases are required. Experimental structures are available at the Protein Data Bank and many new links and software tools are now present at the PDB to facilitate drug discovery [97]. Experimental structures and predicted proteins have, however, to be used with care and detailed investigation of the structures is always required prior to run virtual screening computations (e.g., search for missing residues, alternative side-chain orientations, etc.) [98–101]. Some PPI databases (or databases of hot spots) are listed in Table 16.2, while some tools to analyze interfaces or predict binding pockets and hot spots are listed in Table 16.3. Some protein docking engines can also help in predicting interfaces, and some tools easily accessible online are listed in Table 16.4.

16.4 PPIMs' Chemical Space and ADME/Tox Properties

Historically, peptides, nucleic acids, and antibodies have been considered the primary molecular classes capable of modulating protein–protein interactions [58, 102]. Yet, it is in most cases desirable to modulate PPIs with small organic molecules. Depending on the goals and the targets, in many drug discovery projects, compounds used for screening have to be druglike, but many purchasable compounds or virtual compounds may not have satisfactory ADME/Tox properties to be considered as promising drug candidates while they could be useful chemical probes to help understand some molecular mechanisms. With regard to drug discovery project, it is possible to remove from the libraries some molecules that are likely to be problematic in the hit-to-lead step and further using *in silico* strategies [41, 103, 104]. To probe further the chemical space of PPIMs, a set of inhibitors have been investigated by Pagliaro *et al.* using chemoinformatics protocols and compared to

Table 16.2 List of freely accessible PPI databases.

Database	URL	Short summary
DIP	http://dip.doe-mbi.ucla.edu/	This database catalogues experimentally determined interactions between proteins
DOMINE	http://domine.utdallas.edu/cgi-bin/Domine	DOMINE is a database of known and predicted protein domain (domain–domain) interactions
MINT	http://mint.bio.uniroma2.it/mint	MINT focuses on experimentally verified protein–protein interactions mined from the scientific literature
PRISM	http://prism.ccbb.ku.edu.tr/	PRISM is a web server that can be used to explore protein interfaces and predict protein–protein interactions
PIBASE	http://pibase.janelia.org/	PIBASE is a collection of all protein structural interfaces extracted from the Protein Data Bank and PQS structure databases
DOCKGROUND	http://dockground.bioinformatics.ku.edu/index.shtml	The DOCKGROUND resource implements a comprehensive database of cocrystallized (bound–bound) protein–protein complexes, unbound (experimental and simulated) protein–protein complexes, modeled protein–protein complexes and systematic sets of docking decoys
PROTCOM	http://www.ces.clemson.edu/compbio/protcom/	This database is a collection of protein–protein homo- and heterocomplexes as well as domain–domain structures

molecules present in commercial compound collections [105]. The authors found that only 50% of the 19 PPIMs were covered by the chemical space available in these databases suggesting that the physicochemical properties of PPI inhibitors are somewhat different from the ones present in regular compound collections. This certainly illustrates that compound collections have been enriched with molecules aiming at inhibiting catalytic sites rather than at performing other functions such as PPI inhibition. Interestingly, they also found that four protein–protein complexes were well covered by the chemical space in the commercial databases investigated (International Diversity Collection from Jan. 2004, Maybridge from Feb. 2004, and Asinex from Oct. 2003, thus over 400 000 molecules), namely, the Bak-BH3/Bcl-xl, MDM2/p53, NGF/p75, and LFA/ICAM-1 systems. Furthermore, with regard to the druglikeness characteristics of these 19 published PPI inhibitors as investigated via the Lipinski rule of five (i.e., estimation not only of oral bioavailability but also of some

Table 16.3 Tools to analyze interfaces, predict hot spots, or binding pockets.

Interface analysis, pockets, and hot spot predictions	URL	Short summary
PROFACE	http://resources.boseinst.ernet.in/resources/bioinfo/interface/	Analysis of the physico-chemical features of PPIs
Morphology of protein–protein interfaces	http://mgl.scripps.edu/people/goodsell/interface/interface.html	A visual survey of homodimeric proteins
PROTORP	http://www.bioinformatics.sussex.ac.uk/protorp	Analyze interface properties
Q-siteFinder	http://www.modelling.leeds.ac.uk/qsitefinder/	Probe-mapping method for the prediction of ligand binding site
SURFNET	http://www.biochem.ucl.ac.uk/~roman/surfnet/surfnet.html	The program generates surfaces and void regions between molecules
ODA	http://www.molsoft.com/oda.html	Prediction of protein–protein interaction sites
FoldX	http://foldx.crg.es/	FoldX provides a fast and quantitative estimation of the importance of the interactions contributing to the stability of proteins and protein complexes
Robetta	http://robetta.bakerlab.org/	Interface alanine scanning and numerous other tools
PPI-Pred	http://bmbpcu36.leeds.ac.uk/ppi_pred/	Protein–protein binding site prediction
PROMATE	http://bioinfo.weizmann.ac.il/promate/	Tools to predict the location of potential protein–protein binding sites in unbound proteins
PIER	http://abagyan.ucsd.edu/PIER/	Tool to predict likely protein–protein interaction patches

other pharmacokinetics properties, reviewed in Ref. [41–44]), the authors found that several compounds had a MW around 500, while the others had between 260 and 900. Analysis of these 19 compounds showed that only 8 compounds could survive the rule of five criteria, but molecules inhibiting the Bak-BH3/Bcl-xl, MDM2/p53, and NGF/p75 protein–protein complexes were well covered by the rule-of-five-filtered compound collections, suggesting that at least, some PPIs can be addressed with the available druglike molecules and the way compound collections are traditionally prepared.

Table 16.4 Some protein docking packages and online flexibility investigation.

Protein–protein docking and flexibility	URL	Short summary
FTDock	http://www.sbg.bio.ic.ac.uk/docking/	FTDock (Fourier transform) performs rigid-body docking
Zdock server	http://zdock.bu.edu/	ZDOCK is a fast Fourier transform-based protein docking program
MolFit	http://www.weizmann.ac.il/Chemical_Research_Support//molfit/	The program is based on an algorithm that takes into account geometric recognition (shape complementarity), electrostatic complementarity, and hydrophobic complementarity as well as experimental data from biological, biochemical, and bioinformatics studies
GRAMM-X server	http://vakser.bioinformatics.ku.edu/resources/gramm/grammx	The tool extends the original GRAMM fast Fourier transformation methodology by employing smoothed potentials, refinement stage, and knowledge-based scoring
Hex	http://www.loria.fr/~ritchied/hex/	The tool operates through a novel spherical polar Fourier correlations of protein shape and electrostatic properties
PatchDock server	http://bioinfo3d.cs.tau.ac.il/PatchDock/	PatchDock is a geometry-based molecular docking algorithm
Haddock server	http://haddock.chem.uu.nl/services/HADDOCK/haddockserver-easy.html	HADDOCK (high ambiguity driven protein–protein docking) is an information-driven flexible docking approach for the modeling of biomolecular complexes
RosettaDock server	http://rosettadock.graylab.jhu.edu/	ROSETTA DOCK works by simultaneous optimization of side-chain conformation and rigid-body position of the two docking partners. The former is performed by a packing algorithm and the latter is performed by a rigid-body Monte Carlo minimization strategy

(Continued)

Table 16.4 (*Continued*)

Protein–protein docking and flexibility	URL	Short summary
ClusPro	http://nrc.bu.edu/cluster/	The tool evaluates billions of putative complexes, retaining a preset number with favorable surface complementarities. A filtering method is then applied to this set of structures, selecting those with good electrostatic and desolvation free energies for further clustering
pyDockWeb	http://inb.bsc.es/gn6/PyDock/	The tool generates rigid-body docking orientations by using an FFT-based method and rescores the resulting docking poses by binding electrostatics and desolvation energy
FRODOCK	http://sbg.cib.csic.es/Software/FRODOCK/	The tool performs an exhaustive 6D rigid docking between two protein structures
SKE-DOCK	http://www.pharm.kitasato-u.ac.jp/bmd/files/SKE_DOCK.html	The tool performs docking using molecular dynamics, grid scoring, and a pairwise interaction potential
DFprot	http://sbg.cib.csic.es/Software/DFprot/index.html	The server provides deformability/flexibility analysis of a 3D protein structure
Multiple receptor conformations	http://abagyan.ucsd.edu/MRC/	Generate normal mode-guided multiple receptor conformations

Because the hit rate for the identification of PPIMs tends to be low, the design of specific compound collections (either tuned to PPI family, containing analogues to known PPIMs, or enriched in putative PPIM compounds or in molecules possessing a privileged PPIM structures) is required [7, 18]. A possible way to work around this problem could be to design focused compound collections dedicated to PPIs [7, 106]. Recently, an *in silico* attempt to extract potential PPI inhibitors from compound databases has been reported [107]. The authors extracted known PPI data from the literature (25 representative molecules were selected) and they computed various descriptors (e.g., molecular shape) for each compound. They then used machine-learning methods to try to discriminate PPIs inhibitors from non-PPI inhibitors. The results, although preliminary, show that it is possible to enrich a collection 10-fold in PPI inhibitors with the consideration of essentially a shape descriptor, but it remains to be seen if a database prepared along this line will effectively facilitate the *in vitro* discovery of PPIMs compared to a non-PPI-filtered collection. Extensive analysis of the PPI inhibitor chemical space performed in our laboratory confirms that PPIMs are in general more hydrophobic, aromatic, and larger than other regular oral drugs [7].

With regard to ADME/Tox properties, it is important to underline that some natural products such as paclitaxel, epothilone A, rapamycin, and ascomycin modulate PPIs and so does the synthetic compound ABT 263 [18, 108]. Some of these molecules do not comply with well-known and generally accepted ADME/Tox rules since they, for instance, have a MW over 700 Da, but are yet orally bioavailable (i.e., in some cases with some special formulations) with acceptable pharmaceutical properties. Taken together, these findings and observations emphasize that significant work is needed to define rules able to profile the chemical space of PPIMs while bearing in mind key ADME/Tox properties. For this task, chemoinformatics and chemistry tools are very well suited and should be combined in an appropriate manner. Rationalization of the chemical space could lead, for instance, to the design of focused libraries and could point to regions of the chemical space that need to be explored and/or possibly designed/engineered through oriented synthesis.

16.5
Drug Discovery, Chemical Biology, and *In Silico* Screening Methods: Overview and Suggestions for PPIM Search

Drug discovery is a costly and time-consuming process that critically depends on the identification of disease-modifying proteins and on small molecules acting on these targets (i.e., targets are essentially proteins, but they can be DNA, RNA, etc.). Given the explosion of potential new targets derived from genome research, there is a great need for the development and optimization of technologies assisting the discovery of hit compounds and the hit-to-lead steps, even more so for the so-called difficult targets, including PPIs. Many different skills and methods are needed from biophysics to medicinal chemistry while *in silico* approaches play a critical role, from target identification/preparation to the generation of appropriate compound collections [12, 38, 39, 46, 75, 79–81, 94, 103, 109–124]. Among the *in silico* screening methods used, one can usually distinguish two main strategies: the so-called ligand-based virtual screening and structure-based virtual screening approaches. Ligand-based and structure-based approaches can, however, be combined. To perform *in silico* screening computations, in all cases, a compound collection is needed and often the compounds have to be transformed in 3D while some ADME/Tox computations may have to be performed and often tuned according to the project (i.e., in case of PPIs, most likely the commonly used ADME/Tox parameters will have to be modified to better account for the PPIMs' still ill-defined chemical space). Often several alternative conformations for the ligands have to be generated and care should be taken about addition of hydrogen atoms. The protein also needs to be prepared; this can involve prediction of pockets and hot spots if they are not known, estimation of flexibility, size, and volume of the binding pockets [125], appropriate assignment of formal charges, alternative positioning of some side chains, and so on. As such, both the ligands and the proteins have to be prepared prior to running structure-based screening computations.

With regard to finding PPIMs, as mentioned above, one important problem is the identification and definition of the binding regions, and assessment of the receptor flexibility. If the binding pocket is visible, the task might be easier, but if no pockets are preformed at the interface, simulations will have to be carried out (e.g., molecular dynamics, normal mode analysis, Gaussian network models, and Monte Carlo simulations) most likely prior to the docking step. Although flexible receptor–flexible ligand methods suited for *in silico* screening experiments are emerging, they will need important developments in the case of PPI screening. Indeed, if receptor (and to some extent ligand) flexibility is not properly treated, it can increase the number of false positive instead of facilitating the identification of relevant hits. A practical solution for PPIs (assuming that some 3D structures of the receptors are known) would be to generate *in silico* different structures of the receptor (unless different experimental structures do exist) and possibly to use soft potentials (some atom overlaps are tolerated) to initially assess the binding poses [126]. Yet, one difficulty in performing docking against multiple receptor conformations is to deal with the different ranked lists since for each structure of the receptor, the docking/scoring procedure can propose over 1000 likely molecules. If, for instance, computations are performed on three snapshot structures collected along a molecular dynamic simulation, one may end up with a list of 3000 molecules to test experimentally with possibly very few consensus compounds. The merge-and-shrink procedure has recently been proposed to address this problem [127]. With this approach, for each compound, the best rank –not the best score – is kept. This has been shown to be efficient on some targets, but, in general, to use this approach, one needs known actives to test the protocol and calibrate the computations. The merge-and-shrink protocol or consensus scoring [128] or a consensus docking–scoring approach [123] can be efficient in some cases, while they could dilute the correct results for some targets, the difficulty being that it is not yet known which target would benefit from a given protocol. In most cases, it is important to remember that scoring (independent of the methods used, from force field to fingerprints) remains very challenging in structure-based virtual screening computations [129–135].

A point that could be of particular importance for the design of PPIMs would be to apply the concept of ligand efficiency or related values such as the binding efficiency index [136]. Ligand efficiency, the experimental binding energy per heavy atoms, can be a useful parameter to select molecules that are rich in atoms really contributing to the binding energy and should help in selecting smaller initial hits easier to optimize within a reasonable range of molecular weight values since PPIMs tend to be relatively large. In addition to ligand efficiency, careful scoring, and postprocessing (e.g., the use of free energy of binding via MMPB(GB)SA, interaction fingerprints, and tuned scoring functions), consideration of

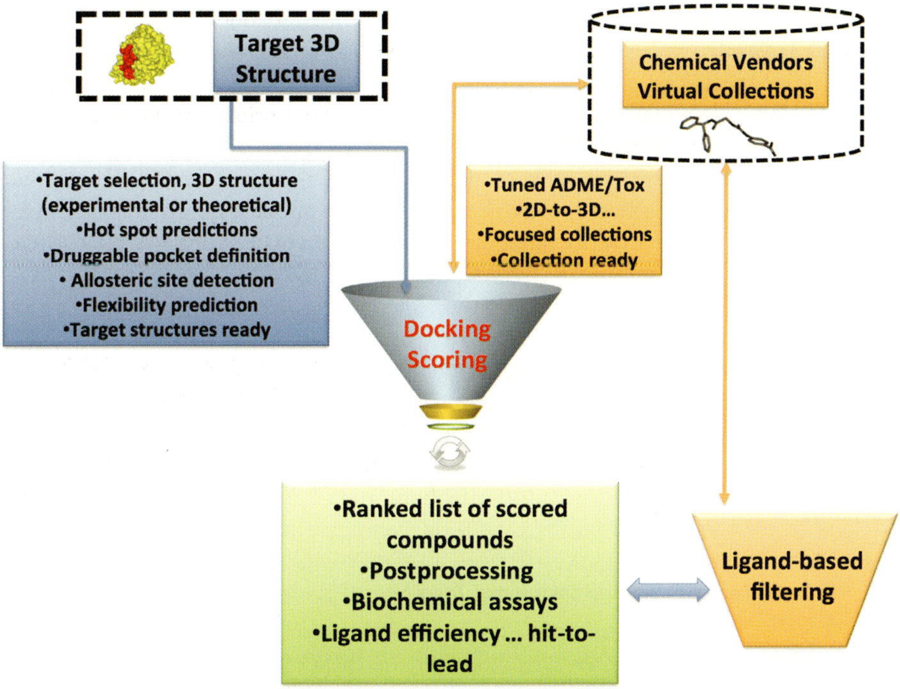

Figure 16.3 Possible structure-based screening flowchart for searching new PPIMs.

flexibility, advanced definition of the binding pocket, and the integration of calorimetry data into the *in silico* procedures [137] is required. In addition, it could certainly be valuable to tune the ADME/Tox filtering rules and design focus libraries enriched in PPIMs either by creating a small screening collection containing molecules that are similar to known PPIMs and/or by using machine-learning methods, selecting appropriate descriptors able to discriminate PPIMs from non-PPIMs, and by designing a mathematical model profiling the input collection such that a focused library gets generated specifically for PPIs [7]. Possibly, enriching the collection in molecules relatively rigid and rich in aromatic rings could be of importance [18, 49]. A specific PPIM structure-based screening scenario integrating some of the above suggestions is depicted in Figure 16.3. There, the users select their favorite docking/scoring engines, some relevant compound collections, while paying great attention to receptor/pocket flexibility and to the compounds present in the chemical collections (many "free tools and compound collections are listed at the following URL: www.vls3d.com [94]). Clearly, this represents a possible protocol that will have to be tuned according to a given project and modified according to the goals (i.e., drug discovery or chemical biology), the targets (e.g., location in the human body), and the pathology under investigation (e.g., cancer or any difficult disease versus diseases for which many "efficient" drugs are already available).

16.6
Case Studies

In the following sections, we present several case studies making use of *in silico/in vitro* methods to design PPIMs. There are debates in the literature about what should be considered a true protein–protein interaction. For instance, GPCR antagonists/ligands are usually believed to allosterically function upon binding and as such they are generally not regarded as authentic inhibitors of protein associations [102]. Along the same line, it is unclear if compounds performing uncompetitive interfacial inhibition (i.e., a compound takes advantage of a transient and dynamic structural conditions) as described in Ref. [138] should be considered as truly PPIMs or if they are more closely related to conventional catalytic site inhibitors. Also, some authors exclude allosteric inhibition and protein–linear–peptide binding domains (e.g., SH2 domains) from the PPI class [91, 139]. We here selected different types of complexes and mechanisms, either fully or partially belonging to the PPIM class, starting with a PPI stabilizer, continuing with PPI inhibitors, and closing with allosteric inhibitors.

16.6.1
PPI Stabilizers: Superoxide Dismutase Type 1

Ray *et al.* performed an interesting study on superoxide dismutase 1 (SOD1), a β-sheet-rich dimeric metalloenzyme that is normally responsible for scavenging superoxide ions and that plays important roles in the health and disease states (diabetes, cancers, liver injury, etc.) [140]. Amyotrophic lateral sclerosis (ALS), or Lou Gehrig's disease, is a fatal motor neuron disease that affects many individuals worldwide. The most common causes of familial ALS (FALS) are point mutations in the gene-encoding SOD1. One or more FALS SOD1 mutations have been linked to decreased metal binding, decreased formation of a stabilizing intermolecular disulfide, decreased structural stability, and increased propensity to monomerize and aggregate. The authors designed a screening strategy with the aim of identifying small druglike molecules that could stabilize the SOD1 native dimer. This strategy was based on the notion that SOD1 monomerization is required for aggregation. The precedent for the discovery of small-molecule stabilizers of a native protein oligomer, as reported by these authors, involves a protein aggregation disease that is analogous to FALS: familial amyloid polyneuropathy (FAP). FAP is caused by mutations in the gene encoding transthyretin (TTR) [53]. Many FAP mutations destabilize the native TTR tetramer, facilitating its dissociation, partial unfolding, and aggregation. The natural ligand of TTR, thyroxine, stabilizes the tetramer and prevents its aggregation *in vitro*. Druglike molecules that are thyroxine analogues bind and stabilize the native TTR tetramer and could potentially be used for the treatment of FAP [141]. However, unlike for TTR, there are no natural ligands of SOD1 to serve as a molecular scaffold for the design of small-molecule stabilizers. Ray *et al.* initiated a virtual screening study using a compound collection of about 1.5 million druglike molecules resulting from the merging of 18 vendor collections (Figure 16.4). They identified a small cavity at the dimer interface

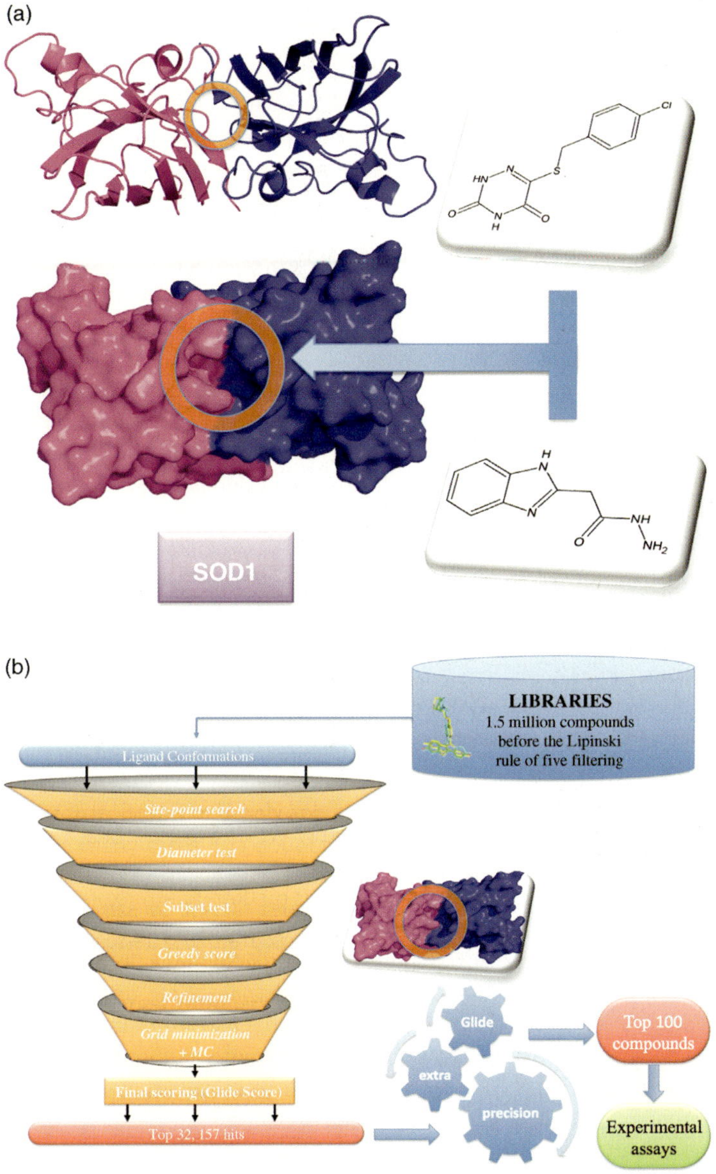

Figure 16.4 (a) SOD1 structure, proposed binding cavity at the dimer interface, and examples of stabilizing compounds; (b) Overview of the SOD1 screening process with Glide (please see http://www.schrodinger.com for detailed information about the Glide algorithm). A first round of docking generated a list of 32 157 potential hits. These molecules were again docked with the "extraprecision" mode of Glide, which penalizes compounds that violate established physicochemical principles of protein–ligand interactions. The compound collections were prepared using a property-based filtering to select molecules that satisfied the Lipinski rule of five, but with relaxed threshold values compared to the original Lipinski values to minimize wastage of compounds. (MC: Monte Carlo.)

that was deemed of sufficient size for SB-VLS. They analyzed the X-ray structures of several SOD1 proteins and did not notice major structural changes among the structure suggesting that a standard protocol could be performed. The database and docking protocol were performed as follow:

First, the authors chose to use property-based filtering to prepare the compound collection in order to select molecules that satisfied the "Lipinski rule of five" but with relaxed threshold values (i.e., MW from 100 to 800; $\log P = 7$). The database was further filtered to remove compounds containing heavy metals and only those compounds were kept that had the elements C, O, N, S, P, F, Cl, Br, I, B, Na, K, Mg, and Ca (Figure 16.4). The compounds were then treated with the LigPrep Schrödinger module to remove counter ions, adjust charge states, and generate tautomers wherever applicable (http://www.schrodinger.com). An energy refinement module was used to generate energy-minimized structure for all the compounds. The wild-type SOD1 structure (PDB entry 1UXM) was energy minimized and one residue in the predicted binding pocket area was chosen as the center of mass for generation of the grid for docking calculation. The program Glide (Schrödinger, http://www.schrodinger.com/) was then used for docking [142]. The first docking computations were carried out by using the default Glide parameters and sorted with GlideScore leading to a focused compound collection containing 32 157 molecules. These molecules were redocked with the "extraprecision" mode of Glide. A maximum of 2000 poses were requested (i.e., exploration of the binding areas). The top 100 compounds were experimentally tested and 15 best hits were identified that have the ability to significantly stabilize FALS variants and prevent its aggregation *in vitro*. These compounds could lead to candidate therapeutics for FALS.

16.6.2
PPI Inhibitors: Lck

The protein p56 lymphoid T-cell tyrosine kinase (Lck) is predominantly expressed in T lymphocytes where it plays a critical role in T-cell-mediated immune response. Lck participates in phosphotyrosine-dependent protein–protein interactions through its modular binding unit, the Src homology-2 (SH2) domain. SH2 domains are noncatalytic modules of about 100 amino acid residues that play important roles in intracellular signal transduction and represent potential targets for pharmacological intervention. Failure of the p56 Lck SH2 domain to bind to immunoreceptor tyrosine-based activation motifs (ITAMs) of CD3 hampers the T-cell receptor (TCR) proximal activation process and suppresses the downstream T-cell activation signaling cascades [143]. Small compounds that would be able to block Lck SH2 domain-dependent protein–protein interactions could find therapeutic utility as immunosuppressants and in the treatment of T-cell leukemias, lymphomas, and autoimmune diseases such as rheumatoid arthritis.

A peptide library was screened and allowed the identification of a phosphopeptide with sequence Ac-pY-E-E-I that binds to the Lck SH2 domain [144]. This tetrapeptide is an attractive lead structure for the rational design of agents to compete with the SH2 domain's natural ligands. However, it was found that the tetrapeptide had several undesirable features that hindered its ability to elicit a response in cell-based assays of T-cell activation. Problems with its metabolic stability were noticed and the five negative charges created additional pharmacokinetic problems including difficulties to cross membranes. High-resolution X-ray structures of the Lck SH2 domain cocrystallized with the phosphopeptide have been solved underlining the presence of two cavities, referred to as the pY and pY + 3 binding sites (Figure 16.5) [145]. Experimental data suggested that pY + 3 binding pocket is important for specific binding. Thus, the pY + 3 site was considered to be a novel target site for rational drug design approaches and structure-based virtual screening experiments with the aim of identifying nonpeptidic and specific inhibitors of the p56 Lck SH2 domain.

Huang *et al.* applied virtual screening techniques followed by experimental assays to identify low MW nonpeptidic compounds targeting the pY + 3 binding site that would be potent inhibitors of the Lck SH2 domain while omitting the phosphotyrosine site and related chemical moieties in the structure of the ligand [146]. First, they generated a compound collection of about 2000 000 compounds and analyzed in depth the X-ray structure of the Lck SH2 domain in complex with a phosphopeptide (PDB code 1lkk), removed water molecules, and added appropriate charges and hydrogen atoms to the system. The docking was performed with DOCK [147], sphere sets were created in the pY + 3 binding site area with SPHGEN routine for initial positioning of the ligands in the binding pocket. The ligand–receptor interaction energies were approximated by the sum of electrostatic and van der Waals components as calculated by the grid method implemented in DOCK. To avoid exploring the phosphotyrosine pocket, this modified amino acid was kept in the structure of the protein while the rest of the peptide was deleted. A fast docking– scoring approach was used first. Because most scoring functions including the one present in DOCK tend to be biased toward the selection of high molecular weight compounds, a normalization procedure was applied. This first round selected about 25 000 compounds that were then screened again with a more rigorous docking method that included simultaneous energy minimization of the so-called anchor fragment. Two sets of 1000 compounds were selected, one on the basis of the total computed interaction energy and the second one on the basis of the MW normalized total energy score. The compounds were clustered in order to define families and most dissimilar structures via computations of descriptors as included in the MOE package (www.chemcomp.com). Compounds for biological assays were selected from the dissimilar sets. Several clusters were generated and two compounds were selected from each cluster. In total, 210 + 218 diverse compounds were selected *in silico* from the two energy sets. Comparisons between these molecules revealed a significant number of identical compounds, finally leading to a list of 288 unique molecules. From this list, 196 compounds were available from the commercial vendors and 34 hits were identified experimentally *in vitro* and 13 functioning in cellular assays. The molecules were analyzed on the computer screen using different packages including VMD (http://www.ks.uiuc.edu/Research/vmd/) and Chimera (e.g., to compute hydrogen bond networks with the FindHBond utility; http://www.cgl.ucsf.edu/chimera/). These molecules were then used as starting point for further

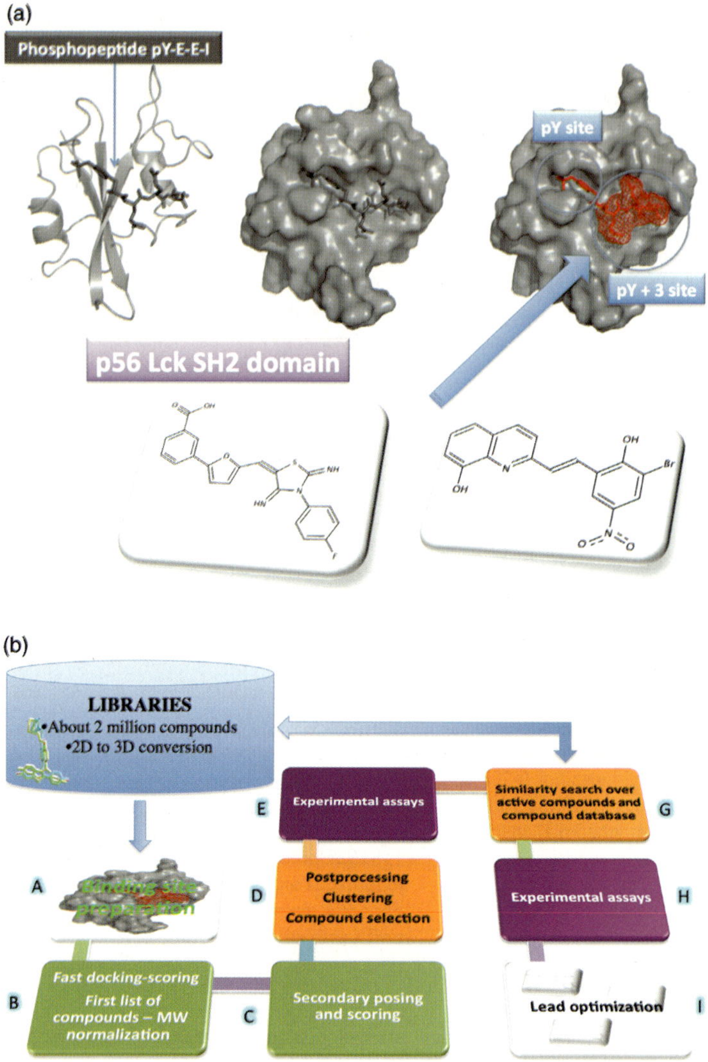

Figure 16.5 (a) Binding pocket and some small compounds binding to the pY + 3 site of the Lck SH2 domain. The phosphotyrosine residue was present in the structure during virtual screening in order to favor compounds that do not fit into this pocket in an attempt to gain selectivity and to explore this specific region of the structure. Computations were performed with DOCK. (b) Key *in silico* screening steps (preparation of the collection and steps A–I) to search for PPIMs interacting with the Lck SH2 domain [146, 148].

hit to lead optimizations via ligand-based similarity approaches and could become novel immunosupressant drugs [148].

16.6.3
Allosteric Inhibitors: Antitrypsin Polymerization

Proteins are dynamic polymers and their conformational flexibility is critical for function. Ability to trap alternate states through binding of small compounds at remote locations from the interface areas could be valuable in many situations [149]. Thus, the concept of allosteric inhibitors of protein–protein interactions that may not totally fit into the absolute definition of PPIMs is exemplified in the following paragraph with the antitrypsin polymerization case. Alpha1-antitrypsin is the archetypal member of the serine proteinase inhibitor or serpin superfamily. Most individuals carry a normal allele, but 4% of the Northern European population are heterozygous for the severe Z deficiency variant that translates into a Glu342Lys substitution and subsequent perturbations both of the secondary structure elements and of the mobile reactive center loop. The resulting unstable intermediate serpin molecules then link to form loop-sheet polymers in which the reactive loop of one protein inserts as strand 4 of the so-called β-sheet A of another α1-antitrypsin molecule. It is the accumulation of polymers that predisposes the Z α1-antitrypsin homozygote to hepatitis, cirrhosis, and hepatocellular carcinoma. Other mutations in the serpin family also lead to polymer formation leading to thrombosis, angioedema, emphysema, or familial encephalopathy. With regard to α1-antitrypsin structural problem, the only curative treatment available today is liver transplantation. Recently, Mallya *et al.* performed structure-based *in silico* screening computations with the ICM package against a nonredundant library of about 1.2 million commercial druglike compounds (resulting from 10 vendors) in a hydrophobic pocket present in this serpin that is remote from this abnormal protein–protein interaction site (Figure 16.6) [150]. The pocket was predicted using the ICM PocketFinder analysis tool and this lateral cavity was identified as being "druggable" in terms of pocket volume and shape, and was present in several X-ray structures. Its allosteric role was not known at the beginning of the study, but the overall plasticity of this region supported the idea that a compound there could modify the behavior of the protein. An initial screen was performed on the crystal structure of α1-antitrypsin (PDB code 1qlp), but none of the nominated compounds was effective in impeding polymerization. It should be noted that this pocket is very challenging as it is located in a flexible region ("allosteric cavity"). Amino acid side-chain simulation was performed (biased probability Monte Carlo simulation) to identify the most flexible residues lining the cavity and one Asn residue was found to be very flexible. A low-energy conformation for this residue was generated through Monte Carlo simulation. *In silico* screening was repeated on this modified cavity and 68 compounds were selected for further characterization *in vitro*. One compound completely blocked polymerization while another one presented interesting activity as it allowed the formation of only dimeric structures. Ligand-induced changes were then modeled for these two best compounds prior to an additional round of *in silico* screening

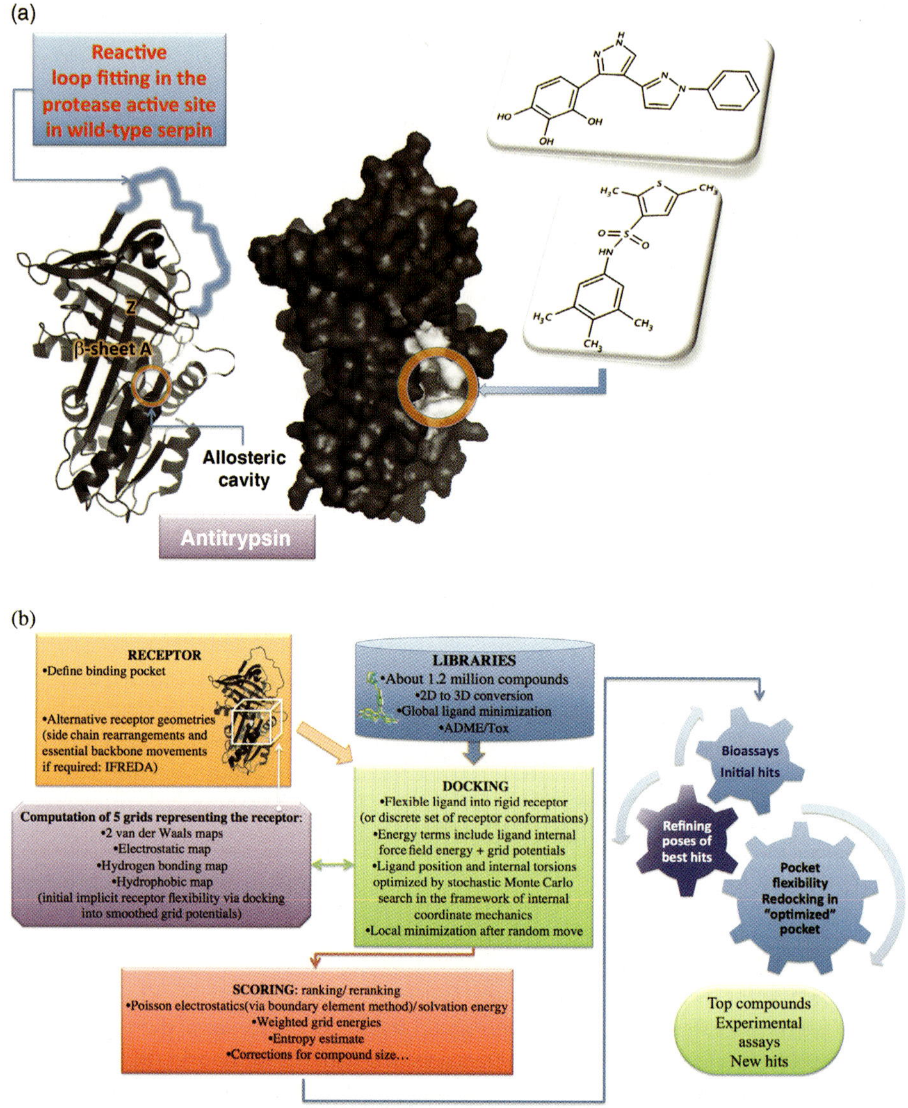

Figure 16.6 (a) Antitrypsin polymerization: design of allosteric inhibitors with the ICM package. The Z mutation and the so-called β-sheet A are highlighted in orange and the reactive center loop is labeled for orientation and painted blue. The allosteric binding pocket is colored white, some compounds identified in that study are shown to the right-hand side of the figure, and the molecule that blocks polymerization is the bottom compound [150]. (b) Overview of the ICM structure-based virtual screening process for antitrypsin.

experiments. These changes were achieved by performing internal coordinate Monte Carlo side-chain simulations in the presence of each ligand in its predicted binding pose. Nineteen extra compounds were selected after redocking on this modified receptor structure, ten of them were structurally similar to the original two active compounds, suggesting that ligand-based approaches could also have been performed instead of docking–scoring. Some of these molecules were as active as the best molecule identified in the previous screen. Thus, several compounds were found by combining rounds of *in silico* screening and *in vitro* testing with the desired biological activity, opening new ways of blocking polymer formation. Interestingly, the compound appears to be specific to α1-antitrypsin and does not act on other members of the serpin family.

16.7 Conclusions and Future Directions

The pharmaceutical industry or public sector is looking for new opportunities outside the enzyme field. PPIs are thus an attractive new class of potential therapeutic targets that have just started to be investigated in a high-throughput manner. Very few of the designed molecule inhibitors of protein–protein interactions have been clinically tested. One example is a synthetic cyclic heptapeptide that inhibits interaction between CD4 and MHC class II proteins and that has been approved by the FDA for a phase I clinical trial in graft-versus-host disease prophylaxis in bone marrow transplant patients [85]. Another example is a new thrombopoetic growth factor, eltrombopag (or SB-497 115), which is actually in phase III clinical trials as an oral and nonpeptide thrombopoetin receptor agonist for the treatment of idiopathic thrombocytopenic purpura [85]. Other molecules in clinical trials are being developed by Genentech and Abott [6, 83, 85]. Systematic efforts to identify PPIMs and to chart complex and dynamic interaction networks are thus definitively needed.

Several challenges for *in silico* methods have to be faced:

a) Some interfaces are rather flat and may appear as undruggable; however, cavities suitable to bind a small druglike compound may exist and could be investigated using simulation methods such as molecular dynamics or normal modes analysis. Tools to predict and define druggable pockets even in the absence of a visible cavity will have to be developed.
b) Better incorporation of flexibility during docking, specific scoring functions, and better postprocessing tools could be devised.
c) It will be important to answer one crucial question: is it possible to achieve the levels of potency and selectivity required for a drug for PPIMs while still remaining within the limits of the acceptable ADME/Tox properties for oral administration? This suggests that investigations on the chemical space of PPIMs and comparisons with other drugs are needed. Knowledge about the chemical space of PPIMs could lead to the design of focused libraries enriched in molecules displaying such a profile [7].

A possible strategy before initiating the screening of a PPI is to follow the decision tree model as proposed by Chene, where one asks specific PPI questions before moving to the next step [49]. For instance, is the 3D structure of the system known? Is there a cavity or is it possible to find one? What is the physical nature of this cavity? Is it compatible with binding of a small druglike compound? At the end of the process, the protein complex under study could be classified as tractable or not by a small molecule. Recent success stories and advances in virtual screening computations [151–153] suggest that PPIs can be screened and we envision that many new complexes will be targeted and drugged in the coming years.

References

1 Stumpf, M.P., Thorne, T., de Silva, E., Stewart, R., An, H.J., Lappe, M., and Wiuf, C. (2008) Estimating the size of the human interactome. *Proceedings of the National Academy of Sciences of the United States of America*, **105**, 6959–6964.

2 Kelly, W. and Stumpf, M. (2008) Protein–protein interactions: from global to local analyses. *Current Opinion in Biotechnology*, **19**, 396–403.

3 Morsy, M., Gouthu, S., Orchard, S., Thorneycroft, D., Harper, J.F., Mittler, R., and Cushman, J.C. (2008) Charting plant interactomes: possibilities and challenges. *Trends in Plant Science*, **13**, 183–191.

4 Ruffner, H., Bauer, A., and Bouwmeester, T. (2007) Human protein–protein interaction networks and the value for drug discovery. *Drug Discovery Today*, **12**, 709–716.

5 Stockwell, B.R. (2006) Preventing protein secretion with chemical glue. *Nature Chemical Biology*, **2**, 7–8.

6 Wells, J.A. and McClendon, C.L. (2007) Reaching for high-hanging fruit in drug discovery at protein–protein interfaces. *Nature*, **450**, 1001–1009.

7 Sperandio, O., Reynes, C.H., Camproux, A.C., and Villoutreix, B.O. (2009) Rationalizing the chemical space of protein–protein interaction inhibitors. *Drug Discovery Today*, **15** (5–6), 220–229.

8 Hopkins, A.L. and Groom, C.R. (2002) The druggable genome. *Nature Reviews. Drug Discovery*, **1**, 727–730.

9 Imming, P., Sinning, C., and Meyer, A. (2006) Drugs, their targets and the nature and number of drug targets. *Nature Reviews. Drug Discovery*, **5**, 821–834.

10 Zheng, C., Han, L., Yap, C.W., Xie, B., and Chen, Y. (2006) Progress and problems in the exploration of therapeutic targets. *Drug Discovery Today*, **11**, 412–420.

11 Landry, Y. and Gies, J.P. (2008) Drugs and their molecular targets: an updated overview. *Fundamental & Clinical Pharmacology*, **22**, 1–18.

12 Stockwell, B.R. (2004) Exploring biology with small organic molecules. *Nature*, **432**, 846–854.

13 Newman, R.H. and Zhang, J. (2008) Small molecules and chemical tools at the interface. *Nature Chemical Biology*, **4**, 382–386.

14 Ma, P. and Zemmel, R. (2002) Value of novelty? *Nature Reviews. Drug Discovery*, **1**, 571–572.

15 Betz, U.A. (2005) How many genomics targets can a portfolio afford? *Drug Discovery Today*, **10**, 1057–1063.

16 Betz, U.A., Farquhar, R., and Ziegelbauer, K. (2005) Genomics: success or failure to deliver drug targets? *Current Opinion in Chemical Biology*, **9**, 387–391.

17 Barnes, M.R., Harland, L., Foord, S.M., Hall, M.D., Dix, I., Thomas, S., Williams-Jones, B.I., and Brouwer, C.R. (2009) Lowering industry firewalls: pre-competitive informatics initiatives in drug discovery. *Nature Reviews. Drug Discovery*, **8** (9), 701–708.

18 Whitty, A. and Kumaravel, G. (2006) Between a rock and a hard place? *Nature Chemical Biology*, **2**, 112–118.

19 Mazuc, E., Villoutreix, B.O., Malbec, O., Roumier, T., Fleury, S., Leonetti, J.P., Dombrowicz, D., Daeron, M., Martineau, P., and Dariavach, P. (2008) A novel druglike spleen tyrosine kinase binder prevents anaphylactic shock when administered orally. *The Journal of Allergy and Clinical Immunology*, **122**, 188–194. 194 e1-3.

20 Fletcher, S. and Hamilton, A.D. (2007) Protein–protein interaction inhibitors: small molecules from screening techniques. *Current Topics in Medicinal Chemistry*, **7**, 922–927.

21 Robinson, J.A., Demarco, S., Gombert, F., Moehle, K., and Obrecht, D. (2008) The design, structures and therapeutic potential of protein epitope mimetics. *Drug Discovery Today*, **13**, 944–951.

22 Baines, I.C. and Colas, P. (2006) Peptide aptamers as guides for small-molecule drug discovery. *Drug Discovery Today*, **11**, 334–341.

23 Goncalves, V., Gautier, B., Coric, P., Bouaziz, S., Lenoir, C., Garbay, C., Vidal, M., and Inguimbert, N. (2007) Rational design, structure, and biological evaluation of cyclic peptides mimicking the vascular endothelial growth factor. *Journal of Medicinal Chemistry*, **50**, 5135–5146.

24 Neduva, V. and Russell, R.B. (2006) Peptides mediating interaction networks: new leads at last. *Current Opinion in Biotechnology*, **17**, 465–471.

25 Shiau, A.K., Massari, M.E., and Ozbal, C.C. (2008) Back to basics: label-free technologies for small molecule screening. *Combinatorial Chemistry & High Throughput Screening*, **11**, 231–237.

26 Congreve, M., Murray, C.W., and Blundell, T.L. (2005) Structural biology and drug discovery. *Drug Discovery Today*, **10**, 895–907.

27 Blundell, T.L., Jhoti, H., and Abell, C. (2002) High-throughput crystallography for lead discovery in drug design. *Nature Reviews. Drug Discovery*, **1**, 45–54.

28 Colas, P. (2008) High-throughput screening assays to discover small-molecule inhibitors of protein interactions. *Current Drug Discovery Technologies*, **5**, 190–199.

29 Neumann, T., Junker, H.D., Schmidt, K., and Sekul, R. (2007) SPR-based fragment screening: advantages and applications. *Current Topics in Medicinal Chemistry*, **7**, 1630–1642.

30 Jhoti, H., Cleasby, A., Verdonk, M., and Williams, G. (2007) Fragment-based screening using X-ray crystallography and NMR spectroscopy. *Current Opinion in Chemical Biology*, **11**, 485–493.

31 Congreve, M., Chessari, G., Tisi, D., and Woodhead, A.J. (2008) Recent developments in fragment-based drug discovery. *Journal of Medicinal Chemistry*, **51**, 3661–3680.

32 Chessari, G. and Woodhead, A.J. (2009) From fragment to clinical candidate: a historical perspective. *Drug Discovery Today*, **14**, 668–675.

33 Bartoli, S., Fincham, C.I., and Fattori, D. (2007) Fragment-based drug design: combining philosophy with technology. *Current Opinion in Drug Discovery & Development*, **10**, 422–429.

34 Tintelnot-Blomley, M. and Lewis, R.A. (2006) A critical appraisal of structure-based drug design. *Investigational Drugs*, **9**, 114–118.

35 Klebe, G. (2006) Virtual ligand screening: strategies, perspectives and limitations. *Drug Discovery Today*, **11**, 580–594.

36 Willett, P. (2006) Similarity-based virtual screening using 2D fingerprints. *Drug Discovery Today*, **11**, 1046–1053.

37 Clackson, T. and Wells, J.A. (1995) A hot spot of binding energy in a hormone–receptor interface. *Science*, **267**, 383–386.

38 B.-Rao, C., Subramanian, J., and Sharma, S.D. (2009) Managing protein flexibility in docking and its applications. *Drug Discovery Today*, **14**, 394–400.

39 Cozzini, P., Kellogg, G.E., Spyrakis, F., Abraham, D.J., Costantino, G., Emerson, A., Fanelli, F., Gohlke, H., Kuhn, L.A., Morris, G.M., Orozco, M., Pertinhez, T.A., Rizzi, M., and Sotriffer, C.A. (2008) Target flexibility: an emerging consideration in drug discovery and design. *Journal of Medicinal Chemistry*, **51**, 6237–6255.

40 Teague, S.J. (2003) Implications of protein flexibility for drug discovery. *Nature Reviews. Drug Discovery*, **2**, 527–541.

41 Lipinski, C.A., Lombardo, F., Dominy, B.W., and Feeney, P.J. (2001) Experimental and computational approaches to estimate solubility and permeability in drug discovery and development settings. *Advanced Drug Delivery Reviews*, **46**, 3–26.

42 van de Waterbeemd, H. and Gifford, E. (2003) ADMET *in silico* modelling: towards prediction paradise? *Nature Reviews. Drug Discovery*, **2**, 192–204.

43 Blake, J.F. (2000) Chemoinformatics: predicting the physicochemical properties of "drug-like" molecules. *Current Opinion in Biotechnology*, **11**, 104–107.

44 Blake, J.F. (2005) Identification and evaluation of molecular properties related to preclinical optimization and clinical fate. *Journal of Medicinal Chemistry*, **1**, 649–655.

45 Fry, D.C. (2006) Protein–protein interactions as targets for small molecule drug discovery. *Biopolymers*, **84**, 535–552.

46 Villoutreix, B.O., Bastard, K., Sperandio, O., Fahraeus, R., Poyet, J.L., Calvo, F., Deprez, B., and Miteva, M.A. (2008) In *silico–in vitro* screening of protein–protein interactions: towards the next generation of therapeutics. *Current Pharmaceutical Biotechnology*, **9**, 103–122.

47 Fry, D.C. (2008) Drug-like inhibitors of protein–protein interactions: a structural examination of effective protein mimicry. *Current Protein & Peptide Science*, **9**, 240–247.

48 Domling, A. (2008) Small molecular weight protein–protein interaction antagonists: an insurmountable challenge? *Current Opinion in Chemical Biology*, **12**, 281–291.

49 Chene, P. (2006) Drugs targeting protein–protein interactions. *ChemMedChem*, **1**, 400–411.

50 Blazer, L.L. and Neubig, R.R. (2009) Small molecule protein–protein interaction inhibitors as CNS therapeutic agents: current progress and future hurdles. *Neuropsychopharmacology*, **34**, 126–141.

51 Kern, J.T., Hannink, M., and Hess, J.F. (2007) Disruption of the Keap1-containing ubiquitination complex as an antioxidant therapy. *Current Topics in Medicinal Chemistry*, **7**, 972–978.

52 Rochet, J.C. (2007) Novel therapeutic strategies for the treatment of protein-misfolding diseases. *Expert Reviews in Molecular Medicine*, **9**, 1–34.

53 Almeida, M.R., Gales, L., Damas, A.M., Cardoso, I., and Saraiva, M.J. (2005) Small transthyretin (TTR) ligands as possible therapeutic agents in TTR amyloidoses. *Current Drug Targets. CNS Neurological Disorders*, **4**, 587–596.

54 Arkin, M. (2005) Protein–protein interactions and cancer: small molecules going in for the kill. *Current Opinion in Chemical Biology*, **9**, 317–324.

55 Archakov, A.I., Govorun, V.M., Dubanov, A.V., Ivanov, Y.D., Veselovsky, A.V., Lewi, P., and Janssen, P. (2003) Protein–protein interactions as a target for drugs in proteomics. *Proteomics*, **3**, 380–391.

56 Yin, H. and Hamilton, A.D. (2005) Strategies for targeting protein–protein interactions with synthetic agents. *Angewandte Chemie – International Edition in English*, **44**, 4130–4163.

57 Thanos, C.D., DeLano, W.L., and Wells, J.A. (2006) Hot-spot mimicry of a cytokine receptor by a small molecule. *Proceedings of the National Academy of Sciences of the United States of America*, **103**, 15422–15427.

58 Berg, T. (2008) Small-molecule inhibitors of protein–protein interactions. *Current Opinion in Drug Discovery & Development*, **11**, 666–674.

59 Stauffer, S.R. (2007) Small molecule inhibition of the Bcl-X(L)-BH3 protein–protein interaction: proof-of-concept of an *in vivo* chemopotentiator ABT-737. *Current Topics in Medicinal Chemistry*, **7**, 961–965.

60 Schimmer, A.D., Dalili, S., Batey, R.A., and Riedl, S.J. (2006) Targeting XIAP for the treatment of malignancy. *Cell Death and Differentiation*, **13**, 179–188.

61 Arkin, M.R. and Whitty, A. (2009) The road less traveled: modulating signal transduction enzymes by inhibiting

their protein–protein interactions. *Current Opinion in Chemical Biology*, **13**, 284–290.

62 Betzi, S., Restouin, A., Opi, S., Arold, S.T., Parrot, I., Guerlesquin, F., Morelli, X., and Collette, Y. (2007) Protein–protein interaction inhibition (2P2I) combining high throughput and virtual screening: application to the HIV-1 Nef protein. *Proceedings of the National Academy of Sciences of the United States of America*, **104**, 19256–19261.

63 Soulere, L. (2009) Toward docking-based virtual screening for discovering antitubulin agents by targeting taxane and colchicine binding sites. *ChemMedChem*, **4**, 161–163.

64 Xu, X., Kasembeli, M.M., Jiang, X., Tweardy, B.J., and Tweardy, D.J. (2009) Chemical probes that competitively and selectively inhibit Stat3 activation. *Public Library of Science One*, **4**, e4783.

65 Hachet-Haas, M., Balabanian, K., Rohmer, F., Pons, F., Franchet, C., Lecat, S., Chow, K.Y., Dagher, R., Gizzi, P., Didier, B., Lagane, B., Kellenberger, E., Bonnet, D., Baleux, F., Haiech, J., Parmentier, M., Frossard, N., Arenzana-Seisdedos, F., Hibert, M., and Galzi, J.L. (2008) Small neutralizing molecules to inhibit actions of the chemokine CXCL12. *The Journal of Biological Chemistry*, **283**, 23189–23199.

66 Bahadur, R.P. and Zacharias, M. (2008) The interface of protein–protein complexes: analysis of contacts and prediction of interactions. *Cellular and Molecular Life Sciences*, **65**, 1059–1072.

67 Janin, J., Bahadur, R.P., and Chakrabarti, P. (2008) Protein–protein interaction and quaternary structure. *Quarterly Reviews of Biophysics*, **41**, 133–180.

68 Keskin, O., Gursoy, A., Ma, B., and Nussinov, R. (2007) Towards drugs targeting multiple proteins in a systems biology approach. *Current Topics in Medicinal Chemistry*, **7**, 943–951.

69 Keskin, O. and Nussinov, R. (2007) Similar binding sites and different partners: implications to shared proteins in cellular pathways. *Structure (London, England: 1993)*, **15**, 341–354.

70 Keskin, O., Tuncbag, N., and Gursoy, A. (2008) Characterization and prediction of protein interfaces to infer protein–protein interaction networks. *Current Pharmaceutical Biotechnology*, **9**, 67–76.

71 Reichmann, D., Rahat, O., Cohen, M., Neuvirth, H., and Schreiber, G. (2007) The molecular architecture of protein–protein binding sites. *Current Opinion in Structural Biology*, **17**, 67–76.

72 de Vries, S.J. and Bonvin, A.M. (2008) How proteins get in touch: interface prediction in the study of biomolecular complexes. *Current Protein & Peptide Science*, **9**, 394–406.

73 Bonvin, A.M. (2006) Flexible protein–protein docking. *Current Opinion in Structural Biology*, **16**, 194–200.

74 Wells, J.A. (1996) Binding in the growth hormone receptor complex. *Proceedings of the National Academy of Sciences of the United States of America*, **93**, 1–6.

75 Gonzalez-Ruiz, D. and Gohlke, H. (2006) Targeting protein–protein interactions with small molecules: challenges and perspectives for computational binding epitope detection and ligand finding. *Current Medicinal Chemistry*, **13**, 2607–2625.

76 Reynolds, C., Damerell, D., and Jones, S. (2009) ProtorP: a protein–protein interaction analysis server. *Bioinformatics (Oxford, England)*, **25**, 413–414.

77 Jones, S. and Thornton, J.M. (1996) Principles of protein–protein interactions. *Proceedings of the National Academy of Sciences of the United States of America*, **93**, 13–20.

78 Mintseris, J., Wiehe, K., Pierce, B., Anderson, R., Chen, R., Janin, J., and Weng, Z. (2005) Protein–protein docking benchmark 2.0: an update. *Proteins*, **60**, 214–216.

79 Cavasotto, C.N. and Singh, N. (2008) Docking and high throughput docking: successes and the challenge of protein flexibility. *Current Computer-Aided Drug Design*, **4**, 221–234.

80 Alonso, H., Bliznyuk, A.A., and Gready, J.E. (2006) Combining docking and molecular dynamic simulations in drug design. *Medicinal Research Reviews*, **26**, 531–568.

81 Zhong, S., Macias, A.T., and MacKerell, A.D., Jr. (2007) Computational identification of inhibitors of protein–protein interactions. *Current Topics in Medicinal Chemistry*, **7**, 63–82.

82 Carlson, H.A. (2002) Protein flexibility and drug design: how to hit a moving target. *Current Opinion in Chemical Biology*, **6**, 447–452.

83 Grosdidier, S. and Fernandez-Recio, J. (2009) Docking and scoring: applications to drug discovery in the interactomics era. *Expert Opinion on Drug Discovery*, **4**, 673–686.

84 Brown, S.P. and Hajduk, P.J. (2006) Effects of conformational dynamics on predicted protein druggability. *ChemMedChem*, **1**, 70–72.

85 Grosdidier, S., Totrov, M., and Fernandez-Recio, J. (2009) Computer applications to prediction of protein–protein interactions and rational drug design. *Journal of Advances and Application in Bioinformatics and Chemistry*, **2009** (2), 101–123.

86 Arkin, M.R., Randal, M., DeLano, W.L., Hyde, J., Luong, T.N., Oslob, J.D., Raphael, D.R., Taylor, L., Wang, J., McDowell, R.S., Wells, J.A., and Braisted, A.C. (2003) Binding of small molecules to an adaptive protein–protein interface. *Proceedings of the National Academy of Sciences of the United States of America*, **100**, 1603–1608.

87 Sugaya, N. and Ikeda, K. (2009) Assessing the druggability of protein–protein interactions by a supervised machine-learning method. *BMC Bioinformatics*, **10**, 263.

88 Sugaya, N., Ikeda, K., Tashiro, T., Takeda, S., Otomo, J., Ishida, Y., Shiratori, A., Toyoda, A., Noguchi, H., Takeda, T., Kuhara, S., Sakaki, Y., and Iwayanagi, T. (2007) An integrative *in silico* approach for discovering candidates for drug-targetable protein–protein interactions in interactome data. *BMC Pharmacology*, **7**, 10.

89 Eyrisch, S. and Helms, V. (2009) What induces pocket openings on protein surface patches involved in protein–protein interactions? *Journal of Computer-Aided Molecular Design*, **23**, 73–86.

90 Eyrisch, S. and Helms, V. (2007) Transient pockets on protein surfaces involved in protein–protein interaction. *Journal of Medicinal Chemistry*, **50**, 3457–3464.

91 Fuller, J.C., Burgoyne, N.J., and Jackson, R.M. (2009) Predicting druggable binding sites at the protein–protein interface. *Drug Discovery Today*, **14**, 155–161.

92 Luque, I. and Freire, E. (2000) Structural stability of binding sites: consequences for binding affinity and allosteric effects. *Proteins* (Suppl. 4), 63–71.

93 Tuncbag, N., Kar, G., Keskin, O., Gursoy, A., and Nussinov, R. (2009) A survey of available tools and web servers for analysis of protein–protein interactions and interfaces. *Briefings in Bioinformatics*, **10**, 217–232.

94 Villoutreix, B.O., Renault, N., Lagorce, D., Sperandio, O., Montes, M., and Miteva, M.A. (2007) Free resources to assist structure-based virtual ligand screening experiments. *Current Protein & Peptide Science*, **8**, 381–411.

95 Martin, J., Regad, L., Lecornet, H., and Camproux, A.C. (2008) Structural deformation upon protein–protein interaction: a structural alphabet approach. *BMC Structural Biology*, **8**, 12.

96 Cho, K.I., Kim, D., and Lee, D. (2009) A feature-based approach to modeling protein–protein interaction hot spots. *Nucleic Acids Research*, **37**, 2672–2687.

97 Kirchmair, J., Markt, P., Distinto, S., Schuster, D., Spitzer, G.M., Liedl, K.R., Langer, T., and Wolber, G. (2008) The Protein Data Bank (PDB), its related services and software tools as key components for *in silico* guided drug discovery. *Journal of Medicinal Chemistry*, **51**, 7021–7040.

98 Anderson, A.C. (2003) The process of structure-based drug design. *Chemistry & Biology*, **10**, 787–797.

99 Davis, A.M., Teague, S.J., and Kleywegt, G.J. (2003) Application and limitations of X-ray crystallographic data in structure-based ligand and drug design. *Angewandte Chemie – International Edition in English*, **42**, 2718–2736.

100 Davis, A.M., St-Gallay, S.A., and Kleywegt, G.J. (2008) Limitations and lessons in the use of X-ray structural information in drug design. *Drug Discovery Today*, **13**, 831–841.

101 Wlodawer, A., Minor, W., Dauter, Z., and Jaskolski, M. (2008) Protein crystallography for non-crystallographers, or how to get the best (but not more) from published macromolecular structures. *FEBS Journal*, **275**, 1–21.

102 Toogood, P.L. (2002) Inhibition of protein–protein association by small molecules: approaches and progress. *Journal of Medicinal Chemistry*, **45**, 1543–1558.

103 Lipinski, C. and Hopkins, A. (2004) Navigating chemical space for biology and medicine. *Nature*, **432**, 855–861.

104 Li, A.P. (2001) Screening for human ADME/Tox drug properties in drug discovery. *Drug Discovery Today*, **6**, 357–366.

105 Pagliaro, L., Felding, J., Audouze, K., Nielsen, S.J., Terry, R.B., Krog-Jensen, C., and Butcher, S. (2004) Emerging classes of protein–protein interaction inhibitors and new tools for their development. *Current Opinion in Chemical Biology*, **8**, 442–449.

106 Orry, A.J., Abagyan, R.A., and Cavasotto, C.N. (2006) Structure-based development of target-specific compound libraries. *Drug Discovery Today*, **11**, 261–266.

107 Neugebauer, A., Hartmann, R.W., and Klein, C.D. (2007) Prediction of protein–protein interaction inhibitors by chemoinformatics and machine learning methods. *Journal of Medicinal Chemistry*, **50**, 4665–4668.

108 Park, C.M., Bruncko, M., Adickes, J., Bauch, J., Ding, H., Kunzer, A., Marsh, K.C., Nimmer, P., Shoemaker, A.R., Song, X., Tahir, S.K., Tse, C., Wang, X., Wendt, M.D., Yang, X., Zhang, H., Fesik, S.W., Rosenberg, S.H., and Elmore, S.W. (2008) Discovery of an orally bioavailable small molecule inhibitor of prosurvival B-cell lymphoma 2 proteins. *Journal of Medicinal Chemistry*, **51**, 6902–6915.

109 Shoichet, B.K. (2004) Virtual screening of chemical libraries. *Nature*, **432**, 862–865.

110 Abagyan, R. and Totrov, M. (2001) High-throughput docking for lead generation. *Current Opinion in Chemical Biology*, **5**, 375–382.

111 Jorgensen, W.L. (2004) The many roles of computation in drug discovery. *Science*, **303**, 1813–1818.

112 Jain, A.N. (2004) Virtual screening in lead discovery and optimization. *Current Opinion in Drug Discovery & Development*, **7**, 396–403.

113 Krovat, E.M., Steindl, T., and Langer, T. (2005) Recent advances in docking and scoring. *Current Computer-Aided Drug Design*, **1**, 93–102.

114 Sperandio, O., Miteva, M.A., and Villoutreix, B.O. (2008) Combining ligand and structure-based methods in drug design projects. *Current Computer-Aided Drug Design*, **4**, 250–258.

115 Moitessier, N., Englebienne, P., Lee, D., Lawandi, J., and Corbeil, C.R. (2008) Towards the development of universal, fast and highly accurate docking/scoring methods: a long way to go. *British Journal of Pharmacology*, **153** (Suppl. 1), S7–S26.

116 Cavasotto, C.N. and Orry, A.J. (2007) Ligand docking and structure-based virtual screening in drug discovery. *Current Topics in Medicinal Chemistry*, **7**, 1006–1014.

117 Sperandio, O., Miteva, M.A., Delfaud, F., and Villoutreix, B.O. (2006) Receptor-based computational screening of compound databases: the main docking-scoring engines. *Current Protein & Peptide Science*, **7**, 369–393.

118 Kitchen, D.B., Decornez, H., Furr, J.R., and Bajorath, J. (2004) Docking and scoring in virtual screening for drug discovery: methods and applications. *Nature Reviews. Drug Discovery*, **3**, 935–949.

119 Cavasotto, C.N. and Phatak, S.S. (2009) Homology modeling in drug discovery: current trends and applications. *Drug Discovery Today*, **14**, 676–683.

120 Auer, J. and Bajorath, J. (2008) Molecular similarity concepts and search calculations. *Methods in Molecular Biology (Clifton, NJ)*, **453**, 327–347.

121 Tanrikulu, Y. and Schneider, G. (2008) Pseudoreceptor models in drug design:

bridging ligand- and receptor-based virtual screening. *Nature Reviews. Drug Discovery*, **7**, 667–677.
122 Stahura, F.L. and Bajorath, J. (2005) New methodologies for ligand-based virtual screening. *Current Pharmaceutical Design*, **11**, 1189–1202.
123 Miteva, M.A., Lee, W.H., Montes, M.O., and Villoutreix, B.O. (2005) Fast structure-based virtual ligand screening combining FRED, DOCK, and Surflex. *Journal of Medicinal Chemistry*, **48**, 6012–6022.
124 Sauton, N., Lagorce, D., Villoutreix, B.O., and Miteva, M.A. (2008) MS-DOCK: accurate multiple conformation generator and rigid docking protocol for multi-step virtual ligand screening. *BMC Bioinformatics*, **9**, 184.
125 An, J., Totrov, M., and Abagyan, R. (2005) Pocketome via comprehensive identification and classification of ligand binding envelopes. *Molecular & Cellular Proteomics*, **4**, 752–761.
126 Totrov, M. and Abagyan, R. (2008) Flexible ligand docking to multiple receptor conformations: a practical alternative. *Current Opinion in Structural Biology*, **18**, 178–184.
127 Cavasotto, C.N. and Abagyan, R.A. (2004) Protein flexibility in ligand docking and virtual screening to protein kinases. *Journal of Molecular Biology*, **337**, 209–225.
128 Feher, M. (2006) Consensus scoring for protein–ligand interactions. *Drug Discovery Today*, **11**, 421–428.
129 Gilson, M.K. and Zhou, H.X. (2007) Calculation of protein–ligand binding affinities. *Annual Review of Biophysics and Biomolecular Structure*, **36**, 21–42.
130 Brewerton, S.C. (2008) The use of protein–ligand interaction fingerprints in docking. *Current Opinion in Drug Discovery & Development*, **11**, 356–364.
131 Jain, A.N. (2006) Scoring functions for protein–ligand docking. *Current Protein & Peptide Science*, **7**, 407–420.
132 Rajamani, R. and Good, A.C. (2007) Ranking poses in structure-based lead discovery and optimization: current trends in scoring function development. *Current Opinion in Drug Discovery & Development*, **10**, 308–315.
133 Huang, N. and Jacobson, M.P. (2007) Physics-based methods for studying protein–ligand interactions. *Current Opinion in Drug Discovery & Development*, **10**, 325–331.
134 Leach, A.R., Shoichet, B.K., and Peishoff, C.E. (2006) Prediction of protein–ligand interactions. Docking and scoring: successes and gaps. *Journal of Medicinal Chemistry*, **49**, 5851–5855.
135 Corbeil, C.R., Therrien, E., and Moitessier, N. (2009) Modeling reality for optimal docking of small molecules to biological targets. *Current Computer-Aided Drug Design*, **5**, 242–263.
136 Orita, M., Ohno, K., and Niimi, T. (2009) Two "Golden Ratio" indices in fragment-based drug discovery. *Drug Discovery Today*, **14**, 321–328.
137 Ladbury, J.E., Klebe, G., and Freire, E., (2010) Adding calorimetric data to decision making in lead discovery: a hot tip. *Nature Reviews. Drug Discovery*, **9**, 23–27.
138 Pommier, Y. and Cherfils, J. (2005) Interfacial inhibition of macromolecular interactions: nature's paradigm for drug discovery. *Trends in Pharmacological Sciences*, **26**, 138–145.
139 Berg, T. (2003) Modulation of protein–protein interactions with small organic molecules. *Angewandte Chemie – International Edition in English*, **42**, 2462–2481.
140 Ray, S.S., Nowak, R.J., Brown, R.H., Jr., and Lansbury, P.T., Jr. (2005) Small-molecule-mediated stabilization of familial amyotrophic lateral sclerosis-linked superoxide dismutase mutants against unfolding and aggregation. *Proceedings of the National Academy of Sciences of the United States of America*, **102**, 3639–3644.
141 Adamski-Werner, S.L., Palaninathan, S.K., Sacchettini, J.C., and Kelly, J.W. (2004) Diflunisal analogues stabilize the native state of transthyretin. Potent inhibition of amyloidogenesis. *Journal of Medicinal Chemistry*, **47**, 355–374.
142 Repasky, M.P., Shelley, M., and Friesner, R.A. (2007) Flexible ligand docking with Glide, *Current Protocols in Bioinformatics*, John Wiley & Sons, Inc.

143 Broadbridge, R.J. and Sharma, R.P. (2000) The Src homology-2 domains (SH2 domains) of the protein tyrosine kinase p56lck: structure, mechanism and drug design. *Current Drug Targets*, **1**, 365–386.

144 Cousins-Wasti, R.C., Ingraham, R.H., Morelock, M.M., and Grygon, C.A. (1996) Determination of affinities for lck SH2 binding peptides using a sensitive fluorescence assay: comparison between the pYEEIP and pYQPQP consensus sequences reveals context-dependent binding specificity. *Biochemistry*, **35**, 16746–16752.

145 Tong, L., Warren, T.C., King, J., Betageri, R., Rose, J., and Jakes, S. (1996) Crystal structures of the human p56lck SH2 domain in complex with two short phosphotyrosyl peptides at 1.0 A and 1.8 A resolution. *Journal of Molecular Biology*, **256**, 601–610.

146 Huang, N., Nagarsekar, A., Xia, G., Hayashi, J., and MacKerell, A.D., Jr. (2004) Identification of non-phosphate-containing small molecular weight inhibitors of the tyrosine kinase p56 Lck SH2 domain via *in silico* screening against the pY + 3 binding site. *Journal of Medicinal Chemistry*, **47**, 3502–3511.

147 Shoichet, B.K. and Kuntz, I.D. (1991) Protein docking and complementarity. *Journal of Molecular Biology*, **221**, 327–346.

148 Macias, A.T., Mia, M.Y., Xia, G., Hayashi, J., and MacKerell, A.D., Jr. (2005) Lead validation and SAR development via chemical similarity searching: application to compounds targeting the pY + 3 site of the SH2 domain of p56lck. *Journal of Chemical Information and Modeling*, **45**, 1759–1766.

149 Hardy, J.A. and Wells, J.A. (2004) Searching for new allosteric sites in enzymes. *Current Opinion in Structural Biology*, **14**, 706–715.

150 Mallya, M., Phillips, R.L., Saldanha, S.A., Gooptu, B., Brown, S.C., Termine, D.J., Shirvani, A.M., Wu, Y., Sifers, R.N., Abagyan, R., and Lomas, D.A. (2007) Small molecules block the polymerization of Z alpha1-antitrypsin and increase the clearance of intracellular aggregates. *Journal of Medicinal Chemistry*, **50**, 5357–5363.

151 Koppen, H. (2009) Virtual screening: what does it give us? *Current Opinion in Drug Discovery & Development*, **12**, 397–407.

152 Rester, U. (2008) From virtuality to reality – virtual screening in lead discovery and lead optimization: a medicinal chemistry perspective. *Current Opinion in Drug Discovery & Development*, **11**, 559–568.

153 Clark, D.E. (2008) What has virtual screening ever done for drug discovery. *Expert Opinion on Drug Discovery*, **8**, 841–851.

17
Fragment-Based Approaches in Virtual Screening

Danzhi Huang and Amedeo Caflisch

17.1
Introduction

Fragment-based screening (FBS) as a method to identify starting points for small-molecule drug discovery has become increasingly popular in recent years [1]. As a complementary and alternative approach to the traditional high-throughput screening (HTS), FBS starts from molecules whose molecular weights typically range from 150 to 250 Da. This approach is more routinely undertaken in therapeutic areas such as infectious disease, for which conventional screening has usually resulted in low hit rates [2]. The theoretical basis regarding the benefits of the fragment linking approach has already been reported about 30 years ago [3]. Interestingly, the importance of molecular fragments has been first recognized and exploited by computational approaches [4–6], which share similar aspects with experimental techniques that have been developed afterward, such as structure–activity relationship by nuclear magnetic resonance (NMR) [7]. More recently, fragment-based drug discovery strategies have been developed using X-ray crystallography [8], NMR spectroscopy [9], surface plasmon resonance [10], mass spectrometry [11, 12], substrate activity screening (where the fragments are substrates later converted into inhibitors [13–15]), and tethering [16, 17]. Experimental techniques for fragment-based drug discovery have been discussed in previous reviews that contain a large number of applications [1, 18–22]. Successful *in vitro* screening campaigns have been reported for several targets, and a nonexhaustive list includes β-secretase [10, 18, 23, 24], several protein kinases [25–29], DNA gyrase [30], caspase [31, 32], anthrax lethal factor [33], and phosphodiesterase [34].

The advantages of FBS over HTS have been reported [1], the main benefit being that a larger degree of chemical space can be explored using fragment libraries. HTS handles compounds up to millions but this amount only covers a tiny amount of the chemical space accessible to the small druglike molecules, which is estimated in the range of 10^{60}–10^{100} [35, 36]. Fragment-based approaches, however, allow sampling of a much larger amount of chemical diversity using a much smaller number of starting molecules. It has been estimated that the number of stable and synthetically

Virtual Screening. Edited by C. Sotriffer

ISBN: 978-3-527-32636-5

accessible molecular fragments is around 50 million [37]. This number is only about one order of magnitude larger than what is tested with HTS but covers a much vaster part of the chemical space, for example, up to 10^{25} if connecting combinatorially three fragments [38]. Second, fragments often bind to the target protein with higher "ligand efficiency" [39] than leadlike "hits." Third, fragment-based approaches lead to higher hit rates. Since the likelihood of unfavorable ligand–protein interactions increases exponentially with the size and complexity of the molecule [37], the small and simple molecules have more chances to bind to the protein, even if their affinity is usually low. The hit rates can be 30–40% for simple fragments [40].

In this chapter, we focus on the computational methods for fragment-based docking and particularly in Section 17.3 present the methods developed by our research group with applications to proteases and protein kinases. Notably, it has been possible to identify single-digit micromolar inhibitors for all enzymes by fragment-based docking of large libraries of small molecules. We also give possible reasons for the difficulties encountered in discovering submicromolar inhibitors by *in silico* fragment-based screening of collections of available compounds. Finally, we discuss the challenges that may be faced in fragment-based approaches.

17.2 *In Silico* Fragment-Based Approaches

In silico fragment-based approaches have been pioneered by Martin Karplus [4]. His paper with Andrew Miranker on the simultaneous minimization of multiple copies of small and mainly rigid functional groups in the protein force field (MCSS) can be considered as the first fragment-based procedure for drug discovery. It is based on a combination of Monte Carlo and energy minimization/quenched dynamics techniques and makes possible the efficient determination of energetically favorable positions and orientations of functional groups in the binding site of a protein with known three-dimensional structure. Preliminary tests of the MCSS method were made on the influenza coat protein hemagglutinin, and it showed that certain functional group minima correspond to those of the bound sialic acid ligand [4]. The approach was further validated on HIV-1 protease [6]. A set of functional groups corresponding to the protein main chain (*N*-methylacetamide) and to protein side chains (e.g., ethanol, ethylguanidinium) were used. The most favorable positions of these functional groups were used to derive the binding mode of a hexapeptide inhibitor. Notably, the result not only was in agreement with a published X-ray structure but also discovered an alternative binding mode that was confirmed a posteriori by further refinement of the X-ray structure. In another case, the binding sites of three fragments to protein FKBP12 were investigated by MCSS combined with energy evaluations using a physics-based scoring function that includes contributions from CHARMM [41, 42] and implicit solvation [43]. The computational results agreed with the NOE constraints from NMR spectroscopy [44]. Recently, MacKerell and Guvench have used explicit water molecular dynamics simulations to sample the positions of small aliphatic and aromatic molecules on the protein surface [45]. Their approach has the twofold advantage of accurate treatment of solvent and protein flexibility but is computationally more expensive than MCSS. The methodology was evaluated on BCL-6 oncoprotein and key binding interactions of the fragments used were in agreement with crystal structures [45].

Fragment-based approaches exist also for de novo design. LUDI is the first program developed for such a purpose [5]. Programs with similar functions include HOOK [46], PRO_ligand [47], Skelgen [48], CCLD [49], BREED [50], Lea3D [51], and GANDI [52]. These programs mainly differ in the design strategy (ligand- or receptor-based), the building blocks used to construct the ligands (atoms or fragments), the strategy used to sample the chemical and structural space, and the scoring function used to rank the putative ligands [53].

The effectiveness of virtual FBS at accurately docking fragment-like small molecules is less well studied compared to usual virtual screening. Recently, a critical assessment of virtual FBS has been reported by Joseph-McCarthy and coworkers who have used the program Glide [54] with nine different scoring schemes [55] for docking fragments in prostaglandin D synthase and DNA ligase [56]. Self-docking and cross-docking (docking ligands back into their cocrystal structure and a structure from a complex with a different compound, respectively) as well as enrichment studies were performed. They reported that even for difficult test cases, fragment docking yields higher enrichment than random selection [56]. Another interesting *in silico* FBS approach called replica generation has been developed by Fukunishi *et al.* [57]. For each fragment in the library, a set of replica molecules of different size are generated by adding side chains to the fragment and these molecules are used in docking. With the virtual chemical modification, potentially active fragments have more chances to be selected than just considering the original form of the fragment. This procedure was validated in the screening of inhibitors of six target proteins using known active compounds.

Hits from virtual FBS are usually weak but they can be further improved via structure-based designs and chemical editions. Metz and coworkers performed FBS using FlexX [58] to screen about 10 000 fragments with a pharmacophore-constrained docking against dipeptidyl peptidase IV. A range of β-phenethylamine-based compounds were identified and the results were also confirmed by X-ray crystallography. On the basis of the virtual FBS results and crystal structure, further structure-based optimization resulted in the discovery of a series of potent inhibitors [59, 60]. Hurley and coworkers screened a virtual fragment library of about 70 000 compounds against Aurora A kinase. Subsequent optimization was carried out by linking two *in silico* identified fragments of micromolar affinity resulting in an inhibitor of nanomolar potency [28].

Most of the approaches mentioned above make use of virtual FBS for identifying binders that consist of more than one fragment. In contrast, virtual FBS has been routinely carried out in pharmaceutical industry to generate focused subsets of large libraries for experimental screening with the aim of increasing the hit rate [54]. Jhoti and coworkers have used *in silico* FBS to construct target-specific fragment sets for their high-throughput X-ray crystallography using the program GOLD [61]. Docking with a variety of scoring functions was performed for relevant protein targets to select suitable fragments from 3.6 million unique compounds. With this approach, they have succeeded in identifying fragments for various proteins, for example, ribonuclease A, and confirmed their *in silico* findings by X-ray structures [62]. Hubbard and coworkers have used pharmacophore triangle approaches to design a diverse fragment library. Since their aim is to use NMR spectroscopy to screen against a wide range of targets [63, 64], a library that contains as much chemical diversity as possible has to be prepared. A measure of diversity was determined by molecular fingerprints based on 2D three-point pharmacophores. The presence or the absence of the encoding fingerprint components can be used to assess the uniqueness of a fragment for its putative recognition pattern. The resulting library was used to screen against 12 different protein targets using NMR spectroscopy and rather high hit rates (average 3.2%) have been achieved [63].

17.3 Our Approach to High-Throughput Fragment-Based Docking

Two essential elements of our *in silico* screening approach are the fragment-based docking procedure and the scoring based on force field energy [65] with continuum electrostatics solvation [66–70]. The pipeline for high-throughput docking consists of four consecutive steps (Figure 17.1): (1) automatic decomposition of each molecule of the library into fragments [71], (2) fragment docking and ranking of poses [68, 69], (3)

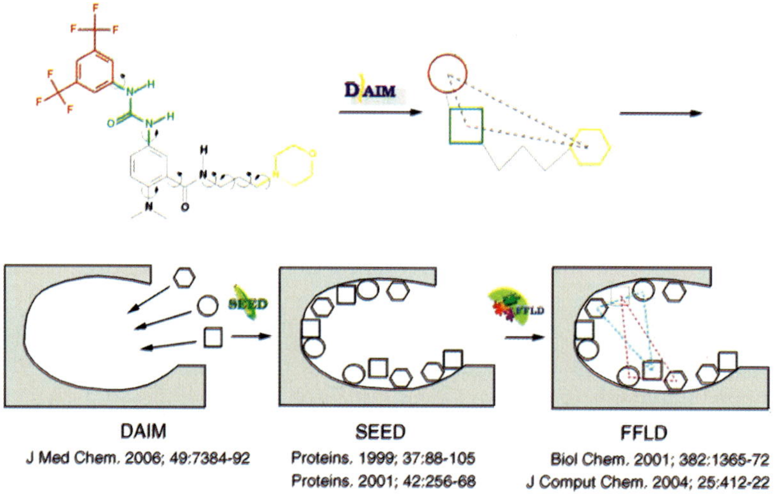

Figure 17.1 Schematic picture of the pipeline for automatic docking developed by our group. The automatic decomposition of the molecules into rigid fragments is carried out by the program DAIM [71]. The fragments are docked by the program SEED that evaluates the binding free energy including electrostatic solvation effects [68]. The program FFLD [72] is used for flexible ligand docking using positions and orientations of fragment triplets (dashed triangles).

flexible docking of each molecule of the library using the best poses of its fragments as anchors [72], and (4) evaluation of the binding free energy of multiple poses of each compound by the LIECE method (linear interaction energy with continuum electrostatics [73]). The first three steps are performed by computer programs developed by our research group. In the fourth step, CHARMM [41, 42] is used for the energy minimization and finite-difference Poisson calculations. In general, our FBS approach uses the fragment docking information only *in silico* and this information ultimately leads to larger hits, which are then used for experimental validation. With this strategy, the searchable conformational space in docking can be significantly reduced, which allows us to use accurate approaches for the evaluation of binding affinity, including solvation.

17.3.1
Decomposition of Compounds into Fragments

The automatic fragmentation of a molecule into substructures and the selection of the three anchor fragments for docking (see below) are performed by the program DAIM (Decomposition and Identification of Molecules [71]). The decomposition generates mainly rigid fragments that can be docked very efficiently (as explained in the next subsection). The decomposition of a molecule consists of four steps: ring identification, fragment definition, functional group merging, and completion of the valences. (i) Rings are identified by successively enumerating all neighbors (i.e., directly covalently bound atoms) of every atom, similar to a breadth-first search. (ii) A fragment is defined as a set of atoms connected by unbreakable bonds. The basic definition of unbreakable bonds includes terminal, double, triple, aromatic bonds, and bonds in rings. (iii) To form chemically relevant fragments and avoid the generation of many small groups, small functional groups (e.g., $-OH$, $-CH_3$, $-CX_3$ (where X can be any halogen), $-SO_3$, $-CHO$, $-NO_2$, $-NH_2$, and $-SH$) are merged with the fragment they are connected to. Unbreakable bonds and functional groups (points ii and iii, respectively) can be defined by the user. (iv) In the final step, missing atom neighbors are added. An atom will lack a neighbor atom whenever the bond connecting them has been cut. These missing neighbors are replaced by hydrogen atoms to reconstitute the correct valence for every atom. A methyl group is used to fill valences where a hydrogen atom would result in an unwanted additional hydrogen bond direction (e.g., a hydrogen replacing a carbon atom bound to an sp^3 nitrogen).

17.3.2
Docking of Anchor Fragments

The docking approach implemented in the program SEED determines optimal positions and orientations of small and rigid molecular fragments in the binding site of a protein target [68, 69]. Apolar fragments are docked into hydrophobic regions of the receptor while polar fragments are positioned such that at least one intermolecular hydrogen bond is formed. Each fragment is placed at several thousand different positions with multiple orientations (on the order of 10^6 poses in total) and the binding energy is estimated whenever severe clashes are not present (usually about 10^5 poses). The binding energy is the sum of the van der Waals interaction and the electrostatic energy. The latter consists of screened receptor–fragment interaction as well as receptor and fragment desolvations calculated by an efficient numerical implementation of the generalized Born approach [67].

17.3.3 Flexible Docking of Library Compounds

The flexible ligand docking approach FFLD uses a genetic algorithm and a very efficient scoring function [72, 74]. The random perturbations (i.e., sampling) in the genetic algorithm affect only the conformation of the ligand; its placement in the binding site is determined by the SEED anchors and a least square fitting method [75]. In this way, the position and orientation of the ligand in the binding site are determined by the best binding modes of its fragments previously docked by SEED. On the other hand, the scoring function used in FFLD is based on van der Waals and hydrogen bond terms and does not explicitly include solvation for efficiency reasons. Solvation effects are implicitly accounted for because the poses of the fragments are previously sorted according to force field energy with electrostatic solvation in SEED. FFLD requires three not-necessarily different fragments to place a flexible ligand unambiguously in the binding site, for example, the fluorobenzene, morpholine, and benzoic acid of compound **2** (Table 17.1 and Figure 17.2). The automatic definition of the three anchor fragments for each molecule of the library is performed by DAIM using the chemical richness, that is, the sum of all entries in the DAIM fingerprint [71].

17.3.4 LIECE Binding Energy Evaluation

The essential idea of linear interaction energy (LIE) models is that the free energy of complex formation can be calculated by considering only the end points of the thermodynamic cycle of ligand binding, that is, bound and free states. For this purpose, one usually calculates average values of interaction energies from molecular dynamics simulations of the isolated ligand and the ligand–protein complex [76, 77]. The free energy of binding is approximated by

$$\Delta G = \alpha(\langle E^{\mathrm{vdW}}\rangle_{\mathrm{bound}} - \langle E^{\mathrm{vdW}}\rangle_{\mathrm{free}}) + \beta(\langle E^{\mathrm{elec}}\rangle_{\mathrm{bound}} - \langle E^{\mathrm{elec}}\rangle_{\mathrm{free}}) \tag{17.1}$$

where E^{vdW} and E^{elec} are the van der Waals and electrostatic interaction energies between the ligand and its environment, respectively. The environment is either the solvent (free) or both the protein and solvent (bound). $\langle\,\rangle$ denotes an ensemble average sampled over a molecular dynamics [76] or Monte Carlo [78] trajectory. The coefficient α is determined empirically [76]. Originally, β was fixed to a value of 1/2, as predicted by the linear response approximation [76]. Later studies have shown, however, that improved models for a large variety of systems could be obtained by

Table 17.1 The library screening campaigns by fragment-based docking performed at the University of Zurich.

Protein	Enzyme class	Most potent inhibitor				Hit rate[a)]	Size of library	Scoring method	Reference
		Compound	Affinity (μM)	Ligand efficiency (kcal/mol per non-hydrogen atom)	MW (g/mol)				
Proteases									
β-Secretase	Asp protease	1	3.0[b)]	0.19	561	17% (12/72)	512 000	LIECE	[95]
β-Secretase	Asp protease	2	7.1[c)]	0.19	538	10% (9/88)	316 000	LIECE	[96]
Plasmepsin	Asp protease	3	2[c)]	0.25	500	32% (6/19)	40 000	Consensus scoring	[89]
NS3 protease	Ser protease	4	40[d)]	0.33	282	5% (1/22)	12 000	LIECE	[90]
NS3 protease	Ser protease	5	2.8[c)]/90[d)]	0.34/0.25	298	40% (2/5)	19 000	Pose filtering	[97]
Cathepsin B	Cys protease	6	4.8/6.7[c)]	0.29/0.28	369	3% (1/29)	48 000	Consensus scoring	[98]
Kinases									
EphB4	Tyr kinase	7	1.5[c)]	0.32	337	19% (8/43)	728 000	LIECE	[99]
CDK2	Ser/Thr kinase	8	7.8[c)]	0.32	321	3% (1/30)	40 000	LIECE	[91]

a) The ratio in parentheses is the number of compounds with a value of the measured affinity below 100 μM divided by the number of molecules tested experimentally.
b) Cell-based assay.
c) Enzymatic assay with purified protein in solution.
d) Binding affinity measured by nuclear magnetic resonance spectroscopy. Compounds **1–8** are listed in Figure 17.2.

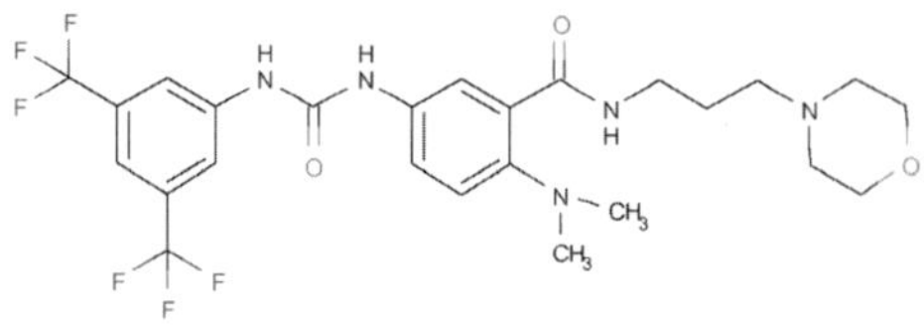

1

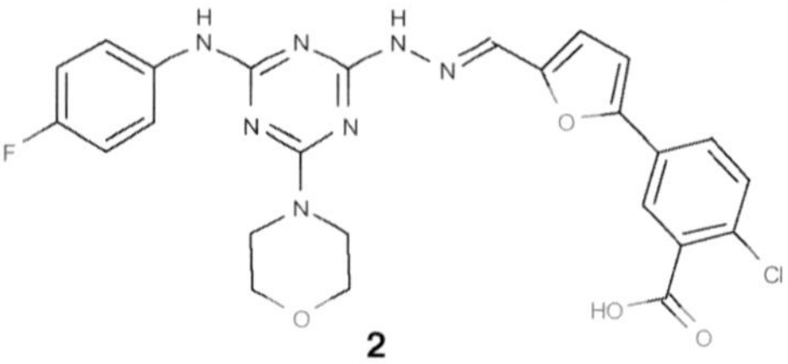

2

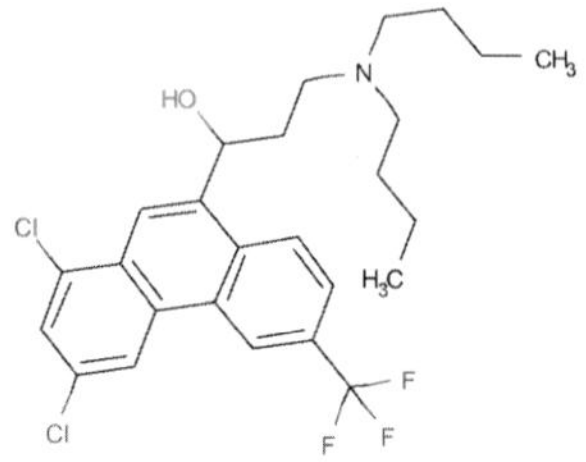

3

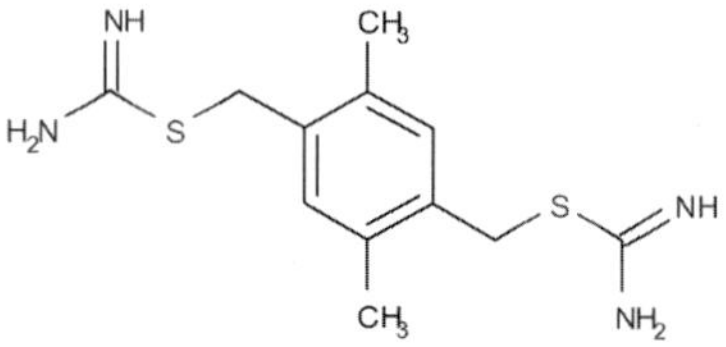

4

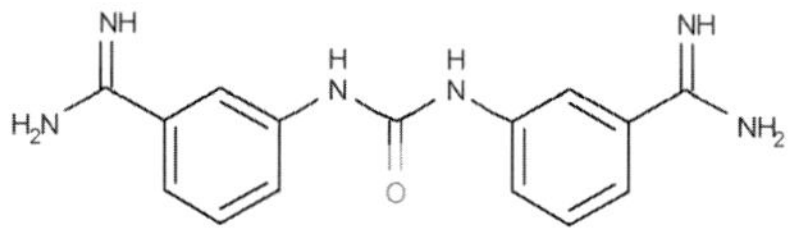

5

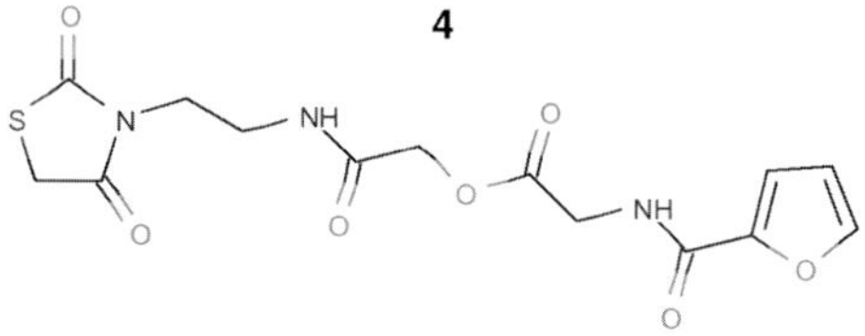

6

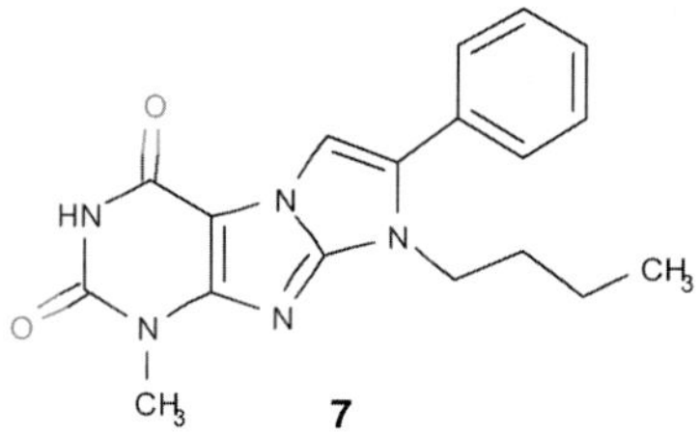

7

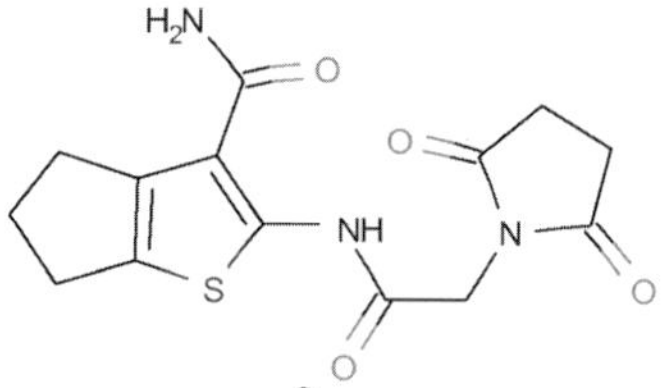

8

Figure 17.2 Low micromolar inhibitors discovered by high-throughput fragment-based docking into β-secretase (compounds **1** and **2**), plasmepsin II (**3**), West Nile virus NS3 protease (**4** and **5**), cathepsin B (**6**), EphB4 tyrosine kinase (**7**), and CDK2 Ser/Thr kinase (**8**). See Figure 17.1 for the programs used for docking and Table 17.1 for hit rates, sizes of libraries screened, and experimentally measured affinities.

considering β as a free parameter [79]. Consequently, both coefficients are obtained by a fit of experimentally determined values of ΔG to the calculated values of E^{elec} and E^{vdW} for a training set of known ligands.

The original LIE method and modifications thereof have been applied to a large number of existing inhibitor/protein data sets [76, 80–85]. Moreover, LIE-based scorings of ligands were shown to perform better than established scoring functions [86]. Interestingly, recent applications to pharmaceutically relevant enzyme targets have documented the predictive ability and usefulness in lead discovery projects. As an example, the LIE method with explicit water molecular dynamics sampling was successfully used in the design of a series of inhibitors of the malarial aspartic proteases plasmepsin I and II [87]. Unfortunately, LIE cannot be used for high-throughput docking because of its computational requirements (the currently fastest implementation needs about 6 h for each compound [86]). Therefore, we have replaced the explicit water molecular dynamics (or Monte Carlo) simulations with a simple energy minimization and combined the LIE method with a rigorous treatment of solvation within the continuum electrostatics approximation [73], that is, the numerical solution of the Poisson equation by the finite-difference technique [88]. The LIECE approach, where the last two letters stand for continuum electrostatics, is about two orders of magnitude faster than previous LIE methods and shows a similar precision on the targets tested. In fact, we have observed an error of about 1 kcal/mol for 13 and 29 peptidic inhibitors of β-secretase and HIV-1 protease, respectively [73]. Similar accuracy has been reported for other proteases [89, 90] and five kinases [91].

17.3.5 Consensus Scoring

It has been reported that consensus scoring is generally preferable to the use of a single scoring function [92]. Furthermore, the median rank is more suitable than the average rank in consensus scoring because the former is less sensitive to outliers [93]. Rank by median consensus scoring was used in the *in silico* screening against plasmepsin and cathepsin B (Table 17.1). For plasmepsin, consensus scoring was preferred to ranking by LIECE because visual inspection of the best LIECE poses revealed several unlikely binding modes. In the case of cathepsin B, the lack of experimental data on inhibitors binding outside the catalytic center was the reason for not using LIECE, which requires at least 10–15 binding affinity data points for fitting the 2–3 parameters of the linear model.

17.3.6 *In Silico* Screening Campaigns

During 2004–2008, our suite of programs for fragment-based docking [68, 71, 72] has been employed in eight *in silico* screening campaigns on six different enzymes that play a key role in a variety of diseases (Table 17.1) [94]. Four of these enzymes are proteases of three different classes (aspartic, serine, and cysteine proteases), while the remaining two are a tyrosine kinase and a Ser/Thr kinase. The 2D structures of the most potent inhibitors discovered in the eight high-throughput docking campaigns are shown in Figure 17.2. Here we present the results obtained on two of the six enzymes, West Nile virus NS3 protease and EphB4 tyrosine kinase, while more details can be found in a recent review [94] and the original publications [89–91, 95–99].

17.3.7 West Nile Virus NS3 Protease (Flaviviral Infections)

The pathogenic members of the flavivirus family, for example, West Nile virus and the closely related dengue virus, are transmitted by mosquito bites. Although an estimated 2.5 billion people are potential victims of encephalitis and other fatal maladies caused by flaviviruses [100], these diseases have received much less attention than other tropical diseases such as avian influenza. Their status as "neglected" diseases is in part due to the fact that flaviviruses are widespread mainly in poor countries, and mosquitoes can fly only much shorter distances than migratory birds, so they do not represent a threat in developed countries. Recently, the nonstructural 3 (NS3) protease has been shown to be responsible for cleavage of the viral polyprotein precursor and to play a pivotal role in the replication of flaviviruses [101, 102]. In fact, site-directed mutagenesis focused on the NS3 protease cleavage sites in the polyprotein precursor abolishes viral infectivity [102]. Therefore, the NS3 protease is one of the most promising targets for drug development against Flaviviridae infections. In this context, it is important to note that two inhibitors of the closely related hepatitis C virus protease are under late-stage clinical development [103–106].

We have run two *in silico* screening campaigns to identify inhibitors of the West Nile virus NS3 protease. The first high-throughput docking campaign (Figure 17.3a) was performed on the X-ray structure of the protease [90], and only compounds with at least five hydrogen bond donors or one positive charge were used. After docking, poses with less than three intermolecular hydrogen bonds were filtered out. The selection of compounds for docking and the filter is justified by the strong polar character of the pockets. Then the poses that passed the filter were further evaluated by LIECE. Finally, the 1000 poses (354 unique compounds) with most favorable LIECE energies and the 1000 poses (297 unique compounds) with most intermolecular hydrogen bonds were selected for visual inspection. In the second campaign

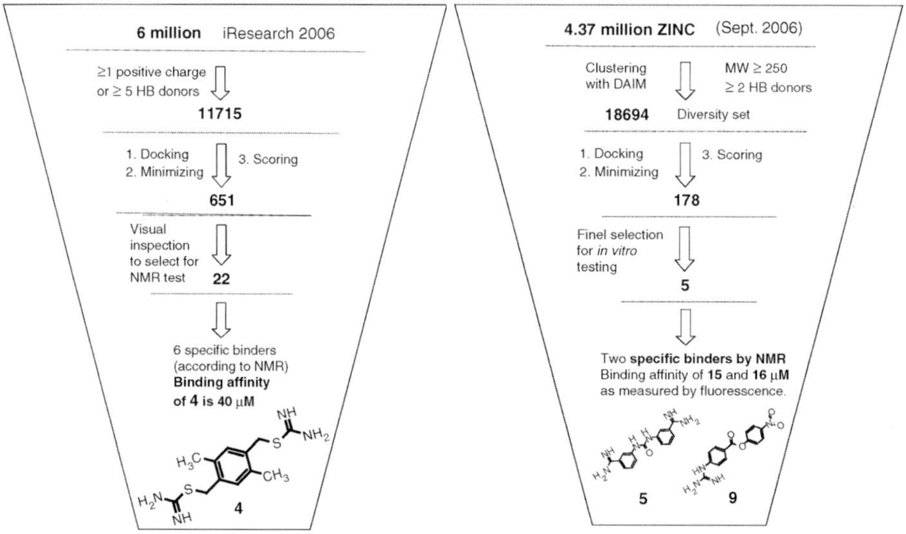

Figure 17.3 Schematic picture of the two *in silico* screening campaigns against West Nile virus NS3 protease. Docking of the compounds was performed by DAIM/SEED/FFLD using the 2fp7 structure of the WNV protease as explained in the text and Refs [90, 97].

(Figure 17.3b), the screening made use of a snapshot selected along a 1 ns explicit solvent molecular dynamics simulation started from the crystal structure [97]. This snapshot was chosen from a set of 100 as it optimally accommodates three representative molecular fragments: benzene and two functional groups with a positive charge. The former is the most common ring in the known drugs, while the latter were employed because the active site of the NS3 protease has a large amount of hydrogen bond acceptors. A diversity set with at least two hydrogen bond donors and molecular weight larger than 250 Da was used. The docked poses were filtered according to thresholds in van der Waals efficiency (the ratio of the van der Waals energy and the molecular weight), intermolecular hydrogen bonds, and unfavorable interactions between the small molecule and the protein [97]. A total of 480 poses (of 178 compounds) passed all filters and were visually inspected. No scoring function was used in ranking the compounds. In both docking campaigns, the final selection of compounds for testing was based on visual inspections. Poses with poor shape or electrostatic complementarity and/or bad geometry of the intermolecular hydrogen bonds were removed. Interestingly, the hit rate was high in both campaigns (5 and 40%, Table 17.1). Most importantly, inhibitors **4** and **5** are candidate lead compounds. They occupy only the S1 and S2 pockets of the substrate binding site (Figure 17.4), so that additional substituents are expected to improve their affinity and, at the same time, retain good druglike properties as they both have very favorable ligand efficiency (which is defined as the experimentally measured free energy of binding divided by the number of non-hydrogen atoms [39]). The *in silico* discovery of compounds **4** and **5** is remarkable because the West Nile virus NS3 protease is a very difficult target. Very few nonpeptidic inhibitors have been reported. Moreover, less than 10 molecules emerged as inhibitors (in the micromolar range) from a library of more than one million compounds submitted to a high-throughput *in vitro* screening campaign [108].

It is interesting to note that compound **5**, as well as another inhibitor of the West Nile virus NS3 protease discovered by docking into the molecular dynamics snapshot (the diphenyl ester **2** in [97]), would not have been identified by docking into the X-ray structure, as the S1 pocket in the latter does not accommodate the benzene ring in an energetically favorable way [97].

17.3.8
EphB4 Tyrosine Kinase (Cancer)

The protein kinase EphB4 (erythropoietin producing human hepatocellular carcinoma receptor tyrosine kinase B4) is a highly attractive angiogenic target involved in many types of cancer [109]. It seems to be rather recalcitrant to inhibition because, despite its potential therapeutic importance, very few inhibitors have been reported in the literature up to date.

We have developed and applied the ALTA (anchor-based library tailoring) approach to identify ATP-competitive inhibitors of EphB4 [99] (Figure 17.5). ALTA is an automatic fragment-based procedure for focusing libraries of compounds. First, molecular fragments are docked and prioritized (i.e., anchors are selected based on a

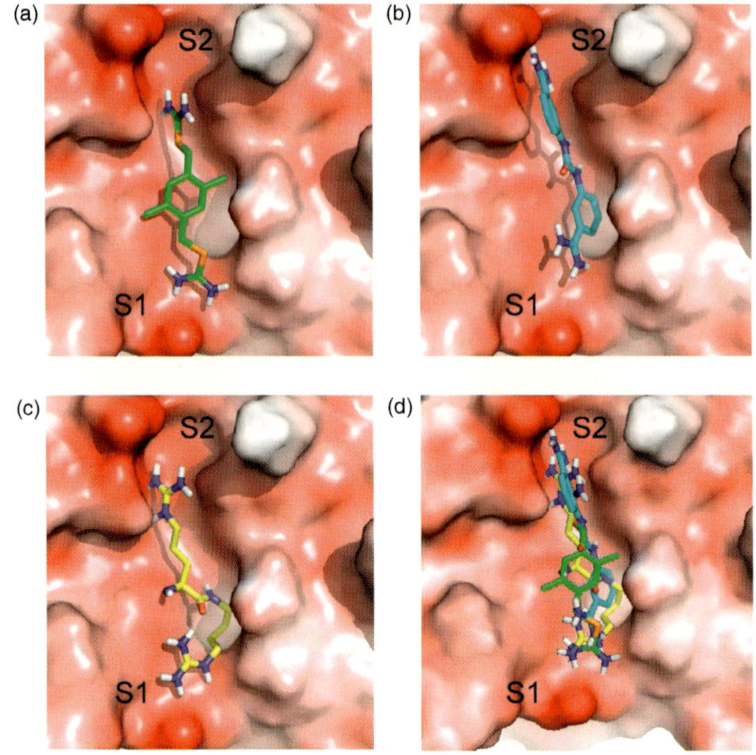

Figure 17.4 The guanidinium groups of inhibitors **4** (a) and **5** (b) are involved in electrostatic interactions with hydrogen bond acceptors in the S1 and S2 pockets of the West Nile virus NS3 protease, as observed in the X-ray structure of the aldehyde peptidic inhibitor benzoyl-Nle-Lys-Arg-Arg-H (PDB code 2fp7). (c) Only the C-terminal dipeptide Arg-Arg-H of the aldehyde inhibitor is shown for clarity. (d) Overlap of the poses of compounds **4** and **5**, which were generated by fragment-based docking, with the binding mode of the peptidic inhibitor. The inhibitors are shown by sticks colored by atom type with carbon atoms in green, cyan, and yellow for compounds **4**, **5**, and the peptidic inhibitor, respectively. The surface of WNV NS2B-NS3 pro is colored by electrostatic potential with red and blue for negative and positive potentials, respectively. The figure was prepared using PyMOL (Delano Scientific, San Carlos, CA) and the APBS program [107] was used for calculation of the electrostatic surface.

ranking) according to force field energy that includes continuum electrostatics solvation [67, 68]. Large collections of molecules can then be effectively reduced in size by selecting only the compounds that have one (or more) fragment among the top-ranking anchors. In principle, ALTA does not require any information about known inhibitors but in the application to the EphB4 kinase pharmacophore knowledge (hydrogen bonds to the hinge region) was additionally used to efficiently reduce the size of the original library from about 728 000 to 21 418 molecules. These molecules are docked and the docking poses are filtered according to thresholds in van der Waals energy and van der Waals efficiency. A general LIECE model [99] is

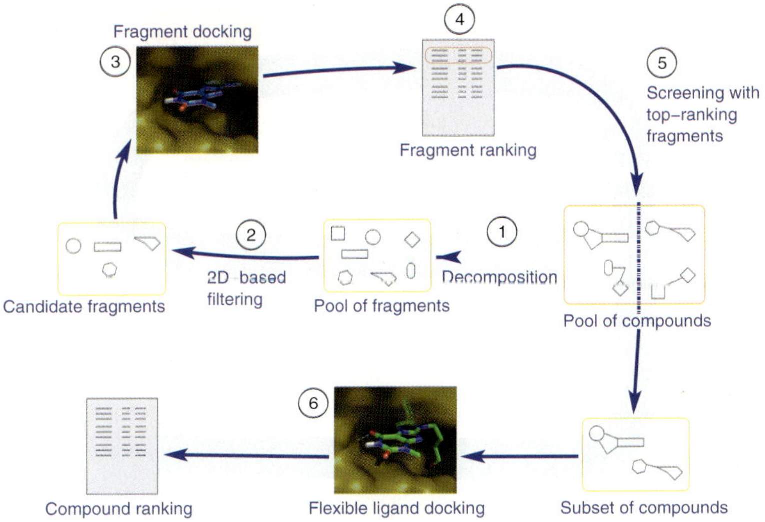

Figure 17.5 Graphical representation of the workflow of the ALTA procedure [99]. The first step is the automatic decomposition [71] of a library of compounds (orange rectangle) to obtain the pool of fragments. Afterward, fragments selected based on the binding site features (step 2) are docked [68] (step 3) and ranked according to their binding energy [69] (step 4). Poses for molecules that contain at least one of the top-ranking fragments (step 5) are then generated by flexible ligand docking [72] (step 6).

used for the final ranking and selection of compounds for testing and two series of novel EphB4 inhibitors have been identified by ALTA. Compound **7** (Figure 17.2) is a potential candidate for further development because of its low micromolar affinity and molecular weight of only 337 Da, which result in a very favorable ligand efficiency (Table 17.1). Moreover, the kinetic characterization of a very similar compound (**2** in Table I of Ref. [99]) indicates that this series of molecules bind to the ATP binding site, as predicted by the docking calculations [99]. Recently, single-digit nanomolar affinities have been reached by chemical synthesis of derivatives of compound **7** that were designed on the basis of the binding mode obtained by docking [110].

17.4 Lessons Learned from Our Fragment-Based Docking

Low micromolar inhibitors of four proteases and two protein kinases have been identified by high-throughput screening using fragment-based docking of large libraries of compounds. The substrate binding sites of the proteases have very different shape from the ATP binding sites of the protein kinases. Moreover, the former show a broad range of surface hydrophilicity ranging from mainly hydrophobic (β-secretase) to a strong electrostatic potential (NS3 protease). It is thus encouraging that docking finds inhibitors for all of them. The six enzymes are involved in key biological processes in humans or human parasites. Therefore, they are relevant drug targets: β-secretase in Alzheimer's disease, cathepsin B in cancer and rheumatic disorders, EphB4 tyrosine kinase in cancer-related angiogenesis, CDK2 Ser/Thr kinase in several types of cancer, plasmepsin II in malaria, and NS3 protease in infections caused by flaviviruses, in particular West Nile virus and dengue virus. Recently, a series of 50 derivatives of the inhibitor **7** of the EphB4 tyrosine kinase have been synthesized. These 50 compounds were designed using the binding mode obtained by automatic docking. Notably, six of these compounds are active in the submicromolar range and one of them has an IC_{50} value of about 5 nM [110]. It is likely that medicinal chemistry optimization of all of the inhibitors presented in this chapter (i.e., discovered by high-throughput docking) might yield (low) nanomolar inhibitors but it is very difficult to predict in advance the eventual improvement in potency.

One essential component of our scoring approach is the use of a force field energy supplemented by the evaluation of electrostatic solvation effects. The latter are calculated by models of aqueous solvent based on the continuum dielectric approximation. For fragment docking, the generalized Born approximation is used for evaluating the electrostatic component of the binding free energy that includes screened electrostatic interaction, and protein and fragment desolvation terms [68, 69]. The finite-difference Poisson equation is employed to calculate electrostatic solvation effects for the poses of the compounds obtained by flexible ligand docking. The poses are then usually ranked by the LIECE approach [73, 91].

The two main outcomes of our *in silico* screening campaigns on six different enzymes are that the hit rate is rather high (between 3 and 40%) and the most potent inhibitors have low micromolar affinity and favorable ligand efficiency (Table 17.1). It is difficult to compare hit rates reported in different studies due to differences in the libraries employed for screening and in the affinity thresholds adopted for the definition of hits. Yet, our hit rates compare favorably with those reported for experimental high-throughput screening (0.01–0.1%) and fragment-based screening (0.1–1%) techniques. Moreover, *in silico* screening involves much smaller time, consumables, and labor costs than *in vitro* screening.

It was not possible to identify submicromolar inhibitors in the eight high-throughput docking campaigns (for six different enzymes), probably because of one or more of the three following reasons. First, the libraries of available compounds cover a very small fraction of the potential druglike molecules. In fact, it has been estimated that the number of potential fragments with up to 11 heavy atoms (under constraints due to chemical stability and synthetic feasibility) is on the order of 10^7 [37], while the number of druglike molecules with less than 30 heavy atoms is larger than 10^{60} [111]. Furthermore, it is likely that the coverage of chemical space is very heterogeneous in the libraries of compounds that are available. A recent analysis of commercially available compounds suggests that the chemical space is skewed mainly toward ligands of G-protein-coupled receptors (10.6% of the compounds in a database of about 1 million small molecules resemble known ligands of these receptors) with fewer kinase-like ligands (4.2%) and an even smaller number of compounds resembling protease inhibitors (2.3%) [112]. On the other hand, one should note that an 80 nM ATP-competitive inhibitor of casein kinase II has been identified directly by high-throughput docking (of a subset of the Novartis collection of compounds, about 400 000 molecules, which are not in the public domain) [113].

Second, there are significant sources of errors in both the force field and continuum dielectric model used to approximate solvation effects. As an example, polarization effects are neglected in force fields based on fixed partial charges. A recent extension of the LIECE model has emphasized the importance of quantum mechanics to capture these effects, in particular for sets of inhibitors with significant differences in the number of formal charges [114].

Third, all docking studies presented in this chapter were performed with a rigid protein. The rigid protein approximation, which is required for efficiency reasons, dramatically restricts the number of favorable poses and results in false negatives. As an example, two small molecule inhibitors of the NS3 protease have been identified by docking into a molecular dynamics snapshot, which would not have been possible by using the X-ray structure [97].

17.5 Challenges of Fragment-Based Approaches

In silico and *in vitro* FBS techniques are increasingly being used to identify hits as starting points to develop leads for specific pharmaceutical targets. Despite the recent growth and successes of FBS approaches, there are several challenges. First, most of the docking programs and scoring functions are optimized for screening molecules consisting of several fragments rather than isolated fragments. The effectiveness of these approaches at accurately docking small fragments has recently been studied [56] but more investigations with different docking programs, scoring functions, and targets are essential for shedding light on the weak points and potential improvements. Second, the fragment hits from virtual or experimental screening are usually rather weak (mM range), and therefore the binding has to be validated carefully. The false positive issue is especially problematic because the follow-up requires intensive chemical synthesis efforts. Relatively complicated (and sometimes expensive) biophysical approaches, for example, NMR spectroscopy, X-ray crystallography, and mass spectrometry, are usually required to validate the hits. Third, fragments may have multiple binding modes with similar binding free energy, which is a challenge even for the most accurate methods for calculating relative affinities. Therefore, a crystal structure is highly desired for the follow-up optimization. However, even for protein targets with robust crystallographic systems in place, it can be difficult to obtain structures of fragment–protein complexes if the affinity is too weak [56]. Finally, synthetic accessibility to further develop the fragments, for example, by linking and growing, is not always possible. Several strategies may be used to overcome this problem. The simplest way is to search for commercially available compounds with substructures or scaffolds similar to the fragments identified by virtual FBS [52]. Alternatively, experienced medicinal chemists can be involved for trying to improve synthetic accessibility while preserving the key interactions with the protein target.

Acknowledgments

A.C. thanks the talented and dedicated PhD students and postdocs who have developed and applied the methods for fragment-based docking and scoring. The computer programs have been developed mainly by three PhD students: N. Budin (FFLD), P. Kolb (DAIM), and N. Majeux (SEED), with the help of J. Apostolakis, M. Cecchini, F. Dey, C. Ehrhardt, and the late M. Scarsi. The *in silico* screening campaigns have been carried out by P. Alfarano (cathepsin B), M. Convertino (β-Secretase), D. Ekonomiuk (NS3 protease), R. Friedman (plasmepsin II), and F. Dey and P. Kolb (kinases). We thank Peter Kollo for preparing Figure 17.1. Very generous financial support has been provided by the innovation promotion agency (KTI) of the Swiss government and the Canton of Zürich.

Availability of programs for fragment-based docking: All of our software packages for docking are available for free at http://www.biochem-caflisch.uzh.ch/download/.

References

1 Congreve, M., Chessari, G., Tisi, D., and Woodhead, A.J. (2008) Recent developments in fragment-based drug discovery. *Journal of Medicinal Chemistry*, **51** (13), 3661–3680.

2 Payne, D.J., Gwynn, M.N., Holmes, D.J., and Pompliano, D.L. (2007) Drugs for bad bugs: confronting the challenges of antibacterial discovery. *Nature Reviews. Drug Discovery*, **6**, 29–40.

3 Jencks, W.P. (1981) On the attribution and additivity of binding energies. *Proceedings of the National Academy of Sciences of the United States of America*, **78**, 4046–4050.

4 Miranker, A. and Karplus, M. (1991) Functionality maps of binding sites: a multiple copy simultaneous search method. *Proteins: Structure, Function and Genetics*, **11**, 29–34.

5 Boehm, H.J. (1992) The computer program LUDI: a new method for the de novo design of enzyme inhibitors. *Journal of Computer-Aided Molecular Design*, **6** (1), 61–78.

6 Caflisch, A., Miranker, A., and Karplus, M. (1993) Multiple copy simultaneous search and construction of ligands in binding sites: application to inhibitors of HIV-1 aspartic proteinase. *Journal of Medicinal Chemistry*, **36**, 2142–2167.

7 Shuker, H., Hajduk, P., Meadows, R., and Fesik, S.W. (1996) Discovering high affinity ligands for proteins: SAR by NMR. *Science*, **274**, 1531–1534.

8 Nienaber, V.L., Richardson, P.L., Klighofer, V., Bouska, J.J., Giranda, V.L., and Greer, J. (2000) Discovering novel ligands for macromolecules using X-ray crystallographic screening. *Nature Biotechnology*, **18**, 1105–1108.

9 Pellecchia, M., Bertini, I., Cowburn, D., Dalvit, C., Giralt, E., Jahnke, W., James, T.L., Homans, S.W., Kessler, H., Luchinat, C., Meyer, B., Oschkinat, H., Peng, J., Schwalbe, H., and Siegal, G. (2008) Perspectives on NMR in drug discovery: a technique comes of age. *Nature Reviews. Drug Discovery*, **7** (9), 738–745.

10 Geschwindner, S., Olsson, L.-L., Albert, J.S., Deinum, J., Edwards, P.D., de Beer, T., and Folmer, R.H.A. (2007) Discovery of a novel warhead against beta-secretase through fragment-based lead generation. *Journal of Medicinal Chemistry*, **50** (24), 5903–5911.

11 Swayze, E.E., Jefferson, E.A., Sannes-Lowery, K.A., Blyn, L.B., Risen, L.M., Arakawa, S., Osgood, S.A., Hofstadler, S.A., and Griffey, R.H. (2002) SAR by MS: a ligand based technique for drug lead discovery against structured RNA targets.

Journal of Medicinal Chemistry, **45**, 3816–3819.

12 Ockey, D.A., Dotson, J.L., Struble, M.E., Stults, J.T., Bourell, J.H., Clark, K.R., and Gadek, T.R. (2004) Structure–activity relationships by mass spectrometry: identification of novel MMP-3 inhibitors. *Bioorganic and Medicinal Chemistry*, **12**, 37–44.

13 Wood, W.J.L., Patterson, A.W., Tsuruoka, H., Jain, R.K., and Ellman, J.A. (2005) Substrate activity screening: a fragment-based method for the rapid identification of nonpeptidic protease inhibitors. *Journal of the American Chemical Society*, **127** (44), 15521–15527.

14 Patterson, A.W., Wood, W.J.L., Hornsby, M., Lesley, S., Spraggon, G., and Ellman, J.A. (2006) Identification of selective, nonpeptidic nitrile inhibitors of cathepsin S using the substrate activity screening method. *Journal of Medicinal Chemistry*, **49** (21), 6298–6307.

15 Patterson, A.W., Wood, W.J.L., and Ellman, J.A. (2007) Substrate activity screening (SAS): a general procedure for the preparation and screening of a fragment-based non-peptidic protease substrate library for inhibitor discovery. *Nature Protocols*, **2** (2), 424–433.

16 Erlanson, D.A., Lam, J.W., Wiesmann, C., Luong, T.N., Simmons, R.L., DeLano, W.L., Choong, I.C., Burdett, M.T., Flanagan, W.M., Lee, D., Gordon, E.M., and O'Brien, T. (2003) In *situ* assembly of enzyme inhibitors using extended tethering. *Nature Biotechnology*, **21**, 308–314.

17 Erlanson, D.A., Wells, J.A., and Braisted, A.C. (2004) Tethering: fragment-based drug discovery. *Annual Review of Biophysics and Biomolecular Structure*, **33**, 199–223.

18 Hajduk, P.J. and Greer, J. (2007) A decade of fragment-based drug design: strategic advances and lessons learned. *Nature Reviews. Drug Discovery*, **6** (3), 211–219.

19 Jhoti, H., Cleasby, A., Verdonk, M., and Williams, G. (2007) Fragment-based screening using X-ray crystallography and NMR spectroscopy. *Current Opinion in Chemical Biology*, **11**, 485–493.

20 Siegal, G., Ab, E., and Schultz, J. (2007) Integration of fragment screening and library design. *Drug Discovery Today*, **12**, 1032–1039.

21 Fattori, D., Squarcia, A., and Bartoli, S. (2008) Fragment-based approach to drug lead discovery: overview and advances in various techniques. *Drugs in R&D*, **9**, 217–227.

22 Hesterkamp, T. and Whittaker, M. (2008) Fragment-based activity space: smaller is better. *Current Opinion in Chemical Biology*, **12**, 260–268.

23 Murray, C.W., Callaghan, O., Chessari, G., Cleasby, A., Congreve, M., Frederickson, M., Hartshorn, M.J., McMenamin, R., Patel, S., and Wallis, N. (2007) Application of fragment screening by X-ray crystallography to beta-secretase. *Journal of Medicinal Chemistry*, **50**, 1116–1123.

24 Congreve, M., Aharony, D., Albert, J., Callaghan, O., Campbell, J., Carr, R.A.E., Chessari, G., Cowan, S., Edwards, P.D., Frederickson, M., McMenamin, R., Murray, C.W., Patel, S., and Wallis, N. (2007) Application of fragment screening by X-ray crystallography to the discovery of aminopyridines as inhibitors of beta-secretase. *Journal of Medicinal Chemistry*, **50**, 1124–1132.

25 Furet, P., Bold, G., Hofmann, F., Manley, P., Meyer, T., and Altmann, K.-H. (2003) Identification of a new chemical class of potent angiogenesis inhibitors based on conformational considerations and database searching. *Bioorganic & Medicinal Chemistry Letters*, **13** (18), 2967–2971.

26 Gill, A. (2004) New lead generation strategies for protein kinase inhibitors: fragment based screening approaches. *Mini-Reviews in Medicinal Chemistry*, **4** (3), 301–311.

27 Szczepankiewicz, B.G., Liu, G., Hajduk, P.J., Abad-Zapatero, C., Pei, Z., Xin, Z., Lubben, T.H., Trevillyan, J.M., Stashko, M.A., Ballaron, S.J., Liang, H., Huang, F., Hutchins, C.W., Fesik, S.W., and Jirousek, M.R. (2003) Discovery of a potent, selective protein tyrosine phosphatase 1B inhibitor using a linked-fragment strategy. *Journal of the*

American Chemical Society, **125**, 4087–4096.

28 Warner, S.L., Bashyam, S., Vankayalapati, H., Bearss, D.J., Han, H., Mahadevan, D., Hoff, D.D.V., and Hurley, L.H. (2006) Identification of a lead small-molecule inhibitor of the Aurora kinases using a structure-assisted, fragment-based approach. *Molecular Cancer Therapeutics*, **5**, 1764–1773.

29 Wyatt, P.G., Woodhead, A.J., Berdini, V., Boulstridge, J.A., Carr, M.G., Cross, D.M., Davis, D.J., Devine, L.A., Early, T.R., Feltell, R.E., Lewis, E.J., McMenamin, R.L., Navarro, E.F., O'Brien, M.A., O'Reilly, M., Reule, M., Saxty, G., Seavers, L.C.A., Smith, D.-M., Squires, M.S., Trewartha, G., Walker, M.T., and Woolford, A.J.-A. (2008) Identification of *N*-(4-piperidinyl)-4-(2,6-dichlorobenzoylamino)-1*H*-pyrazole-3-carboxamide (AT7519), a novel cyclin dependent kinase inhibitor using fragment-based X-ray crystallography and structure based drug design. *Journal of Medicinal Chemistry*, **51**, 4986–4999.

30 Boehm, H.J., Boehringer, M., Bur, D., Gmuender, H., Huber, W., Klaus, W., Kostrewa, D., Kuehne, H., Luebbers, T., Meunier-Keller, N., and Mueller, F. (2000) Novel inhibitors of DNA gyrase: 3D structure based biased needle screening, hit validation by biophysical methods, and 3D guided optimization. A promising alternative to random screening. *Journal of Medicinal Chemistry*, **43** (14), 2664–2674.

31 Choong, I.C., Lew, W., Lee, D., Pham, P., Burdett, M.T., Lam, J.W., Wiesmann, C., Luong, T.N., Fahr, B., DeLano, W.L., McDowell, R.S., Allen, D.A., Erlanson, D.A., Gordon, E.M., and O'Brien, T. (2002) Identification of potent and selective small-molecule inhibitors of caspase-3 through the use of extended tethering and structure-based drug design. *Journal of Medicinal Chemistry*, **45**, 5005–5022.

32 O'Brien, T., Fahr, B.T., Sopko, M.M., Lam, J.W., Waal, N.D., Raimundo, B.C., Purkey, H.E., Pham, P., and Romanowski, M.J. (2005) Structural analysis of caspase-1 inhibitors derived from Tethering. *Acta Crystallographica Section F: Structural Biology and Crystallization Communications*, **61**, 451–458.

33 Forino, M., Johnson, S., Wong, T.Y., Rozanov, D.V., Savinov, A.Y., Li, W., Fattorusso, R., Becattini, B., Orry, A.J., Jung, D., Abagyan, R.A., Smith, J.W., Alibek, K., Liddington, R.C., Strongin, A.Y., and Pellecchia, M. (2005) Efficient synthetic inhibitors of anthrax lethal factor. *Proceedings of the National Academy of Sciences of the United States of America*, **102**, 9499–9504.

34 Card, G.L., Blasdel, L., England, B.P., Zhang, C., Suzuki, Y., Gillette, S., Fong, D., Ibrahim, P.N., Artis, D.R., Bollag, G., Milburn, M.V., Kim, S.-H., Schlessinger, J., and Zhang, K.Y.J. (2005) A family of phosphodiesterase inhibitors discovered by cocrystallography and scaffold-based drug design. *Nature Biotechnology*, **23**, 201–207.

35 Lipinski, C. and Hopkins, A. (2004) Navigating chemical space for biology and medicine. *Nature*, **432**, 855–861.

36 Dobson, C.M. (2004) Chemical space and biology. *Nature*, **432**, 824–828.

37 Fink, T., Bruggesser, H., and Reymond, J.-L. (2005) Virtual exploration of the small-molecule chemical universe below 160 Daltons. *Angewandte Chemie – International Edition in English*, **44** (10), 1504–1508.

38 Zoete, V., Grosdidier, A., and Michielin, O. (2009) Docking, virtual high throughput screening and *in silico* fragment-based drug design. *Journal of Cellular and Molecular Medicine*, **13**, 238–248.

39 Hopkins, A.L., Groom, C.R., and Alex, A. (2004) Ligand efficiency: a useful metric for lead selection. *Drug Discovery Today*, **9** (10), 430–431.

40 Hann, M.M., Leach, A.R., and Harper, G. (2001) Molecular complexity and its impact on the probability of finding leads for drug discovery. *Journal of Chemical Information and Computer Sciences*, **41** (3), 856–864.

41 Brooks, B.R., Bruccoleri, R.E., Olafson, B.D., States, D.J., Swaminathan, S., and Karplus, M. (1983) CHARMM: a program for macromolecular energy, minimization, and dynamics calculations. *Journal of Computational Chemistry*, **4**, 187–217.

42 Brooks, B.R., Brooks, C.L., III, Mackerell, A.D.J., Nilsson, L., Petrella, R.J., Roux, B., Won, Y., Archontis, G., Bartels, C., Boresch, S., Caflisch, A., Caves, L., Cui, Q., Dinner, A.R., Feig, M., Fischer, S., Gao, J., Hodoscek, M., Im, W., Kuczera, K., Lazaridis, T., Ma, J., Ovchinnikov, V., Paci, E., Pastor, R.W., Post, C.B., Pu, J.Z., aefer, M.S., Tidor, B., Venable, R.M., Woodcock, H.L., Wu, X., Yang, W., York, D.M., and Karplus, M. (2009) CHARMM: the biomolecular simulation program. *Journal of Computational Chemistry*, **30** (10), 1545–1614.

43 Davis, M.E., Madura, J.D., Sines, J., Luty, B.A., Allison, S.A., and McCammon, J.A. (1991) Diffusion-controlled enzymatic reactions. *Methods in Enzymology*, **202**, 473–497.

44 Sirockin, F., Sich, C., Improta, S., Schaefer, M., Saudek, V., Froloff, N., Karplus, M., and Dejaegere, A. (2002) Structure activity relationship by NMR and by computer: a comparative study. *Journal of the American Chemical Society*, **124**, 11073–11084.

45 Guvench, O. and MacKerell, A.D.J. (2009) Computational fragment-based binding site identification by ligand competitive saturation. *PLoS Computational Biology*, **5**, e1000435.

46 Eisen, M.B., Wiley, D.C., Karplus, M., and Hubbard, R.E. (1994) HOOK: a program for finding novel molecular architectures that satisfy the chemical and steric requirements of a macromolecule binding site. *Proteins: Structure, Function, and Bioinformatics*, **19**, 199–221.

47 Clark, D.E., Frenkel, D., Levy, S.A., Li, J., Murray, C.W., Robson, B., Waszkowycz, B., and Westhead, D.R. (1995) PRO-LIGAND: an approach to de novo molecular design. 1. Application to the design of organic molecules. *Journal of Computer-Aided Molecular Design*, **9**, 13–32.

48 Todorov, N.P. and Dean, P.M. (1997) Evaluation of a method for controlling molecular scaffold diversity in de novo ligand design. *Journal of Computer-Aided Molecular Design*, **11**, 175–192.

49 Caflisch, A. (1996) Computational combinatorial ligand design: application to human α-thrombin. *Journal of Computer-Aided Molecular Design*, **10**, 372–396.

50 Pierce, A.C., Rao, G., and Bemis, G.W. (2004) BREED: generating novel inhibitors through hybridization of known ligands. Application to CDK2, p38, and HIV protease. *Journal of Medicinal Chemistry*, **47**, 2768–2775.

51 Douguet, D., Munier-Lehmann, H., Labesse, G., and Pochet, S. (2005) LEA3D: a computer-aided ligand design for structure-based drug design. *Journal of Medicinal Chemistry*, **48**, 2457–2468.

52 Dey, F. and Caflisch, A. (2008) Fragment-based de novo ligand design by multiobjective evolutionary optimization. *Journal of Chemical Information and Modeling*, **48**, 679–690.

53 Schneider, G. and Fechner, U. (2005) Computer-based de novo design of drug-like molecules. *Nature Reviews. Drug Discovery*, **4**, 649–663.

54 Friesner, R.A., Banks, J.L., Murphy, R.B., Halgren, T.A., Klicic, J.J., Mainz, D.T., Repasky, M.P., Knoll, E.H., Shelley, M., Perry, J.K., Shaw, D.E., Francis, P., and Shenkin, P.S. (2004) Glide: a new approach for rapid, accurate docking and scoring. 1. Method and assessment of docking accuracy. *Journal of Medicinal Chemistry*, **47**, 1739–1749.

55 Friesner, R.A., Murphy, R.B., Repasky, M.P., Frye, L.L., Greenwood, J.R., Halgren, T.A., Sanschagrin, P.C., and Mainz, D.T. (2006) Extra precision glide: docking and scoring incorporating a model of hydrophobic enclosure for protein–ligand complexes. *Journal of Medicinal Chemistry*, **49**, 6177–6196.

56 Kawatkar, S., Wang, H., Czerminski, R., and Joseph-McCarthy, D. (2009) Virtual fragment screening: an exploration of various docking and scoring protocols for

fragments using Glide. *Journal of Computer-Aided Molecular Design*, **23**, 527–539.

57 Fukunishi, Y., Mashimo, T., Orita, M., Ohno, K., and Nakamura, H. (2009) *In silico* fragment screening by replica generation (FSRG) method for fragment-based drug design. *Journal of Chemical Information and Modeling*, **49**, 925–933.

58 Rarey, M., Kramer, B., Lengauer, T., and Klebe, G. (1996) A fast flexible docking method using an incremental construction algorithm. *Journal of Molecular Biology*, **261**, 470–489.

59 Rummey, C., Nordhoff, S., Thiemann, M., and Metz, G. (2006) *In silico* fragment-based discovery of DPP-IV S1 pocket binders. *Bioorganic & Medicinal Chemistry Letters*, **16**, 1405–1409.

60 Nordhoff, S., Cerezo-Galvez, S., Feurer, A., Hill, O., Matassa, V.G., Metz, G., Rummey, C., Thiemann, M., and Edwards, P.J. (2006) The reversed binding of beta-phenethylamine inhibitors of DPP-IV: X-ray structures and properties of novel fragment and elaborated inhibitors. *Bioorganic & Medicinal Chemistry Letters*, **16**, 1744–1748.

61 Jones, G., Willett, P., and Glen, R.C. (1995) Molecular recognition of receptor sites using a genetic algorithm with a description of desolvation. *Journal of Molecular Biology*, **245**, 43–53.

62 Hartshorn, M.J., Murray, C.W., Cleasby, A., Frederickson, M., Tickle, I.J., and Jhoti, H. (2005) Fragment-based lead discovery using X-ray crystallography. *Journal of Medicinal Chemistry*, **48**, 403–413.

63 Chen, I.-J. and Hubbard, R.E. (2009) Lessons for fragment library design: analysis of output from multiple screening campaigns. *Journal of Computer-Aided Molecular Design*, **23**, 603–620.

64 Baurin, N., Aboul-Ela, F., Barril, X., Davis, B., Drysdale, M., Dymock, B., Finch, H., Fromont, C., Richardson, C., Simmonite, H., and Hubbard, R.E. (2004) Design and characterization of libraries of molecular fragments for use in NMR screening against protein targets. *Journal of Chemical Information and Computer Sciences*, **44**, 2157–2166.

65 Momany, F. and Rone, R. (1992) Validation of the general purpose QUANTA 3.2/CHARMm force field. *Journal of Computational Chemistry*, **13**, 888–900.

66 Caflisch, A., Fischer, S., and Karplus, M. (1997) Docking by Monte Carlo minimization with a solvation correction: application to an FKBP–substrate complex. *Journal of Computational Chemistry*, **18**, 723–743.

67 Scarsi, M., Apostolakis, J., and Caflisch, A. (1997) Continuum electrostatic energies of macromolecules in aqueous solutions. *Journal of Physical Chemistry A*, **101**, 8098–8106.

68 Majeux, N., Scarsi, M., Apostolakis, J., Ehrhardt, C., and Caflisch, A. (1999) Exhaustive docking of molecular fragments on protein binding sites with electrostatic solvation. *Proteins: Structure, Function, and Bioinformatics*, **37**, 88–105.

69 Majeux, N., Scarsi, M., and Caflisch, A. (2001) Efficient electrostatic solvation model for protein–fragment docking. *Proteins: Structure, Function, and Bioinformatics*, **42**, 256–268.

70 Scarsi, M., Majeux, N., and Caflisch, A. (1999) Hydrophobicity at the surface of proteins. *Proteins: Structure, Function, and Bioinformatics*, **37**, 565–575.

71 Kolb, P. and Caflisch, A. (2006) Automatic and efficient decomposition of two-dimensional structures of small molecules for fragment-based high-throughput docking. *Journal of Medicinal Chemistry*, **49**, 7384–7392.

72 Budin, N., Majeux, N., and Caflisch, A. (2001) Fragment-based flexible ligand docking by evolutionary optimization. *Biological Chemistry*, **382**, 1365–1372.

73 Huang, D. and Caflisch, A. (2004) Efficient evaluation of binding free energy using continuum electrostatic solvation. *Journal of Medicinal Chemistry*, **47**, 5791–5797.

74 Cecchini, M., Kolb, P., Majeux, N., and Caflisch, A. (2004) Automated docking of highly flexible ligands by genetic

algorithms: a critical assessment. *Journal of Computational Chemistry*, **25**, 412–422.

75 Kabsch, W. (1976) A solution for the best rotation to relate two sets of vectors. *Acta Crystallographica Section A: Foundations of Crystallography*, **32**, 922–923.

76 Åqvist, J., Medina, C., and Samuelsson, J.-E. (1994) A new method for predicting binding affinity in computer-aided drug design. *Protein Engineering*, **7**, 385–391.

77 Hansson, T. and Åqvist, J. (1995) Estimation of binding free energies for HIV proteinase inhibitors by molecular dynamics simulations. *Protein Engineering*, **8**, 1137–1144.

78 Jones-Hertzog, D.K. and Jorgensen, W.L. (1996) Binding affinities for sulfonamide inhibitors with human thrombin using Monte Carlo simulations with a linear response method. *Journal of Medicinal Chemistry*, **40**, 1539–1549.

79 Hansson, T., Marelius, J., and Åqvist, J. (1998) Ligand binding affinity prediction by linear interaction energy methods. *Journal of Computer-Aided Molecular Design*, **12**, 27–35.

80 Wang, J., Dixon, R., and Kollman, P. (1999) Ranking ligand binding affinities with avidin: a molecular dynamics-based interaction energy study. *Proteins: Structure, Function, and Bioinformatics*, **34**, 69–81.

81 Carlson, H.A. and Jorgensen, W.L. (1995) An extended linear response method for determining free energies of hydration. *The Journal of Physical Chemistry*, **99**, 10667–10673.

82 Wall, I.D., Leach, A.R., Salt, D.W., Ford, M.G., and Essex, J.W. (1999) Binding constants of neuraminidase inhibitors: an investigation of the linear interaction energy method. *Journal of Medicinal Chemistry*, **42**, 5142–5152.

83 Zhou, R., Friesner, R.A., Ghosh, A., Rizzo, R.C., Jorgensen, W.J., and Levy, R.M. (2001) New linear interaction method for binding affinity calculations using a continuum solvent model. *The Journal of Physical Chemistry. B*, **102**, 10388–10397.

84 Tounge, B.A. and Reynolds, C.H. (2003) Calculation of the binding affinity of β-secretase inhibitors using the linear interaction energy method. *Journal of Medicinal Chemistry*, **46**, 2074–2082.

85 Tominaga, Y. and Jorgensen, W.L. (2004) General model for estimation of the inhibition of protein kinases using Monte Carlo simulations. *Journal of Medicinal Chemistry*, **47**, 2534–2549.

86 Stjernschantz, E., Marelius, J., Medina, C., Jacobsson, M., Vermeulen, N.P.E., and Oostenbrink, C. (2006) Are automated molecular dynamics simulations and binding free energy calculations realistic tools in lead optimization? An evaluation of the linear interaction energy (LIE) method. *Journal of Chemical Information and Modeling*, **46**, 1972–1983.

87 Ersmark, K., Nervall, M., Hamelink, E., Janka, L.K., Clemente, J.C., Dunn, B.M., Blackman, M.J., Samuelsson, B., Åqvist, J., and Hallberg, A. (2005) Synthesis of malarial plasmepsin inhibitors and prediction of binding modes by molecular dynamics simulations. *Journal of Medicinal Chemistry*, **48**, 6090–6106.

88 Warwicker, J. and Watson, H.C. (1982) Calculation of the electric potential in the active site cleft due to α-helix dipoles. *Journal of Molecular Biology*, **157**, 671–679.

89 Friedman, R. and Caflisch, A. (2009) Discovery of plasmepsin inhibitors by fragment-based docking and consensus scoring. *ChemMedChem*, **4**, 1317–1326.

90 Ekonomiuk, D., Su, X.-C., Ozawa, K., Bodenreider, C., Lim, S.P., Yin, Z., Keller, T.H., Beer, D., Patel, V., Otting, G., Caflisch, A., and Huang, D. (2009) Discovery of a non-peptidic inhibitor of West Nile virus NS3 protease by high-throughput docking. *PloS Neglected Tropical Diseases*, **3**, e356.

91 Kolb, P., Huang, D., Dey, F., and Caflisch, A. (2008) Discovery of kinase inhibitors by high-throughput docking and scoring based on a transferable linear interaction energy model. *Journal of Medicinal Chemistry*, **51**, 1179–1188.

92 Charifson, P.S., Corkery, J.J., Murcko, M.A., and Walters, W.P. (1999) Consensus scoring: a method for

obtaining improved hit rates from docking databases of three-dimensional structures into proteins. *Journal of Medicinal Chemistry*, **42**, 5100–5109.

93 Klon, A.E., Glick, M., and Davies, J.W. (2004) Combination of a naive Bayes classifier with consensus scoring improves enrichment of high-throughput docking results. *Journal of Medicinal Chemistry*, **47**, 4356–4359.

94 Huang, D. and Caflisch, A. (2009) Library screening by fragment-based docking. *Journal of Molecular Recognition*, doi: .

95 Huang, D., Lüthi, U., Kolb, P., Edler, K., Cecchini, M., Audetat, S., Barberis, A., and Caflisch, A. (2005) Discovery of cell-permeable non-peptide inhibitors of β-secretase by high-throughput docking and continuum electrostatics calculations. *Journal of Medicinal Chemistry*, **48**, 5108–5111.

96 Huang, D., Lüthi, U., Kolb, P., Cecchini, M., Barberis, A., and Caflisch, A. (2006) In *silico* discovery of β-secretase inhibitors. *Journal of the American Chemical Society*, **128**, 5436–5443.

97 Ekonomiuk, D., Su, X.-C., Bodenreider, C., Lim, S.P., Otting, G., Huang, D., and Caflisch, A. (2009) Flaviviral protease inhibitors identified by fragment-based library docking into a structure generated by molecular dynamics. *Journal of Medicinal Chemistry*, **52** (15), 4860–4868.

98 Schenker, P., Alfarano, P., Kolb, P., Caflisch, A., and Baici, A. (2008) A double-headed cathepsin B inhibitor devoid of warhead. *Protein Science: A Publication of the Protein Society*, **17** (12), 2145–2155.

99 Kolb, P., Berset, C., Huang, D., and Caflisch, A. (2008) Structure-based tailoring of compound libraries for high-throughput screening: discovery of novel EphB4 kinase inhibitors. *Proteins: Structure, Function, and Bioinformatics*, **73**, 11–18.

100 Division of Vector-Borne Infectious Disease (2007) West Nile virus homepage. Centers for Disease Control and Prevention, http://www.cdc.gov/ncidod/dvbid/westnile.

101 Mukhopadhyay, S., Kuhn, R.J., and Rossmann, M.G. (2005) A structural perspective of the flavivirus life cycle. *Nature Reviews Microbiology*, **3**, 13–22.

102 Chappell, K.J., Stoermer, M.J., Fairlie, D.P., and Young, P.R. (2006) Insights to substrate binding and processing by West Nile virus NS3 protease through combined modeling, protease mutagenesis, and kinetic studies. *The Journal of Biological Chemistry*, **281**, 38448–38458.

103 Perni, R.B., Almquist, S.J., Byrn, R.A., Chandorkar, G., Chaturvedi, P.R., Courtney, L.F., Decker, C.J., Dinehart, K., Gates, C.A., Harbeson, S.L., Heiser, A., Kalkeri, G., Kolaczkowski, E., Lin, K., Luong, Y.-P., Rao, B.G., Taylor, W.P., Thomson, J.A., Tung, R.D., Wei, Y., Kwong, A.D., and Lin, C. (2006) Preclinical profile of VX-950, a potent, selective, and orally bioavailable inhibitor of hepatitis C virus NS3-4A serine protease. *Antimicrobial Agents and Chemotherapy*, **50**, 899–909.

104 Tomei, L., Failla, C., Santolini, E., Francesco, R.D., and Monica, N.L. (1993) NS3 is a serine protease required for processing of hepatitis C virus polyprotein. *Journal of Virology*, **67**, 4017–4026.

105 Malcolm, B.A., Liu, R., Lahser, F., Agrawal, S., Belanger, B., Butkiewicz, N., Chase, R., Gheyas, F., Hart, A., Hesk, D., Ingravallo, P., Jiang, C., Kong, R., Lu, J., Pichardo, J., Prongay, A., Skelton, A., Tong, X., Venkatraman, S., Xia, E., Girijavallabhan, V., and Njoroge, F.G. (2006) SCH 503034, a mechanism-based inhibitor of hepatitis C virus NS3 protease, suppresses polyprotein maturation and enhances the antiviral activity of alpha interferon in replicon cells. *Antimicrobial Agents and Chemotherapy*, **50**, 1013–1020.

106 Seiwert, S.D., Andrews, S.W., Jiang, Y., Serebryany, V., Tan, H., Kossen, K., Rajagopalan, P.T.R., Misialek, S., Stevens, S.K., Stoycheva, A., Hong, J., Lim, S.R., Qin, X., Rieger, R., Condroski, K.R., Zhang, H., Do, M.G., Lemieux, C., Hingorani, G.P., Hartley, D.P., Josey, J.A., Pan, L., Beigelman, L., and Blatt, L.M.

(2008) Preclinical characteristics of the hepatitis C virus NS3/4A protease inhibitor ITMN-191 (R7227). *Antimicrobial Agents and Chemotherapy,* **52** (12), 4432–4441.

107 Baker, N.A., Sept, D., Joseph, S., Holst, M.J., and McCammon, J.A. (2001) Electrostatics of nanosystems: application to microtubules and the ribosome. *Proceedings of the National Academy of Sciences of the United States of America,* **98**, 10037–10041.

108 Bodenreider, C. *et al.* (2009) Identification of leadlike and nonleadlike inhibitors for the dengue virus NS2B/NS3 protease by tryptophan fluorescence. *Analytical Biochemistry,* **395** (2), 195204.

109 Cheng, N., Brantley, D.M., and Chen, J. (2002) The ephrins and Eph receptors in angiogenesis. *Cytokine & Growth Factor Reviews,* **13** (1), 75–85.

110 Lafleur, K., Huang, D., Zhou, T., Caflisch, A., and Nevado, C. (2009) Structure-based optimization of potent and selective inhibitors of the tyrosine kinase Ephb4. *Journal of Medicinal Chemistry,* **52** (20), 6433–6446.

111 Bohacek, R.S., McMartin, C., and Guida, W.C. (1996) The art and practice of structure-based drug design: a molecular modeling perspective. *Medicinal Research Reviews,* **16** (1), 3–50.

112 Kolb, P. *et al.* (2009) Structure-based discovery of β_2-adrenergic receptor ligands. *Proceedings of the National Academy of Sciences of the United States of America,* **106**, 6843–6848.

113 Vangrevelinghe, E., Zimmermann, K., Schoepfer, J., Portmann, R., Fabbro, D., and Furet, P. (2003) Discovery of a potent and selective protein kinase CK2 inhibitor by high-throughput docking. *Journal of Medicinal Chemistry,* **46** (13), 2656–2662.

114 Zhou, T., Huang, D., and Caflisch, A. (2008) Is quantum mechanics necessary for predicting binding free energy? *Journal of Medicinal Chemistry,* **51**, 4280–4288.

Appendix A: Software Overview

The following table provides a brief compilation of databases, programs, and functions mentioned in the chapters of this book. The software tools are grouped in different classes and listed alphabetically within each class. Where possible, a Web site address is provided from which the software itself or further information about the software can be obtained. References to the literature are provided in cases where no suitable Web site could be identified (and generally for all listed scoring functions). For all other items, the original references are available in the chapters in which the corresponding software is mentioned, as listed in the last column.

With respect to the list of scoring functions, most of the functions are not available as "stand-alone" program, but implemented in docking programs or related software. For availability, refer to the provided references and/or contact the corresponding authors. One representative reference is selected where multiple references would be available. Refer to Section 7.3.2 for further comments about this compilation.

Type	Software name	Developed at or provided by	Reference/ Web site	Cited in Chapter
Databases				
(A) Compounds				
	ACD	Symyx	www.symyx.com	9, 14
	ChemBridge	ChemBridge	www.chembridge.com	12, 14, 15
	ChemDiv	ChemDiv	www.chemdiv.com	14
	ChemDB	University of California, Irvine	cdb.ics.uci.edu	1
	ChemSpider	Royal Society of Chemistry	www.chemspider.com	1, 2
	CSD	CCDC	www.ccdc.cam.ac.uk/products/csd	4
	eMolecules	eMolecules, Inc.	www.emolecules.com	1
	GDB-13	University of Berne	www.dcb-server.unibe.ch/groups/reymond/gdb/home.html	1

(Continued)

Virtual Screening. Edited by C. Sotriffer

ISBN: 978-3-527-32636-5

Type	Software name	Developed at or provided by	Reference/ Web site	Cited in Chapter
	InterBioScreen	InterBioScreen	www.ibscreen.com	14
	Maybridge	Maybridge	www.maybridge.com	14, 15
	NCI/DTP	National Cancer Institute	dtp.nci.nih.gov/docs/3d_database/Structural_information/structural_data.html	9, 12, 14, 15
	SPECS	Specs	www.specs.net	12
	SureChem	SureChem Inc.	www.surechem.org	1
	VEHICLe	UCB Celltech	*J. Med. Chem.* **2009**, *52*, 2952.	1
	ZINC	UCSF	zinc.docking.org	1, 2, 11, 12, 14
(B) Interactions and targets				
	AurSCOPE	Aureus Pharma	www.aureus-pharma.com	1
	BioPrint	Cerep	www.cerep.fr	1
	ChEMBLdb	EMBL-EBI	www.ebi.ac.uk/chembldb	1, 5
	ChemBank	Broad Institute	chembank.broadinstitute.org	1
	DIP	University of California, Los Angeles	dip.doe-mbi.ucla.edu	16
	DOCKGROUND	University of Kansas	dockground.bioinformatics.ku.edu/index.shtml	16
	DOMINE	University of Texas at Dallas	domine.utdallas.edu/cgi-bin/Domine	16
	DrugBank	University of Alberta	www.drugbank.ca	1
	DUD	University of California, San Francisco	dud.docking.org	2, 7, 10
	MDDR	MDL	www.symyx.com	2, 12, 14
	MINT	University of Rome	mint.bio.uniroma2.it/mint	16
	MUV	University of Braunschweig	www.pharmchem.tu-bs.de/lehre/baumann/MUV.html	5
	PDB	RCSB, Rutgers, UCSD	www.pdb.org	1, 4, 7, 10, 12, 14, 16
	PDBbind	University of Michigan and Shanghai Institute of Organic Chemistry	www.pdbbind.org and www.pdbbind.org.cn	7, 10
	PIBASE	Janelia Farm	pibase.janelia.org	16
	PRISM	Koc University, Istanbul	prism.ccbb.ku.edu.tr	16
	PROTCOM	Clemson University	*Nucleic Acids Res.* **2007**, *35*, D575.	16
	PubChem	NIH, NCBI	pubchem.ncbi.nlm.nih.gov	1, 5
	ReliBase	CCDC	relibase.ccdc.cam.ac.uk	4, 7

(Continued)

Type	Software name	Developed at or provided by	Reference/ Web site	Cited in Chapter
	SCORPIO	University of London	scorpio.biophysics.ismb.lon.ac.uk	10
	WOMBAT	Sunset Molecular	www.sunsetmolecular.com	1, 5
	World Drug Index	Thomson Reuters	thomsonreuters.com	5, 15
Chemoinformatic tools and workflow toolkits				
	ChemAxon	ChemAxon	www.chemaxon.com	6
	Filter	OpenEye	www.eyesopen.com	6
	Inforsense	Inforsense	www.inforsense.com	2
	KNIME	KNIME.com GmbH	www.knime.org	2
	LigPrep	Schrödinger	www.schrodinger.com	16
	OEChem	OpenEye	www.eyesopen.com	2
	OpenBabel	OpenBabel community project	openbabel.org	2
	PipelinePilot	Accelrys	accelrys.com	2, 5, 6, 13
	Taverna	myGrid	taverna.sourceforge.net	2
	Topomers (dbtop)	Tripos	tripos.com	13
Similarity analysis				
	ACCS-FP	University of Bonn	*ChemMedChem* **2008**, *3*, 67.	11
	ChemGPS	University of Uppsala	chemgps.bmc.uu.se	1
	Dragon	TALETE srl	www.talete.mi.it	1
	DynaMAD	University of Bonn	*J. Chem. Inf. Model.* **2006**, *46*, 1623.	11
	EON	OpenEye	www.eyesopen.com	13
	Fieldscreen	Cresset	www.cresset-bmd.com	13
	FLAP	Molecular Discovery	*J. Chem. Inf. Model.* **2007**, *47*, 279.	5, 12
	FTrees, FTrees-FS	BioSolveIT	www.biosolveit.de	1, 3
	GRIND (Almond/ Pentacle)	Molecular Discovery	www.moldiscovery.com	12
	Meqi	Pannanugget Consulting	www.pannanugget.com	1
	MoBSS	Pfizer	*J. Chem. Inf. Model.* **2009**, *49*, 745.	1
	ROCS	OpenEye	www.eyesopen.com	3, 12, 13
	Scaffold Hunter	TU Dortmund/MPI Dortmunt	www.scaffoldhunter.com	1
	Volsurf	Molecular Discovery	www.moldiscovery.com	12
Conformer generation				
	Caesar	Accelrys	accelrys.com	6
	Concord	Tripos	tripos.com	13, 14
	Corina	Molecular Networks	www.molecular-networks.com	6
	DS Catalyst CONFIRM	Accelrys	accelrys.com	5, 6

(Continued)

Type	Software name	Developed at or provided by	Reference/ Web site	Cited in Chapter
	Omega	OpenEye	www.eyesopen.com	5, 6
	ROTATE	Molecular Networks	www.molecular-networks.com	5
Pharmacophore modeling				
	DS Catalyst	Accelrys	accelrys.com	5, 12, 13, 15
	GALAHAD	Tripos	tripos.com	5
	GASP	Tripos	tripos.com	5
	LigandScout	inte:ligand	www.inteligand.com	5, 10, 15
	MOE	Chemical Computing Group	www.chemcomp.com	5, 13
	PHASE	Schrödinger	www.schrodinger.com	5, 12
	UNITY	Tripos	tripos.com	5, 10, 12–14
***De novo* design**				
	BREED	Chemical Computing Group	www.chemcomp.com	17
	CCLD	University of Zurich	*J. Comp. Aided Mol. Des.* **1996**, *10*, 372.	17
	GANDI	University of Zurich	www.biochem-caflisch.uzh.ch/download	17
	HOOK	Harvard University	*Proteins* **1994**, *19*, 199.	17
	LEA3D	University of Nice	bioinfo.ipmc.cnrs.fr/lea.html	17
	LUDI	Accelrys	accelrys.com	12, 17
	PRO_ligand	Proteus Molecular Design	*J Comp. Aided Mol. Des.* **1995**, *9*, 13.	17
	Skelgen	De Novo Pharmaceuticals	www.denovopharma.com/page2.asp	17
Protein analysis (binding sites, flexibility, hot spots, interfaces, water sites, etc.)				
	Chimera	University of California, San Francisco	www.cgl.ucsf.edu/chimera	16
	Consolv	Michigan State University	www.bch.msu.edu/~kuhn/software/consolv	4, 10
	CS-Map	Boston University	*Proteins* **2003**, *51*, 340.	10
	DFprot	Centro de Investigaciones Biológicas	sbg.cib.csic.es/Software/DFprot	16
	Electron Density Server	University of Uppsala	eds.bmc.uu.se/eds/	4, 10
	FoldX	EMBL	foldx.crg.es	10, 16
	GRID	Molecular Discovery	www.moldiscovery.com	4, 5, 10, 15
	Harmony	NCBS, Bangalore	caps.ncbs.res.in/harmony	14
	HINT	eduSoft	www.edusoft-lc.com	4, 10
	MCSS	Accelrys	accelrys.com	17

(Continued)

Type	Software name	Developed at or provided by	Reference/ Web site	Cited in Chapter
	Mogul	CCDC	www.ccdc.cam.ac.uk/products/csd_system/mogul/	4
	Molprobity	Duke University	molprobity.biochem.duke.edu	4
	MRC	University of California, San Diego	abagyan.ucsd.edu/MRC	16
	ODA	MolSoft	www.molsoft.com/oda.html	16
	PIER	University of California, San Diego	abagyan.ucsd.edu/PIER	16
	PPI-Pred	University of Leeds	bmbpcu36.leeds.ac.uk/ppi_pred	16
	PQS	EMBL/EBI	www.ebi.ac.uk/pdbe/pqs/	4
	PROCHECK	EMBL/EBI	www.biochem.ucl.ac.uk/~roman/procheck/procheck.html	4, 14
	PROFACE	Bose Institute, Kolkata	resources.boseinst.ernet.in/resources/bioinfo/interface	16
	PROMATE	Weizmann Institute of Science	bioinfo.weizmann.ac.il/promate	16
	PROTORP	University of Sussex	www.bioinformatics.sussex.ac.uk/protorp	16
	Q-siteFinder	University of Leeds	www.modelling.leeds.ac.uk/qsitefinder	16
	Relibase, Waterbase	CCDC	relibase.ccdc.cam.ac.uk	4, 7
	Robetta	University of Washington	robetta.bakerlab.org	16
	SuperStar	CCDC	www.ccdc.cam.ac.uk/products/life_sciences/superstar/	4, 10
	SURFNET	University College London	www.biochem.ucl.ac.uk/~roman/surfnet/surfnet.html	16
	UniProt	UniProt Consortium	www.uniprot.org	4
	VMD	University of Illinois at Urbana-Champaign	www.ks.uiuc.edu/Research/vmd	16
	Watermap	Schrödinger	www.schrodinger.com	10
	WaterScore	University of Cambridge/De Novo Pharmaceuticals	*J. Mol. Model.* **2003**, *9*, 172.	4, 10
	WHAT_CHECK	CMBI	swift.cmbi.ru.nl/gv/whatcheck/	4
Homology modeling				
	CODA, FREAD, PETRA	Tripos	tripos.com	14

(Continued)

Type	Software name	Developed at or provided by	Reference/ Web site	Cited in Chapter
	COILS	EMBnet	www.ch.embnet.org/software/COILS_form.html	14
	MOBILE	University of Marburg	*J. Mol. Biol.* **2003**, *334*, 327.	14
	Modeller	University of California, San Francisco	salilab.org/modeller	14
	MOE	Chemical Computing Group	www.chemcomp.com	2, 14
	PLOP	University of California, San Francisco	www.jacobsonlab.org	14
	PSIPRED	University College London	bioinf.cs.ucl.ac.uk/psipred	14
	SCWRL	Fox Chase Cancer Center	dunbrack.fccc.edu/scwrl4	15
	Sybyl Biopolymer	Tripos	tripos.com	14
	Whatif	CMBI	swift.cmbi.kun.nl/whatif/	14
MD Simulations				
	Amber	UCSF, Scripps	ambermd.org	6, 7, 9
	CHARMM	Harvard University/ Accelrys	www.charmm.org	6, 7, 17
	Gromacs	University of Groningen	www.gromacs.org	14
Docking				
	ADAM	IMMD, Toyko	*Proteins* **2006**, *63*, 878.	8
	ADDock	Biodelight Biotech Inc.	www.biodelight.com.tw/ English	6
	ASEDock	Tokai University School of Medicine	*J. Chem. Inf. Model.* **2008**, *48*, 583.	6
	Autodock	The Scripps Research Institute	autodock.scripps.edu	6, 9, 10, 14, 15
	CDOCKER	Accelrys	accelrys.com	9
	ClusPro	Boston University	nrc.bu.edu/cluster	16
	CombiDOCK	University of California, San Francisco	*J. Comp.-Aided Mol. Des.* **1998**, *12*, 597.	1
	CombiGlide	Schrödinger	www.schrodinger.com	1
	DOCK	University of California, San Francisco	dock.compbio.ucsf.edu	6, 7, 9, 12, 14, 16
	DREAM ++	University of California, San Francisco	*J. Comp.-Aided Mol. Des.* **1999**, *13*, 513.	1
	eHiTS	SimBioSys	www.simbiosys.ca	6

(Continued)

Type	Software name	Developed at or provided by	Reference/ Web site	Cited in Chapter
	EUDOC	Mayo Foundation for Medical Education and Research	*J. Comput. Chem.* **2001**, *22*, 1750.	12
	FITTED	McGill University/ Forecaster	fitted.ca	6, 10
	FlexE	BioSolveIT	www.biosolveit.de	6, 12, 15
	FlexNovo	BioSolveIT	www.biosolveit.de	1
	FlexScreen	BioSolveIT	www.biosolveit.de	6, 8
	FlexX	BioSolveIT	www.biosolveit.de	3, 6, 8–10, 12, 14, 17
	$FlexX^C$	BioSolveIT	www.biosolveit.de	1
	FlexX-Pharm	BioSolveIT	www.biosolveit.de	6, 14
	FLIPDock	The Scripps Research Institute	flipdock.scripps.edu	6, 8
	FRED	OpenEye	www.eyesopen.com	6, 10, 14
	FRODOCK	Centro de Investigaciones Biológicas	sbg.cib.csic.es/Software/ FRODOCK	16
	FTDock	Imperial College London	www.sbg.bio.ic.ac.uk/ docking	16
	GasDock	Dalian University of Technology	*Bioorg. Med. Chem. Lett.* **2004**, *14*, 4671.	12
	GlamDock	$Chil^2$	www.chil2.de	6
	Glide	Schrödinger	www.schrodinger.com	6, 9, 10, 12, 14–17
	GOLD	CCDC	www.ccdc.cam.ac.uk/products/life_sciences/gold	4, 6, 7, 9, 10, 12, 14, 15, 17
	GRAMM-X	University of Kansas	vakser.bioinformatics.ku.edu/resources/gramm/grammx	16
	Haddock	University of Utrecht	haddock.chem.uu.nl/services/HADDOCK/haddockservereasy.html	16
	Hex	INRIA	www.loria.fr/~ritchied/hex	14, 16
	ICM	MolSoft	www.molsoft.com	6, 12, 14, 16
	ISE-dock	Hebrew University of Jerusalem	*Proteins* **2008**, *71*, 1373.	6
	LibDock	Accelrys	accelrys.com	14
	Ligandfit	Accelrys	accelrys.com	14
	LIGIN	Weizmann Institute of Science	*Proteins* **1996**, *25*, 120.	12
	MOE	Chemical Computing Group	www.chemcomp.com	14, 15

(Continued)

Type	Software name	Developed at or provided by	Reference/ Web site	Cited in Chapter
	MolFit	Weizmann Institute of Science	www.weizmann.ac.il/Chemical_Research_Support//molfit	16
	PatchDock	Tel-Aviv University	bioinfo3d.cs.tau.ac.il/PatchDock	16
	PLANTS	University of Konstanz	www.tcd.uni-konstanz.de/research/plants.php	6
	Pso@autodock	University of Leipzig	biophys.biow.uni-leipzig.de/psoatautodock.html	6
	QXP/FLO	Colin McMartin	*J. Comp.-Aided Mol. Des.* **1997**, *11*, 333.	10, 12
	rDock	York Structural Biology Laboratory	www.ysbl.york.ac.uk/rDock	12
	RosettaDock	Johns Hopkins University	rosettadock.graylab.jhu.edu	16
	SEED, FFLD	University of Zurich	www.biochem-caflisch.uzh.ch	17
	SKE-DOCK	Kitasato University	www.pharm.kitasato-u.ac.jp/bmd/files/SKE_DOCK.html	16
	SLIDE	Michigan State University	www.bch.msu.edu/~kuhn/software/slide	8–10
	Sodock	National Chiao Tung University	iclab.life.nctu.edu.tw/sodock	6
	Surflex	Tripos	tripos.com	6, 12, 14
	ZDOCK	Boston University	zdock.bu.edu	16
Scoring functions (SF)				
(A) Empirical SF				
	AIScore	Raub *et al.*, *J. Chem. Inf. Model.* **2008**, *48*, 1492.		7
	AutoDock3 SF	Morris *et al.*, *J. Comput. Chem.* **1998**, *19*, 1639.		(7)
	AutoDock4 SF	Huey *et al.*, *J. Comput. Chem.* **2007**, *28*, 1145.		(7)
	ChemScore	Eldridge *et al.*, *J. Comp.-Aided Mol. Des.* **1997**, *11*, 425.		7, 12, 14
	eHITS SF	Zsoldos *et al.*, *J. Mol. Struct. Theochem.* **2003**, *666–667*, 659.		7
	FlexX SF	Rarey *et al.*, *J. Mol. Biol.* **1996**, *261*, 470.		(7)
	Fresno	Rognan *et al.*, *J. Med. Chem.* **1999**, *42*, 4650.		(7)
	GlideScore/GlideXP	Friesner *et al.*, *J. Med. Chem.* **2006**, *49*, 6177.		7, 16
	Giordanetto's SF	Giordanetto *et al.*, *J. Chem. Inf. Comput. Sci.* **2004**, *44*, 882.		7
	Jain's SF	Jain, *J. Comp. Aided Mol. Des.* **1996**, *10*, 427.		(7)
	LigScore	Krammer *et al.*, *J. Mol. Graph. Model.* **2005**, *23*, 395.		(7)
	PLP	Gehlhaar *et al.*, *Chem. Biol.* **1995**, *2*, 317.		6, 7
	RankScore	Moitessier *et al.*, *J. Med. Chem.* **2006**, *49*, 5885.		7
	SCORE	Wang *et al.*, *J. Mol. Model.* **1998**, *4*, 379.		(7)
	SCORE 3.0	Pei *et al.*, *Proteins* **2006**, *62*, 934.		(7)

(Continued)

Type	Software name	Developed at or provided by	Reference/ Web site	Cited in Chapter
	SCORE1	Boehm, *J. Comp. Aided Mol. Des.* **1994**, *8*, 243.		(7)
	SCORE2	Boehm, *J. Comp. Aided Mol. Des.* **1998**, *12*, 309.		(7)
	ScreenScore	Stahl *et al., J. Med. Chem.* **2001**, *44*, 1035.		(7)
	SFCscore	Sotriffer *et al., Proteins* **2008**, *73*, 395.		7
	SIE (FF)	Naim, *J. Chem. Inf. Model.* **2007**, *47*, 122.		(7)
	SLIDE SF	Schnecke *et al., Perspect. Drug Discov. Des.* **2000**, *20*, 171.		7
	Surflex-Dock	Pham *et al., J. Med. Chem.* **2006**, *49*, 5856.		7
	X-Score	Wang *et al., J. Comp.-Aided Mol. Des.* **2002**, *16*, 11.		(7)
(B) Knowledge-based SF				
	ASP	Mooij *et al., Proteins* **2005**, *61*, 272.		7
	BLEEP	Mitchell *et al., J. Comput. Chem.* **1999**, *20*, 1165.		7
	DFIRE	Zhang *et al., J. Med. Chem.* **2005**, *48*, 2325.		(7)
	$DrugScore^{PDB}$	Gohlke *et al., J. Mol. Biol.* **2000**, *295*, 337.		7
	$DrugScore^{CSD}$	Velec *et al., J. Med. Chem.* **2005**, *48*, 6296.		7
	ITScore	Huang *et al., J. Comput. Chem.* **2006**, *27*, 1866.		(7)
	M-Score	Yang *et al., J. Med. Chem.* **2006**, *49*, 5903.		7
	PMF	Muegge, *J. Med. Chem.* **2006**, *49*, 5895.		7
	SMoG	Ishchenko *et al., J. Med. Chem.* **2002**, *45*, 2770.		7
(C) Other approaches				
	AFMoC	Gohlke *et al., J. Med. Chem.* **2002**, *45*, 4153.		7
	AutoShim	Martin *et al., J. Chem. Inf. Model.* **2008**, *48*, 861.		7
	BBCS	Fukunishi *et al., J. Chem. Inf. Model.* **2008**, *48*, 988.		7
	COMBINE	Ortiz *et al., J. Med. Chem.* **1995**, *38*, 2681.		7
	CScore	Clark *et al., J. Mol. Graph. Model.* **2002**, *20*, 281.		14
	GFScore	Betzi *et al., J. Chem. Inf. Model.* **2006**, *46*, 1704.		7
	HINT	Cozzini *et al., J. Med. Chem.* **2002**, *45*, 2469.		4, 7, 10
	HYDE	Reulecke *et al., ChemMedChem* **2008**, *3*, 885.		7
	LIE	Åqvist *et al., Protein Eng.* **1994**, *7*, 385.		6, 7, 10, 17
	LIECE	Huang *et al., J. Med. Chem.* **2004**, *47*, 5791.		7, 17
	MM-GBSA	Huang *et al., J. Chem. Inf. Model.* **2006**, *46*, 243.		7, 9, 10
	MM-PBSA	Kollman *et al., Acc. Chem. Res.* **2000**, *33*, 889.		7, 9, 10
	ROTA	Hartmann *et al.,, Proteins* **2009**, *74*, 712.		14
	SeleX-CS	Bar-Haim *et al., J. Chem. Inf. Model.* **2009**, *49*, 623.		7
	SIFt	Deng *et al., J. Med. Chem.* **2004**, *47*, 337.		1, 5–7
	SSM	Teramoto *et al., J. Chem. Inf. Model.* **2007**, *47*, 1858.		7
	TOP	Seifert, *J. Comp. Aided Mol. Des.* **2009**, *23*, 633.		7
	TScore	Matter *et al., J. Med. Chem.* **2005**, *48*, 3290.		7
Miscellaneous				
	AMSOL (solvation free energies)	University of Minnesota	comp.chem.umn.edu/amsol	12
	DAIM (molecule decomposition)	University of Zurich	www.biochem-caflisch.uzh.ch	17
	Fragment – RECAP method (molecule fragmentation)	ChemAxon	chemaxon.com	1, 3

Appendix B: Virtual Screening Application Studies

The following table provides a brief compilation of virtual screening application studies mentioned in the chapters of this book. Additional case studies not mentioned in the book are taken from the following review and are denoted with (*): H. Kubinyi, Success Stories of Computer-Aided Design, in *Computer Applications in Pharmaceutical Research and Development*, edited by Sean Ekins, John Wiley & Sons, Inc., 2006.

Only prospective virtual screenings are shown; purely retrospective studies or enrichment studies, as well as studies without experimental testing, are not included. The targets are grouped in different protein classes and sorted alphabetically within each class (first column). Where possible, the number of tested compounds, the number of detected active compounds, and activity data of the most potent hits are reported in the third column (n.a., not available). In general, the results refer to the primary screening hits; secondary screens and optimizations are not considered.

Targets	Cited in Chapter	Tested/actives/ highest affinity	References
GPCRs			
Adenosine A_{2A} R.	12	17/17/1.6 nM (K_i)	Schneider, G. *et al., J. Comb. Chem.* **2003**, *5*, 233.
α_{1A} Adrenergic R.	12	80/37/1.4 nM (K_i)	Evers, A. *et al., J. Med. Chem.* **2005**, *48*, 1088.
β_2 Adrenergic R.	12	25/6/9 nM (K_i)	Kolb, P. *et al., Proc. Natl. Acad. Sci. USA* **2009**, *106*, 6843.
		56/19/0.11 nM (K_i)	Sabio, M. *et al., Bioorg. Med. Chem. Lett.* **2008**, *18*, 5391.
Cannabinoid CB1 R.	5, 12	420/5/53 nM (K_i)	Wang, H. *et al., J. Med. Chem.* **2008**, *51*, 2439.
Cannabinoid CB2 R.	5	n.a./n.a./93 nM (EC_{50})	Cheng, Y. *et al., J. Med. Chem.* **2008**, *51*, 5019.
Cannabinoid CB2 R.	5	14/7/1.35 μM (K_i)	Markt, P. *et al., J. Med. Chem.* **2009**, *52*, 369.

(Continued)

Virtual Screening. Edited by C. Sotriffer

ISBN: 978-3-527-32636-5

Targets	Cited in Chapter	Tested/actives/ highest affinity	References
Complement C3AR1	5	157/4/310 nM (EC_{50})	Klabunde, T. *et al.*, *J. Med. Chem.* **2009**, *52*, 2923.
Chemokine CCR3 R.	12	43/5/12 μM (K_i)	Becker, O.M. *et al.*, *Proc. Natl. Acad. Sci. USA* **2004**, *101*, 11304.
Chemokine CCR5 R.	6, 12, 14, 15	59/10/17 μM (IC_{50})	Kellenberger, E. *et al.*, *J. Med. Chem.* **2007**, *50*, 1294.
Corticotropin releasing factor 1 R.	13	655/10/>20% inhib. at 10 μM	Tresadern, G. *et al.*, *J. Mol. Graph. Des.* **2009**, *27*, 860.
CRTH2	1	600/60/≤10 μM (IC_{50})	Frimurer, T.M. *et al.*, *Bioorg. Med. Chem. Lett.* **2005**, *15*, 3707.
Dopamine D_2 R.	12	42/7/58 nM (K_i)	Becker, O.M. *et al.*, *Proc. Natl. Acad. Sci. USA* **2004**, *101*, 11304.
Dopamine D_3 R.	12, 14	20/8/11 nM (K_i)	Varady, J. *et al.*, *J. Med. Chem.* **2003**, *46*, 4377.
Endothelin A R.	(*)	383/n.a./9 μM (IC_{50})	Astles, P.C. *et al.*, *Eur. J. Med. Chem.* **1997**, *32*, 409.
		6/4/220 nM (IC_{50})	Funk, O.F. *et al.*, *J. Med. Chem.* **2004**, *47*, 2750.
FFAR1	14	52/6/10 μM (EC_{50})	Tikhonova, I.G. *et al.*, *J. Med. Chem.* **2008**, *51*, 625.
Histamine H3 R.	15	7/7/79 nM (IC_{50})	Schlegel, B. *et al.*, *Comput.-Aid. Mol. Des.* **2007**, *21*, 437.
Histamine H4 R.	12, 14	255/16/85 nM (K_i)	Kiss, R. *et al.*, *J. Med. Chem.* **2008**, *51*, 3145.
LPA_{-3} R.	5	36/3/24 nM (IC_{50})	Fells, J.I. *et al.*, *Bioorg. Med. Chem.* **2008**, *16*, 6207.
Melanin-concentrating hormone 1 R.	12, 14	795/62/55 nM (IC_{50})	Clark, D.E. *et al.*, *J. Med. Chem.* **2004**, *47*, 3962.
	9, 14	129/6/7.5 μM (K_i)	Cavasotto, C.N. *et al.*, *J. Med. Chem.* **2008**, *51*, 581.
mGlu1R	13	28/13/0.74 μM (IC_{50})	Noeske, T. *et al.*, *Bioorg. Med. Chem.* **2009**, *17*, 5708.
	15	23/13/0.36 nM (IC_{50})	Noeske, T. *et al.*, *ChemMedChem.* **2007**, *2*, 1763.
mGlu4R	5, 12, 14	38/6/n.a.	Triballeau, N. *et al.*, J. *Med. Chem.* **2005**, *48*, 2534.
Muscarinic M_3 R.	12	172/3/0.2 μM (K_B)	Marriot D.P. *et al.*, *J. Med. Chem.* **1999**, *42*, 3210.
Neurokinin-1 R.	6, 9, 12, 14, 15	7/1/251 nM (K_i)	Evers, A. *et al.*, *Angew. Chem., Int. Ed.* **2004**, *43*, 248. Evers, A. *et al.*, *J. Med. Chem.* **2004**, *47*, 5381.
NPY5 R.	12	632/31/40 nM (IC_{50})	Guba, W. *et al.*, *Bioorg. Med. Chem. Lett.* **2005**, *15*, 1599.
Rhodopsin R.	14	9/2/15 μM (IC_{50})	Taylor, C.M. *et al.*, *J. Med. Chem.* **2008**, *51*, 5297.

(Continued)

Targets	Cited in Chapter	Tested/actives/ highest affinity	References
Serotonin $5\text{-}HT_{1A}$ R.	12	78/16/1 nM (K_i)	Becker, O.M. *et al.*, *Proc. Natl. Acad. Sci. USA* **2004**, *101*, 11304.
Serotonin $5\text{-}HT_4$ R.	12	93/19/1.6 nM (K_i)	Becker, O.M. *et al.*, *Proc. Natl. Acad. Sci. USA* **2004**, *101*, 11304.
Serotonin $5\text{-}HT_{2C}$ R.	14	21/9/424 nM (IC_{50})	Ahmed, A. *et al.*, *Bioorg. Med. Chem.* **2009**, *17*, 4559.
Sigma-1 R.	5	11/9/1.3 nM (K_i)	Laggner, C. *et al.*, *J. Med. Chem.* **2005**, *48*, 4754.
SST5R	1	31/27/13 nM (K_i)	Martin, R.E. *et al.*, *J. Med. Chem.* **2007**, *50*, 6291.
Tachykinin NK1 R.	12	53/8/56 nM (K_i)	Becker, O.M. *et al.*, *Proc. Natl. Acad. Sci. USA* **2004**, *101*, 11304.
TRH-R1	12	100/5/0.29 μM (IC_{50})	Engel, S. *et al.*, *J. Am. Chem. Soc.* **2008**, *130*, 5115.
Urotensin II R.	12	500/10/400 nM (IC_{50})	Flohr, S. *et al.*, *J. Med. Chem.* **2002**, *45*, 1799.
Nuclear receptors			
CAR (constitutive androstane receptor)	15	30/17/7.76-fold CAR activation	Küblbeck, J. *et al.*, *Biochem. Pharmacol.* **2008**, *76*, 1288.
ERα	12	7/3/1.4 μM (IC_{50})	Knox, A.J.S. *et al.*, *J. Med. Chem.* **2007**, *50*, 5301.
LXRβ	12	1290/n.a./0.21 μM (EC_{50})	Bakir, F. *et al.*, *Bioorg. Med. Chem. Lett.* **2007**, *17*, 3473.
		1308/69/n.a.	Cheng, J.-F. *et al.*, *J. Med. Chem.* **2008**, *51*, 2057.
PPAR(α,γ,δ)	12	10/5/1 μM (IC_{50})	Markt, P. *et al.*, *J. Med. Chem.* **2008**, *51*, 6303.
PPARγ	9	29/6/2.9 μM (EC_{50})	Salam, N. K. *et al.*, *Chem. Biol. Drug Des.* **2008**, *71*, 57.
	5	8/2/15 μM (EC_{50})	Tanrikulu, Y. *et al.*, *ChemBioChem* **2009**, *10*, 75.
	5	4/3/0.24 μM (K_i)	Fakhrudin, N. *et al.*, *Mol. Pharmacol.* **2010**, *77*, 559.
RARα	12	32/2/55% inhib. at 20 μM	Schapira, M. *et al.*, *Proc. Natl. Acad. Sci. USA* **2000**, *97*, 1008.
Thyroid hormone receptor	12	100/14/20 μM (IC_{90})	Schapira, M. *et al.*, *Proc. Natl. Acad. Sci. USA* **2003**, *100*, 7354.
Other receptors			
$\alpha_4\beta_1$-Integrin R.	12	12/12/1.3 nM (IC_{50})	Singh, J. *et al.*, *J. Med. Chem.* **2002**, *45*, 2988.
LFA-1 (integrin)	11, 12	25/1/70 μM (IC_{50})	Shoda, M. *et al.*, *ChemMedChem* **2007**, *2*, 515.
Oxidoreductases			
Aldose reductase	12	9/6/2.4 μM (IC_{50})	Krämer, O. *et al.*, *Proteins Struct. Funct. Genet.* **2004**, *55*, 814.

(Continued)

Targets	Cited in Chapter	Tested/actives/ highest affinity	References
	9	6/4/8 μM (IC_{50})	Ferrari, A.M. *et al.*, *J. Med. Chem.* **2004**, *47*, 5076.
	9	25/5/42 μM (IC_{50})	Rastelli, G. *et al.*, *Bioorg. Med. Chem.* **2002**, *10*, 1437.
Aromatase	5	10/4/0.266 μM (IC_{50})	Neves, M.A.C. *et al.*, *Eur. J. Med. Chem.* **2009**, *44*, 4121.
COX-1	5	9/3/10.3 μM (IC_{50})	Rollinger, J.M. *et al.*, *Planta Medica* **2005**, *71*, 399.
COX-2	12	12/4/60% inhib. at 1 μM	Mozziconacci, J.-C. *et al.*, *J. Med. Chem.* **2005**, *48*, 1055.
CYP 2D6	10	16/14/0.06 μM (IC_{50})	De Graaf, C. *et al.*, *J. Med. Chem.* **2006**, *49*, 2417.
Dihydrofolate reductase	(*)	21/2/0.54 μM (IC_{50})	Toyoda, T. *et al.*, *Biochem. Biophys. Res. Commun.* **1997**, *235*, 515.
	12	252/54/2.8 nM (IC_{50})	Wyss, P.C. *et al.*, *J. Med. Chem.* **2003**, *46*, 2304.
Enoyl-acyl-carrier-protein reductase	12	169/16/4.2 μM (IC_{50})	Nicola, G. *et al.*, *Biochem. Biophys. Res. Commun.* **2007**, *358*, 686.
11β-HSD1	5	12/4/1.9 μM (IC_{50})	Rollinger, J.M. *et al.*, *Bioorg. Med. Chem.* **2010**, *18*, 1507.
	12	30/7/0.14 μM (IC_{50})	Schuster, D. *et al.*, *J. Med. Chem.* **2006**, *49*, 3454.
17β-HSD1	5, 12	14/4/5.7 μM (IC_{50})	Schuster, D. *et al.*, *J. Med. Chem.* **2008**, *51*, 4188.
Human lipoxygenase	12, 14	20/3/6.8 μM (IC_{50})	Kenyon, V. *et al.*, *J. Med. Chem.* **2006**, *49*, 1356.
5-lipoxygenase	5, 12, 13	18/2/0.8 μM (IC_{50})	Franke, L. *et al.*, *J. Med. Chem.* **2007**, *50*, 2640.
	13	23/4/0.8 μM (IC_{50})	Schwarz, O. *et al.*, *J. Comb. Chem.* **2007**, *9*, 1104.
	5	5/2/14 μM (IC_{50})	Aparoy, P. *et al.*, *Bioorg. Med. Chem. Lett.* **2010**, *20*, 1013.
IMP	(*)	74/7/31 μM (IC_{50})	Pickett, S.D. *et al.*, *Bioorg. Med. Chem. Lett.* **2003**, *13*, 1691.
Trypanothione reductase TryR	12	29/10/11.5 μM (IC_{50})	Perez-Pineiro, R. *et al.*, *J. Med. Chem.* **2009**, *52*, 1670.
Kinases			
Akt1	(*)	100/2/2.6 μM (IC_{50})	Forino, M. *et al.*, *J. Med. Chem.* **2005**, *48*, 2278.
Aurora A	17	7/4/3 μM (IC_{50})	Warner, S.L. *et al.*, *Mol. Cancer Ther.* **2006**, *5*, 1764.
Bcr-Abl	12	15/8/24 μM (IC_{50})	Peng, H. *et al.*, *Bioorg. Med. Chem. Lett.* **2003**, *13*, 3693.
Cdk2	(*)	120/17/0.9 μM (IC_{50})	Wu, S.Y. *et al.*, *Structure* **2003**, *11*, 399.

(Continued)

Targets	Cited in Chapter	Tested/actives/ highest affinity	References
	17	30/1/7.8 μM (IC_{50})	Kolb, P. *et al.*, *J. Med. Chem.* **2008**, *51*, 1179.
Cdk4	(*)	382/18/14 μM (IC_{50})	Honma, T. *et al.*, *J. Med. Chem.* **2001**, *44*, 4615.
Chk-1	12	103/36/110 nM (IC_{50})	Lyne, P. D. *et al.*, *J. Med. Chem.* **2004**, *47*, 1962.
	12	1179/10/13.4 μM (IC_{50})	Foloppe, N. *et al.*, *Bioorg. Med. Chem.* **2006**, *14*, 4792.
Casein kinase 2 (CK2)	12, 14, 17	12/4/80 nM (IC_{50})	Vangrevelinghe, E. *et al.*, *J. Med. Chem.* **2003**, *46*, 2656.
EphB4	17	43/8/1.4 μM (IC_{50})	Kolb, P. *et al.*, *Proteins* **2008**, *73*, 11.
GSK-3β	5	56/3/1.6 μM (IC_{50})	Kim, H.-J. *et al.*, *Bioorg. Med. Chem.* **2008**, *16*, 636.
IKKβ	14	75/6/1.76 μM (IC_{50})	Nagarajan, S. *et al.*, *Bioorg. Med. Chem.* **2009**, *17*, 2759.
JAK 2	14	7/1/1 μM (IC_{50})	Sandberg, E.M. *et al.*, *J. Med. Chem.* **2005**, *48*, 2526.
		39/5/60 nM (IC_{50})	Kiss, R. *et al.*, *Bioorg. Med. Chem. Lett.* **2009**, *19*, 3598.
JAK 3	12	79/4/1 nM (IC_{50})	Chen, X. *et al.*, *J. Med. Chem.*, **2008**, *51*, 7015.
RSK2	14	19/2/1 μM (IC_{50})	Nguyen, T.L. *et al.*, *Bioorg. Med. Chem.* **2006**, *14*, 6097.
Syk	5	30/6/63% inhib. at 10 μM	Xie, H.-Z. *et al.*, *Bioorg. Med. Chem. Lett.* **2009**, *19*, 1944.
TβRI	(*)	87/n.a./27 nM (IC_{50})	Singh, J. *et al.*, *Bioorg. Med. Chem. Lett.* **2003**, *13*, 4355.
Other transferases			
AICAR transformylase	(*)	16/8/4.1 μM (IC_{50})	Li, C. *et al.*, *J. Med. Chem.* **2004**, *47*, 6681.
Farnesyl transferase	12	21/4/25 μM (IC_{50})	Perola, E. *et al.*, *J. Med. Chem.* **2000**, *43*, 401.
	(*)	718/5/0.7 μM (IC_{50})	Kaminski, J. J. *et al.*, *J. Med. Chem.*, **1997**, *40*, 4103.
Guanine phosphoribosyl transferase	(*)	6/4/52 μM (IC_{50})	Aronov, A.M. *et al.*, *Antimicr. Agents Chemother.* **2001**, *45*, 2571.
Histone arginine methyltransferase	15	36/7/1.7 μM (IC_{50})	Spannhoff, A. *et al.*, *J. Med. Chem.* **2007**, *50*, 2319.
PRMT1	14, 15	9/9/13 μM (IC_{50})	Heinke, R. *et al.*, *ChemMedChem* **2009**, *4*, 69.
HIV-1 integrase	12	29/10/2 μM (IC_{50})	Hong, H. *et al.*, *J. Med. Chem.* **1997**, *40*, 930.
	5	234/2/35 μM (IC_{50})	De Luca, L. *et al.*, *ChemMedChem* **2009**, *4*, 1311.

(Continued)

Targets	Cited in Chapter	Tested/actives/ highest affinity	References
HIV-1 RT	12	4/0/–	Barreiro, G. *et al., J. Med. Chem.* **2007**, *50*, 5324.
KAS III	5	16/3/0.02 μM (K_d)	Lee, J.Y. *et al., Bioorg. Med. Chem.* **2009**, *17*, 1506.
Nonnucleosidic DNA alkyltransferase MGMT	12	17/4/10 μM (IC_{50})	Ruiz, F.M. *et al., J. Chem. Inf. Model.* **2008**, *48*, 844.
Poly(ADP-ribose)-polymerase-1 (PARP1)	13	n.a./n.a./40 nM (IC_{50})	Branca, D. *et al., Bioorg. Med. Chem. Lett.* **2009**, *15*, 4042.
Sirtuin	15	5/5/9.1 μM (IC_{50})	Uciechowska, U. *et al., ChemMedChem* **2008**, *3*, 1965.
Sirtuin type 2	12	11/4/51 μM (IC_{50})	Tervo, A.J. *et al., J. Med. Chem.* **2006**, *49*, 7239.
Thymidylat synthase	12	33/29/3 μM (IC_{50})	Shoichet, B.K. *et al., Science* **1993**, *259*, 1445.
	12	5/3/300 μM (IC_{50})	Tondi, D. *et al., Chem. Biol.* **1999**, *6*, 319.
t-RNA-guanine transglycosylase	10, 12	9/9/0.25 μM (K_i)	Brenk, R. *et al., J. Med. Chem.* **2003**, *46*, 1133.
Proteases			
β-Secretase	17	72/12/2.6 μM (EC_{50})	Huang, D. *et al., J. Med. Chem.* **2005**, *48*, 5108.
	17	88/11/7.1 μM (IC_{50})	Huang, D. *et al., J. Am. Chem. Soc.* **2006**, *128*, 5436.
	5	11/9/18 μM (IC_{50})	Huang, W. *et al., Bioorg. Med. Chem.* **2008**, *16*, 10190.
Cathepsin-B	17	29/1/4.8 μM (K_i)	Schenker, P. *et al., Protein Sci.* **2008**, *17*, 2145.
Cathepsin-K (S, L)	11	16/3/31 μM (IC_{50})	Stumpfe, D. *et al., ChemMedChem* **2008**, *4*, 52.
Cercarial elastase	12	52/5/3 μM (K_i)	Ring, C.S. *et al., Proc. Natl. Acad. Sci.USA* **1993**, *90*, 3583.
Dipeptidyl peptidase IV (DPP-IV)	12	4000/51/81.9% inhib. at 30 μM	Ward, R.A. *et al., J. Med. Chem.* **2005**, *48*, 6991.
	17	12/10/2.3 μM (IC_{50})	Rummey, C. *et al., Bioorg. Med. Chem. Lett.* **2006**, *16*, 1405.
Falcipain-2	14	84/24/1.0 μM (IC_{50})	Desai, P. V. *et al., J. Med. Chem.* **2004**, *47*, 6609.
		100/18/1.4 μM (IC_{50})	Desai, P. V. *et al., J. Med. Chem.* **2006**, *49*, 1576.
	12	81/28/2.4 μM (IC_{50})	Li, H. *et al., J. Med. Chem.* **2009**, *52*, 4936.
HIV protease	(*)	15/5/10 μM (K_i)	Rutenber, E. *et al., J. Biol. Chem.* **1993**, *268*, 15343.

(Continued)

Targets	Cited in Chapter	Tested/actives/ highest affinity	References
	12	50/15/0.32 μM (IC_{50})	Wang, S. *et al.*, *J. Med. Chem.* **1996**, *39*, 2047.
	5	1/1/18 μM (IC_{50})	Damm, K.L. *et al.*, *Biopolymers* **2008**, *89*, 643.
NS3 protease	17	5/2/90 μM (K_d)	Ekonomiuk, D. *et al.*, *J. Med. Chem.* **2009**, *52*, 4860.
	17	22/6/40 μM (K_d)	Ekonomiuk, D. *et al.*, *PloS Negl. Trop. Dis.* **2009**, *3*, e356.
Plasmepsin	17	59/13/2 μM (IC_{50})	Friedman, R. *et al.*, *ChemMed-Chem* **2009**, *4*, 1317.
Plasmepsin II	9	30/26/4.3 nM (IC_{50})	Degliesposti, G.V. *et al.*, *Chem-MedChem* **2009**, *4*, 1164.
SARS CoV 3C-like protease	14	40/3/(61 μM) (K_i)	Liu, Z. *et al.*, *J. Chem. Inf. Model.* **2005**, *45*, 10.
Thrombin	12	10/5/95 nM (K_i)	Böhm, H. J. *et al.*, *J. Comput.-Aid. Mol. Des.* **1999**, *13*, 51.
Trophozoite cysteine protease	12	31/4/6 μM (IC_{50})	Ring, C. S. *et al.*, *Proc. Natl. Acad. Sci. USA* **1993**, *90*, 3583.
Other hydrolases			
AChE	5	2/2/3.2 μM (IC_{50})	Rollinger, J. M. *et al.*, *J. Med. Chem.* **2004**, *47*, 6248.
Adenylyl cyclase	(*)	24/2/40 μM (IC_{50})	Soelaiman, S. *et al.*, *J. Biol. Chem.* **2003**, *278*, 25990.
α-Glucosidase	14	188/13/71.4 % at 50 μM	Park, H. *et al.*, *Bioorg. Med. Chem.* **2008**, *16*, 284.
AmpC β-lactamase	(*)	56/3/26 μM (K_i)	Powers, R. A. *et al.*, *Structure* **2002**, *10*, 1013.
	6	48/23/0.7 mM (K_i)	Teotico, D.G. *et al.*, *Proc. Natl. Acad. Sci. USA* **2009**, *106*, 7455.
Autotaxin (NPP-2)	15	94/19/59% inhib. at 10 μM	Parrill, A.L. *et al.*, *Bioorg. Med. Chem.* **2008**, *16*, 1784.
Cdc25 phosphatase	14	182/16/0.82 μM (IC_{50})	Park, H. *et al.*, *J. Med. Chem.* **2008**, *51*, 5533.
CTX-M β-lactamase	6	69/10/0.19 mM (K_i)	Chen, Y. *et al.*, *Nature Chem. Biol.* **2009**, *5*, 358.
Human ubiquitous kinesin ATPase	12	65/9/1.4 μM (K_i)	Hopkins, S.C. *et al.*, *Biochemistry* **2000**, *39*, 2805.
Leukotrien A4 hydrolase	5	n.a./3/n.a.	Grice, C.A. *et al.*, *J. Med. Chem.* **2008**, *51*, 4150.
Neuraminidase	5	105/83/1.8 μM (IC_{50})	Hammad, A.M.A. *et al.*, *J. Chem. Inf. Model.* **2009**, *49*, 978.
Phosphodiesterase 4	(*)	9/5/0.9 nM (IC_{50})	Krier, M. *et al.*, *J. Med. Chem.* **2005**, *48*, 3816.
Protein tyrosine phosphatase 1B	5, 12	365/127/1.7 μM (IC_{50})	Doman, T.N. *et al.*, *J. Med. Chem.* **2002**, *45*, 2213.
T4 Lysozyme	9	18/14/1 mM (K_i)	Wei, B.Q. *et al.*, *J. Mol. Biol.* **2004**, *337*, 1161.

(Continued)

Targets	Cited in Chapter	Tested/actives/ highest affinity	References
Other enzymes			
Asparaginyl-tRNA synthetase	9	45/7/low μM (IC_{50})	Sukuru, S.C. *et al., J. Comput.-Aid. Mol. Des.* **2006**, *20*, 159.
Carbonic anhydrase II	12	13/3/0.6 nM (IC_{50})	Grüneberg, S. *et al., J. Med. Chem.* **2002**, *45*, 3588.
Carbonic anhydrase IX	5	6/6/0.3 μM (IC_{50})	Thiry, A. *et al., Bioorg. Med. Chem.* **2009**, *17*, 553.
DNA gyrase	(*)	3000/150/5 μg/ml (MNEC)	Boehm, H.J. *et al., J. Med. Chem.* **2000**, *43*, 2664.
RNA-editing ligase	9	8/2/57% inhib. at 10 μM	Amaro, R.E. *et al., Proc. Natl. Acad. Sci. USA* **2008**, *105*, 17278.
RmlC epimerase	(*)	94/30/70.5% inhib. at 2 μM (IC_{50})	Babaoglu, K. *et al., Bioorg. Med. Chem. Lett.* **2003**, *13*, 3227.
Ion channels			
Calcium channel	12	20/7/8.21 μM (IC_{50})	Carosati, E. *et al., J. Med. Chem.* **2006**, *49*, 5206.
Kv1.5 potassium channel	(*)	75/1/9.5 μM (IC_{50})	Peukert, S. *et al., J. Med. Chem.* **2003**, *46*, 486.
NR2B/NMDA-R.	5	3/1/86% inhib. at 10 μM	Gitto, R. *et al., ChemMedChem* **2008**, *3*, 1539.
Pankreatic K_{ATP} channel	12	32/3/0.94 μM (IC_{50})	Carosati, E. *et al., J. Med. Chem.* **2007**, *50*, 2117.
Shaker K^+ channel	(*)	4/4/3.8 μM (IC_{50})	Liu, H. *et al., Chem. Biol.* **2003**, *10*, 1103.
Protein–protein and protein–RNA interactions			
Bcl-2	12	35/7/1.6 μM (IC_{50})	Enyedy, I.J. *et al., J. Med. Chem.* **2001**, *44*, 4313.
c-Myc–Max	5	9/4/10 μM (K_d)	Mustata, G. *et al., J. Med. Chem.* **2009**, *52*, 1247.
Lck	16	196/34/4 μM (K_d)	Huang, N. *et al., J. Med. Chem.* **2004**, *47*, 3502.
MDM2	9	23/4/110 nM (K_i)	Bowman, A.L. *et al., J. Am. Chem. Soc.* **2007**, *129*, 12809.
p53-HDM2	2	6/4/0.4 μM (IC_{50})	Cummings, M.D. *et al., Chem. Biol. Drug Des.* **2006**, *67*, 201.
Rac1 GTPase	(*)	15/1/50 μM (IC_{50})	Gao, Y. *et al., Proc. Natl. Acad. Sci. USA* **2004**, *101*, 7618.
Superoxide dismutase	16	100/15/n.a.	Ray, S.S. *et al., Proc. Natl. Acad. Sci. USA*, **2005**, *102*, 3639.
VLA-4	12	12/12/1.3 nM (IC_{50})	Singh, J. *et al., J. Med. Chem.* **2002**, *45*, 2988.
Z alpha1-antitrypsin	16	68/6/active at 10 μM	Mallya, M. *et al., J. Med. Chem.* **2007**, *50*, 5357.
Other protein targets			
Dvl PDZ domain	5	116/15/8.6 μM (K_d)	Shan, J. *et al., J. Comput.-Aid. Mol. Des.* **2009**, *23*, 37.

(Continued)

Targets	Cited in Chapter	Tested/actives/ highest affinity	References
Influenza hemagglutinin	12	43/1/0.5 μM (IC_{50})	Bodian, D.L. *et al.*, *Biochemistry* **1993**, *32*, 2967.
HRV coat protein	5	4/2/2.5 μM (IC_{50})	Rollinger, J.M. *et al.*, *J. Med. Chem.* **2008**, *51*, 842.
HSP90	5	122/5/2.1 μM (IC_{50})	Sanam, R. *et al.*, *J. Mol. Graph. Mod.* **2010**, *28*, 472.
Penicillin binding protein PBP2x	12	55/3/70 μM (IC_{50})	Miguet, L. *et al.*, *J. Med. Chem.* **2009**, *52*, 5926.
Thrombospondin-1	5	19/3/1.3 μM (IC_{50})	Colombo, G. *et al.*, *J. Biol. Chem.* **2010**, *285*, 8733.
Tubulin	5	142/4/187 nM (IC_{50})	Chiang, Y.K. *et al.*, *J. Med. Chem.* **2009**, *52*, 4221.

Index

Virtual Screening. Edited by C. Sotriffer

ISBN: 978-3-527-32636-5